Purchased : A.C. Un. Library

April 1906

Property of

Dr. Wenifreto M. Iglecia

Surgery of the Breast

Diagnosis and Treatment of Breast Diseases

Edited by
Jan Olof Strömbeck and Francis E. Rosato

335 Illustrations by K.-H. Seeber
46 Tables

With Contributions by

K. I. Bland
H. Bohmert
R. S. Boova
R. Cantor
K. Carlström
L. Clodius
A. Costa
R. W. Crichlow
R. A. Egeli
M. Földi
S. Franzén
H.-J. Frischbier
Karin Gyllensköld
L. S. Heuser

C. E. Horton
N. T. Johansson
C. Johnsén
A. Kratochwil
H. P. Leis, Jr.
J. B. McCraw
Martha D. McDaniel
W. P. Maier
W. H. Messerschmidt
W. Mühlbauer
R. R. Olbrisch
H. C. Polk, Jr.
P. Regnault
F. E. Rosato

G. P. Rosemond
R. Saccozzi
H. Sköldefors
J. S. Spratt
H.-E. Stegner
J. O. Strömbeck
N. O. Theve
L. Uddströmer
J. A. Urban
U. Veronesi
L. Wallenberg
A. Wallgren
N. Wilking

1986
Georg Thieme Verlag Stuttgart · New York
Thieme Inc. New York

Library of Congress Cataloging-in-Publication Data

Main entry under title:

Surgery of the breast.

Includes bibliographies and index.
1. Breast--Surgery. 2. Breast--Cancer--Surgery.
I. Strömbeck, Jan Olof. II. Rosato, Francis E.
III. Bland, K. I. [DNLM: 1. Breast--surgery. 2. Breast
Diseases. 3. Mastectomy. 4. Surgery, Plastic.
WP 910 S961]
RD539.8.S87 1986   618.1'9   85-24672

© 1986 Georg Thieme Verlag, Rüdigerstrasse 14,
D-7000 Stuttgart 30, FRG
Printed in Germany
Typesetting (System 5, Linotron 202) by Druckhaus Dörr,
Ludwigsburg
Printing by K. Grammlich, Pliezhausen

ISBN 3-13-657301-3 (Georg Thieme Verlag Stuttgart · New York)
ISBN 0-86577-188-X (Thieme Inc. New York)
1 2 3 4 5 6

Preface

At first consideration there might be some question as to the need for a book devoted to surgery of the breast. Several excellent works on the same subject exist already. However, on close inspection, most of these books are written with a particular emphasis and usually a single discipline point of view. If there has been any major trend in the improved care of patients with breast cancer, it has been a development of the multi-disciplinary approach involving, at different stages, oncologists, surgeons, gynecologists, plastic surgeons, pathologists and radio-therapists. A major purpose of this book is to integrate and review the contributions of all the specialties in the management of diseases of the breast, with the hopeful result that doctors involved in one phase or another may become more knowledgeable of what is possible and available through the other disciplines as well. If this purpose is served there is bound to be a broader, more comprehensive view taken of the problems – to the ultimate benefit of the patient.

The second purpose is obviously to update the information base on all aspects of breast disease treatment. There have been rapid advances particularly in the areas of adjuvant chemotherapy, new and effective surgical approaches in reconstructive surgery, and further advances in diagnostic methods as well. It is hoped that this book will stand at least for some time as a statement of the current available therapies.

This book is a joint effort with contributors from both sides of the Atlantic Ocean, from North America and many European countries as well. Such a broad-based contributorship should also add to the scope of the work.

There has been some overlap in the materials covered by the various contributors. Although the editors have attempted to minimize this, we have allowed a fair amount in the hope that such expanded coverage will be viewed favorably by the reader. At times the contributors may even hold differing viewpoints, which certainly reflects the changing and evolving approaches to breast disease.

The editors have tried to confer a unity of style, but the rigors of translating the contributions were such that we worked primarily to retain the authors' original and exact sense, even at the expense of smooth style. The editors are most appreciative of the excellent chapters submitted by each of the authors.

We also extend our thanks to Tord Sundberg, M. D. who helped in the editorial work and our secretaries Miss Kathie Wood, Miss Karen Cahill and Miss Ingegerd Ahlin. We are also grateful to Georg Thieme Verlag for its help, forebearance, and support and to K.-H. Seeber whose excellent illustrations add so much to the value of this book.

Stockholm/Philadelphia, Summer 1985

Jan Olof Strömbeck
Francis E. Rosato

Contributors

Bland, K. I., M.D., Department of Surgery, Box J-286, JHMHC, University of Florida, College of Medicine, Gainesville, Florida 32610, USA

Bohmert, H., Prof. Dr., Chirurgische Klinik und Poliklinik am Klinikum Großhadern, Marchioninistr. 15, D-8000 München 70

Boova, R. S., M.D., Department of Surgery, Jefferson Medical College, 1025 Walnut Street, Philadelphia, Penn 19107, USA

Cantor, R., M.D., Jefferson Medical College, 1025 Walnut Street, Philadelphia, Penn 19107, USA

Carlström, K., M.D., Hormonlaboratoriet, Kvinnokliniken K 57, Huddinge sjukhus, S-141 86 Huddinge

Clodius, L., Dr., Abteilung für Plastische Chirurgie, Universitätsspital Zürich, Rämistr. 100, CH-8091 Zürich

Costa, A., M.D., Instituto Nazionale, Per Lo Studio E La Cura Dei Tumori, Via Venezian 1, I-20133 Milano

Crichlow, R. W., William and Bessie Allyn Professor and Chairman, Department of Surgery, Dartmouth Medical School, Hanover, New Hampshire 03756, USA

Egeli, R. A., M.D., Department of Surgery Hospital Cantonal, 1211 Geneva 4, Switzerland

Földi, M., Prof. Dr., Haus am Kurpark, Haslachstr. 1, D-7821 Feldberg 1

Franzén, S., Prof. M.D., Kevingestrand 45, S-182 13 Danderyd

Frischbier, H.-J., Prof. Dr., Direktor der Strahlenabteilung der Frauenklinik der Universität, Martinistr. 52, D-2000 Hamburg 20

Gyllensköld, Karin, Dr., Department of Psychotherapeutic Training, Karolinska Institutet, St. Görans Sjukhus Psykiatriska Klinik, Box 12500, S-112 81 Stockholm

Heuser, L. S., M.D., University of Louisville, School of Medicine, Health Sciences Center, Louisville, Ky 40232, USA

Horton, C. E., M.D., 400 W Brambleton Avenue, Suite 300, Norfolk, Virginia 23510, USA

Johansson, N. T., M.D., Kirurgiska Kliniken, Lasarettet, S-521 01 Falköping

Johnsén, Chr., M.D., Kirurgiska Kliniken, Sahlgrenska sjukhuset, S-413 45 Göteborg

Kratochwil, A., Prof. Dr., Vorstand der gebh. gyn. Abteilung des Allgemein öffentlichen Krankenhauses der Kurstadt Baden bei Wien, Wimmergasse 19, A-2500 Baden

Leis, H. P., Jr., M.D., Clinical Professor of Surgery, University of South Carolina School of Medicine, Columbia, 113 11th Avenue North, North Myrtle Beach, South Carolina 29582, USA

McDaniel, Martha D., M.D., Assistant Professor of Surgery, Department of Surgery, Dartmouth Medical School, Hanover, New Hampshire 03756, USA

McGraw, J. B., M.D., 400 W Brambleton Avenue, Suite 300, Norfolk, Virginia 23510, USA

Maier, W. P., M.D., Department of Surgery, Temple University Hospital Health Sciences Center, Philadelphia, Pa 19140, USA

Messerschmidt, W. H., M.D., Department of Surgery, Jefferson Medical College, 1025 Walnut Street, Philadelphia, Pa 19107, USA

Mühlbauer, W., Prof. Dr., Abteilung für Plastische Chirurgie, Städtisches Krankenhaus München-Bogenhausen, Englschalkinger Str. 77, D-8000 München 81

Olbrisch, R. R., Priv.-Doz. Dr., Chefarzt der Klinik für Plastische Chirurgie, Diakoniekrankenhaus Kaiserswerth, Kreuzbergstr. 79, D-4000 Düsseldorf 31

Polk, H. C., Jr., M.D. Professor of Surgery and Chairman of the Department of Surgery, University of Louisville, Health Sciences Center, Louisville, Ky 40232, USA

Regnault, P., M.D., Chirurgie Plastique, 300 Léo Parizeau, Suite 901, Montreal, H2W 2N1, Canada

Rosato, F. E., M.D., Chairman of the Department of Surgery, Jefferson Medical College of Thomas Jefferson University, 1025 Walnut Street, Philadelphia, Pa, 19107, USA

Rosemond, G. P., M.D., Professor of Surgery, Emeritus Chairman of the Department of Surgery, Temple University, 3400 N. Broad Street, Philadelphia, Pa 19140, USA

Saccozzi, R., M.D., Instituto Nazionale, Per Lo Studio, E La Cura Dei Tumori, Via Venezian 1, I-20133 Milano

Sköldefors, H., M.D., Kirurgiska kliniken, Sabbatsbergs sjukhus, S-113 82 Stockholm

Spratt, J. S., M.D., University of Louisville, School of Medicine, Raymond Meyers Hall, Cancer Center, Louisville, Ky 40292, USA

Stegner, H.-E., Prof. Dr., Direktor der Abteilung für gynäkologische Histopathologie und Elektronenmikroskopie, Universitäts-Frauenklinik, Martinistr. 52, D-2000 Hamburg 20

Strömbeck, J. O., M.D., Plastikkirurgiska Kliniken, Sabbatsbergs sjukhus, S-11382 Stockholm

Theve, N. O., M.D., Kirurgiska Kliniken, Sabbatsbergs sjukhus, S-11382 Stockholm

Uddströmer, L., M.D., Kirurgiska Kliniken, Sjukhuset, S-800 87 Gävle 7

Urban, J. A., M.D., Professor of Clinical Surgery, 215 East 68th Street, New York, N.Y. 10021, USA

Veronesi, U., Prof. M.D., Instituto Nazionale, Per Lo Studio, E La Cura Dei Tumori, Via Venezian 1, I-20133 Milano

Wallenberg, L., Prof. M.D., Plastikkirurgiska Kliniken, Sabbatsbergs sjukhus, S-113 82 Stockholm

Wallgren, A., M.D., University of Gothenburg, Department of Oncology, Sahlgrenska sjukhuset, S-413 45 Gothenburg

Wilking, N., M. D., Kirurgiska Kliniken, Sabbatsbergs sjukhus, S-11382 Stockholm

Contents

Chapter 5

Excisional Biopsy 40

L. Uddströmer

Chapter 6

Inflammatory Lesions of the Breast 48

C. Johnsén

Chapter 7

Pathology of Potentially Malignant Diseases 53

H.-E. Stegner

Chapter 8

Pathology of Malignant Diseases of the Breast 66

H.-E. Stegner

Contents

Chapter 9

Epidemiology in Breast Cancer 100

H. P. Leis, Jr.

Chapter 10

Prognosis in Breast Cancer 110

H. P. Leis, Jr.

Contents

Contents

Contents

Chapter 27

Reduction Mammaplasty 277

J. O. Strömbeck

Chapter 28

Breast Augmentation 312

P. Regnault

Chapter 29

The Inverted Nipple 321

J. O. Strömbeck and L. Wallenberg

Chapter 30

Male Breast Carcinoma 325

W. H. Messerschmidt and F. E. Rosato

Contents

Chapter 1

Clinical Examination and Aspiration Biopsy Cytology (ABC) of the Breast

S. Franzén

Introduction

When a woman seeks help for a breast lesion, the first step is to reach a correct diagnosis. This is based on the foundations of clinical examination, mammography, and microscopy of an aspirate or piece of tissue (Frischbier 1977). This involves a microscopic definition and in cases of cancer, malignancy grading as a basis for therapy. A team consisting of an oncologist, a radiologist, a cytologist, and a surgeon who evaluate the patient at a regular "breast conference" provides the necessary expertise.

In the last decade, the therapy of mammary cancer has become more complex as many women have become informed about this topic through the lay press. The patient should have the right to an exact diagnosis and the opportunity to share in the final decision about treatment. Discussion with the team is most valuable, providing the patient with accurate information and advice about different types of treatment.

Clinical Examination

When a patient is referred to our department for a diagnostic aspiration biopsy, we listen to her description of how she became aware that something has appeared in her breast, and we then ask her to point her finger to the actual site of the lump (Fig. 1.**1**).

We rely on the patient's description of her findings. Most women seek advice with insignificant symptoms and signs, a circumstance that should not, however, exclude a thorough examination.

The first step in the examination is a careful inspection. Changes of contour are most easily observed when the patient is seated and raises and lowers both arms simultaneously (Fig. 1.**2**A, B). Most lumps can be reliably palpated with the patient first seated and then lying supine (Fig. 1.**3**A, B).

Women themselves often discover a change in the glandular tissue with their soapy fingers under the shower or in the bath. Our experience is that palpation, with the patient supine, gives the best results when using lubricated fingers (we prefer Hibitane solution). The friction between the examining hand and the patient's skin is thus eliminated and even very slight irregularities can be detected and evaluated. (Fig. 1.**4**).

The next step is to wipe away the lubricant and determine whether there is any dimpling of the skin over the lesion by compressing the breast with the examining hands over the lump. This so-called "plateau test" is very important since dimpling is not rare and is observed even in small cancers when they are superficial. This "plateau test" can also be positive in cases of fat necrosis, simple cysts, and granular cell tumors (myoblastomas) (Fig. 1.**5**). Routinely, the axillary and supraclavicular node regions are meticulously palpated (Fig. 1.**6**A, B).

Fine Needle Aspiration Biopsy Cytology (ABC)

Technique

Any palpable lesion can be aspirated. The lump is fixed between the index finger and the thumb. A disposable needle with an external diameter of 0.6 to 0.7 mm (23 to 22 gauge) is fixed on a disposable syringe (which is

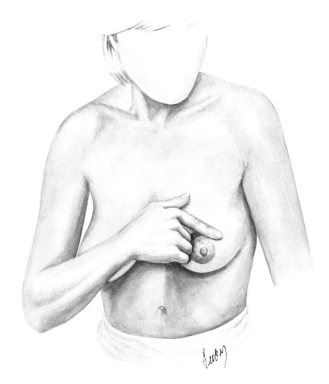

Fig. 1.**1** The patient is asked to point to the lump or to the site of discomfort.

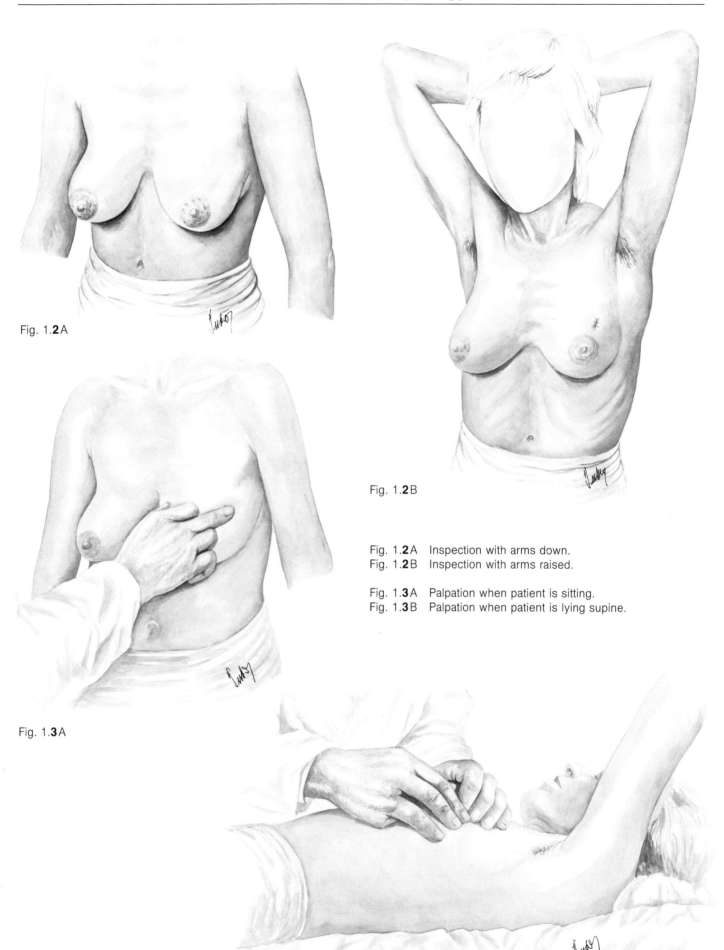

Fig. 1.**2**A

Fig. 1.**2**B

Fig. 1.**2**A   Inspection with arms down.
Fig. 1.**2**B   Inspection with arms raised.

Fig. 1.**3**A   Palpation when patient is sitting.
Fig. 1.**3**B   Palpation when patient is lying supine.

Fig. 1.**3**A

Fig. 1.**3**B

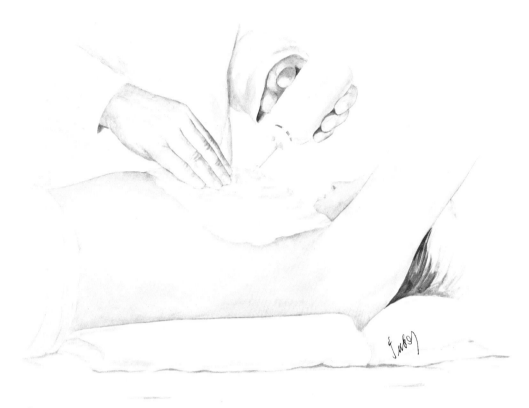

Fig. 1.4 Palpation with soaped fingers.

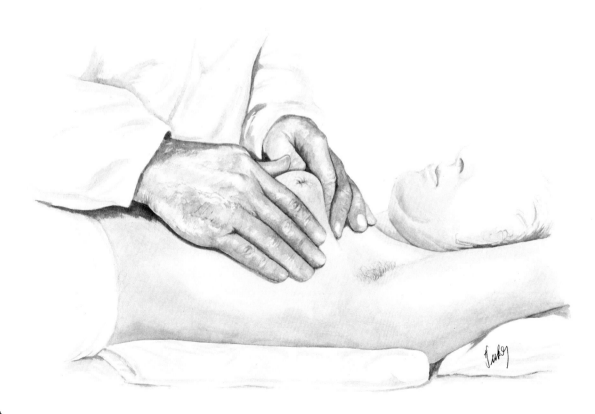

Fig. 1.5 Plateau test.

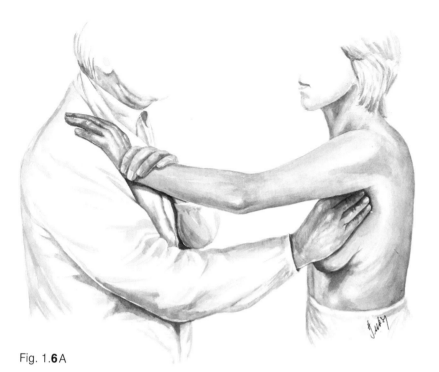

Fig. 1.**6**A

Fig. 1.**6**B

Fig. 1.**6**A Palpation of lymph nodes in the left axilla.
Fig. 1.**6**B Palpation of lymph nodes in the supraclavicular region.

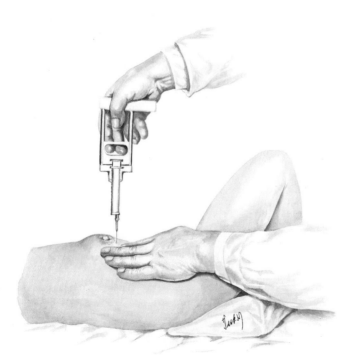

Fig. 1.**7** Aspiration with the Cameco pistol.

inserted in a one-hand grip, for example, the Cameco-pistol) and applied at right angles to the skin, then inserted into the lump. Local anesthesia is not required (Fig. 1.**7**).

Under a negative pressure created by completely withdrawing the plunger of the syringe, the needle is moved forward and backward four or five times in the same channel. After releasing the pressure, the needle is removed from the lump. The material in the needle is spread on glass slides by first removing the needle from the syringe and filling the syringe with air, then blowing the aspirated material from the needle with the air in the syringe. The material in the needle is spread on glass slides and smeared in the manner of peripheral blood. The smear is air-dried and can be stained immediately by the May-Grünwald-Giemsa (MGG) method (Zajicek 1974). If there are some doubts as to whether the material is sufficient for diagnostic purposes, a rapid-staining procedure can be performed within five minutes, while the patient waits. Sometimes, it is necessary to repeat the procedure to obtain cellular material sufficient for an accurate report.

In cases where a patient seeks help for an obviously palpable and well-defined lump, the aspiration should be performed prior to mammography. This is especially practical if the lump is a cyst, which can be easily and totally emptied. The presence of one or more cysts can be troublesome at mammography causing pain on examination and concealing structures of interest. In addition, it is helpful for the mammographer to know whether the aspirated lesion was solid or cystic. It is very unusual that a thin-needle puncture of a distinct palpable lump gives rise to a hematoma, which is large enough to complicate the interpretation of the mammogram. If the patient, however, has no well-defined mass, mammography can serve as a guide for aspiration. If mammography is negative and palpation is inconclusive, there is no reason for an aspiration (Fig. 1.**8**).

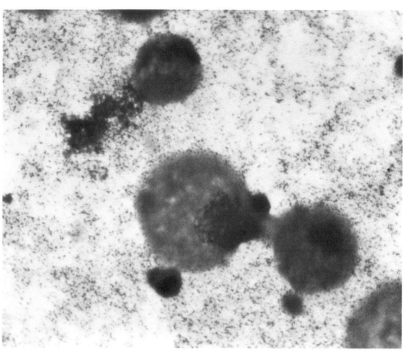

Fig. 1.**10**

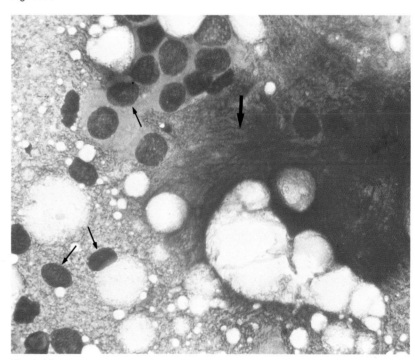

Fig. 1.**11**

Fig. 1.**10** Cystic disease. The smear from the aspirated liquid contains macrophages ("cyst cells"). The background shows amorphous stippled debris.

Fig. 1.**11** Aspirated material from a fibroadenoma. The smear shows a mixture of mesenchymal mucous substance (dark pink in MGG) indicated by the thick arrow and small epithelial cells with oval nuclei (thin arrows). The material includes fat droplets (the pale areas) aspirated from the adjacent breast tissue.

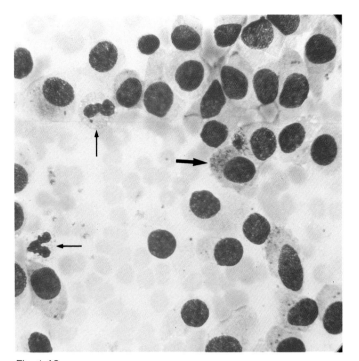

Fig. 1.**12**

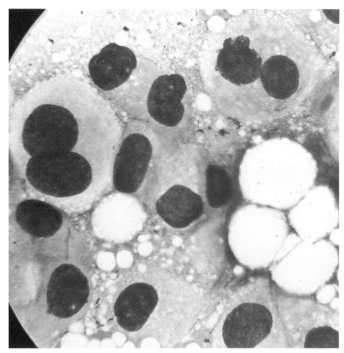

Fig. 1.**13**

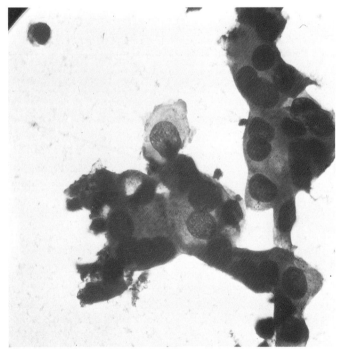

Fig. 1.**14**

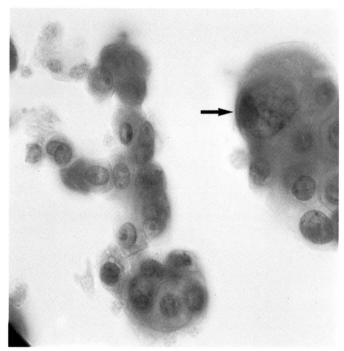

Fig. 1.**15**

Fig. 1.**12** Aspirated material from a small cell duct carcinoma. The cell-rich smear shows a monotonous pattern of a small cell carcinoma. The cytoplasma of some cells contains a fine reddish granulation (see thick arrow). The size of the malignant cells equals that of leukocytes (fine arrows).

Fig. 1.**13** Aspirated material from an apocrine carcinoma. Enlarged irregular epithelial cells with abundance of cytoplasma (the same magnification in all figures presented).

Fig. 1.**14** Smear from nipple discharge in duct papilloma. A cluster of uniform cells showing a papillary pattern.

Fig. 1.**15** Smear from nipple discharge in a case of intraductal carcinoma. Papillary pattern with atypical duct cells (see arrow).

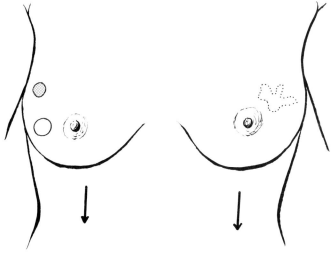

Fig. 1.8 Well defined lump
1. Aspiration
2. Mammography

Inconclusive palpation
1. Mammography
2. Aspiration, if needed

Accuracy

When a patient is referred to our department, the clinical examination, the aspiration, and the making of the smear are all performed by the same physician who reads the slides and gives the final report. For this routine, one physician must have the experience necessary to reach an optimal result.

At the beginning of the 1970s, our diagnostic results were good, with a frequency of approximately 10% false negative and 0.1% false positive results in breast cancer (Franzén and Zajicek 1968). A closer cooperation with the department of radiology (mammography) has helped us to decide more precisely on the area for aspiration and our accuracy has improved in regard to the incidence of false-negative results. A prerequisite for this is a good relationship between the clinical oncologist, the cytologist, and the specialist in mammography (Kreuzer and Boquoi 1981). Thus with good palpation, mammography, and aspiration, it is possible today to diagnose cancer preoperatively in nearly every case. Today the incidence of false-positive results is less than 0.1% and usually is due to the misinterpretation of cellular material from florid sclerosing adenosis, papillomas, or fibroadenomas. The mammographic finding of a round, well-defined lesion typical for fibroadenoma should make the cytologist aware of this benign lesion and thus avoid the misdiagnosis of cancer based solely on the findings in the smear. False-positive results are never accepted, although this cannot be totally eliminated.

It should be kept in mind that false positive cancer diagnoses might as likely happen with excision biopsy histology (frozen sections!) (Wallgren et al. 1977). In our experience the incidence of false-positives by the ABC technique is not any higher than by histology.

Despite a good technical routine and experience, the material obtained in some cases can be meager, for instance in the case of scirrhous cancer or when the lesion is small. A clinically suspicious, palpable lesion must therefore always be excised even when the mammogram and the fine-needle aspiration are negative. Too much reliance is placed on a negative mammogram. Cancer in premenopausal women shows, in 10% to 15% of patients, no typical changes or even a completely normal mammogram. Estrogen treatment may alter tissue so that malignant changes are hidden on the mammogram.

Because of fine-needle aspiration, operative interventions have been found unnecessary in our experience in many benign lesions (cysts, fibroadenomas, and sclerosing adenosis to name several). An additional advantage in avoiding an operation is that scars often make palpation and mammography more difficult. Still, in many institutions where this technique is not so well refined, a diagnosis of benign disease by ABC would in fact require subsequent excision of a well-defined lump. Aspirates can be used for special studies such as an analysis of estrogen receptors (ER) and a quantitative analysis of cellular DNA.

Nonpalpable Lesion

Because of the increasing use of mammographic screening procedures in regular physical check-ups, minimally suspicious lesions have become a clinical problem. The choice has been between further mammography (four months later) or an operative biopsy. A stereotactic method has been devised that makes possible a precise location for aspiration of nonpalpable lesions (Nordenström et al. 1981).

Our equipment consists of an adjustable examination table, two compression plates, an attachable instrument for biopsy, and a roentgenographic tube. The tube can be

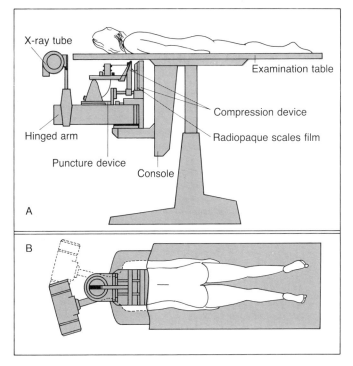

Fig. 1.9 Breast examination.
A: position of the patient during the examination.
B: x-ray tube angulation.
(From Nordenström et al. 1981.)

angulated and by this means two stereoradiographs are exposed (Fig. 1.**9**). The exact position of the actual minimal lesions can be calculated from the films with the help of a computer in which the true co-ordinates (x, y, z) are found. The instrument for aspiration consists of a cannula with an outer diameter of 0.8 mm and an inner screw needle, which is rotated through the lesion. The material thus obtained mostly consists of fragments of tissue, which are squeezed on slides, air-dried, and stained with MGG.

About 1,500 cases have been examined by this technique and the preliminary results are promising. With intensive co-operation between the radiologist and the cytologist, minimal mammographic lesions have been evaluated using this technique. With increased experience in the stereotactic ABC technique, we now are able to reach a preoperative diagnosis in about 70% of nonpalpable lesions that later proved to be cancers. In addition to aspiration biopsies, preoperative markings are made for the surgeon by the injection of an aqueous solution of medical carbon particles.

Cytologic Diagnostic findings

The cytologic diagnosis is based on the microscopic appearance of the cellular details in the smear (Kline and Neal 1976; Schöndorf 1978; Grubb 1981; Linsk and Franzén 1983). The decisive characteristics are listed in Table 1.**1**.

The intention here is not to write a textbook on clinical cytology, but to give some examples of the possibility of cytological tumor diagnosis. Four examples of benign and malignant tumors are shown Figs. 1.**10** to 1.**13**.

Paget's disease of the nipple can be diagnosed by scraping with a scalpel and preparing a smear from the scrapings. A bloody discharge from the nipple must always be subjected to a cytologic examination; and it is often possible to differentiate between fragments of benign papillomas and clusters of intraductal carcinomas in these discharges. However, exfoliated cells from papillomas may be so atypical as to be mistaken for a malignancy (Figs. 1.**14**, 1.**15**).

Needle Aspiration Technique for Estrogen Receptor Determination

The prognostic value of the determination of ER in mammary adenocarcinoma is well established (compare p. 115). Thus, tumors with a high ER content are likely to respond to endocrine therapy (Auer et al. 1980a), and knowledge of the ER content will facilitate the choice between endocrine therapy and chemotherapy.

Estrogen receptor determinations are usually performed on operative biopsies, and thus adequate samples can be a problem to obtain from many cases of inoperable or recurrent adenocarcinomas. A method for ER analysis on material from fine-needle aspirates was therefore developed in our department (Silfverswärd 1979; Silfverswärd and Humla 1980; Silfverswärd et al. 1980; Benyahia et al. 1982). The following procedure is used: double aspirations are performed with a 0.7 mm (outer diameter) or 22 gauge needle, and the material is injected into an ice-cold buffer solution containing ^{3}H-estradiol. The needles are rinsed with the same solution and a sample (one drop) is smeared on a slide for microscopic control to identify the cancer cells. The ER content is analyzed by isoelectric focusing and the value is expressed as femtomole/µg DNA (for details see reference number). With our technique, we usually obtain around 20 µg of DNA, which corresponds to approximately 2×10^6 cells. Receptor determinations on aspirates containing less than 10 µg of DNA tend to give erroneously low values and are accordingly interpreted cautiously. At present we have more than four years experience with ER analysis in material obtained by fine-needle aspiration. We find the method quick, inexpensive, and readily acceptable to the patient; at the Radiumhemmet in Stockholm, the ER values obtained by this technique are often the basis for the choice of therapy.

Table 1.**1** Aspiration biopsy cytology (ABC) of breast lesions. A short guide for microscopy

Diagnostic guidelines		
Benign features	Malignant features	Benign neoplasia
Scanty cells	Cellular smears	Duct papilloma
Cell dispersion discrete	Cell dispersion prominent	High cellularity
Free cells: Naked oval monomorphic nuclei	Free cells: Round or irregular nuclei with preserved dense cytoplasm	Papillary structures Degenerative cell changes Macrophages
Nuclei normochromatic	Nuclei hyperchromatic	Debris
Regular mono/dilayered sheets	Multilayered clusters	Elongated cells Moderate nuclear hypercromasia
Apocrine cells/phagocytes	Apocrine cells/phagocytes infrequent	
Fat/glandular cells separated	Fat/glandular cells mixed	Fibroadenoma
		High cellularity Branching mono/dilayered sheets Free cells: Oval round normochromatic Loose stroma fragments

Needle Aspiration Technique for DNA Analysis

Smears of aspirated material from mammary cancers can be used for *quantitative* DNA analysis for the estimation of the grade of malignancy, but not for diagnosis of cancer (Auer et al. 1980a). Air-dried smears are fixed in a 10% neutral solution of formaldehyde and stained according to the method of Feulgen, a reaction that is specific for the nuclear DNA. The amount of Feulgen-DNA can then be measured quantitatively, cell by cell, using a scanning spectromicrophotometer set at a wavelength of 546 nm. With this technique, aspirated material was studied from 112 patients with comparable carcinomas of the breast, diagnosed and treated more than ten years ago. Results of the study are summarized in Fig. 1.**16**. By comparing these with survival, a significant correlation between DNA content of the neoplastic cells and survival was found. Patients showing DNA-histogram type 1 or type 2 (diploid or polyploid patterns) exhibited a good prognosis, whereas type 3 and especially type 4 were indicative of a poor prognosis. We believe that this method of grading will be of great importance in the choice of therapy in the future (Auer et al. 1983).

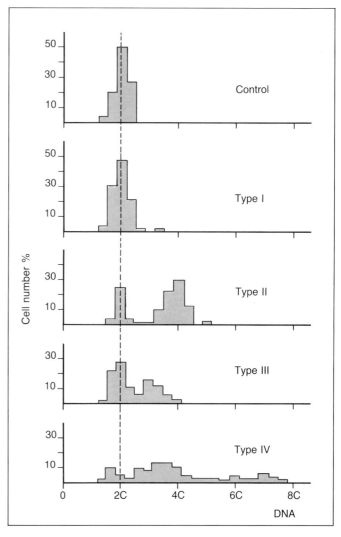

Fig. 1.**16** DNA distribution patterns, determined by Feulgen cytophotometry, from nonproliferating normal mammary epithelial cells (control) and from a series of mammary carcinomas (types I to IV). (From Auer et al. 1980).

References

Auer, G. U., T. O. Caspersson, A. S. Wallgren: DNA content and survival in mammary carcinoma. Anal. Quant. Cytol. 2: 161–165, 1980a

Auer, G. U., T. O. Caspersson, S. A. Gustafsson, S. A. Humla, B.-M. Ljung, B. A. Nordenskjöld, C. Silfverswärd, S. A. Wallgren: Relationship between nuclear DNA distribution and estrogen receptors in human mammary carcinomas. Anal. Quant. Cytol. 2: 280–284, 1980b

Auer, G. U., J. Ono, T. O. Caspersson: Determination of the fraction of G_o cells in cytologic samples by means of simultaneous DNA and nuclear protein analyses. Anal. Quant. Cytol. 5: 1–4, 1983

Benyahia, B., H. Magdelenat, A. Zajdela, J. R. Vilcoq: Ponction-aspiration à l'aiguille fine et dosage des récepteurs d'aestrogènes dans le cancer du sein. Bull. Cancer (Paris) 69: 456–460, 1982

Frischbier, H.-J., H. U. Lohbeck: Frühdiagnostik des Mammakarzinoms. Georg Thieme Verlag, Stuttgart 1977

Franzén, S., J. Zajicek: Aspiration biopsy in diagnosis of palpable lesions of the breast. Critical review of 3479 consecutive biopsies. Acta Radiol. Ther. 7: 241–262, 1968

Grubb, Ch.: Colour Atlas of Breast Cytopathology. HM + M Publishers, London 1981

Kline, T. S., H. S. Neal: Needle aspiration of the breast – Why bother? Acta Cytol. 20: 324, 1976

Kreuzer, G., E. Boquoi: Zytologie der weiblichen Brustdrüse. Thieme, Stuttgart–New York 1981

Linsk, J. A., S. Franzén: Breast aspiration. In Linsk, J. A., S. Franzén: Clinical Aspiration Cytology. Lippincott, Philadelphia 1983

Nordenström, B., H. Rydén, G. Svane: Breast. In Zornosa, J.: Percutaneous Needle Biopsy. Williams & Wilkins, Baltimore–London 1981

Schöndorf, H.: Aspiration Cytology of the Breast. W. B. Saunders Co, Philadelphia–London–Toronto 1978

Silfverswärd, C.: Estrogen Receptors in Human Breast Cancer. Dissertation, Institute for Tumor Pathology–Karolinska Institute, Stockholm 1979

Silfverswärd, C., S. A. Humla: Estrogen receptor analysis on needle aspirates from human mammary cancer. Acta Cytol. 24: 54–57, 1980

Silfverswärd, C., J.-Å. Gustafsson, S. A. Gustafsson, B. Nordenskjöld, A. Wallgren, Ö. Wrange: Estrogen receptor analysis on fine needle aspirates and on histologic biopsies from human breast cancer. Eur. J. Cancer 16: 1351–1357, 1980

Wallgren, A., C. Silfverswärd, A. Hultborn: Carcinoma of the breast in women under 30 years of age. Cancer 40: 916–923, 1977

Zajicek, J.: Aspiration Biopsy Cytology, Part 1. Karger, Basel 1974

Chapter 2

Mammography

H.-J. Frischbier

Introduction

Since it is apparent that palpation and inspection of the female breast are only crude measures for the diagnosis of a mammary carcinoma, new methods have been developed that have been widely introduced in clinical practice within the last two decades. Of these, mammography is the oldest and most widely used. The clinical value of this method has been proved in many collective studies. Numerous monographs have been published covering technique, diagnostic criteria for benign and malignant diseases, and clinical efficiency (Leborgne 1953; Ingleby and Gershon-Cohen 1960; Buttenberg and Werner 1962; Gross 1963; Egan 1964; Baclesse and Willemin 1967; Witt and Burger 1968; Witten 1969; Gerson-Cohen 1970; Willemin 1972; Hoeffken and Lanyi 1973; Picard 1974; Seifert 1975; Frischbier and Lohbeck 1977; Barth 1977; Logan and Muntz 1979; Otto 1980).

Although mammography is without question the current method with the highest accuracy in the diagnosis of a carcinoma, a number of more specialized radiologic procedures have been developed for different indications. In the case of pathologic secretion from the breast, a better diagnosis of intraductal changes can be obtained with the injection of a contrast medium and a subsequent x-ray picture (galactography). In cysts, the inner wall of the cysts can be clearly seen if puncture and subsequent air injection is used (pneumocystography). Another special x-ray method is the xeroradiography. The information on the x-ray film is reproduced by charge distribution of a semiconductor plate made from selenium.

Also widely used is breast thermography either as electronic thermography or contact (plate) thermography. Since the clinical value of thermography is limited for early diagnosis, thermography is of no value in the early detection of a mammary carcinoma, this method must be considered as an adjunctive method to mammography in special cases, but certainly not as an equal alternative method to mammography.

The value of mammasonography cannot currently be fully evaluated. Existing data have been obtained only in a small number of patients. In addition, the technological development is still in progress. For these reasons, it cannot be judged whether sonography will become an adjunctive method or will develop into an alternative method to mammography. (See Chapter 3 for a full review of breast sonography).

Examination Technique

The female breast is not a good object for an x-ray examination since it has different thicknesses between the thoracic wall and the nipple and since the thoracic base of the breast is not a straight line. In addition, different tissues such as connective tissue, fat, glands, and tumor-like formations show only small differences in x-ray absorption. For this reason, a high difference in contrast among these tissues is necessary to allow for the recognition of the necessary details.

Mammography must always be performed under standardized conditions. These include a craniocaudal projection with the upper torso of the patient turned to the opposite side so that the parenchyma of the lateral quadrant is fully visible. The nipple must be located in the center of the circumference of the breast. A second projection is the mediolateral.

With good technique, no additional films are necessary. An additional view of the axilla is of no diagnostic importance. A single oblique projection, according to Lundgren (1975), in which only one oblique is obtained with a 45° tilted x-ray tube is still under discussion. Although Lundgren emphasized that x-ray examinations with only one picture are more economical and more rapid, it seems to be clear that the interpretation and accuracy using views in two planes is better.

Technical Equipment for Mammography

The industry manufactures special equipment for mammography carries a rotating molybdenum anode and can use an anode voltage of 25 to 35 kV. The current apparatus has a movable arm holding the tube and plate holder that can be rotated around the horizontal axis. If this arm cannot be adjusted for height, then a chair adjustable for height is necessary. The use of a special tube and the ability to compress the breast to narrow the x-ray bundle are absolutely necessary.

An automatic light meter has proved advantageous since measurement of the thickness of the breast is not a good measure for proper lighting (Hoeffken et al. 1970).

Contrast and picture sharpness depend on the x-ray quality and the film material used. The film for mammography must fulfill three criteria. It must:

1. Be fine-grained in order to produce fine detail
2. Have sufficient range to cover all structures in one picture from the skin to the dense glandular portion
3. Show a steep gradient in order to give high contrast (Otto 1980)

For many years it was felt that a special industrial film was necessary for mammographic purposes. This film was particularly fine-grained with high silver content. These films show a steep gradient in spite of a low sensitivity and a high contrast. The relatively high x-ray dose necessary for sufficient contrast was, however, considered a disadvantage.

In order to reduce the doses for safety reasons, the use of intensifying screens was investigated about ten years ago. However, unclearness and loss of details are recognized as disadvantages of these screens. Large phantom examinations led to the conclusion that the use of different commercially available film and intensifying systems did not improve the recognition of details and that significant differences in resolution could not be compensated for. These systems are not alternatives to the special industrial film in spite of a lower x-ray load (Frischbier et al. 1977).

The introduction of grid is one of the important improvements of the mammographic technique. A grid increases the sharpness of details by reducing scattered radiation. Based on the detailed examinations by Friedrich (1975, 1977, 1978), the technical necessities were developed to fit standard machines for mammography with additional equipment for grid technique. The advantages of grid mammography are summarized by Friedrich (1982) as follows:

1. Increased general picture contrast with clear transparency and structure differentiation in dense glandular areas
2. Better recognition of detailed structures as well as microcalcium and connective tissue septa
3. A reduction in dosage to one quarter to one half depending on the film and intensifying system

The technique of grid mammography can be considered the optimal standard procedure for mammography today. Based on a two-year clinical evaluation of grid mammography, we could show that the diagnosis of clinically occult carcinomas and preinvasive tumors was considerably improved through the detection of smaller dust-like microcalcifications (Frischbier and Bernauer, 1982b).

Another technique also tested in the United States as an alternative to the grid technique is enlargement mammography as described and advocated by Stickler (1979).

Xeroradiography

A special x-ray technique for the breasts is xeroradiography (Wolfe 1972; Bonilla-Musoles et al. 1979; Luzatti et al. 1979). This technique does not use the distribution of black areas as does the common film mammography, but uses as information the charge distribution of a semiconductor plate made of selenium.

The advantage of xeroradiography compared with standard x-ray examination of the breast rests in the physical process that is characteristic for the system and is called an "edge enhancement effect." This effect is based on the fact that high-potential differences occur at boundaries that lead to the pile up of toner at electrostatic boundaries. Thus, the boundaries of areas with uneven densities are particularly well seen. This effect makes calcifications or rough edges and lines particularly clear. In addition to the edge effect, the broad area contrast is lacking in xeroradiograms. The resolution should be identical to that of the film mammogram as based on experimental comparative investigations.

Another advantage is the reduced exposure to radiation. This advantage exists only if the exposure to radiation is compared with a technique using industrial film. The currently used grid mammography, which uses only 20% to 30% of the radiation dose, shows the same radiation exposure as does the xeroradiogram.

In the literature, the xeroradiogram is often compared on a competitive basis with the mammogram. Compared with the industrial film mammography and in particular with the low-dose technique, xeroradiography excels in a better reproduction of microcalcifications and radial structures. These advantages are particularly apparent in the case of a shadow-rich mastopathy, so that under these circumstances the xeroradiogram is superior to the mammogram.

A decisive disadvantage of xeroradiography in comparison to mammography is in the reproduction of unclear, limited densities behind which a solid carcinoma can be hiding. If the local mass does not show radial extensions, but only an unclear border, then the reproduction of such mass is considerably less accurate with xeroradiography as compared with mammography. Once in a while, the difference in contrast is so low with the xeroradiogram that such limited masses do not reproduce at all.

In Germany, these disadvantages have led to the assumption that xeroradiography is only an adjunctive technique to mammography. Even this place as an adjunctive technique has currently been lost since the character of the picture of the mammogram with the help of the grid technique and its reduced peripheral radiation is very comparable to that of the xeroradiogram. The grid mammogram shows equally clearly very fine radial structures such as microcalcifications in the range of 120 to 150 μm. In the United States, however, xeroradiography is the preferred technique in most medical centers, even totally replacing film mammography.

Electron Radiography

A newer technical procedure for x-ray examination of the breast is electron radiography, a procedure based on the fact that ions are generated when x-rays are absorbed in tissue. The result is a transparent x-ray picture with moderate edge effect and good area contrast. This technique has not yet found widespread clinical application.

Computer Tomography

Another new, but also little-tested mammographic procedure is computerized tomography. A computer tomography of the breast using contrast substance can show static, anatomical changes of the breast. Pathologic iodide concentrations in the tissue of the breast give a better differentiation, which is of interest since it has been shown that a higher iodide content is found in mammary carcinoma.

In the United States, the General Electric Company has developed a "computed tomographic breast scanner." The computer tomography may have the highest accuracy in diagnosing breast cancers according to the investigations of Chang (1982), who compared this approach with film mammography, thermography, and physical examinations in 100 patients with breast cancer. Although he feels that the computer tomography is no substitute for the conventional mammography, the procedure did have a better diagnostic accuracy in the case of dense and dysplastic breasts.

X-Ray Exposure by Mammography

Since the examinations by Wanebo (1968) of the atomic bomb victims from Hiroshima and Nagasaki, by Mackenzie (1965) of patients in a tuberculosis hospital in Nova Scotia who were frequently exposed to x-rays, and by Mettler (1969) of x-ray-exposed mastitis patients, there can be no doubt that ionizing radiation, even in relatively small doses, is carcinogenic in people. In particular, these three investigations have shown that the mammary parenchyma is relatively x-ray sensitive. Since mammography is now more and more used in the early diagnosis of breast cancer and since the breast is exposed to radiation during mammography, one must consider that this procedure has not only beneficial effects but also possible detrimental aspects through cancer induction.

It has to be recognized that the above cited three investigations allow only a qualitative judgment. Based on differences among the investigations, with respect to age, race, radiation field, dose fractionation, and exact radiation dosage, it is impossible to evaluate the results statistically. Thus, the data on dosage in the atomic bomb explosions could only be obtained through model calculations so that the actual x-ray exposure of the individuals could only be roughly estimated. Similarly, in the case of the tuberculosis patients, exposures occurred many decades ago so that incomplete data were available on the doses used. Further uncertainties exist in extrapolating these radiologic-biologic facts to mammography.

A judgment of the extent of the risk must contain the consideration that not every radiation-induced cancer is lethal but can itself be cured by early diagnosis. In the United States, benefit versus risk analysis as performed by Bailar (1976) and Thomas (1977) led to the NIH/NCI Consensus Development Meeting on Breast Cancer Screening. This group recommended that routine mammographic examinations should not be conducted as a screening procedure in women 50 years or younger who were free of breast symptoms since a definite benefit could not be ascertained.

All discussion about the benefits and risks of mammography can be considered closed today for three reasons:

1. Extensive investigations from Boice and Monson (1977) have shown that the induction of carcinomas is mostly concentrated in the younger age groups who were younger than 30 years at the time of exposure. In this age group, routine mammographic examination is not necessary since the spontaneous incidence of mammary carcinomas is so small.
2. Worldwide discussions about the danger of mammography with its high x-ray exposure have lead to a drastic reduction in the x-ray dose through development of special mammography films and the grid technique. As had been shown through extensive examinations (Würthner 1982), the radiologic dose can be considerably reduced.
3. The benefit analysis was mainly based on the results of the HIP study, which included very few mammary carcinomas in women under the age of 50 and accordingly no reduction in the mortality for such young women. However, in the BCDDP study, a different benefit analysis can be made (Lester 1979).

This investigation has shown that no marked differences exist in the rate of mammographically diagnosed, clinically occult carcinomas in the age groups 35 to 50 compared with 50 to 70 years. They concluded that the value of mammography is equal in women under 50 years compared with older women and that it would be irresponsible not to use this important technique in women between the ages of 35 to 50. We believe that routine mammographic examinations of women from age 35 in one- or two-year intervals is the safest method to recognize an early breast carcinoma.

Galactography

Galactography is a special radiologic examination that uses injection of water-soluble contrast media into secreting milk ducts. Through a long, blunt cannula or a thin polyethylene tube, a water-soluble contrast medium is injected. When the milk ducts are filled with contrast medium, the patient does notice a feeling of fullness or tension. Immediately, x-ray pictures are taken in two planes as is done in mammography. Complications caused by the contrast media are extremely rare. Intraductal changes that cannot be detected by palpation or mammography can be seen with galactography. In the diagnosis of a pathologic secretion, the galactogram may be the superior diagnostic method today as compared with clinical examination, mammography, and cytology. (See Chapter 16.)

A collective statistical evaluation of the literature (Frischbier and Lohbeck 1977) showed that in the intraductal mammary carcinomas diagnosed through galactography, one half were detected through galactography alone. In our experience with galactography, we found intraductal changes in 94 cases of unilateral pathologic secretion. Histologic examination showed a preinvasive carcinoma in eight of these cases and an invasive cancer in nine.

Galactography is not specific and cannot distinguish between benign and malignant duct changes. Nevertheless, this procedure must be considered the safest method for the early detection of a duct carcinoma in the case of pathologic secretions where examination and mammograms are negative. For this reason, galactography should be employed in the case of a unilateral pathologic secretion except during pregnancy and lactation.

Filling defects, irregularities of the duct wall, or narrowing and obstruction are important findings. The benign duct papillomas usually produce a round filling defect in the milk duct (Fig. 2.1). If the papilloma grows, it can completely close the duct. In the case of an incomplete closure of the duct, size and extension of the papillomatosis can be seen.

The intraductal carcinoma with pathologic secretion often produces duct ectasia. Depending on the extent of the carcinoma, the duct system can be reduced or replaced (Fig. 2.2). An extension of the carcinoma along the wall of the duct leads radiographically to filling defects or even to a complete obstruction. It is our experience that it is impossible to distinguish a papillary intraductal carcinoma from a benign papilloma with galactography.

Pneumocystography

When a cyst has been aspirated, it may immediately be injected with air. X-ray pictures in two planes are then obtained to judge the cavity of the cyst.

The technique of pneumocystography is very easy: the skin at the punction site is disinfected while the patient lies or sits. Local anesthesia is not necessary. The cyst is fixed with two fingers and tapped with a thick needle adapted to a syringe. Sometimes the wall of the cyst is very tough and more pressure must be exerted to puncture the cystic wall to reach the inside of the cyst. It is very important to empty the cyst completely. No fluid should remain in the cyst. After puncture, air equal to the amount of fluid withdrawn is injected; after removal of the needle, x-ray pictures are made of the breast in two planes.

The cysts appear in the mammogram as smoothly outlined, homogenous, round-to-oval densities that occasionally show a "safety rim" (Fig. 2.3A, B). Significant findings are changes in the inner wall of the cyst and impressions from the outside (Fig. 2.4A, B).

Intracystic carcinomas are extremely rare. Fassin and Jeanmart (1972) observed six intracystic growths with 112 pneumocystographic examinations that showed histologically a malignant papilloma in two cases. Tabar (1973) observed 11 cases of a histologically identified intracystic carcinoma. We saw only one case among about 1000 pneumocystographic examinations. This was a carcinoma in a pseudocyst that presented itself in the pneumocystography as a necrotic cavity.

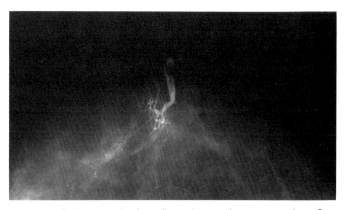

Fig. 2.1 Galactography in unilateral sanguinous secretion. One dilated milk duct with almost complete filling defect. In the periphery, the milk ducts are of fine caliber. Histology: Papilloma.

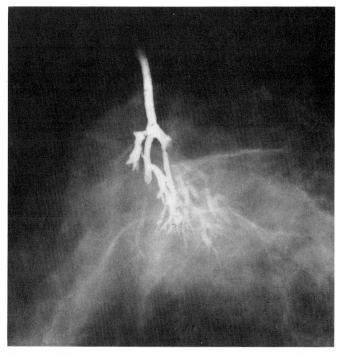

Fig. 2.2 Galactography in sanguinous secretion shows intraductal filling defects. Palpation inconclusive. Cytology: negative. Histology: Malignant degeneration of duct papilloma with development into adenocarcinoma.

The value of the pneumocystogram is to diagnose clinically occult mammary carcinomas and to reduce the number of unnecessary breast biopsies.

Mammographic Examination

Results and Symptomatology

To properly evaluate the results of mammography, the radiologist must know the general clinical condition of the patient, especially the details of the physical examination of the breast.

The mammographic picture changes considerably with age. In younger women, the individual glandular lobes are seen as confluent densities in the surrounding fatty

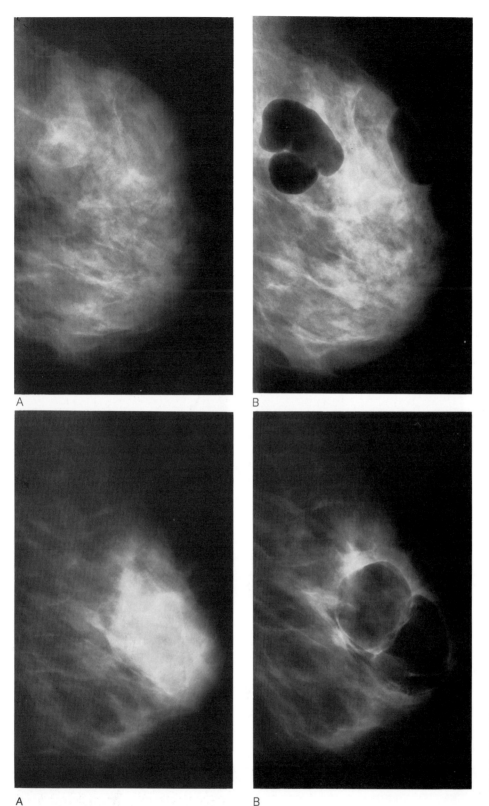

Fig. 2.**3** Palpatory finding: Nodular mastopathy. A: Mammography: Multiple smoothly outlined, homogenous densities in both upper quadrants. B: Pneumocystography: After punction and injection with air, multiple cysts with smooth walls are seen.

Fig. 2.**4** Palpation: Hard, smooth egg-sized tumor above the nipple. A: Mammography: Partly smooth-lined homogenous mass. B: Pneumocystography: After punction and injection with air a multichambered cyst with smooth walls is visualized.

tissue. The glandular parenchyma absorbs the soft x-rays much more than does the fatty tissue. The ducts are not recognizable in the mammogram and they can only be seen with galactography. Whereas the fatty tissue appears as a lighter area, the connective tissue appears as hair-fine structures that proceed from the glandular areas to the skin (Cooper's ligaments). During pregnancy and lactation, the density of the glandular area increases, they grow larger, and the lighter areas of fatty tissue disappear completely.

After pregnancy and as one approaches menopause, an atrophy of the glandular acini occurs. The connective tissue becomes more pronounced and the fatty tissue occupies larger areas. Only weak reminders of the parenchyma are recognizable in older age; the breast becomes predominantly fatty and the connective tissue structures clearer by contrast.

Solid fibroadenomas or isolated cysts appear in the mammogram as smoothly outlined, homogenous foci, sometimes lobular. A radiologic differentiation between a fibroadenoma and a cyst is not possible in many cases. Needle aspiration with cytologic studies and pneumocystography can often help differentiate these lesions.

The different preinvasive or invasive malignant growths of the breast that originate either from the ducts or from the glandular tissue differ radiologically in many aspects. In general, the radiologic manifestations of malignant growths can be divided as follows:

1. Calcifications
2. Localized densities
3. Structural changes
4. Indirect criteria such as skin findings, retractions of the breast surface, and vascular signs

The four groups of pathologic criteria that can appear by themselves or in combination will be the basis of the remainder of this chapter.

Calcifications

Mammographically demonstrable calcifications constitute the most important criteria in the diagnosis of a mammary carcinoma. The incidence of calcifications in cancers depend strongly on the x-ray technique. After the introduction of the molybdenum target tube, the incidence of radiologically recognizable calcifications in breast cancer was reported at 20% to 50% (Fig. 2.5A–F). With the further reduction of scattered radiation, duct-like calcifications can now be seen so that about 70% of all diagnosed carcinomas mammographically show calcium. Shephard et al. (1962) found microcalcifications in 75% of all carcinomas when x-ray pictures were taken of the paraffin-fixed tumors. Black and Young (1965), also x-raying excised tumors, reported calcifications in 13% of histologically identified mastitis and 12% of fibroadeno-

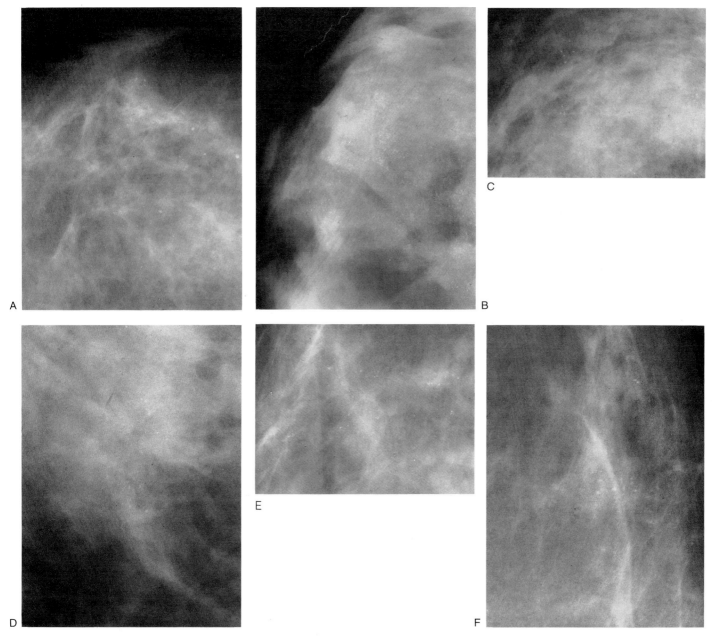

Fig. 2.5 Microcalcifications of different types in mastopathic densities (magnification x 2). Histology: A: Paget's disease with intraductal carcinoma. B: Noninfiltrating comedocarcinoma. C: Intraductal comedocarcinoma. D: Invasive ductal carcinoma.

E: Invasive ductal carcinoma adjacent to atypical intraductal foci. F: Early invasion of ductal carcinoma emanating from a comedocarcinoma.

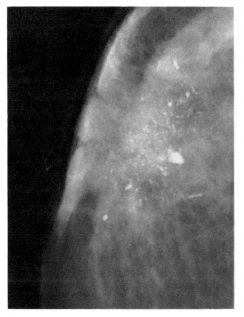

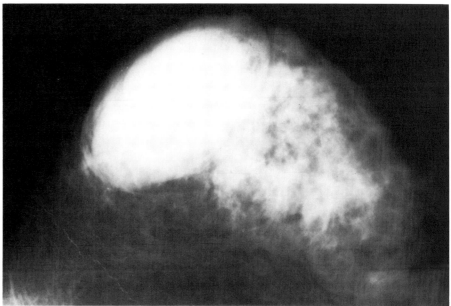

Fig. 2.**6**   Fig. 2.**7**

Fig. 2.**6** Aggregations of calcifications of different size and of bizarre shape in an isolated density with engagement of the overlying skin. Histology: Lobular carcinoma.

Fig. 2.**7** Palpation: Hard, smooth tumor the size of a goose egg, freely movable under the skin. Mammography: Smoothly outlined, ellipsoid, homogenous density with coarse calcifications and retromamillary lightning area. Histology: Fibroadenoma.

mas. Large, millimeter-long calcifications were found by Hamperl (1968) in the hyaline stroma of mastitis and cancer; he also found them in hyaline-poor cancers. Granular calcifications, 1 to 2 mm, were seen in carcinomas that grew in ducts and large lymph vessels.

Microcalcifications refer to those calcium accumulations that are seen in smaller or larger groupings. These accumulations show an amorphous, bizarre shape and differ in size. The smallest, just to be recognized with a magnifying glass, have a size of about 0.1 mm in diameter. Such microcalcifications can be situated intracellularly or interstitially. Whereas the interstitial calcifications appear most frequently by scirrhous carcinomas, the intraductal detritus foci are found in particular by pre-invasive and milk duct carcinomas.

The large, coarse calcifications occur only in fibroadenomas and carcinomas. (Figs. 2.**6**, 2.**7**). In the case of the fibroadenoma, they have particularly bizarre shapes and are often divided into different centers. During longer times of observation, only limited increase in size is noted. Coarse calcifications can also occur in the core of a solid cancer. Such calcifications are then the result of necrosis of tumors and are similarly bizarre and flaky, similar to the necrotic areas of a fibroadenoma.

Ring- or blister-like calcifications are always signs of a benign process. They can be found in cysts, fibroadenomas, fatty tissue necrosis, sebaceous cysts, chronically inflamed, enlarged cuts, enlarged glands of the skin, or as artifacts after the use of zinc ointment. Calcifications in a sebaceous cyst are mostly seen in surgical scars and have a transparent center on x-ray.

Oval or lance-like calcifications, which are always multiple and often in radial formations deep in the breast, are characteristic of a plasma cell mastitis. More typical,

however, are line-like calcifications. Similar calcium arrangements can be found in the walls of arteries on which they occur as double lines. Periductal calcifications in secretory disease can be the result of enlarged duct walls.

We find diffuse microcalcifications mostly in fibroadenosis, fibrous mastopathy, ductal carcinomas, and multicentric lobular carcinoma in situ.

In deciding the need for diagnostic procedures, the following criteria must be considered regarding intra-mammary calcifications:

1. Number
2. Size
3. Shape
4. Arrangement
5. Site

The larger the *number* of clustered calcifications, the greater is the risk for malignancy. If the calcifications are diffuse and if there are less than five calcifications in the densest accumulations that can just be seen with a magnifying lens in the area of 1 cm^2, a biopsy may not be necessary. In respect to the *size*, malignant growths are characterized by calcifications that can range from just visible to very large. The larger the difference in size, the more suspect the finding. The calcifications are relatively uniform in benign disease. The *shape* of the calcification is most varied in malignant processes. The more bizarre and irregular the calcifications are, the more likely is the presence of a malignant process. Ring-like, half circle, and line-like calcifications are generally not suspicious. Point-like and smooth, rounded calcifications are mostly found in sclerosing adenosis. Every irregular *arrangement* of calcifications is suspicious. In terms of the *site*, intracutaneous calcifications, which are harmless, must be evaluated with the help of additional pictures. Similarly, calcifications within fatty tissue are of no consequence. Outlined focal masses with calicifications, particularly where the borders are irregular and perhaps combined with radial extensions, must be biopsied. Calcifications of a scar can be the expression of a scar granuloma. Cancer-related calcifications can occupy a part of a quadrant, an entire quadrant, or the entire breast. Calcifications that are retroareolar, even if they look unsuspicious, must be biopsied if found in a patient with Paget's disease.

Localized Densities

Excluding multicentric cancer that presents diagnostic difficulties, the localized carcinoma is characterized by one defined mass. Small tumors, detected usually through microcalcifications and representing preinvasive

and early invasive carcinomas, present a small shadow that often cannot be differentiated from parenchyma. In the presence of cystic disease or in a youthful breast, even larger focal growth might not be recognizable in the mammogram.

According to Wolfe (1966), 40% of all mammographically misdiagnosed carcinomas present a single circumscribed mass because this looks the most like a benign tumor. Thus, it is recommended that all single, palpable, and circumscribed masses with a homogenous density should be biopsied.

The carcinomas with localized densities in the mammogram can be classified as follows Figs. 2.8–2.12:

1. Circumscribed mass
   a. completely smooth, rounded
   b. partly smooth, rounded
   c. unclear circumscribed
   d. with radial extensions
2. Diffuse densities

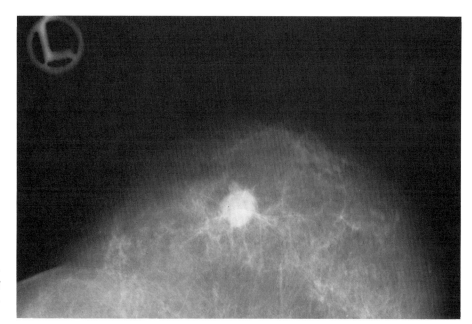

Fig. 2.**8** Smooth rounded density. Histology: Invasive solid, ductal carcinoma. Fairly sharp tumor border, lineal by lymphocytes. Diameter 12 mm.

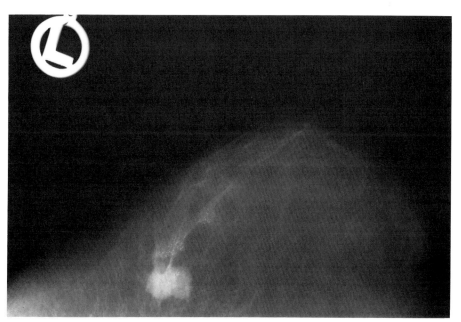

Fig. 2.**9** Nodulous tumor, partly smoothly lined and partly showing irregular lining with microcalcifications. In addition, calcifications in adjacent parenchyma. Histology: Solid cancer with adenoid differentiation.

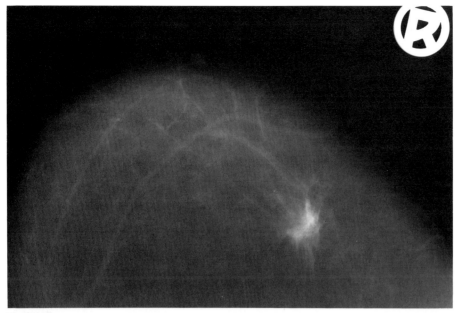

Fig. 2.**10**

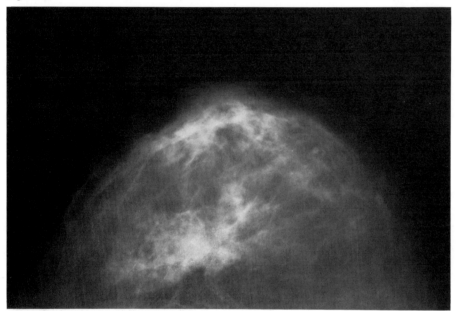

Fig. 2.**11**

Fig. 2.**12**

Fig. 2.**10**   Circumscribed mass with radial extensions. Histology: Solid cancer with pronounced fibrosis.

Fig. 2.**11**   Diffuse density close to the chest wall. Microcalcifications centrally. Histology: Invasive ductal carcinoma.

Fig. 2.**12**   In the lower part of the breast is a mass 1 cm in diameter surrounded by mastopathic densities, which makes it difficult to detect the tumor mass. Histology: Solid fibrous lobular carcinoma with a diameter of 17 mm. Lymphangitic growth in the periphery of the tumor.

The completely smooth, rounded masses are the ones that cause the most difficulties in mammographic differential diagnosis since they are mostly caused by benign processes such as fibroadenomas, cysts, papillomas, or lymph nodes, but although can be expression of a malignant process. In the case of the partially smooth, rounded mass, difficulties with the diagnosis result only when part of the rim structure is covered by the parenchyma so that a complete judgment of the contour is impossible. The unclear circumscribed masses in the mammogram are typical for carcinoma. Pathognomic for a carcinoma are unclear densities that show radial extension caused by the typical scirrhous cancer development.

Difficult to diagnose are the diffuse densities that can often only be recognized by a comparison of both breasts. Shadows often can be found in only one plane if the shadows are covered by parenchyma in the second plane.

Structural Changes

The largest number of mammary cancers are combined with a more or less strong fibrosis. These scirrhous carcinomas show a pattern of fibrotic extensions, of different length radiating from the tumor nucleus. In differential diagnosis these extensions, often called "cancer legs," are very important. They can also be produced by scars or by mastopathy. The radial extensions can be of different width. They range from very fine lines to wide pointed stripes. These radial extensions break through the normal structure of the connective tissue. They can often be very long and when situated close to the skin cause corresponding retraction of breast or nipple (Fig. 2.**13**).

To judge these stellate formations in an x-ray film, it is important to have pictures in two planes and if necessary with compression. To exclude a summation effect of normal tissue structures, the second plane is necessary; in the presence of a summation effect, this star formation is only seen in one plane.

It is difficult to recognize scirrhous carcinomas when the nucleus of the tumor is hidden behind a mastopathy. In such cases the fibrotic component, in the shape of the radial structure, could be seen without the presence of a tumor shadow.

These cases established the great value of xeroradiography, but can today also more easily be recognized in grid mammography. They teach us not only to look for localized densities, but also that every change of the parenchymal structure should be regarded as a suspicious finding indicating additional examinations.

Indirect Criteria of Malignancies

A mammographically recognizable circumscribed skin enlargement that is not caused by scar formation must be looked at as a suspicious finding. Often, skin retraction, caused by scirrhous carcinomas, can be detected earlier with x-ray than with clinical examination (Fig. 2.**14**). If there is a tumor nucleus shadow and if there are fine fibrotic extensions between tumor and the skin enlargement, the finding is always to be interpreted as that of a malignancy.

Mammographic thickening of the skin suggests a diffuse inflammatory carcinoma or a lymphangitic carcinoma. These changes are usually combined with a diffuse, reticular pattern of the mammary parenchyma. In most such cases, no direct shadow of the tumor nucleus can be seen.

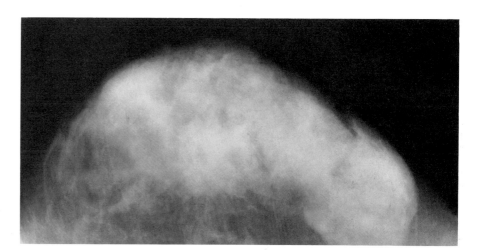

Fig. 2.**13** Pronounced mastopathic densities close to the thoracic wall with fine radial extensions. Histology: Scirrhous carcinoma.

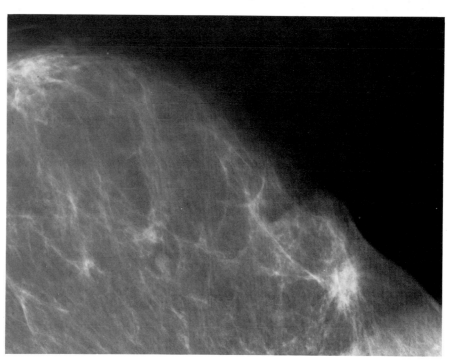

Fig. 2.**14** Diffuse mass with retraction and infiltration of the skin. Histology: Fibrous carcinoma.

To differentiate these findings from an acute mastitis is very difficult and one must assess other clinical signs such as fever, leukocytosis, or lactation. Thermography is also important here since this technique differentiates relatively accurately a mastitis from a lymphangitic carcinoma.

Further indirect criteria are enlargement of the veins with a cork-screw-like course of the arteries. According to our experience, these differential diagnostic criteria do not appear to be carcinoma specific since they may occur in benign space-requiring processes.

Examination Results

Hoeffken and Lanyi in 1973 compiled collective statistics about the accuracy of mammography based on 20 reports involving more than 25,000 cases. They showed the accuracy of mammography to be between 46% and 98.9%. Of course, the accuracy depends on the expertise of the examiner and the technique used. In addition, the statistics are influenced by the fact that the borderline between positive and suspicious findings could be drawn differently and whether or not clinical criteria are used in the evaluations. It thus becomes evident that it is impossible to compare the statistics even from large centers among themselves.

It is clear that every diagnostic technique becomes more efficient with increasing size of the tumor. In the frame of screening studies where mostly small cancers are diagnosed, the accuracy becomes less as shown by Moskowitz (1982).

In general, then, the accuracy of mammography in the diagnosis of a breast carcinoma is between 85% and 95%. Mammography will not produce a 100% accuracy level even with large cancers. In about 5% of clinically obvious mammary cancers, the mammogram will not be positive.

The accuracy of mammography depends on tumor size. We showed in our study of mammary carcinomas (Table 2.1) that the rate of mammographically suspicious findings is between 88% and 98% for all tumor stages. The rate of suspicious findings increased clearly with the size of the tumor. The clinical difference between physical examination and mammography is particularly clear in stages T0 and T1. In these two early tumor stages, the superiority of mammography is very apparent as compared with physical examination and all other diagnostic procedures.

The graphic representations of Feig (1982) demonstrate impressively the importance of mammography in the early detection of mammary carcinoma. He compares the tumor sites of cancers diagnosed by mammography with those found by palpation (Fig. 2.15). The fraction of

Table 2.1 Accuracy of mammographic and clinical diagnosis of breast cancer related to tumor stage for the years 1969 to 1975 at the Universitäts-Frauenklinik Hamburg-Eppendorf

Clinical tumor stage	No. of patients	Clinically suspicious Number	%	Mammographically suspicious Number	%
T_0	53 ⎱ 163	0	0 ⎱ 45%	52	98 ⎱ 96%
T_1	110 ⎰	74	68 ⎰	104	95 ⎰
T_2	432	362	84	401	93
T_3	180	176	98	159	88
T_4	13	13	100	12	92
T_0–T_4	788	625	79	728	92

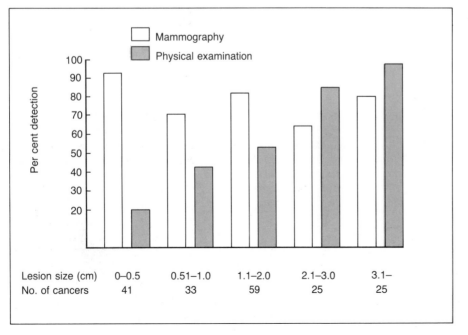

Lesion size (cm)	0–0.5	0.51–1.0	1.1–2.0	2.1–3.0	3.1–
No. of cancers	41	33	59	25	25

Fig. 2.15 Tumor distribution according to tumor size and diagnostic modality (Feig 1982).

diagnosed carcinomas by physical examination becomes less as the tumor becomes smaller. The accuracy of the mammogram was about equal for all tumor sizes. Further, if one reviews the carcinomas without lymph node metastases (Fig. 2.**16**), one finds that 80% of all cases were diagnosed by mammography, whereas only 40% were judged positive or suspicious by physical examination.

The superiority of mammography over physical examination is most obvious in health control examinations.

The best known and largest such experience in the world literature is the HIP Study (Health Insurance Plan of Greater New York) by Strax and Shapiro started in New York in 1963 (Strax et al. 1967). In this study, 31,000 women, aged 40 to 65 years, were randomly selected from the population registry and subjected to mammography and palpation. This study underlines the importance of mammography by the fact that of 44 women in whom a cancer was detected by mammography, only three died of breast cancer in the following eight years. In this HIP study, one third of the mammary cancers were solely detected by mammography. In these cases, the cancers were clinically occult. However, two fifths of the cancers were only detected by physical examination and were mammographically occult. It has to be mentioned further that a high percentage of the cancers detected by only one method – by mammography or palpation – did not show lymph node metastases. There were no lymph node metastases in 79% of the mammographically diagnosed and 75% of the clinically diagnosed cancer patients. The authors could show that the HIP study resulted in not only a longer survival time, but also in a reduction of the mortality rate of cancer patients found in this program. Of importance was the finding that the reduction of mortality did not apply to women under the age of 50, explained by the fact that the accuracy of the mammogram was hindered by the denser breasts of the younger women.

Further supportive is the American BCDDP study (Breast Cancer Detection Demonstration Project), which has existed in the United States since 1973 and in which 27 centers participated; in 1978, the examination results were reported from 270,000 women. Of great importance in the BCDDP study was the conclusion that the same high frequency of clinically occult carcinomas could be diagnosed in younger aged groups as in older women (Fig. 2.**17**). In the course of the BCDDP study, mammary cancers were diagnosed in 15,097 women through 1976. About 40% were clinically occult, about 50% of the examined women were under 50 years of age, and 31% of all the mammary cancers were found in this age group (Table 2.**2**).

Thirty-seven percent of the detected cancers were "minimal cancer" that is either not infiltrating or invasive but smaller than 1 cm in diameter. They are found mostly by mammography (Table 2.**3**). Compared with the HIP study, the BCDDP study detected seven times more "minimal cancers." Although the background of the patients cannot be completely compared, in both studies these results nevertheless show that an improved mam-

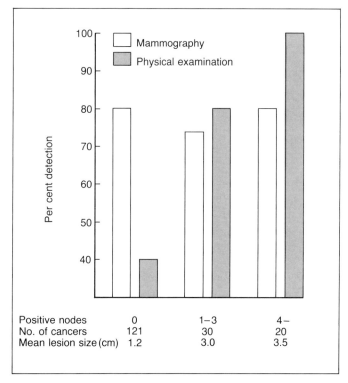

Fig. 2.**16** Incidence of axillary metastasis in breast cancer correlated to the method of diagnosing the cancer (Feig 1982).

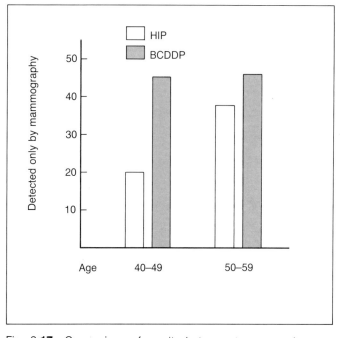

Fig. 2.**17** Comparison of results between two screening programs: HIP = Health Insurance Plan of Greater New York (1963–1967). BCDDP = Breast Cancer Detection Demonstration Projects (1973–1976). Percentage of cancers detected only by mammography in women aged 40 to 49 and 50 to 59 (Feig 1982).

mographic technique not only reduces the mortality by 40% as compared with the HIP study, but also that the benefits apply equally to women under the age of 59.

Based on experiences from the literature, Moskowitz (1982) reported a revealing analysis of the value of the mammography in comparison with palpation and ther-

Diagnostic modality	Age (years)					
	35–39	40–49	50–59	60–64	65–74	Total
Mammography alone	48%	43.5%	48 %	39.5%	38.5%	43.9%
Physical examination alone	4%	9.1%	8.1%	5.8%	5.4%	7.4%
Mammography and physical examination	48%	46.4%	42.1%	54.7%	55.4%	47.7%
Unknown						1.1%

Table 2.**2** Results of BCDDP-study. Percentage of diagnosed cancers in different age groups correlated to the diagnostic modality (Lester 1979)

mography. He analyzed the accuracy of different centers in three single modalities and compared this with the different frequency of carcinomas in each collective. Based on the graphical analysis, he could show that the accuracy of all three methods increases with the number of mammary carcinomas in the collective. Although the three mentioned examination procedures are relatively close where there is a high cancer frequency, it becomes apparent that mammography is superior to palpation the smaller the number of mammary carcinomas in a collective. The statistical analysis is the first evidence that thermography has the least importance in the early detection of a mammary carcinoma.

Indications for Mammography

Due to its clinical significance a mammography should be performed:
1. For any clinically suspicious breast finding
2. For equivocal breast findings on palpation
3. For cancer preventive screening

In the case of clinically suspected findings in the breast that necessitates a biopsy for histologic examination, a mammographic examination of both breasts should be generally performed before surgery. Against this statement critical counter arguments can be raised because it appears that a mammogram is unnecessary when biopsy is to be done. The clinical importance of the mammogram in this setting rests mainly on the fact that a mammogram before histologic results increases the suspicion and supports the criteria for a biopsy with frozen section. According to our experience, a frozen section biopsy is not justified if the possibility is higher that the growth is

benign. Patients should not be asked to sign an agreement for mastectomy unless the clinical suspicion is fully supported by mammographic result.

In addition, the mammogram can preoperatively exclude or disclose the presence of suspicious lesions in a different quadrant of the same breast or in the contralateral breast which could be biopsied at the same time.

On the other hand, a negative mammogram or a mammographic result indicative of a benign disease should not negate a biopsy. We always have to remember that at least 5% of all clinically detected carcinomas can not be seen mammographically. Therefore, the most important rule is that a palpable, isolated clinically suspicious mass must be histologically examined even in the case of a negative mammogram.

In addition, palpable masses that do not appear to be necessarily a carcinoma but remain a palpable suspicious finding should be surgically removed. In these cases, a mammographically indicated malignancy criterion can support the decision to perform a biopsy or can show that the palpable growth is a cyst that can be identified by pneumocystography making a surgical procedure unnecessary and avoidable.

The greatest value of mammography is for breast cancer screening. Only through the use of mammography in screening procedures will it be possible to diagnose invasive carcinomas with smaller diameters. The risk of x-ray exposure is minimal, but the high cost to third party payers is used as an argument against the use of screening mammography on all women of cancer-dangerous age.

It is also argued that the mammography is not specific enough in the early detection of cancer, which yields to a high false-positive quota in clinically normal women that yields many biopsies that are found to be unnecessary.

However, the specificity for palpations is estimated to be 30% to 40%; three clinically indicated biopsies will thus result in one carcinoma and two benign lesions. For all mammographically indicated biopsies, the yield is 20%; that is, five biopsies result in one malignant finding, but these are generally earlier lesions.

As can be seen from Table 2.**4**, we have conducted a mammographic study in our hospital on 543 women in a period of two years and have used the mammogram as the sole indicator for a biopsy. In all cases, the results of palpation were negative. We found only 20% invasive and preinvasive carcinoma. The accuracy could have been raised to 40% if we included all cases with a proliferative mastopathy. Since we can assume that the

Table 2.**3** Results of the BCDDP-study. Percentage of diagnosed cancers and "minimal cancers" detected by different diagnostic modalities (Lester 1979)

Diagnostic modality	Percentage of positive findings	
	Total	"Minimal cancers"
Mammography alone	43.9	55.0
Mammography and physical examination	47.7	34.9
Physical examination alone	7.4	9.0
Unknown	1.1	1.1

Table 2.**4** Histologic findings in excisional biopses (n= 543) made exclusively because of mammography (nonpalpable lesions) 1980 and 1981 at the Universitäts-Frauenklinik Hamburg-Eppendorf

Histology	Number (%)	
Proliferating mastopathy (Prechtel type II)	117 (21.6%)	
Proliferating mastopathy with atypies (Prechtel type III)		41,3%
Intralobulare carcinoma (LCIS) Intraductal carcinoma (DCIS)	45 (8.3%)	
Invasive carcinoma	62 (11.4%)	

proliferative mastopathy and in particular the mastopathy with atypical cells is properly a precursor for malignant disease, then these cases cannot be classified as false positive. Thus, the specificity of the mammography equals that of palpation and inspection.

Unfortunately, valid data are still missing today for sufficient characterization of high-risk patients in whom screening mammography shows a higher efficacy. It is certain that age is an important factor. The incidence increases from the age of 30. Compared with this factor, all the other risk factors are almost neglible: nulliparity, late first pregnancy, and family history, unless mother or a sister were diseased before the menopause. The only true risk group is the one which consists of patients with existing mammary carcinoma of the other breast. The observations that risk groups can be identified through thermography (Stark 1982) or through mammographically determined parenchymal patterns (Wolfe 1982) could not be sufficiently supported in larger studies. If we want to improve the early diagnosis, then we have to perform preventive mammography in women over 35 or at least 40 every two years and in women over 50 at high risk every year. In Hamburg we could show in a screening study in which more than 13,000 women from age 30 on were examined mammographically every two years that the size of the diagnosed cancer decreased with routine mammography and the number with axillary lymph node metastasis decreased also in the diagnosed carcinomas (Frischbier and Bernauer, 1982).

It cannot be expected that the application of mammography to women with suspicious or questionable findings will lead to a decisive improvement in the early diagnosis and cure rate. The value of mammography is much more in the area of routine, preventive screening examinations.

References

Baclesse, F., A. Willemin: Atlas of Mammography. Libraire Facultes, Paris 1967

Bailar, I. C. III: Mammography: A contrary view. Ann. Intern. Med. 84: 77, 1976

Barth, V.: Atlas der Brustdrüsenerkrankungen. Enke, Stuttgart 1977

Black, D. W., B. Young: A radiological and pathological study of the breast and neoplasms of other tissues. Br. J. Radiol. 38: 596, 1965

Boice, I. D., R. Monson: Breast cancer in women after repeated fluoroscopic examinations of the chest. J. Natl. Cancer Inst. 59: 823, 1977

Bonilla-Musoles, F. M., J. R. Romero, J. J. Gil: Xerorradiografia y termografia de placa de la mamma. Editorial Jims, Barcelona 1979

Buttenberg, D., K. Werner: Die Mammographie. Schattauer, Stuttgart 1962

Chang, C. H. J.: Die Computertomographie der Brust. In: Die Erkrankungen der weiblichen Brustdrüse. Hrsg.: H.-J. Frischbier, Thieme, Stuttgart, New York 1982

Egan, R. L.: Mammography. Thomas, Springfield, Ill. 1964

Fassin, Y., I. Jeanmart: La ponction des kystes du sein apport de la pneumocystographie. J. Belge Radiol. 55: 39, 1972

Feig, St. A.: Apparative Verbesserungen zur Dosisreduzierung bei der Mammographie. In: Die Erkrankungen der weiblichen Brustdrüse. Hrsg.: H.-J. Frischbier, Thieme, Stuttgart, New York 1982

Friedrich, M.: Der Einfluß der Streustrahlung auf die Abbildungsqualität bei der Mammographie. Fortschr. Röntgenstr. 123: 556, 1975

Friedrich, M.: Bildqualität in der Mammographie. Einfluß der Streustrahlung und der Bildaufzeichnungssysteme. Fortschr. Röntgenstr. 36: 4, 1977

Friedrich, M.: Neuere Entwicklungstendenzen der Mammographie Technik: Die Rastermammographie. Fortschr. Röntgenstr. 128: 207, 1978

Friedrich, M., P. Weskamp: A Comparison of Direct Film Mammography with Screen Film Mammography. In: Reduced Dose Mammography. Ed.: W. Logan, E. P. Muntz, Masson, New York 1979

Friedrich, M.: Apparative Verbesserungen zur Dosisreduzierung bei der Mammographie. In: Die Erkrankungen der weiblichen Brustdrüse. Hrsg.: H.-J. Frischbier, Thieme, Stuttgart, New York 1982

Frischbier, H.-J., H. U. Lohbeck: Frühdiagnostik des Mammakarzinoms. Klinische, röntgenologische, thermographische und zytologische Untersuchungsmethoden und ihre Wertigkeit. Thieme, Stuttgart 1977

Frischbier, H.-J., A. Gregl, W. Hoeffken, J. R. Hüppe: Vorschläge zur Qualitätsnormierung der Mammographie. Radiologe, 17: 193, 1977

Frischbier, H.-J., M. Bernauer: Zehnjährige Ergebnisse einer Mammographie-Studie zur Brustkrebsfrüherkennung bei klinisch gesunden Frauen. In: Die Erkrankungen der weiblichen Brustdrüse. Hrsg.: H.-J. Frischbier, Thieme, Stuttgart, New York 1982

Gershon-Cohen, J.: Atlas of Mammography. Springer, Berlin 1970

Gros, Ch. M.: Les maladies du sein. Masson, Paris 1963

Hamperl, H.: Zur Frage der pathologisch-anatomischen Grundlagen der Mammographie. Geburtsh. Frauenheilk. 28: 901, 1968

Hoeffken, W., K. Heuss, E. Rödel: Die Notwendigkeit einer Belichtungsautomatik für die Mammographie. Radiologe 10: 154, 1970

Hoeffken, W., M. Lanyi: Röntgenuntersuchung der Brust. Technik, Diagnostik, Differentialdiagnose, Ergebnisse. Thieme, Stuttgart 1973

Ingleby, H., J. Gershon-Cohen: Comparative anatomy, pathology and roentgenology of the breast. University of Pennsylvania Press, Philadelphia 1960

Leborgne, R. A.: The Breast on Roentgen Diagnosis. Constable, London 1953

Lester, R. G.: The Breast Cancer Detection Demonstration Project: An Analysis of the Data. In: Reduced Dose Mammography. Ed.: W. Logan, E. P. Muntz. Masson, New York 1979

Logan, W., E. P. Muntz: Reduced Dose Mammography. Masson, New York 1979

Lundgren, B. O.: One-view x-ray breast cancer screening in a Swedish city. Vortrag IIIrd Congress of European Association of Radiology, Edinburgh 1975

Luzatti, G., B. Salvadori, E. Tavani: La xeromammografia. Excerpta Medica, Amsterdam 1979

MacKenzie, I.: Breast Cancer following multiple fluoroscopies. Br. J. Cancer 19: 1, 1965

Mettler, F. A., Fr.: Breast neoplasms in women treated with x-rays for acute postpartum mastitis. A pilot study. J. Natl. Cancer Inst. 43: 803, 1969

Moskowitz, M.: Reihenuntersuchungen zur Diagnostik des Mammakarzinoms: Wie wirksam sind unsere Untersuchungsmethoden? Ein kritischer Überblick. In: Die Erkrankungen der weiblichen Brustdrüse. Hrsg.: H.-J. Frischbier. Thieme, Stuttgart, New York 1982

Otto, R. Ch.: Aktuelle Röntgendiagnostik im Kampf gegen den Brustkrebs. Huber, Bern, Stuttgart, Wien 1980

Schreer, M., M. Demelt, K. Würthner: Phantomuntersuchungen und erste klinische Erfahrungen an einem Raster Mammographiegerät. Fortschr. Röntgenstr. 129: 357, 1978

Seifert, J.: Das Mammogramm und seine Deutung. 2. Aufl. Steinkopff, Darmstadt 1975

Shapiro, S., P. Strax, L. Venet: Periodic breast cancer screening in reducing mortality from breast cancer. J. Am. Med. Assoc. 215: 1777, 1971

Shepard, J., G. Crile, W. C. Strittmatter: Roentgenographic evaluation of calcifications seen in paraffin block specimens of mammary tumors. Radiology 78: 967, 1962

Sickles, E. A.: Microfocal spot magnification mammography using xeroradiographic and screen-film recording systems. Radiology 131: 347, 1979

Stark, A. M.: Die Bestimmung des Brust-Krebs-Risikos mit der Thermographie. In: Die Erkrankungen der weiblichen Brustdrüse. Hrsg.: H.-J. Frischbier. Thieme, Stuttgart, New York 1982

Strax, P., L. Venet, S. Shapiro, S. Gross: Mammography and clinical examination in mass screening for cancer of the breast. Cancer 20: 2184, 1967

Strax, P.: Die Zielsetzung bei der Durchführung von Reihenuntersuchungen zur Früherkennung des Mammakarzinoms. In: Die Erkrankungen der weiblichen Brustdrüse. Hrsg.: H.-J. Frischbier. Thieme, Stuttgart, New York 1982

Tabár, L., Z. Márton, I. Kádas: Die Pneumocystographie der Brust. Chirurg 44: 428, 1973

Thomas, L. B., et al.: Pathology Review Report. In: Final reports of the National Cancer Institute ad hoc working groups on mammography screening for breast cancer and a summary report of their findings and recommendations. U. S. Department of Health, Education and Welfare; Public Health Service; National Institutes of Health DHEW-Publication No (NIH) 77–1400, March 1977

Wanebo, C. K., G. Johnson, K. Sato, T. W. Thotslung: Breast cancer after exposure to the atomic bombing of Hiroshima and Nagasaki. N. Engl. J. Med. 279: 667, 1968

Logan, W., E. P. Muntz: Reduced Dose Mammography. Masson, New York 1979

Willemin, A.: Les Images Mammographiques. Karger, Basel 1972

Witt, H., H. Bürger: Mammadiagnostik im Röntgenbild. de Gruyter, Berlin 1968

Witten, D. M.: The Breast. Year Book Medical Publishers, Chicago 1969

Wolfe, J. N.: Mammography: Errors in diagnosis. Radiology 87: 214, 1966

Wolfe, J. N.: Xeroradiography of the breast. Thomas, Springfield, Ill. 1972

Wolfe, J. N.: Zusammenhang zwischen Parenchymmuster und der Entstehung von Brustkrebs. In: Die Erkrankungen der weiblichen Brustdrüse. Hrsg.: H.-J. Frischbier. Thieme, Stuttgart, New York 1982

Würthner, K.: Zitiert bei Frischbier u. Lohbeck: Frühdiagnostik des Mammakarzinoms. Thieme, Stuttgart 1977

Würthner, K.: Dosisverteilung und Strahlenbelastung bei der Mammographie. In: Die Erkrankungen der weiblichen Brustdrüse. Hrsg. H.-J. Frischbier. Thieme, Stuttgart, New York 1982

Chapter 3

Diagnostic Ultrasound in Breast Diseases

A. Kratochwil

Introduction

Over the last 20 years, ultrasound has been used with great success in different disciplines of medicine in order to visualize the soft tissue and to detect pathologic changes. This technique is well suited for visualizing changes in the female breast because of its superficial position and tissue structure that seem to be ideal for diagnostic ultrasound.

The first reports in this field date back to 1951 when Wild and Reid tried to discriminate benign from malignant tumors of the female breast by means of ultrasound. Their results stimulated other investigators including, in Japan, Wagai et al. (1972) and Kobayashi et al. (1973), in the United States, Baum (1977) and Kelly-Fry and Harper (1979), and in Europe, Kratochwil et al. (1968, 1975), Ossoinig et al. (1968), and later Gros et al. (1974, 1978). Recently, the most interesting pictures giving a high degree of information were published by Kossoff et al. (1975) and Jellins et al. (1977).

Principles of Technique

The principle of the technique is that of SONAR, which stands for *sound navigation ranging*. The sound waves produced by a transducer are conducted into the tissue. At the border surfaces of different tissues, a partial reflection of the sound waves occurs depending on the difference in impedance. Since the transducer only produces short sound waves, it can be used as a receiver during the interval. The reflected sound waves may be visualized in different ways, either by amplitude technique on a cathode-ray tube (CRT) (A-mode) or as a two-dimensional cross-section picture of the examined region. Presently, gray scale pictures are used; that is, controlling the degree of brightness in the picture by the echo amplitudes. In echo tomography, one can distinguish between compound and real-time techniques. In the compound technique a cross-section picture is produced on the screen.

In real-time technique, immediately after the application of the transducer, a live cross-section picture of the glandular region is produced on the screen. In compound technique, the complete organ is simultaneously visualized, whereas real-time technique gives partial cross-section pictures.

Depending on the physical qualities it is impossible to record the structures lying just beneath the skin by direct application of the transducer to the skin of the breast. This is impossible specifically for the compound scanner, but not when using a real time scanner with a high frequency.

In order to establish a sufficient distance between the transducer and the examined region and to avoid deformation of the breast by the manually applied transducer, a waterbath scanner is used. The first equipment described by Wild and Reid (1952) used such a technique. The transducer was within a water tank where the border on the side of the patient was made of a sound-transparent (transonic) membrane.

Similar methods were used by the Japanese group which used water tanks open upwards and molded by a polyvinyl envelope. During the examination, the patient was placed on her back and the water tank with its transducer was placed on the region to be examined.

The movement of the transducer was curved and automatic, and at the end of each step the scan surface was moved according to a previously decided length (Kobayashi et al. 1973; Wagai et al. 1972). In their first attempts, the Australian authors used a similar principle. The base diameter of the breast was cut out of an adhesive plastic sheet. The sheet was taped around the breast and the surplus part of the sheet made in to a bag. After filling it with degassed water, the breasts were floating in the bag according to their fat content and were examined from above. In further developments the patient was examined lying on her abdomen with her breasts hanging down into a water tank (Kossoff et al. 1975). This permits images without mechanical deformity.

Normal Echography of the Female Breast

The first structure recognized is the skin and the nipple (Fig. 3.1). Under the skin the subcutaneous fat tissue is poorly seen or even empty of echoes. In this area, cords that reflect strongly could be seen corresponding to the Cooper's ligaments that fixate the relatively tense, and in younger females, triangularly shaped parts of the gland to the skin. Within the gland, the papillary ducts could be recognized. Dorsally, the gland is bordered by the retromammary fat tissue or the pectoral fascia. Further dorsally is the muscle tissue that gives considerably less reflection and behind that is the thoracic wall where sections of ribs can be recognized.

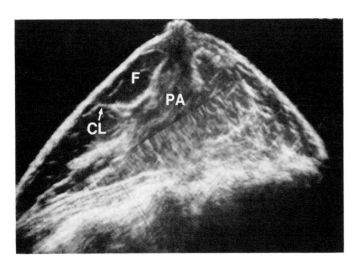

Fig. 3.**1** Normal breast showing triangular-shaped parenchyma (PA) and subcutaneous fat (F) with Cooper's ligaments (CL).

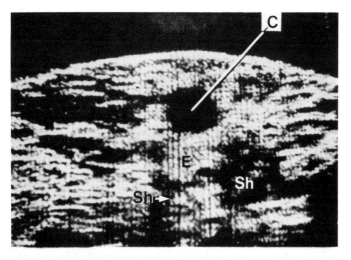

Fig. 3.**2** Cyst (C) within the breast. Behind the cyst, clear echo enhancement (E) and bilateral shadows (Sh) are seen.

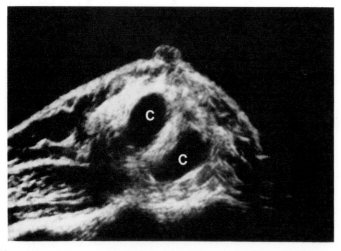

Fig. 3.**3** Multiple cysts (C) in the breast. Longitudinal section. At the border of the cysts, clear enhancement is seen, caused by compression.

This normal picture could be changed through physiologic processes such as lactation or age, but also by pathologic conditions.

Physical Properties

The ultrasound waves lose energy on their way from the transducer through the tissue. The size of this loss of sound energy in addition to the distance to the transducer depend also on the frequency used and the tissue to be examined (Gros et al. 1978; Jellins et al. 1977; Kobayashi et al. 1974; Kossoff 1977; Kossoff et al. 1978; Reeve et al. 1979; Wagai et al. 1972). The higher the frequency, the smaller the wave length of the ultrasound. This gives better discrimination but shorter penetration. The thicker the tissue, the more sound energy is absorbed; fluids produce little sound absorption.

Cysts

Cysts (Figs. 3.**2**, 3.**3**) are seen as distinctly bordered echofree areas. Behind the dorsal cyst wall is a central echorich area. This phenomenon, called "enhancement", depends on the high difference in impedance between the liquid and the neighboring solid tissue, (brake effect). This zone of multiplied reflection is bordered on both sides by two areas of shadow (Jellins et al. 1977; Kobayashi et al. 1973, 1974).

These shadow areas are caused by a refraction of the ultrasonic waves in the sides of the cyst walls, whereby the reflected sound waves no longer return to the receiver. These shadow areas are referred to as refractive shadows.

Solid Tumors

Solid tumors can be relatively sharp bordered. Their wall is usually thicker than that of cysts and often shows a more jagged ("saw toothed") outline. Since solid structures internally contain border surfaces, even central reflections of different intensity are to be seen (Griffiths 1978; Hackelöer et al. 1980; Kobayashi et al. 1973; Kossoff 1977; Reeve et al. 1979; Wagai et al. 1972) (Fig. 3.**4**).

On the dorsal border of solid tumors is a central shadow area in contrast to what could be seen in cysts (Fig. 3.**5**). This shadow area is caused by the sound absorption of the tissue. The shadow areas are also dependent on the technique used (Fig. 3.**6**). In a compound technique where the different sectors overlap, the shadow could be missing. For this reason, a scanning examination with single sweep technique is necessary to interpret the findings (Jellins et al. 1979; Kossoff 1978; Kossoff et al. 1978). The sound attenuation caused by the tumor may also be regarded as a further criterion in tumor differentiation (Gros et al. 1978).

If the tumor is examined in the same view with diminishing sound intensity (sensitivity-graded method), it is possible to distinguish between cystic and solid tumors

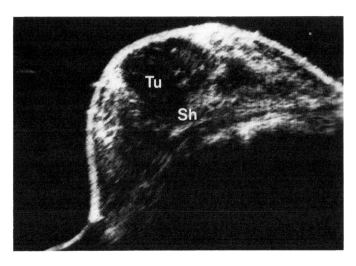

Fig. 3.**4** Solid tumor (Tu) within the breast, with small central echo formations (Sh).

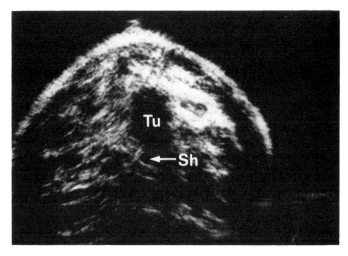

Fig. 3.**5** Solid tumor (Tu) within the breast with clear dorsal shadow formation (Sh).

because of different appearance of the echo from the back wall of the tumor (Kobayashi et al. 1973, 1974; Wagai et al. 1975) (Fig. 3.**7**). In cysts, which absorb a relatively small amount of sound, the amplification can be greatly reduced until the dorsal echo of the cyst is no longer recognized. In solid tumors, however, the baseline echo will disappear after a relatively small reduction of the amplification.

Changes in Shape

Small cysts are always round. When their size increases, they achieve more of an oval shape (Jellins et al. 1977). Solid tumors could be either oval, round, or show a completely irregular border. To estimate the pathologic changes of the female breast, the following criteria are considered:

1. Position and border – distinct or not distinct
2. Central echo – present or not present
3. Dorsal sound enhancement
4. Shadows present – lateral, central
5. Sound impairment – sensitivity-graded method
6. Assessment of tissue architecture
7. Assessment of skin changes – thickening, retractions

(Jellins et al. 1979; Kobayashi et al. 1974; Kossoff 1978; Wagai et al. 1975, 1979) (Table 3.**1**) Further, for instance, semiquantitative ways of assessment were used by Jellins according to the scedule given in Table 3.**1** (Jellins et al. 1979).

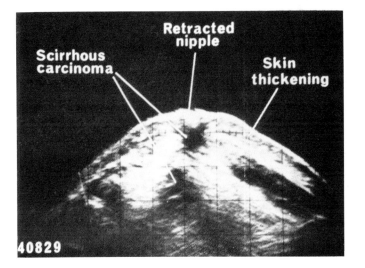

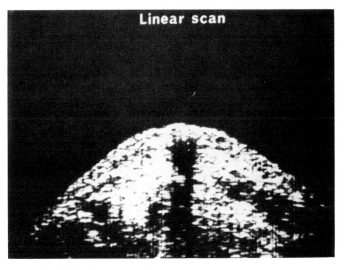

Fig. 3.**6** This shadow could even better be seen in linear scan (lower part). Retracted nipple in scirrhous carcinoma (upper picture). (With kind permission from J. Jellins, Australia.)

Table 3.**1** Echographic criteria for tumor differentiation

	Contour and shape	Internal echoes	Backwell	Shadows	Absorption	Skin involvement
Cyst and Adenoma	smooth, sharp regular	none-weak	pronounced strong enhancement	lateral (refractive)	small	none
Scirrhous carcinoma	irregular	few-weak	slight	central	high	retraction, thickening
Papillary carcinoma	irregular	mixed	slight	central	moderate	
Medullary carcinoma	irregular, sometimes however regular	irregular	often strong with enhancement	central, but often also lateral	moderate to small	

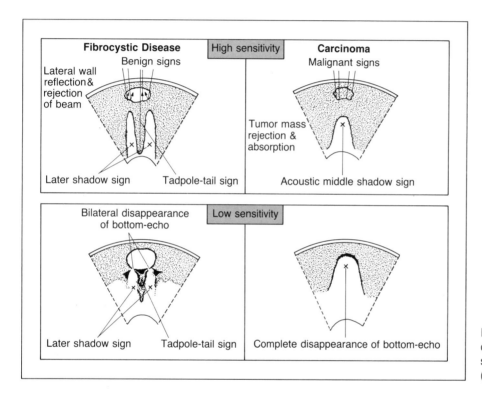

Fig. 3.**7** Difference in behavior between cysts and solid tumors when using different sensitivity: Sensitivity graded method (Kobayashi et al. 1974).

Benign Lesions

With increasing age, the amount of fat in the breast is increased thus reducing the parenchyma (Jellins et al. 1977) (Fig. 3.**8**). Here, areas of reduced echo structure, resembling garlands, can be recognized under the skin. They are lined by strongly reflecting connected tissue septa (Griffiths 1978).

Within the fat tissue, Cooper's ligaments are prominent (Fig. 3.**9**). Isolated conglomerates of fat with strongly reflecting walls but with a weak central reflection may correspond to isolated fat tissue necrosis (Kossoff et al. 1978). The lactating breast is difficult to examine with echography, since the reflecting zone under the skin produces a complete absorption of the ultrasonic waves.

Infections, with abscess formation, can be easily recognized because of their cystic character, with strong central echo complexes. Hematoma after trauma can initially present as echo-free areas without walls. De-

pending on subsequent organization of the clot, central reflections will be seen (Hackelöer et al. 1980; Jellins et al. 1977). The fibroses seen in mastopathy are characterized by abundant reflections.

Fibrous strings replace the parenchyma and cause a complete destruction of the normal architecture (Fig. 3.**10**). In the so-called hormonal fibrocystic mastopathy, a broad semicircular area of reflections can be recognized immediately under the skin. Behind this area is a zone of shadow (Fig. 3.**11**A, B).

Many small cysts, even at 3 to 4 mm, can be recognized with the techniques we have today (Griffiths 1978; Jellins et al. 1977) (Fig. 3.**12**). Isolated cysts can be demonstrated in single scan (Figs. 3.**13**, 3.**14**). Glandular ducts can be demonstrated if they contain fluid and have a diameter of 3 mm (Jellins et al. 1977). They can be seen as parallel echo structures that border a centrally located echo-free area. They are most easily demonstrated in longitudinal sections (Figs. 3.**15**, 3.**16**).

Table 3.**1**

	Characteristics of circumscribed lesions		
Changes of architecture right / left moderate strong	*Posterior details* right / left impaired unchanged in shadow	*Attachment* right / left skin muscels	*Probability of malignancy* right / left 0% 25% 50% 75% 100%
Central echo right / left none fat	*Influence of volume* right / left retraction unchanged expansive	*Skin behavior* right / left normal retraction protrusion thickening	
Borders right / left smooth saw-thoothed not seen	*Surrounding tissue* right / left unchanged reactive compressed	*Size* right / left 1 cm 1 cm, 2 cm 2 cm	

Notes

Table 3.**2**

Size of breast small medium large very large	*Amount of fat tissue* 0–25% 26– 50% 51–75% 76–100%	*Central echo in amplitude* yes no
Cooper's ligament prominent yes no	*Prominent glandular ducts* none some many dilated	*What amount of echoes has shorter amplitude than normal* 0–25% 26– 50% 51–75% 76–100%
Border of fat tissue garland-like flat	*Calcifications* present not present	*What amout of echoes has higher amplitude than normal* 0–25% 26– 50% 51–75% 76–100%
Retromammary fat layer prominent yes no	*Age impression* adequate younger older	*Classification according to Wolfe* N_1 P_1 P_2 D_Y
Notice		*Ultrasound classification* 1 2 3 3a 3b 4 4a 4b 5

In ductal ectasia, numerous glandular ducts can be seen running concentrically toward the nipple. The zone of shadow is recognized immediately under the areola. In cross section, such dilated ducts might be mistaken for small cysts (Jellins et al. 1977). Fibroadenomas show an oval shape in echography (Griffiths 1978; Hackelöer et al. 1980) (Fig. 3.**17**) with a broad and saw-toothed border. Similar to cysts they show a dorsal increase in echo and a lateral shadow zone. In contrast to cysts, however, they show a weak internal structure.

Sarcoma phyllodes (Fig. 3.**18**), which is most commonly seen in younger people, is characterized by its size. The border is sharp and in the neighborhood fibrous reaction can be seen caused by the pressure of the tumor, a phenomenon that also can be seen in larger cysts (Jellins et al. 1977). Centrally, echo structures of different intensity can be demonstrated.

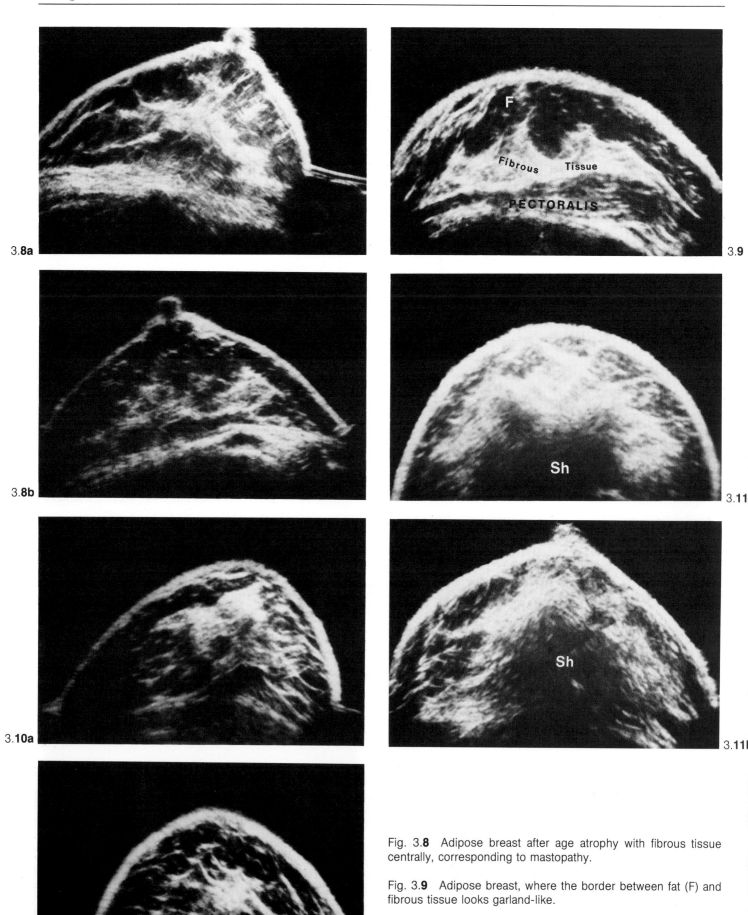

3.8a

3.8b

3.10a

3.10b

3.9

3.11a

3.11b

Fig. 3.8 Adipose breast after age atrophy with fibrous tissue centrally, corresponding to mastopathy.

Fig. 3.9 Adipose breast, where the border between fat (F) and fibrous tissue looks garland-like.

Fig. 3.10 Mastopathy indicated by irregular structure of the fibrous tissue within the breast.

Fig. 3.11A, B So-called endocrine mastopathy showing prominent shadow formation (Sh) behind the fibrous tissue.

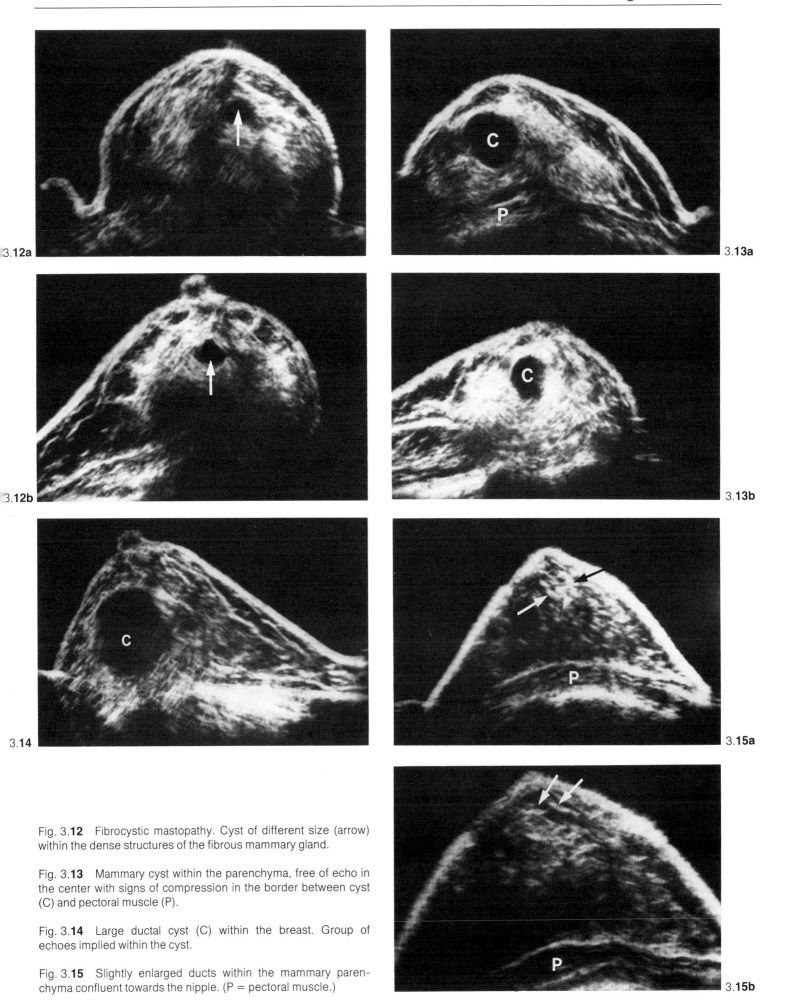

3.12a

3.13a

3.12b

3.13b

3.14

3.15a

3.15b

Fig. 3.**12** Fibrocystic mastopathy. Cyst of different size (arrow) within the dense structures of the fibrous mammary gland.

Fig. 3.**13** Mammary cyst within the parenchyma, free of echo in the center with signs of compression in the border between cyst (C) and pectoral muscle (P).

Fig. 3.**14** Large ductal cyst (C) within the breast. Group of echoes implied within the cyst.

Fig. 3.**15** Slightly enlarged ducts within the mammary parenchyma confluent towards the nipple. (P = pectoral muscle.)

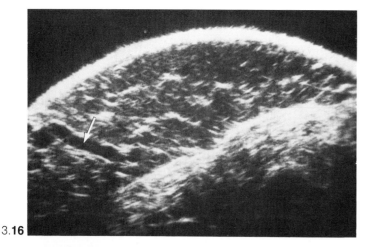

3.16

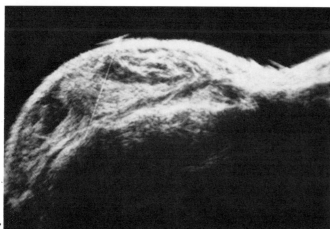

3.17

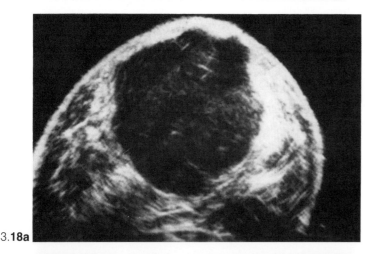

3.18a

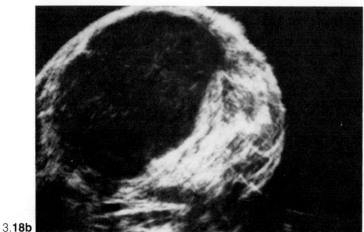

3.18b

Malignant Lesions

Malignant lesions are echographically seen as irregular areas of solid structure (Fig. 3.**19**). Dorsal to the tumors is a central shadow (Hackelöer et al. 1980; Kobayashi 1978). These changes are more easily recognized in a fibrous than a fatty breast (Kossoff 1978; Kossoff et al. 1978; Reeve et al. 1979). Attempts have also been made to correlate the echographic picture to the histology of the tumor based on the content of fibrous tissue (Kobayashi 1978; Kossoff et al. 1978).

The scirrhous carcinoma that is rich in fibrous tissue can always be seen as a solid area with a diffuse border and a radiating structure ("Christmas tree sign") (Hackelöer et al. 1980) (Fig. 3.**20**). Shadows could be demonstrated in about 60% of the tumors (Jellins et al. 1978). The fibrous strings, penetrating through the subcutaneous fat tissue and the skin, might cause changes of the skin such as inversion, thickening, or edema corresponding to the peau d'orange (Fig. 3.**21**).

Smaller changes in the skin might be more easily recognized when the breasts are floating in water as compared with clinical examination. The richer in cells the carcinoma tissue is, the easier it is for the ultrasound to penetrate (Kossoff et al. 1978). This might give a problem in differential diagnoses since the medullary carcinoma and also the mucous carcinoma sometimes give a pattern similar to a fibroadenoma (Kobayashi 1978). The papillary and mucous carcinoma show a very irregular mixed picture consisting of cystic and solid parts. Because of these difficulties of differential diagnoses, it is recommended that the amplitude picture (A-Mode) be used for assessment as different histologic types give different echoes and the findings eventually might be estimated by mathematical calculation.

Further information might be gained from the way the tumor moves. The transducer is pushed against the tissue and the changes of the echo picture are recorded. Malignant tumors generally are more fixed.

A Doppler instrument can be used to detect the vascularity, generally greater in malignant tumors (White and Cledgelt 1978).

Larger calcifications can be demonstrated with ultrasound but usually not microcalcifications (Fig. 3.**22**).

To assess tumors, a scoring system has been devised (Takahayashi et al. 1979) (Fig. 3.**23**).

Fig. 3.**16** Mamma with clearly dilated terminal milk duct (arrow).

Fig. 3.**17** In the lateral quadrant of the breast is a sharply outlined oval area with a few echoes centrally corresponding to an adenoma.

Fig. 3.**18** Sarcoma phyllodes in a young patient. A relatively sharp border of the tumor with signs of compression at the border and echoes centrally.

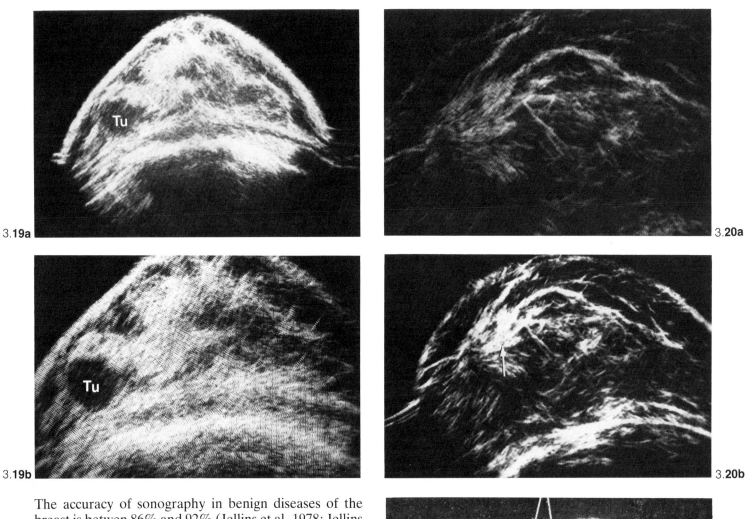

3.19a

3.20a

3.19b

3.20b

The accuracy of sonography in benign diseases of the breast is betwen 86% and 92% (Jellins et al. 1978; Jellins and Reeve 1978; Kobayashi 1978; Kossoff et al. 1978; Pluygers et al. 1977; Reeve et al. 1979), but in cysts is 100%. In the malignant lesions, the correct diagnoses will be between 82% and 90%. The accuracy is, however, strongly dependent on the tumor stage and the histologic type. The accuracy increases from 77% correct findings in stage I to 90% to 100% in stage III.

The smallest carcinoma that could be correctly diagnosed using ultrasound had a diameter of 3 mm (Kossoff et al. 1978). Between the different histologic types, the scirrhous carcinoma showed the best results with 85% to 100% correct diagnoses (Pluyers et al. 1977; Takahayashi et al. 1979; Wagai and Tsutsumi 1979). The poorest results were seen in papillary carcinoma where only 71% to 88% correct diagnoses were made. The medullary carcinoma come between with an accuracy rate of 84% to 95% (Kobayashi 1978; Takahayashi et al. 1979).

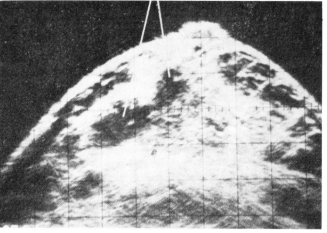

3.21a

Fig. 3.**19**A, B Solid tumor (Tu) within the breast. Carcinoma.

Fig. 3.**20**A, B Centrally strongly reflecting tumor, with irregular border and with radiations into the surroundings (arrow). Typical scirrhous carcinoma.

Fig. 3.**21** Skin changes in carcinoma, in this case marked thickening. (With kind permission from J. Jellins, Australia.)

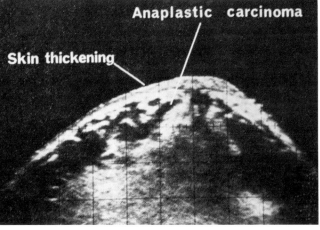

Anaplastic carcinoma

Skin thickening

3.21b

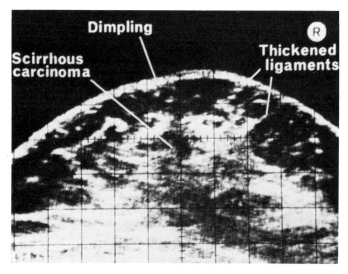

3.**22a**

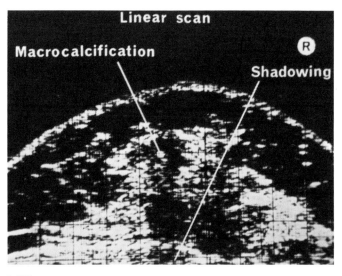

3.**22b**

3.**23**

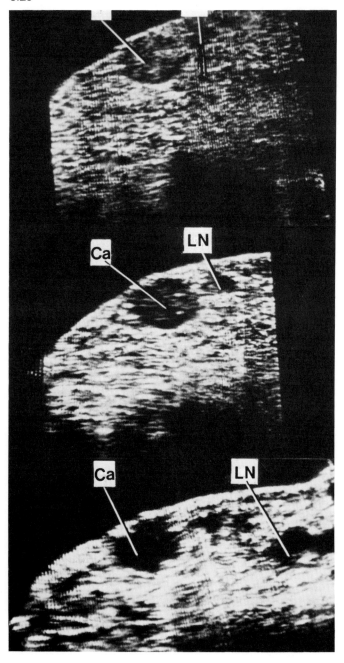

Comparison Between Ultrasound and Mammography

Tumors in very dense fibrous breasts could better be seen by ultrasound than by mammography (Jellins et al. 1978; Jellins and Reeve 1978; Kossoff et al. 1978; Reeve et al. 1979).

This means that ultrasound can offer an additional evaluation to x-ray (Kossoff 1978). Sonography, however, cannot replace mammography especially for screening purposes where microcalcifications are a leading sign of malignancy.

Sonographic examination is presently very time consuming compared with x-ray mammography (Kossoff et al. 1978). By the development of new equipment, the sonographic examination time might be reduced to about 10 to 15 minutes for both breasts (Goldenberg et al. 1979; Jellins et al. 1979).

By use of real-time scanners of high frequency, it might even be possible to guide the fine needle biopsies of suspicious lesions with ultrasound. The patient is then in the same position as at surgery and there are no problems with the water tank covering the breast.

Fig. 3.**22** Macrocalcification within the breast showing marked shadow formation. (With kind permission from J. Jellins, Australia.)

Fig. 3.**23** Carcinoma (Ca) within the breast. Use of the sensitivity grades method. With decreasing amplification, the nodes (LN) in the axilla are more easily seen.

References

Baum, G.: Ultrasound mammography. Radiology 122: 199, 1977

Baum, G.: The need for color coding in ultrasound mammography. J. Clin. Ultrasound 6: 76, 1978

Goldenberg, B. B., C. Cole-Beuglet, A. Kurtz: The evaluation of breast masses and tissue patterns using high resolution ultrasonic equipment. 2nd WFUMB Congress Miyazaki, 1979, p. 119

Griffiths, K.: Ultrasound in the examination of the breast. Med. Ultrasound 2: 13, 1978

Gros, C., P. Haehnel, G. Dale, B. Girard: Echographie mammaire. J. Radiol. Electrol. 55: 611, 1974

Gros, C., G. Dale, B. Girard: Breast Echography. Criteria of malignancy and results. In: Recent Advances in Ultrasound Diagnosis. Ed.: A. Kurjak, Excerpta Medica, 1978, p. 292

Hackelöer, B. J., G. Lauth, K. Duda: Neue Möglichkeiten der Ultraschallmammographie. Geburtsh. Frauenheilkd. 40: 301, 1980

Jellins, K., G. Kossoff, T. S. Reeve: Detection and classification of liquid filled masses in the breast by grey-scale echography. Radiology 125: 205, 1977

Jellins, K., G. Kossoff, B. H. Barraclough: Comparative study of breast imaging by echography and xeroradiography. In: Recent Advances in Ultrasound Diagnosis. Ed.: A. Kurjak, Excerpta Medica, 1978, p. 229

Jellins, J., T. S. Reeve: Breast echography compared with xeroradiography. Ultrasound Med. Biol. 4: 313, 1978

Jellins, J., G. Kossoff, T. S. Reeve: Ultrasonic imaging of breast malignancies. 2nd WFUMB Congress, Miyazaki, 1979, p. 432

Jellins, J., G. Kossoff, T. S. Reeve: Ultrasonic screening of breast diseases. 2nd WFUMB Congress, Miyazaki, 1979, p. 124

Kelly-Fry, E., P. Harper: Multiple approaches to the problem of detection and differential diagnosis of breast pathologies. 2nd WFUMB Congress, Miyazaki, 1979, p. 127

Kobayashi, T., O. Takani, N. Hattori, K. Kimura: Study of sensitivity graded ultrasonography of breast tumor. Med. Ultrason. Jap. 10: 38, 1973

Kobayashi, T., O. Takani, N. Hattori, K. Kimura: Differential diagnosis of breast tumors. Clinical investigation for the differential diagnosis of breast tumors by means of degraded sensitivity. Method ultrasonogram II. Cancer 33: 940, 1974

Kobayashi, T.: Ultrasonic characterization of breast cancer. Correlation of attenuation and echopattern. In: Recent Advances in Ultrasound Diagnosis Ed.: A. Kurjak, Excerpta Medica 1978, p. 281

Kossoff, G., D. A. Carpenter, G. Radamovich, W. J. Garrett: Octoson, a new rapid multitransducer general purpose water coupling ectoscope. Proceedings of the 2nd European Congress on Ultrasonics in Medicine, München 1975, Excerpta Medica, p. 91

Kossoff, G.: Classification of soft tissues by grey-scale echography. Ultrasound Med. Biol. 4: 313, 1977

Kossoff, G.: The view from down under. J. Clin. Ultrasound 6: 144, 1978

Kossoff, G., J. Jellins, T. S. Reeve: Ultrasound in the early detection of breast cancer. Cancer Campaign 1: 149, 1978

Kratochwil, A., P. Kaiser: Die Darstellung der Erkrankungen der weiblichen Brust im Ultraschallschnittbildverfahren. Ultrasonographia Medica 3: 119, 1968

Kratochwil, A., R. Kolb, H. Stöger, B.-E. Dahlberg, K. Brezina, C. Czech: Moderne Methoden der Mammadiagnostik. Wien, Klin. Wochenschr. 87: 47, 1975

Ossoinig, K., P. Kaiser, R. Kolb, G. Lechner: Echographische und röntgenologische Befunde bei Erkrankungen der Mamma. Ultrasonographia Medica 3: 191, 1968

Pluygers, E., M. Rombaut, M. Beauduin, B. Hendricks, F. Dever-Gnies, A. Pieron, G. Tamignaux: Possibilities, results, and indication of breast echography. J. Belge Radiol. 60: 181, 1977

Reeve, T. S., J. Jellins, G. Kossoff, B. H. Barraclough: Ultrasonic visualization of breast cancer. N. Z. J. Surg. 48: 278, 1979

Rubin, C. S., A. Kurtz, B. B. Goldberg, S. Feigl, C. Cole-Beuglet: Ultrasonic mammography patterns. A preliminary report. Radiology 130: 515, 1979

Takahayashi, Y., H. Koyama, S. Sawayama: Echographic diagnosis of breast diseases. 2nd WFUMB Congress, Miyazaki, 1979, p. 330

Wagai, T., M. Tsutsumi, M., A. Ishihara, A. M. Hadidi, S. Hayashi: Detection of breast cancer in the early stages by ultrasound. Ann. Rep. Ultrasonic Center Juntendo Univ. Med. School 1972

Wagai, T.: Sources in ultrasonotomography and its clinical evaluation. Proceedings of the 2nd World Congress on Ultrasonics in Medicine. Rotterdam, Excerpta Medica 1973, p. 186

Wagai, T., M. Tsutsumi, H. Takeuchi: Diagnostic Ultrasound in Breast Diseases. In: Present and Future in Diagnostic Ultrasound. Ed.: I. Donald, S. Levi. Kooyker Scientific Publications, 1975, p. 148

Wagai, T., M. Tsutsumi: Analytical investigation of ultrasonic breast cancer images in relation to the performance of the equipment and histological structure. 2nd WFUMB Congress, Miyazaki, 1979, p. 126

White, D. N., P. R. Cledgelt: Breast carcinoma detection by ultrasonic Doppler signals. Ultrasound Med. Biol. 4: 329, 1978

Wild, J., D. Neal: Use of high frequency ultrasonic waves for detecting changes in living tissue. Lancet I: 656, 1951

Wild, J. J., J. M. Reid: Further pilot echographic studies on the histologic structure of tumors of the living human breast. Am. J. Pathol. 28: 839, 1952

Chapter 4

Thermography

N. T. Johansson

No ideal method for detection of breast cancer is known. In the search for such a method, thermography has been investigated. In 1956, for the first time it was used by Lawson (1956), who considered it promising. He found an increased temperature in the skin over some breast cancers, thereby confirming previous clinical experience. Thermography has since been widely used in clinical work, although its use is based on studies that have often given contradictory results.

Physiology

It is verified that many breast tumors have a higher temperature than the surrounding normal breast tissues (Gullino 1980). The reason for this is not entirely clear. However, all experience is in favor of heat transport from the tumor to the skin either by conduction through the surrounding tissues or by convection with the venous blood draining the tumor (Nilsson et al. 1980).

Conducted heat seems less detectable in most cases. It can be observed only in a limited number of cases; that is, when a high-power output tumor is in close contact with the skin. The convection model will work only if a well-vascularized tumor is draining relatively hot blood directly into subcutaneous veins (Love 1980; Nilsson et al. 1980).

Physics and Technology

Thermography is a method for obtaining a pictorial representation of the infrared radiation from a surface such as human skin. Infrared radiation, which is a part of the continuous electromagnetic spectrum, has wavelengths above the visible radiation; that is, 0.75 to 1 000 μm. The distribution of wavelength and amplitude is proportional to the absolute temperature of the surface (Fig. 4.**1**). This relation is given in the Stefan-Boltzmann law, which in a simplified version says:

$$W_T = \varepsilon\sigma T^4$$

where

W_T = energy radiated per time and per unit area watts/cm^2 × sec.

ε = emissivity = radiation efficiency. For human skin, it is estimated to be 0.98 ± 0.01; that is, close to that of a blackbody. There might be a small variation in emissivity between different parts of the skin and also between different individuals. However, for practical purposes it is judged as a constant.

σ = the Stefan-Boltzmann constant $(5.6697 \pm 0.0029) \times 10^{-12}$ watts/cm^2 × °K^{-4}.

T = absolute temperature Kelvin (°K).

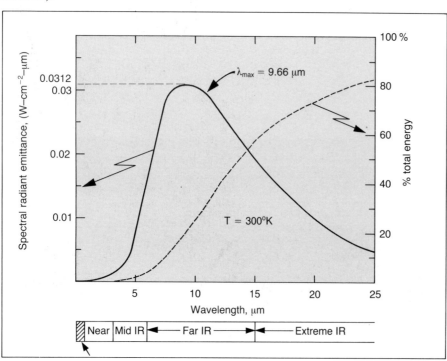

Fig. 4.**1** Infrared emission from a black-body at 300°K. The right hand scale shows the percentage of the total energy that lies below λ.

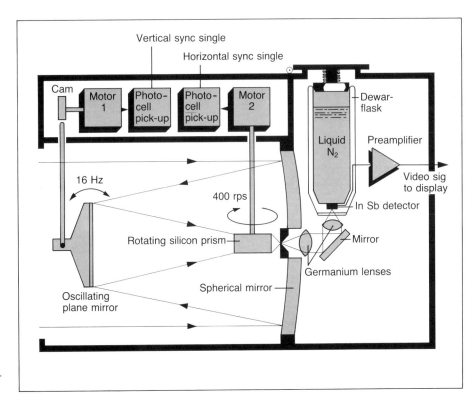

Fig. 4.**2** Schematic diagram of AGA thermovision camera.

This description is very simplified. For details see Johansson, 1976.

A schematic diagram of an AGA Thermovision camera is given in Fig. 4.**2**. The surface under examination is screened by a vertically oscillating mirror and a horizontally rotating prism. Radiation from a large number of small areas is thereby transmitted to a so-called infrared detector, which is designed in various ways in different thermographs. Indium-antimonide is often used as a detector. This requires very low working temperature to eliminate thermal noise. The cooling equipment is made up of a bottle containing liquid nitrogen in the bottom of which the detector is placed. Infrared radiation is converted to electric impulses that are transferred to a display unit – essentially a television set. On the screen, a gray-scale (or color) picture can be seen corresponding to the temperature of the screened surface. Photographs are taken for documentation.

Interpretation of Thermograms

A typical thermogram is seen in Fig. 4.**3**. Hot parts appear black and cold parts are gray or white. Electronic inversion is also possible, giving hot areas in white. This sometimes improves the legibility. In color thermograms, different temperatures are displayed in different colors. It is obviously impossible to make more than crude relative temperature estimations with the naked eye, and still less possible to judge the temperature in degrees centigrade. In order to do this, a so-called isotherm device is used. Using this, all areas in the thermogram with the same temperature can be electronically amplified to saturated white. With the aid of two isotherm devices, temperature differences between corresponding parts of the two breasts can be read from a scale.

Judging a thermogram means a comparison of corresponding areas in the breasts. This is a necessary procedure because even perfectly normal breasts have variable thermic patterns. Temperature varies from point to point on the skin. Further, the subcutaneous veins, often with different patterns in the two breasts, interfere in a nonuniform way.

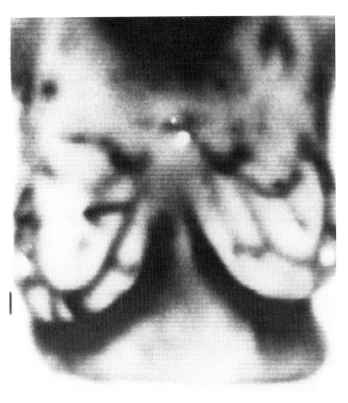

Fig. 4.**3** Thermogram from a woman with healthy breasts.

The Gothenburg Study

In the literature, there is no general agreement about thermographic criteria. Sometimes they are not even mentioned. Neither is there an agreement about the value of thermography for detection of breast cancer. Owing to this, thermography was examined as a part of a joint study of different methods for detection of breast cancer. This was made at the University Hospital of Gothenburg during the years 1968 to 1970 (Bjurstam et al. 1974; Johansson 1976). The thermographic examinations were made by one of two specially trained surgeons, both unbiased by knowledge of the results from other investigations; that is, clinical judgment, mammography, and fine-needle aspiration cytology. When a localized process was found, clinically or on the mammograms, cytology was performed and, finally, surgery.

Performance of Examination and Criteria for Interpretation

It is obviously necessary to standardize the performance of the thermographic examination in order to achieve comparable results between different patients. In this study, (Johansson 1976), all women were equilibrated to the ambient temperature of a specially designed room,
well insulated, and at almost constant temperature (Fig. 4.4). They sat, naked to the waist with their hands clasped behind their neck, in small cabins for ten minutes before the examination. They were not allowed to wear tight clothing or to smoke before the examination in order to avoid thermal artifacts. Other investigations, such as palpation and mammography, were performed later.

When the temperature equilibration was finished, the patient, still with her hands behind her neck, was placed on a chair before the thermograph. After adjustment of the thermograph, a crude ocular estimation was made. Thermal asymmetry was noted. Then the thermogram was examined with the aid of the isotherm device. If a "hot area" in one breast was detected, the isotherm was locked on this area. A second isotherm was locked on the corresponding area in the contralateral breast, and the temperature difference could be read from a scale. A hot area was found to correspond to a subcutaneous vein (veins) or to a smaller or larger part of the breast between the veins. The type of hot area (Fig. 4.5) was noted as well as the vein pattern (Fig. 4.6) in each breast.

This, in my opinion, means that the thermographic examination is an active process of comparison, which must be performed with the patient in front of the camera. Many authors appear to interpret thermograms that were made earlier by an assistant. In my opinion, this is a crude performance.

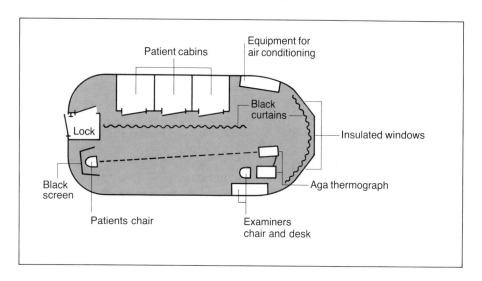

Fig. 4.**4**
Room for thermographic examination.

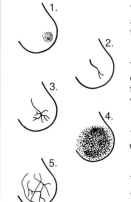

Type 1 means a »hot spot.« This is a rather well defined area of increased temperature confined to one part of the surface without connection with the venous pattern

Type 2 means increased temperature in connection with one single subcutaneous vein, type 3 increased temperature corresponding to an aggregation of subcutaneous veins, limited to a circumscribed part of the breast surface

Type 4 means increased temperature all over the surface, without connection with subcutaneous venous pattern

Type 5 means increased temperature connected with a subcutaneous vein network spread over the entire breast-surface.

Fig. 4.**5**   Types of hot areas.

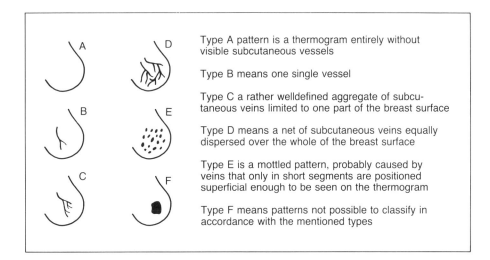

Type A pattern is a thermogram entirely without visible subcutaneous vessels

Type B means one single vessel

Type C a rather welldefined aggregate of subcutaneous veins limited to one part of the breast surface

Type D means a net of subcutaneous veins equally dispersed over the whole of the breast surface

Type E is a mottled pattern, probably caused by veins that only in short segments are positioned superficial enough to be seen on the thermogram

Type F means patterns not possible to classify in accordance with the mentioned types

Fig. 4.**6**   Classification of vein patterns.

Inevitably a thermographic examination is connected with a large subjective influence. Other factors also influence such as distance to the thermograph, focus and angle between surface, and the optic axis. Besides, there are certain imperfections in the function of the thermographs. In the same way, ambient temperature, relative air humidity, circadian temperature rhythms of the patients, phase of the menstrual cycle, pressure artifacts from clothing, medication, smoking, and so on can interfere with the results. For these reasons, temperature differences equal to or exceeding 1.0°C only were judged as "positive thermograms" (Johansson 1976; Møller and Bojsen 1980).

Material

There were 1551 women screened and it was later found that 1456 of these were suitable for thermographic analysis. Of these, 1225 women were consecutively referred to us because of clinical symptoms and/or signs from the breasts. One hundred fifty-five were later found to have unilateral breast cancer, 157 had verified unilateral benign lesions, and 913 were without demonstrable localized lesions. Another 231 women were randomly chosen from a larger sample (in the age groups 38, 46, 50, 54, and 60 years) from the town of Gothenburg in screening for medical diseases (Fig. 4.**7**). The patients were followed for five years and after that an analysis was made for each method separately and for all methods together.

All data from the varying clinical and laboratory evaluations were computerized. This then permitted a detailed evaluation of the thermographic findings in light of the clinical findings in the different patient groups.

Results

It was found that close to 19% of the women with unilateral breast cancer had negative thermograms. Another 10% had a positive thermogram with the hot area in the wrong breast; that is, the healthy breast. Thus, about 72% had positive thermograms with a cancer in the same breast as the hot area.

On the other hand, 47% of women with benign breast disease, for instance a fibroadenoma, had positive thermograms. Most essentially, about 38% without any discernible breast disease had positive thermograms.

In all groups, there was a distinct left dominance of the hot area. The reason for this is unknown, and it is seldom noticed in the literature. The left dominance was present in about 87% in breasts without localized lesions. In the group of fibroadenomas, it was present in 80% and in the cancer group in 69%. On the other hand, there was also a left dominance of the lesions; that is, 60% for the cancers and 70% for the fibroadenomas. The most notable fact is the number of positive thermograms in healthy breasts and the left dominance among these.

In order to find out possible thermogenetic factors, homogenous groups were selected from the total material. These included, for instance, a group of women without demonstrable localized or diffuse lesions. Other groups were formed from women without localized lesions but with different degrees of fibroadenosis (judged both clinically and mammographically). Still other groups contained only a fibroadenoma or a unilateral,

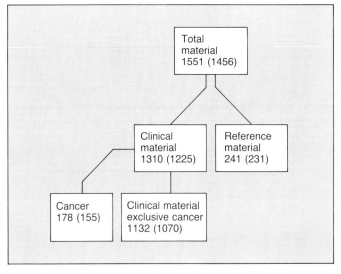

Fig. 4.**7**   Composition of the original material. Number of patients in the thermographic analysis in brackets.

solitary cancer. Precautions were taken not to include patients with bilateral cancers or multiple cancers in the same breast (mammographically found). It was recognized that diffuse fibroadenosis did not influence the frequency of positive thermograms compared with those without it. On the other hand, patients with benign localized lesions or cancer had more positive thermograms than those with healthy breasts.

A comparison of the results of the two investigators was made, thereby comparable groups were created concerning the age of the patient and the type of lesion. Even the healthy breasts were considered. However, no significant difference was found between the investigators.

Special patient factors were also judged, such as size of the breasts, age of the patient, and hormonal function of the ovaries (i. e., premenopausal women, women less than six years postmenopausal or more than six years postmenopausal). No differences were found between these groups. Neither was there any difference between women who were in the preovulatory compared with the postovulatory phase of the menstrual cycle. A small group of women with healthy breasts but on contraceptive pills were compared with a group not taking contraceptive pills. No differences were noted. On the other hand, pregnancy influenced the thermograms by making them hotter, mainly by increasing the number and size of the subcutaneous veins (Fig. 4.8). This makes the examination even more difficult.

Automatic interaction detection (AID) analysis was also performed. This was used to investigate the combined effect of several independant variables. Even this performance failed to explain the results above.

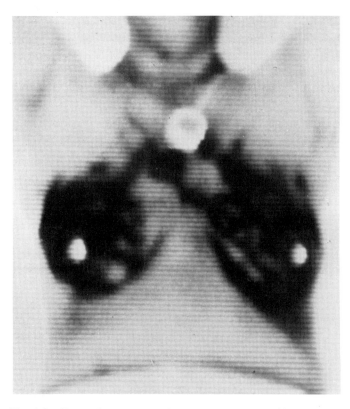

Fig. 4.8 Breast thermogram of a pregnant woman without breast disease.

Discussion

A survey of the literature seems to warrant the conclusion that many papers published up to now are not detailed enough to give a fair basis for scientific judgment and comparison of different materials. It must be stressed that large populations for examination cannot compensate for a nonscientific approach to the analysis. Studies that seem to be properly done often show results that conform to this study, irrespective of various criteria for a "positive thermogram".

This probably means that determination of the temperature difference is most important, and it has also been the main criterion for most authors. It seems natural that temperature differences as small as possible should be recorded, thereby increasing the possibility of also revealing cancers with minor heat production. However, for various reasons discussed above, only temperature differences equal to or above 1.0°C were recorded as "positive thermograms". Most authors also use this limit.

The most important fact to discuss is whether the hot area in a positive thermogram is caused by the underlying lesion or something else. Opinions in the literature vary from those who claim that they have found many clinically occult cancers by thermography. (Dodd et al. 1969) to those who have found normal thermograms for up to 10-cm sized cancers (Gros et al. 1971). In this study, cancers with positive thermograms were as frequent as those with negative thermograms. Neither did the depth of the tumor correlate to the frequency of positive thermograms. This is confirmed by the few authors who have investigated this variable.

Experimental investigations as well as theoretical calculations have been made in order to explore factors necessary for a hot area to develop (Love 1980; Nilsson et al. 1980). They show that only tumors with an energy production above that of the average for breast tissue or a position close to the skin can be detected by thermography. This refers to conducted heat. If convected heat should be discovered, the tumor must be very well vascularized and of course draining to such a vein. Thus, experimental and clinical results correspond to each other, and the former also seem to give a good explanation of the latter.

Screening for Breast Cancer

Much discussion has been devoted to screening for breast cancer. Screening is designed to differentiate women who probably have breast cancer from those who probably do not. Such a method, although not intended to be diagnostic, must be able to detect (almost) all cancers. The Gothenburg study and other studies have shown that thermography does not fulfill these requirements. Besides, the number of false-positive thermograms must not be too large, because other methods must then be applied to solve the problem. From different materials, the conclusion has been drawn that thermography is of no value for screening purposes (Bears et al. 1979; Feig et al. 1977; Isard 1980; Moskowitz et al. 1976; Strax 1977).

Those who claim that it is have often mixed up the thermographic results with those from clinical examination or mammography in a way that no conclusions can be made (Amalric et al. 1976; Gautherie 1980; Stark 1977). In almost all projects presented in the literature, thermography has been abandoned as a method with too low a sensitivity and specificity.

However, there are other methods well suited for breast cancer screening. Mammography has given excellent results in experienced hands. Furthermore, the new low-dose, one-picture technique is said to give little risk of damage to the genetic material of the cells.

Conclusions

In conclusion, there do not seem to be any results in the literature, including this study, that give thermography a place in the diagnostic armamentarium for detection of breast cancer. Nor is there a place for thermography for screening purposes.

Many investigations seem to be under way for improving thermography, such as computerized pattern recognition (Threatt et al. 1980) and examination at other wavelengths or at different ambient temperatures (Edrich et al. 1980; Myers et al. 1980).

But today there are no results pointing to essential improvement. It does not seem to be the technology that limits the ability of thermography as a diagnostic method. It is restricted rather by the thermogenetic factors of the tumors and the isolation properties of the surrounding tissues in the breasts. The complex thermic pattern even in perfectly healthy breasts, with its left-dominant thermic asymmetry, further confuses the picture.

References

Amalric, R., D. Giraud, C. Altschuler, J. M. Spitalier: Value and interest in dynamic telethermography in detection of breast cancer. Acta Thermograph. 1: 89–96, 1976

Beahrs, D. H., S. Shapiro, C. Smart: Report of the working group to review the national cancer institute – American Cancer Society Breast Cancer Detection Demonstration Projects. J. Natl. Cancer Inst. 62: 641–709, 1979

Bjurstam, N., K. Hedberg, K. A. Hultborn, N. T. Johansson, C. Johnsén: Diagnosis of breast carcinoma. Prog. Surg. 13: 1–65, 1974

Dodd, G. D., J. D. Wallace, I. M. Freundlich, L. Marsh, A. Zermino: Thermography and cancer of the breast. Cancer 23: 797–802, 1969

Edrich, J., W. E. Jobe, R. K. Cacak, W. R. Hendee, C. J. Smyth, M. Gautherie, C. Gros, R. Zimmer, J. Robert, P. Thouvenot, J. M. Escanye, C. Itty: Imaging thermograms at centimeter and millimeter wavelengths. Ann. N.Y. Acad. Sci. 335: 456–474, 1980

Feig, S. A., G. S. Shaber, G. F. Schwartz, A. Patchefsky, H. I. Libshitz, J. Edeiken, R. Nerlinger, R. F. Curley, J. D. Wallace: Thermography, mammography, and clinical examination in breast cancer screening. Radiology 122: 123–127, 1977

Gautherie, M.: Thermopathology of breast cancer: Measurement and analysis of in vivo temperature and blood flow. Ann. N. Y. Acad. Sci. 335: 383–415, 1980

Gros, C., M. Gautherie, F. Archer: Séméiologie thermographique des épithéliomas mammaires. Bull. Cancer (Paris) 58: 69–90, 1971

Gullino, P. M.: Influence of blood supply on thermal properties and metabolism of mammary carcinomas. Ann. N. Y. Acad. Sci. 335: 1–21, 1980

Isard, H. J.: Thermography in mass screening of cancer: Success and failures. Ann. N. Y. Acad. Sci. 335: 489–491, 1980

Johansson, N. T.: Thermography of the Breast. Acta Chir. Scand., Suppl. 460: 1–91, 1976

Lawson, R. N.: Implications of surface temperatures in the diagnosis of breast cancer. Can. Med. Assoc. J. 75: 309–310, 1956

Love, T. J.: Thermography as an indicator of blood perfusion. Ann. N. Y. Acad. Sci. 335: 429–437, 1980

Moskowitz, M., J. Milbrath, P. Gartside, A. Zermeno, D. Mandel: Lack of efficacy of thermography as a screening tool for minimal and stage I breast cancer. N. Engl. J. Med. 295: 249–252, 1976

Møller, U. J. Bojsen: Heat transfer and blood flow in experimental tumors in rats compared with the circadian temperature rhythm of the body. Ann. N. Y. Acad. Sci. 335: 22–34, 1980

Myers, P. C., A. H. Barrett, N. L. Sadowsky: Microwave thermography of normal and cancerous breast tissue. Ann. N. Y. Acad. Sci. 335: 443–455, 1980

Nilsson, S. K., S. E. Gustafsson, L. M. Torell: Skin temperature over a heat source: Experimental studies and theoretical calculations. Ann. N. Y. Acad. Sci. 335: 416–428, 1980

Stark, A. M.: The role of thermography in early breast cancer and the socio-economic aspects of screening. Gynäk. Rdsch. 17 (Suppl. 1): 29–38, 1977

Strax, P.: The role of thermography as compared with mammography. Int. J. Radiat. Oncol. Biol. Phys. 2: 751–752, 1977

Threatt, B., J. M. Norbeck, N. S. Ullman, R. Kummer, P. F. Roselle: Thermography and breast cancer: An analysis of a blind reading. Ann. N. Y. Acad. Sci. 335: 501–519, 1980

Chapter 5

Excisional Biopsy

L. Uddströmer

Excisional biopsy has received little attention in the literature and even less by the surgeons performing the operation. It is all too often treated as an undramatic precursor to a mutilating operation.

The size of a tumor when first discovered has tended to diminish with the advent of better education, self-examination, screening techniques, and routine mammography. As a result, 40% of all presented cancers are in our experience nonpalpable. This, together with a wider range of therapy and reconstruction, may lead to better prognosis, less psychosomatic problems, and acceptable cosmetic results.

Changing surgical attitudes have increased the interest shown in a wider variety of problems associated with cancer of the breast, among these being surgical biopsy.

In Scandinavia, the Netherlands, and Germany, aspiration biopsy cytology is an accepted method of diagnosing breast cancer. An accuracy of 92% has been reported (Franzén 1979) with an incidence of only 0.2% of false positives.

The risk of false negatives has resulted in criticism of the method and is the reason why aspiration is less commonly used elsewhere.

Aspiration biopsy is the method of choice when dealing with cystic lesions. However, excision biopsy must follow if aspiration:

1. Fails to produce fluid
2. Produces a sanguinous (bloody) fluid
3. Results in incomplete resolution of the cyst
4. Fails to prevent recurrence of the cyst

Intracystic carcinomas are uncommon, but their presence will be detected if the suggestions above are adhered to. Although aspiration biopsy can be used in cases of palpable and suspicious lesions and is a reliable method of detecting cancer, it will give no information about the invasiveness of a carcinoma and negative cytology does not exclude malignancy.

Indications for Excisional Biopsy

The indications for a diagnostic excisional biopsy are:

1. *The presence of a palpable mass,* remembering that a painful lump does not exclude malignancy. This should also include those cystic lesions discussed earlier.

2. *The presence of nonpalpable masses or microcalcifications* detected by mammography.

3. *A persistent spontaneous discharge* from one or two ducts of the nipple. A discharge is a common sign of breast pathology. In cancer the discharge is usually sanguinous, but in fact any type of fluid discharge may accompany cancer.

4. *Abnormalities of the nipple,* which are commonly an area of suspicious eczema around the nipple or its recent spontaneous retraction.

5. *Breast skin changes,* which may consist of dimpling (peau d'orange) or the presence of inflammatory signs without infection.

6. *Axillary lymph node enlargement.* The female breast is the most common site of a primary cancer when the axillary lymph nodes are involved.

7. *Positive cytology.* In some centers surgical treatment will depend on histologic staging that cannot be obtained by aspiration biopsy.

Information to the Patient

Most women will be alarmed and apprehensive when they first contact the physician. Many patients will ask for more information, whereas others will avoid further discussion. At this stage, their wishes should be observed. However, all patients should be fully informed prior to surgery.

The patient should understand why the biopsy has to be taken, and also the possible surgical consequences of histologic examination of the biopsy material. Thus:

1. If the frozen section is positive then she must realize that immediate mastectomy may follow the biopsy.

2. If the frozen section is negative or inconclusive, or perhaps the facility is unavailable, then it must be explained to her that a histologic paraffin section will determine whether or not a second operation will be necessary at a later date.

Rarely, the patient will be unable to make a decision regarding mastectomy until a final histologic result is available. It is not advisable to force a mastectomy on any woman.

Operative Procedure

Planning the Surgery

When planning the operation, it is wise to remember that excision is often not an isolated procedure, but the means of getting a definite diagnosis with an eye toward further treatment. The choice of anesthesia and site of incision will be influenced by the likelihood of a biopsy being followed by mastectomy. Whether the procedure is carried out on an outpatient or inpatient basis will depend on the likely outcome of histologic inspection, the patient's agreement on treatment, and the available laboratory resources.

Anesthesia

The type of anesthesia used will be influenced by many factors such as past medical history, drug usage, previous operations, age, specific cardiac and pulmonary pathology and allergic problems. It is rare that general anesthesia is contraindicated. However, it is as well to remember that intercostal blockade of the second to the fifth intercostal nerves provides an acceptable alternative for excisional biopsy, but is hardly adequate for a mastectomy. Some surgeons avoid the use of epinephrine with local anesthetics because of the risk of delayed bleeding. There is little evidence to substantiate this fear.

General anesthesia should be used when:

1. There is a strong clinical suspicion of cancer and mastectomy may well follow frozen section examination.
2. There is a small but palpable tumor difficult to define. Every experienced surgeon is aware of the difficulties of "losing" a lump that may well have seemed comparatively large preoperatively. Infiltrating the skin and surrounding parenchyma with local anesthetic solution can disguise the tumor and lead to uncertainty and the removal of voluminous amounts of breast material. This problem can be avoided by using general anesthesia and/or markers.

Local anesthesia can be used when:

1. There is a minimal lesion, localized and marked by the radiologist and considered too small to provide enough material for both a frozen section as well as a paraffin section. Since the latter examination gives a more reliable result, there will be a delay of some days before a possible mastectomy is undertaken.
2. There are large or small tumors that are not clinically suspicious. In these cases the surgeon will not expect further surgical intervention, and the patients may be treated as outpatients. Sometimes histologic examination reveals a carcinoma, but as shown by many authors, a delayed mastectomy does not hold any grave disadvantage.
Local anesthesia for biopsies of nonpalpable lesions can be justified if indicators are used with mammographic control.

Incisions

Fortunately not all tumors are malignant. In our experience 35% are benign, and since no further surgery is envisaged the biopsy scar should be as cosmetically acceptable as possible. The above incidence of benign tumors is low because so many benign lesions are screened before referral (Lundgren 1981).

On the other hand a biopsy may be followed by mastectomy and the mastectomy incision should not be influenced by the site or extent of the biopsy scar.

Therefore, the surgeon should begin any excision biopsy by defining where the mastectomy scar will be, should it ultimately be necessary, and then locate the diagnostic incision inside the planned area. The incisions to be recommended (Fig. 5.1) are arranged in order of cosmetic acceptability.

1. *The periareolar incision.* The skin incision is made just inside the junction between the areola and the surrounding skin. The length of the incision can be extended to more than half the total areolar circumference and, combined with extensive peripheral undermining, it is possible to reach tumors that are 3 to 4 cm distant. Alternatively, central undermining produces an areolar flap and gives good access to subareolar masses.

2. *The submammary incision.* Lesions situated in the lower part of the breast can be reached through an incision placed just above the submammary fold. The incision not only permits access to tumors higher in the breast but also gives better cosmetic results and the incision can be "moved" along and just above the fold to locate lesions that are more lateral or medial.
In the small or normal sized breast, it is possible to remove most tumors in the lower half of the breast using the periareolar or submammary incisions. For

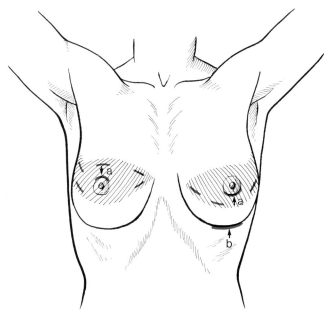

Fig. 5.1 Shows the relationship of biopsy to that of later possible mastectomy incisions.
a: Periareolar incision.
b: Submammary incision.

lumps situated more medially or laterally, or elsewhere in the breast, other types of incisions must be chosen.

3. *Other mammary incisions.* Although all surgeons are conscious of skin tension lines when incising the body surface, few are aware of the direction those lines take. Ignorance of its application in breast surgery has led to a variety of incisions being recommended that are less desirable.

In 1861, Langer published an extensive work on skin tension lines and he suggested, with regard to the breast, that the lines are concentric to the nipple. Since then Langer's work has been repeated and to some extent revised. Kraissl (1951) states that because of the influence of gravity and the constant movement of the mammary glands in the female breast, the tension lines, although still curved, become more horizontal. In other words, the lines are parallel to the incision when performing a horizontal mastectomy.

Personal experience suggests a compromise using the ideas of both Langer and Kraissl. Incisions close to the areola are made in a concentric fashion, whereas the peripheral incisions, while still curved, should be more horizontal (Fig. 5.**1**). However, concentric incisions have limited use since the periareolar approach as already described allows distant excision.

Lesions localized in the axillary tail of the breast are reached through an incision placed just behind and parallel to the lateral border of the pectoralis major muscle.

All the above incisions have the advantage of being placed within the area to be excised if the biopsy is followed by mastectomy, assuming the mastectomy is horizontal. This type of mastectomy should be the rule, because of the increasing demand for secondary breast reconstruction.

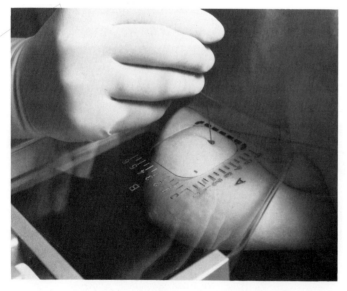

Fig. 5.**2** Craniocaudal mammographic position with pressure applied on the breast. Using these coordinates, the relationship of the tumor to the skin has been calculated and through this point the cannula and wire have been inserted.

In two series (Saltzstein et al. 1974; Moskowitz et al. 1975), 75% to 85% of all biopsies showed no malignant change. With this in mind, it is important to choose an incision that will give minimum scarring.

In summary, it is suggested that the incisions mentioned above, namely the perioareolar, submammary, and peripheral incisions will leave cosmetically acceptable scars, but will lie within the area excised should mastectomy follow biopsy.

Excision

The overall incidence of malignant breast lesions in the female population is increasing. This has occurred despite the fact that the number of large and palpable tumors is decreasing. The difference is the result of an explosive increase in the numbers of small nonpalpable lesions discovered as a result of screening mammography.

This changed ratio of palpable/nonpalpable tumors has raised considerable problems concerning the excision and localization of minimal breast lesions. One is faced with either voluminous and thus cosmetically unacceptable resections, or the development of more refined techniques permitting minimal excision. This means that those hospitals without sufficient expertise should refer their patients to more specialized centers.

These numerous minimal lesions have made fine needle aspiration less feasible at a time when surgical biopsy is becoming more important. The small size of the specimen has also produced a problem for the pathologist in that there is insufficient tissue for both frozen and paraffin sections. Since paraffin section is more reliable, an increasing number of mastectomies are delayed pending histologic examination. However those patients referred to a center for biopsy can return to their local hospital for mastectomy after the paraffin section result becomes available.

Excisional Biopsy in Minimal Breast Tumors

In 1966, Schwartz and Siegelman proposed an elliptical radial incision for nonpalpable microcalcifications, but unfortunately this gave rise to large resections and wrongly placed scars. Simon et al. (1972) inserted a needle under x-ray control and when it was in an acceptable position, small amounts of tissue color were injected together with a radiopaque marker. The latter, however, made it difficult to identify the specimen on x-ray. Different needle methods have also been presented by Rosato et al. (1973) and Cooperman et al. (1976).

Our experience of nonpalpable lesions is mainly the result of a screening project using single-view mammography (Lundgren 1978). In 1969, when Lundgren started his screening (population circa 300,000), only 20% of the malignant cases were free of metastases. Today, more than 85% are clinically free. This early diagnosis has also led to an increasing number of small and nonpalpable lesions being referred for biopsy, of which 55% are 10 mm or less in diameter.

Fig. 5.**3** A schematic drawing showing the identification of a nonpalpable lesion.
A: The needle and hook in place close to the lesion.
B: Extracting the needle leaving the barb at the site of the lesion.

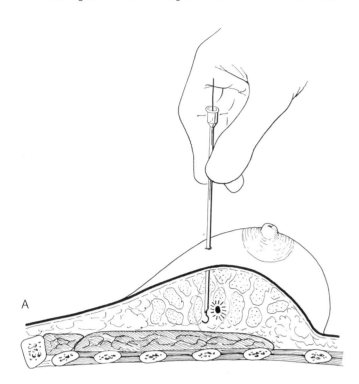

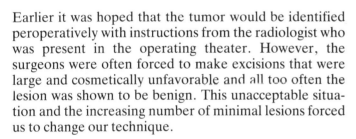

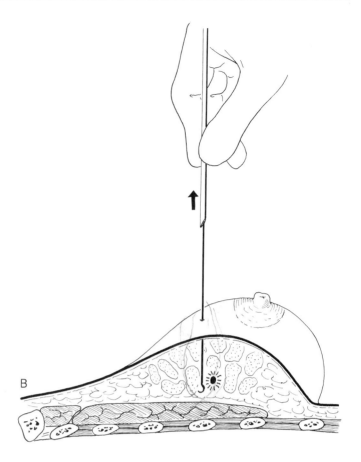

Earlier it was hoped that the tumor would be identified peroperatively with instructions from the radiologist who was present in the operating theater. However, the surgeons were often forced to make excisions that were large and cosmetically unfavorable and all too often the lesion was shown to be benign. This unacceptable situation and the increasing number of minimal lesions forced us to change our technique.

Identification

When a small tumor is found by mammography, further identification of the area is performed preoperatively using two mammographic projections, one craniocaudal and the other a mediolateral view. When x-raying the vertical view, a coordinate system is used (Fig. 5.**2**) allowing a calculation to be made of the exact position of the tumor. This is then marked on the skin and from the lateral view the depth of the lesion can be estimated.

Thereafter the indicating procedure requires a minimum of utensils; one sterilized cannula of 12 cm in length and one piece of steel wire (piano wire) approximately 14 cm long and 0.8 mm in diameter.

The area around the point marked on the skin is then aseptically cleaned, and under sterile conditions the skin is anesthetized using local anesthetic solution. The cannula containing the steel wire, which is angled at the distal end, is now inserted through the marked skin and aimed directly at the tumor (Fig. 5.**3**). The depth of the insertion is calculated from the lateral mammographic view. When the cannula is extracted, the barb remains in the tissue, thereby acting as a marker, its relationship to the tumor being checked by two more x-rays (Fig. 5.**4**). As a further

aid to the surgeon, a minimum amount of methylene blue may be injected before the needle is taken out.

The position of the marker is classified as excellent if its distance from the tumor is within 10 mm. If the displacement exceeds 10 mm, experience has taught us that there may be difficulty excising the tumor. This is especially so if the desired minimum of parenchyma is to be included in the specimen.

Out of 195 nonpalpable lesions identified in the described way, 180 were classified as excellent after only one insertion, and after a repeated insertion 193 cases were excellent (Table 5.**1**).

Technique

After the identification, the steel wire is left outside the skin and covered with a sterile swab and the patient brought to the operating theater to be prepared for surgery. General or local anesthesia is used, depending on the criteria discussed earlier.

Table 5.**1** Locating the lesions. Numbers of identification attempts to get excellent position of the barb (195 nonpalpable breast lesions)

No. of identification attempts	Position of the barb	
	Excellent (< 10 mm)	Poor (> 10 mm)
1	180	15
2	13	2
3	2	0

A sharp and full-thickness incision is made in the locations described earlier. It must be pointed out that this may not necessarily be directly related to the indicator wire. If, for instance, the wire is situated some centimeters from the areolar margin, the incision may still be placed inside the areolar-skin margin (periareolar incision).

Depending on the relationship between the incision and wire, the dissection either follows the wire, or it is found by subcutaneous or parenchymatous undermining. Once contact with the wire is established, it is followed and thus acts as a guide. When the hook or the colored tissue is found, a representative excision is made as calculated from the mammogram; it is at this point that the radiologist's presence is necessary.

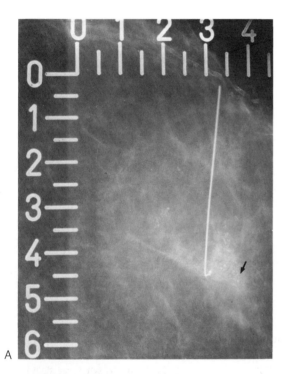

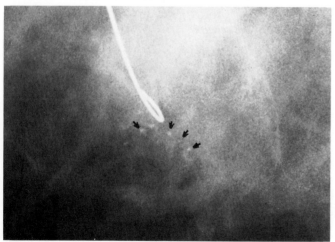

Fig. 5.4 A: A craniocaudal mammographic view with the coordinates projected onto the film. The position of the wire is shown close to the lesion (see arrow).
·B: Lateral mammographic view showing the barb in relationship to microcalcifications (see arrows).

Although the lesion is not palpable from the outside, it is sometimes palpable once the operative cavity has been dissected. In these cases there is little problem removing the whole specimen.

The minimal size of a tumor often makes it difficult to guarantee its location in the excised specimen. This problem can be avoided by taking an x-ray of the excised material before it is sent to the pathologist. Even in the laboratory an x-ray of the smaller embedded specimens can be useful, when this contains microcalcifications.

Wound Closure

After excision, the cavity is treated in the usual way; that is, careful hemostasis and good wound closure. In fatty parenchymatous tissue, electrocautery is preferred.

An acceptable cosmetic scar results from:

1. The correct incision
2. Total hemostasis
3. Closure of the cavity in stages from the bottom

For closure, synthetic absorbable sutures are preferred to catgut, which has a tendency to loosen. The skin is best closed with an intracutaneous continuous nonabsorbable suture.

The wound is dressed with surgical tape and provided there has been adequate hemostasis, little else is necessary. The patient is encouraged to wear her bra as an outer compression bandage and support. She is also advised to wear her bra night and day for some months since it would seem to diminish traction on the scar.

The above technique has markedly reduced the amount of tissue removed at biopsy and yet has increased the accuracy of the excision. Of 195 cases, 192 tumors were excised totally at the first attempt (Table 5.2).

Excisional Biopsy in Palpable Breast Tumors

When dealing with palpable masses, the decision has to be made whether the biopsy is to be excisional or incisional. Excisional biopsy is always preferred since it gives the pathologist more opportunity to examine several sections and thus give a more accurate report – and to give a more precise volume measurement of the tumor. For example, a large tumor does not necessarily mean a large cancer, since the lump may be enlarged by peripheral inflammatory reaction.

Incisional biopsy, a partial excision, is used only for voluminous tumors exceeding 3 cm in diameter. This is particularly true of peripheral masses or when the lump is

Table 5.2 Excision biopsy. Numbers of excisional attemps and frequency of malignancy in 195 nonpalpable breast lesions biopsed with the marker technique

No. of excisional attempts	No. of representative biopsies	No. of malignant diagnosis
1	192	122
2	3	1
	Total 195	123 (63%)

in close contact with the underlying muscle fascia. In these cases, partial removal of the tumor leaves a smaller cavity, which may mean less interference with a subsequent mastectomy. If, however, frozen section does not confirm a malignant diagnosis, the residual mass is excised since security is more important than a cosmetic result.

If the procedure is to be performed under local anesthesia, it is wise to use an identification technique as described above under nonpalpable lesions. However, there is no need to check the position of the barb with x-ray control since the surgeon can feel when the tumor is encountered as he inserts the cannula. The dissection then follows the steel wire or is aimed towards the tumor. In this way, lesions of less than 3 cm in diameter are removed together with a thin shell of normal breast tissue.

Hemostasis and wound closure are similar to that described under nonpalpable lesions.

Excisional Biopsy in Other Breast Tumors

A frequent sign of a breast lesion is a discharge from the nipple, although not more than 10% of these cases are malignant. Serosanguinous or bloody secretions are usually associated with an intraductal carcinoma, but any watery, serous, or even milky secretion does not exclude malignancy.

Since mammography often fails to show a tumor in these cases, and cytologic examination is unreliable, a biopsy is very important. This is easier when performed under general anesthesia. The discharging duct is cannulated and a small amount of methylene blue injected. The areolar area is then explored subcutaneously through a periareolar incision and flap dissection. The tissue around the cannula or the colored area is excised and sent for paraffin section and examination.

If a palpable mass or tumor is visible mammographically, the excision can be performed without cannulation or indicators.

Persistent eczematous changes of the nipple or areola necessitate skin excision. Where there is no underlying mass, this is sufficient, but if present, an associated mass must be removed.

Where the mammary skin is involved in an inflammatory process, and since there is sometimes an underlying carcinoma, skin together with its related parenchymatous tissue must be excised and sent for diagnostic histological examination.

Enlarged axillary nodes in women are most frequently associated with a carcinoma of the breast. It has been shown that mammography will uncover primary lesions in 50% of these cases (Westbrook and Gallager 1971) and also that when mammography fails and no local evidence of carcinoma exists, mastectomies have uncovered in 88% of such patients small or minimal breast carcinomas (Ashikari et al. 1976). In all cases of axillary node enlargement, the nodes should be biopsied and if an adenocarcinoma is revealed, then a radical mastectomy should be performed, assuming no other site is discovered.

In conclusion, whenever breast signs and symptoms are present without proof of a lesion being benign, a biopsy should be performed.

Excisional Biopsy From the Other Breast

It is well known that after mastectomy the remaining breast often develops a carcinoma (Urban 1969; Leis 1971). Recently (Ringberg et al. 1981), a study was presented of 25 women who had undergone a mastectomy and who subsequently underwent a second mastectomy and 37 women with a diagnosed noninvasive carcinoma of the breast that resulted in bilateral subcutaneous mastectomies.

Thus extensive histologic examination of the contralateral breast was possible. This study revealed that in 44% of the breasts studied, invasive and noninvasive carcinomas were present. In addition, 80% contained lesions of a precancerous type.

On the other hand, lesions that are detectable on mammography in the other breast are extremely rare. However, this high incidence of histologically minimal cancerous lesions has induced some surgeons to biopsy the contralateral breast when cancer has been diagnosed (Urban et al. 1977).

In our opinion, biopsies taken in this way are unreliable unless performed as a proper subcutaneous mastectomy.

Frequent mammographic control is preferable and a biopsy is not undertaken unless there is x-ray or clinical evidence of a tumor in the contralateral breast.

Complications of Biopsy

Hematomas and infection may complicate any form of surgery and excision biopsy is no exception.

Hematomas are usually avoided by using a careful hemostatic technique. Electrocautery is preferable and the use of epinephrine supplementing local anesthetics does not give rise to delayed bleeding. The indications for drainage are rare and compression is no alternative to careful hemostasis and certainly does not prevent the formation of a hematoma.

However, despite good technique this complication still occurs. If this happens before an elective mastectomy, it is unimportant, since the hematoma will be removed together with the mass of the breast. If biopsy proves the lesion to be benign, then there is some point in evacuation, since it may prevent a broad and late-maturing scar that might have to be revised at a later date.

Infections are avoided by using aseptic conditions combined with skillful technique. The dissection should be sharp, thereby promoting well-vascularized wound edges. Once an infection is established, it should be treated by drainage and sometimes antibiotics and the wound healed before a mastectomy is performed.

Such a delay is no longer looked on as prognostically unfavorable and wound infections after a benign biopsy are no great problem, except that the scar is likely to be far from cosmetic.

Frozen Section and Paraffin Section Diagnosis

In 1905, Wilson described his frozen section method for rapid histopathologic examination of fresh tissues. With only slight modifications and with few exceptions (Webber 1976), the method is looked on as highly reliable for immediate diagnosis of breast cancer and is used by every trained pathologist.

Ackerman and Ramirez (1959) suggested that the correlation between immediate histologic diagnosis and a later paraffin section was about 98% and this was based on some 1,269 cases. Sparkman (1959), reviewing American reports of more than 3,500 cases, confirmed a diagnostic reliability of the same order. Furthermore, he showed that there were no false positives and only 0.6% false negatives.

Rosen (1978) showed that out of 556 consecutive breast biopsies, 145 (26%) proved to be malignant after frozen section examination. There were no false positives, but after paraffin section 1.4% (8) of the remaining cases proved to be carcinoma, that is, false negative. Thirty cases (5.4%) were questionable on frozen section and referred for paraffin section. Of these, 11 cases were confirmed as malignant.

Frozen section, therefore, is of considerable value and is quite accurate. False negatives are comparatively few, but they do emphasize the importance of informing the patients preoperatively that a final and definitive answer must await the result of the paraffin section.

In general, frozen section enables the pathologist to diagnose or exclude cancer. However, surgeons must accept that not all tumors can be diagnosed histologically in this way. Permanent slides from paraffin sections are used when interpretation is difficult or when there is insufficient material for both frozen and paraffin sections. A detailed histological examination, that is, paraffin section, may be necessary for the surgeon to decide the surgical treatment best suited to the patient. This information may also be of value to a patient who wishes to influence the surgical decision.

Delayed Surgery

From the above discussion it is obvious that some surgery must be delayed after excisional biopsy. This delay has been the subject of criticism in earlier literature (Ewing 1933; Harrington 1933). Their view was that the mechanical trauma of biopsy dislodged malignant cells giving them the opportunity to reach distant lymph nodes.

More recently, numerous authors (Pierce et al. 1956; Jackson and Pitts, 1959; Abramson 1976, among others) have shown convincingly that a short delay of up to one week does not affect the five-year survival rate in any way. Indeed, Donegan (1972) suggests that even longer periods are safe. One explanation may be that cancers in most delayed operations are noninvasive, thereby having a better prognosis.

However, the five-year survival rate in more advanced carcinomas, that is, those with axillary or internal mammary nodes, has been shown to be reduced if treatment is postponed for more than two weeks (Urban 1971). Therefore, since the results of paraffin section are usually available within 24 to 48 hours, there can be no defense for delaying surgery for more than five or six days.

Conclusion

It would seem reasonable to assume that since the diagnosis of tumors is made earlier and that the size of tumors is smaller, the prognosis should improve. This is yet to be proved.

Suffice to say that the surgeon who performs the initial biopsy should be aware of the many problems involved. He should be aware of the limitations of aspiration, the indications for excisional biopsy, be familiar with the technique of identification of minimal lesions, and the problems of frozen section and delayed surgery. Lastly, he should be competent to follow up a malignant diagnosis with the appropriate surgical treatment.

References

Abramson, D. J.: Delayed mastectomy after outpatient breast biopsy. Long-term survival study. Am. J. Surg. 132: 596, 1976

Ackerman, L. V., G. A. Ramirez: The indications for and limitations of frozen section diagnosis. Br. J. Surg. 46: 336, 1959

Ashikari, R., P. P. Rosen, J. A. Urban, T. Senoo: Breast cancer presenting as an axillary mass. Ann. Surg. 183: 415, 1976

Cooperman, A. M., S. A. Cook, R. E. Hermann, C. B. Esselstyn: Preoperative localization of occult lesions of the breast. Surg. Gynecol. Obstet. 142: 917, 1976

Donegan, W. L.: Diagnosis. In W. L. Donegan and J. S. Spratt (Eds.), Cancer of the Breast. Philadelphia, London, Toronto, W. B. Saunders Company, 1979

Ewing, J.: Biopsy in mammary cancer. Bull. Am. Soc. Control Cancer 72: 322, 1933

Franzén, S.: Fine needle aspiration cytology. In Tidig upptäckt av bröstcancer. Symp. arr. by Riksföreningen mot cancer, Stockholm, 1979

Harrington, S. W.: Carcinoma of the breast. Surg. Gynecol. Obstet. 56: 438, 1933

Jackson, P. P., H. H. Pitts: Biopsy with delayed radical mastectomy for carcinoma of the breast. Am. J. Surg. 98: 184, 1959

Kraissl, C. J.: The selection of appropriate lines for elective surgical incisions. Plast. Reconstr. Surg. 8: 1, 1951

Langer, K.: Über die Spaltbarkeit der Cutis. Sitzungab. d., k. Akad. d. Wissensch. Math.-naturw. Cl. 43: 233, 1861

Leis, H. P., Jr., W. L. Mersheimer, M. M. Black, A. de Chabon: The second breast. N. Y. State J. Med. 65: 2460, 1965

Leis, H. P., Jr., S. Pilnik, A. Cammarata: Clinical significance of nipple discharge. Female Patient 1: 22, 1976

Lundgren, B.: Personal communication, 1981

Lundgren, B., S. Jacobsson: Single-view mammography screening. Three-year follow-up interval cancer cases. Radiology 130: 109, 1979

Moskowitz, M., S. Pemmaraju, J. A. Fidler, D. J. Sutorius, P. Russell, J. Holle: On the diagnosis of minimal breast cancer in a screened population. Cancer 37: 2543, 1976

Pierce, E. H., O. T. Clagett, J. R. McDonald, R. P. Gage: Biopsy of the breast followed by delayed radical mastectomy. Surg. Gynecol. Obstet. 105: 559, 1956

Ringberg, A., B. Palmer, F. Linell: The contralateral breast at reconstructive surgery secondary to mastectomy. A histopathological study. To be published in: Trans. IV Congr. Europ. Sect. Int. Conf. Plast. Reconstr. Surg., Athens 1981

Rosato, F. E., J. Thomas, F. E. Rosato: Operative management of nonpalpable lesions detected by mammography. Surg. Gynecol. Obstet. 137: 491, 1973

Rosen, P. P.: Frozen section diagnosis of breast lesions. Recent experience with 556 consecutive biopsies. Ann. Surg. 187:17, 1978

Saltzstein, E. C., R. W. Mann, T. Y. Chua, J. J. de Cosse: Outpatient breast biopsy, Arch. Surg. 109: 287, 1974

Schwartz, A. M., S. S. Siegelman: A technique for biopsy of nonpalpable breast tumors. Surg. Gynecol. Obstet. 123: 1321, 1966

Simon, N., G. J. Lesnick, W. N. Lerer, A. L. Bachman: Roentgenographic localization of small lesions of the breast by the spot method. Surg. Gynecol. Obstet. 134: 572, 1972

Sparkman, R. S.: Reliability of frozen section in the diagnosis of breast lesions. Ann. Surg. 155: 924, 1959

Uddströmer, L., O. Gidlund, A. Helleberg, B. Lundgren: Preoperative localizing of nonpalpable breast lesions. (In Swedish) in Tidig upptäckt av bröstcancer. Symp. arr. by Riksföreningen mot cancer, Stockholm 1979

Uddströmer, L.: Excisional biopsy in minimal breast cancer. To be published in Trans. Int. Symp. on Surg. Treatm. and Research for Breast Cancer. Madrid 1981

Urban, J. A.: Biopsy of the "normal" breast in treating breast cancer. Surg. Clin. North. Am. 49: 291, 1969

Urban, J. A.: The case against delayed operation for breast cancer. Cancer 21: 132, 1971

Urban, J. A., M. D. Papachristou, J. Taylor: Bilateral breast cancer: Biopsy of the opposite breast. Cancer 40: 1968, 1977

Webber, B. M.: Frozen section – frozen attitudes. J. Surg. Oncol. 8: 191, 1976

Westbrook, K. C., H. S. Gallager: Breast carcinoma presenting as an axillary mass. Am. J. Surg. 122: 607, 1971

Wilson, L. B.: A method for the rapid preparation of fresh tissues for the microscope. J. A. M. A. 45: 1737, 1905

Chapter 6

Inflammatory Lesions of the Breast

C. Johnsén

Introduction

The breast may be the site for many types of infections. The frequency of infection probably varies in different countries. In Sweden, and probably in many other western countries, a lactation abscess is now a rather rare condition probably due to a high hygienic standard and early antibiotic treatment at signs of infection. In tropical African countries, however, a breast abscess is relatively common (Ajao and Ajao 1979). It tends to occur primarily during lactation and often interferes with the possibility of breast feeding; therefore, the mother frequently is forced to resort to artificial feeding. This may have serious implications for the infants if the quantity or hygiene of the artificial feeding is unsatisfactory. Since it is now universally accepted that breast feeding is better than artificial feeding for the infants, the importance of breast abscess is at once obvious.

Carcinoma with Inflammatory Reaction

Certain forms of breast carcinoma might be difficult to distinguish from breast infections. The inflammatory type of carcinoma is accompanied by redness, temperature rise, and edema of the skin over the tumor. The

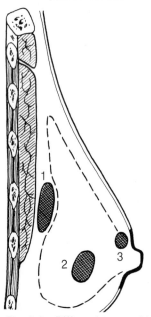

Fig. 6.1   Different types of breast abscesses. (1) Retromammary abscess; (2) intramammary abscess; (3) subareolar abscess.

distinction between infection and malignancy must be kept in mind.

Inflammatory carcinoma in a lactating patient is very rare. Necrotic changes in malignant tumors may also produce inflammatory signs such as edema and redness of the skin simulating a breast abscess. Sometimes the content of a necrotic tumor is thick, yellowish, and very puslike, and such a tumor is macroscopically indistinguishable from an abscess. When incising and draining a breast abscess, it is always wise to perform a biopsy from the abscess wall to rule out malignancy.

Mastitis and Lactation Abscess

These forms of infection are a diminishing problem in the so-called developed countries, but they are relatively common in other parts of the world.

During lactation, the nipple may be macerated and small fissures may appear. These may be the portals for infection. The first sign is tenderness in the breast, accompanied by some degree of induration, slight redness of the skin, and a minimal systemic reaction. Cessation of nursing combined with antibiotics often cures such a limited infection within a few days; nursing may then be resumed. If the inflammatory reaction persists, a tumor will usually appear in the breast representing an abscess. A tumor in the lactating breast with pain and tenderness, redness, and edema of the overlying skin makes the diagnosis obvious. The presence of pus may be demonstrated by needle aspiration. If no pus is obtained, however, an infection is not excluded; even if pus is obtained, it does not eliminate a possible presence of carcinoma.

The most commonly cultured organism in breast abscess is *Staphylococcus aureus*, but *Salmonella, Pseudomonas aeruginosa, Escherichia coli, Proteus mirabilis,* and other organisms may be found (Ajao and Ajao 1979; Rudoy and Nelson 1975).

It is possible to separate three types of abscesses according to their position in the breast: superficial abscess, intramammary abscess, and retromammary abscess (Fig. 6.1). Deep intramammary and retromammary abscesses can sometimes reach a large diameter and lack the typical signs of inflammation such as redness and increased heat of the skin thus simulating, for example, a giant fibroadenoma or a carcinoma. Mammography and needle biopsy may be helpful for diagnosis.

Treatment

Treatment consists of incision and drainage. General anesthesia is to be preferred because the abscess is often more deeply situated than initially suspected. Bacteriologic culture of the pus is routine. Small superficial abscesses are incised just over the lesion and a small drain is left in the abscess. When treating larger abscesses, it is often recommended that an incision be made over the lesion with a complementary incision in the submammary fold; a drain is then placed through the abscess via these two incisions (Fig. 6.2). Systemic antibiotics, chosen according to the bacteriologic findings, may be used, but a circumscribed abscess without systemic symptoms and with adequate drainage does not necessarily need antibiotic treatment.

Recurring Subareolar Abscess

This is a rather common and troublesome disease of the breast in younger women. It usually develops in women between 20 to 40 years of age, but has no relationship to pregnancy or lactation. The author has personally treated more than 30 cases during the last four years. The condition is often unsuccessfully treated by repeated excisions of the central parts of the breast parenchyma by surgeons who do not understand the pathology of this lesion. Chronic subareolar breast abscess, lactiferous duct fistula, or mammary duct fistula are other names of this disease.

The disease has no relation to pregnancy and lactation and often begins as a comparatively localized area of inflammation of the subareolar area, which develops into a small abscess at the edge of the areola. When it is incised and drained or spontaneously drains, the process seemingly subsides only to flare up again in the same region after a few months. A small sinus that intermittently drains often develops. The condition is frequently associated with a congenitally inverted nipple. Sometimes there is simultaneous drainage of pus from the sinus and from the affected duct orifice at the nipple. This cycle is repeated over several years. Unsuccessful treatment by repeated incisions or local excisions of the infected area may lead to unnecessarily radical surgery and cases treated by simple mastectomy have been reported (Kilgore and Fleming 1952). In my personal series of cases, the history of the disease varies from a few months up to ten years (Johnsen 1976, 1982).

A typical case involved a 19-year-old nulliparous woman who appeared with a 10-cm tumor in the left breast. She had no systemic reaction and the lump was hard, rather well circumscribed with the characteristics of a giant fibroadenoma. The nature of this lesion was detected on operation and the abscess was incised and drained. A biopsy from the abscess wall showed inflammatory reaction. The process healed and the tumor disappeared completely, but after 18 months the patient returned with a small subareolar abscess situated at the margin of the areola. This abscess was incised and drained, but recurred after a few months and a fistula developed. The

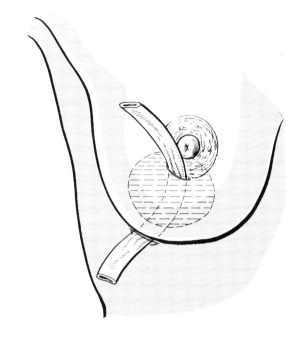

Fig. 6.2 Drainage of a larger breast abscess.

histology of this condition has been described in detail by several authors (Patey and Thackray 1958; Toker 1962; Kleinfeld 1966). To understand the pathology of this disorder, it is important to be familiar with the anatomy of the nipple and the lactiferous ducts. Normally the larger lactiferous ducts are lined with a double-layered low columnar or cuboidal epithelium. Below the surface of the nipple each duct dilates to form a terminal ampulla (milk sinus) and then narrows slightly to open on the surface of the nipple. At the commencement of the ampulla, the columnar epithelium is abruptly replaced by a stratified squamous layer, which lines the remainder of the ampulla up to the duct orifice. In recurring subareolar breast abscess, histologic examination reveals a hugely dilated duct lying within or just beneath the nipple, lined with a stratified squamous epithelium, and plugged by keratinous debris. At some point, there is disruption of the wall of this duct, which communicates with the subareolar abscess (Fig. 6.3).

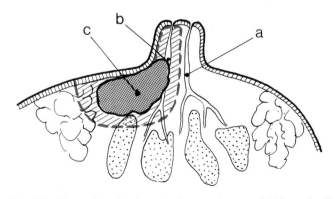

Fig. 6.3 Illustration of subareolar breast abscess. (a) Normal milk duct; (b) pathologically changed duct plugged by keratinous debris, dilated and ruptured to form an abscess (c).

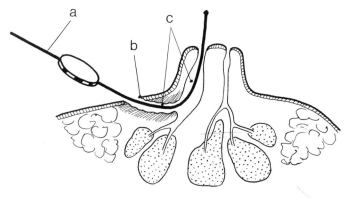

Fig. 6.**4** Operative technique for mammary duct fistula.
A lacrimal duct probe (a) is inserted through the sinus (b) into the fistula and affected milk duct (c).

In this disease the squamous epithelium, normally found only in the wider terminal portion of the ducts within the nipple, lines the affected duct for a considerable distance into the subareolar region. It has been claimed that it is this abnormal squamous metaplasia of the lining of the duct leading to the area of the abscess, which is the key to the natural history of recurring subareolar abscess. Incision and drainage, or local excision of the abscess and the fibrosis surrounding it, does not remove the source of the infection, namely, the duct lined with the abnormal epithelium. The pathogenesis of the disease is not known, but its relation to so-called central invagination of the nipple a congenital anomaly has been emphasized (Caswell and Burnett 1956).

Treatment

Once the underlying pathology is known, the effective treatment is very simple and nonmutilating. The fistulous character of the disease is important. It is often possible to put a lacrimal duct probe through the sinus tract into the affected lactiferous duct and out through the nipple (Fig. 6.**4**). The simplest way of treating the disease is then to incise the affected duct over the probe and excise the granulomatous tissue and leave the scar open to heal by second intension (Fig. 6.**5**). Healing occurs in three to six weeks, often with rather good cosmetic results (Fig. 6.**6**). Sometimes a smaller reconstruction of the nipple may be performed secondarily. It is wise to wait 6 to 12 months after the operation of the fistula before reconstruction is considered.

When a patient comes the first time with a subareolar abscess, it is recommended to treat it with incision and drainage. After two to three recurrences have occurred and the true fistulous character of the disease is recognized, a more radical treatment is then advised.

The key to a successful treatment of this disease is to understand the necessity for excision of the diseased duct within the nipple itself.

Mammary Duct Ectasia

This lesion has been identified by a wide variety of names. The most common is plasma cell mastitis (Haagensen 1971). This is a benign condition in the aging breast usually in patients over 65 years of age. It is important because its clinical picture may simulate carcinoma so closely that it has often been mistaken for it.

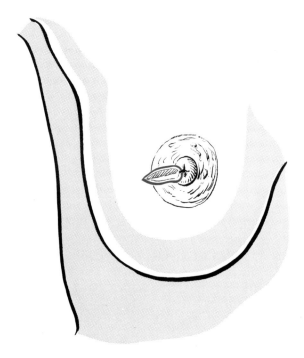

Fig. 6.**5** Operative technique for mammary duct fistula.
The lacrimal duct probe (a) put in position through the sinus (b) and out through the duct orifice at the nipple (c).

Fig. 6.**6** Operative technique for mammary duct fistula.
The tissue is incised over the lacrimal duct probe and all inflammatory changed tissue is excised. The wound is left open for healing.

Mammary duct ectasia begins with dilatation of the terminal collecting ducts beneath the nipple and areola. They become distended with cellular debris and lipid-containing material. At this initial stage, there is no accompanying inflammation or other symptoms and the disease ordinarily escapes detection. In a small number of individuals with mammary duct ectasia, the lesion develops further and gives rise to symptoms such as a yellowish or brownish nipple discharge.

As the disease progresses, the duct walls are greatly thickened by fibrosis and inflammatory infiltration. The fibrosis within the duct walls not only thickens them but also shortens them, so that flattening and eventually retraction of the nipple develops.

With further disease progression, the continuity of the atrophic duct epithelium is broken in places. The irritating lipid material then gives an inflammatory reaction, sometimes similar to that in fat necrosis. In some cases there is a predominance of plasma cells, giving the picture of so-called plasma cell mastitis. This is merely a late phase of mammary duct ectasia.

In the early stages of the disease, there are no symptoms at all. When the fibrosis and inflammatory changes have developed, there might be a spontaneous nipple discharge and later a retraction of the nipple. Eventually an irregular mass develops beneath the areola simulating a carcinoma.

At one time or another during the evolution of the disease, patients with duct ectasia often have clinical signs of inflammation, such as pain or tenderness over the tumor, slight redness or edema of the overlying skin, often intermittent, or elevation of the body temperature.

Sometimes in the final inflammatory stages of duct ectasia, an abscess may form accompanied by all the usual signs: local redness and heat and even edema of the skin. Such abscesses evolving from duct ectasia, however, are usually more indolent and low grade than the more common abscesses associated with lactation.

A rather distinctive feature of duct ectasia is its tendency to manifest itself by repeated episodes of inflammation in the same breast and to develop in both breasts over the course of years. This means that repeated subareolar signs of inflammation and even abscesses in older women are most often due to mammary duct ectasia.

Treatment

Mammary duct ectasia with inflammatory signs is a rather uncommon condition and needs treatment only in exceptional cases. It may be a diagnostic problem, but usually fine needle aspiration biopsy and mammography reveal the true nature of the lesion. If abscesses recur, the treatment of choice is excision of all the subareolar tissue including the terminal ducts.

Tuberculosis of the Breast

This is a very rare disease in western countries, but it still exists in many other parts of the world (Alagarathnam and Ong 1980). Tuberculosis of the breast may be either primary or secondary. The clinical characteristics include a hard, nontender mass with some fixation in the breast tissue and retraction of the nipple and/or skin, thus mimicking carcinoma. There may also be signs of a subacute or chronic breast abscess. A nipple discharge occurs in some cases. The lesion may break down to ulcerate the skin or to form characteristic draining sinuses or fistulas. The diagnosis can be established by biopsy or a positive bacteriologic test.

Early diagnosis is difficult, but tuberculosis should be suspected in a patient who has recurring breast abscess after adequate treatment on previous occasions. Multiple biopsies of the abscess wall are sometimes necessary to confirm the diagnosis. The mammographic picture is not diagnostic, being very similar in some patients to that of fibroadenosis (Alagarathnam and Ong 1980). Essentially, the diagnosis is histological; acid-fast bacilli were present in only 25% of a series of 439 cases (Morgen 1981).

Treatment

Tuberculosis of the breast, when the lesion is small, is treated by local excision with a margin of normal tissue around the lesion. Sometimes a simple mastectomy may be indicated. Antimicrobiologic chemotherapy is then employed after surgical excision.

One must always consider this disease in the patient who presents with a persistent breast abscess following adequate treatment and be aware that it can be the cause of a breast mass, often mimicking a breast carcinoma.

Sarcoid of the Breast

This is a rare condition. It is important to know that this lesion can appear in the breast and may resemble tuberculosis or other granulomas of the breast.

Syphilis of the Breast

This can occur in the breast during any of the three stages of the disease (Shackelford 1968).

Primary syphilis of the breast is usually manifested as an ulcerated lesion in the region of the nipple. The diagnosis is established by finding spirochetes in the ulcer.

Secondary syphilis rarely involves the breast, but when it does it is manifested by the signs of mildly acute mastitis. It is diagnosed by positive serologic findings.

Tertiary or late syphilis of the breast is rare, but when it occurs it is manifested by the formation of gumma, which is a hard, painless, circumscribed mass in the breast and frequently involves and ulcerates the skin. It may be mistaken for carcinoma. The diagnosis is established by serologic tests and biopsy findings. The treatment of syphilis of the breast is by antiluetic therapy.

Unspecified Abscesses

The author has, in several cases, observed breast abscesses that cannot be referred to the more specific type of abscesses described in this chapter. These abscesses are treated like lactation abscesses, and a biopsy from the abscess wall is even more important in these cases.

References

Ajao, O. G., A. O. Ajao: Breast abscess. J. Natl. Med. Assoc. 71: 1197, 1979

Alagarathnam, T. T., G. B. Ong: Tuberculosis of the breast. Br. J. Surg. 67: 125, 1980

Caswell, H. T., W. E. Burnett: Chronic recurrent breast abscess secondary to inversion of the nipple. Surg. Gynecol. Obstet. 102: 439, 1956

Haagensen, C. D.: Diseases of the Breast. W. B. Saunders Co., Philadelphia 1971

Johnsén, C.: Recurring subareolar abscess. Acta Chir. Scand. 142: 393, 1976

Johnsén, C.: Treatment of mammary duct fistula. 1982

Kilgore, A. R., R. Fleming: Abscesses of the breast, recurring lesions in areolar area. Calif. Med. 77: 190, 1952

Kleinfeld, G.: Chronic subareolar breast abscess. J. Fl. Med. Assoc. 53: 21, 1966

Morgen, M.: Tuberculosis of the breast. Surg. Gynecol. Obstet. 53: 593, 1931

Patey, D. H., A. C. Thackray: Pathology and treatment of mammary-duct fistula. Lancet 2: 871, 1958

Rudoy, R. C., J. D. Nelson: Breast abscess during the neonatal period. Am. J. Dis. Child. 129: 1031, 1975

Shackelford, R. T.: Diagnosis of Surgical Disease. W. B. Saunders Philadelphia, p. 544, 1968

Toker, C.: Lactiferous duct fistula. J. Pathol. Bacteriol. 84: 143, 1962

Pathology of Potentially Malignant Diseases of the Breast

H.-E. Stegner

Mastopathy (Cystic disease)

A great number of hormone-dependent proliferative and regressive changes of the glandular tissue of the breast are included under mastopathy. The most important histologic components of mastopathy are shown in Table 7.**1**. The microscopic diagnosis of mastopathy is based on the relative frequency of certain combinations of hormone-dependent features, but it is difficult to differentiate between specific hormonal changes due to a spectrum of mammotropic hormones interacting with changing dominances. Although ill-defined, it seems justified to retain the term mastopathy to describe a structural disorder of high complexity reflecting a disturbed homeostasis. The World Health Organization has chosen to call this "mammary dysplasia," which is an eponym of even wider meaning, including benign as well as potentially malignant lesions, and causes more confusion than enlightment regarding the complex pathomorphology.

Mastopathy is usually bilateral and predominantly found in the upper lateral quadrants of the breast. This predilection cannot be explained only by the relatively large amount of parenchyma in this region. Less frequently, mastopathy is manifested in more discrete, even microscopic foci or isolated nodular areas. The clinical symptoms are determined by vascular congestion, the condition of the connective tissue, increased nodularity and cyst formation.

Cystic Mastopathy (Cystic Disease)

Cysts arise in the terminal and interlobular parts of the ducts because of active proliferation of the epithelium (cystadenoma). Following retention of secretion, pressure atrophy of the epithelium develops secondarily. The escape of retained secretions into the connective tissue causes aseptic inflammation with subsequent granulomatous and sclerotic processes (Fig. 7.**1**).

The epithelium of the mastopathic cysts may show apocrine (eosinophilic) metaplasia or foam-cell transformation. According to Davies (1974), the lipid or hemosiderin-loaded foam cells represent migrating histiocytes and not transformation of the autochthonous epithelial cells. Hamperl (1970) regards the foam cells as a functional type of myoepithelial cell. The secretion of the cysts may contain formed components such as cholesterol crystals or laminated calcium precipitates (microliths) (Fig. 7.**2**).

These concretions are of great importance in mammographic diagnosis of mammary diseases. So-called "duct ectasia" has to be clearly separated from the cyst formation seen in the parenchyma with mastopathy. Duct ectasia represents saccular dilatation of the distal retroareolar ducts and is particularly seen in involution of the breast and in hyperprolactinemia.

Cellular Types in Mastopathy

Functional transformation, degeneration, and metaplasia cause a broad spectrum of cellular types in glandular tissue with mastopathy. A common finding is the so-called apocrine (eosinophilic) metaplasia of the epithelial cells. This change in the epithelium is connected with simple and proliferative mastopathy, fibroadenoma, and sclerosing adenoses and is also seen as an independent neoplasia (apocrine carcinoma). The apocrine cells are recognized by their prism-like appearance with dome-shaped apex, eosinophilic granular cytoplasm, and round basal nuclei (Fig. 7.**3**).

Electron microscopic characteristics include a high content of mitochondria and closely packed osmiophilic granules in the apical part of the cells (Fig. 7.**4**). No

Table 7.**1** Histological components of mastopathy

Microcysts and macrocysts

Precipitation of calcium and cholesterin

Ductal adenosis
  – blunt
  – microglandular
  – sclerosing
  tubular pseudoinfiltration

Epithelial hyperplasia (Epitheliosis)
  – solid
  – pseudopapillary
  – fenestrated

Lobular secretion
Periductal fibrosclerosis
Periductal and perilobular edema
Aseptic "reabsorbing" inflammation
Distorsion of mesenchymal architecture
Apocrine (eosinophilic) metaplasia
Foam-cell transformation
Light-cell transformation (lamprocyts)

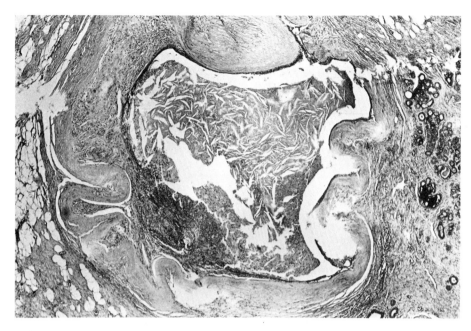

Fig. 7.**1** Mastopathic cysts with retention of secretion. Sclerosis of the wall and aseptic "reabsorbing" inflammation.

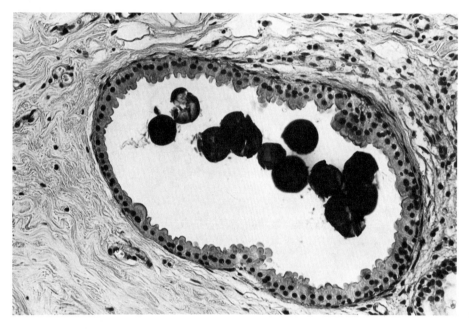

Fig. 7.**2** Intraductal psammomatous calcification (microliths) in simple mastopathy. Apocrine metaplasia of duct epithelium.

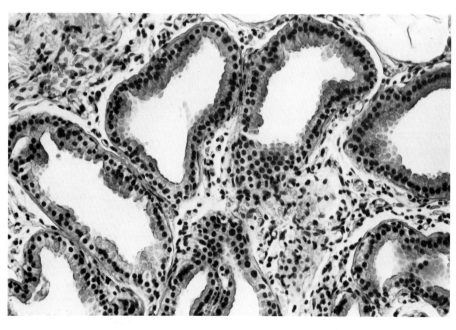

Fig. 7.**3** Apocrine (eosinophilic) metaplasia of duct epithelium.

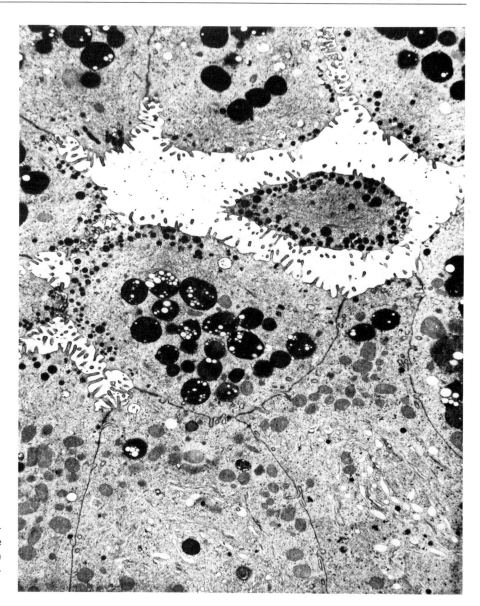

Fig. 7.**4** Accumulation of osmiophilic granules in the dome-shaped apical part of the cells in so-called apocrine (eosinophil) metaplasia of duct epithelium. (Electron microscopy x 10,800.)

specific apocrine secretion mechanism is seen. The ultrastructure of these cells is more like eccrine sweat glands than apocrine secretory cells. Apocrine (eosinophilic) metaplasia is usually a special differentiation of ductal and lobular cells without any relationship to the development of carcinoma although in certain cases the apocrine cell, similar to the normal glandular cell, could be the cell of origin of regular and atypical hyperplasia as well as true apocrine carcinoma. Another feature occasionally found in mastopathy is lobular secretion seen in the lobular compartments. The microscopic picture corresponds to the situation in lactation with retention of secretions in the terminal ducts (Fig. 7.**5**). This change is therefore described as persistent or residual lactation (Bonser et al. 1961; McFarland 1962). According to Theele and Bässler (1981), as well as shown in my own investigations, it is connected with an increased prolactin level (hyperprolactinemia). Possibly this isolated transformation of secretion as seen in a single lobule could be caused by an increased hormonal receptivity.

Other cell types seen in mastopathy are foam cells (Fig. 7.**6**), fluorocytes containing ceroid (Hamperl 1949), and light cells loaded with glycogen (lamprocytes).

Benign Epithelial Hyperplasia

The many different types of benign epithelial hyperplasia might be divided in intraductal and extraductal cell proliferation. The intraductal changes are classified as epitheliosis and the extraductal as adenosis. The recognition of premalignant hyperplasia is mainly based on cytomorphologic criteria.

Epitheliosis

Epitheliosis is a frequent component of cystic mastopathy, but is also seen as a specific microscopic entity.

According to the tissue pattern, different types are recognized such as solid obstructive, pseudopapillary, fenestrated, and cribriform. Papillomatosis does not belong to the entity of epitheliosis. Two types of cells are most commonly seen in epitheliosis; the basal cell type (indeterminate) and the flat or cylindrical secretory cell type.

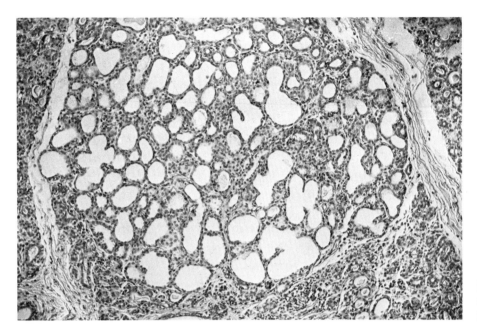

Fig. 7.**5** Terminal ducts and acini with ectasia and secretion of epithelium in hyperprolactinemia. So-called lobular secretion.

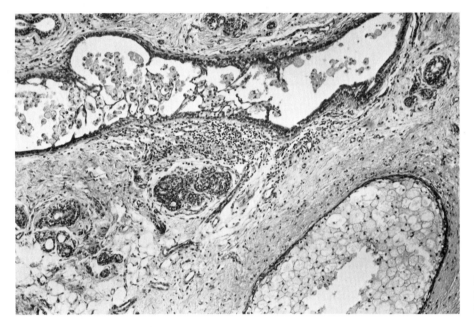

Fig. 7.**6** Foam-cell transformation of duct epithelium and desquamation of foam-cells into the lumen.

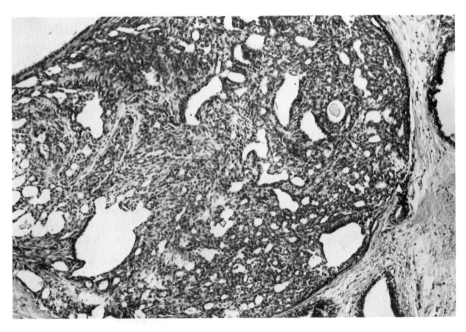

Fig. 7.**7** Intraductal "regular" epithelial hyperplasia with irregularly lined spaces (fenestrated epitheliosis). Polarization of the solid epithelial cell complexes (streaming pattern).

Apocrine cells or foam cells are relatively frequent. In the solid obstructive type of epitheliosis the indeterminate type of cells dominates. Through a parallel orientation of the cells in the solid proliferates, the impression of streaming might appear (Fig. 7.7). The cylindrical secretory cells usually preserve their epithelial arrangement. They may develop secondary lumina within the solid proliferations thus giving rise to a cribriform pattern or may also form irregularly shaped split lumina (fenestrated epitheliosis) (Fig. 7.7). They often show apical secretions. Benign epitheliosis has regular cellular and nuclear structures or shows only mild pleomorphism. Mitoses are rare.

Adenosis

Simple adenosis (blunt duct adenosis) has to be separated from the myoepithelial sclerosing adenosis. Simple adenosis is the most frequent type of extraductal epithelial hyperplasia and a prominent component in mastopathy.

In the area of the lobules, it shows the picture of an organoid hyperplasia. The terminal ducts show ectasia with hypertrophy of both cell layers (Fig. 7.8). The lobules are enlarged throughout, but the total number of terminal units is not increased in contrast to the situation in lobular hyperplasia. Microcystic adenosis could originate from all parts of the duct system, but is more common in the area of the terminal ducts and rare in the different parts of the large ducts.

Myoepithelial adenosis is characterized by hyperplasia of the myoepithelial cells. The spindle shaped, often water-clear myoepithelial cells show diffuse or fascicular growth. The epithelial cells in microglandular formations

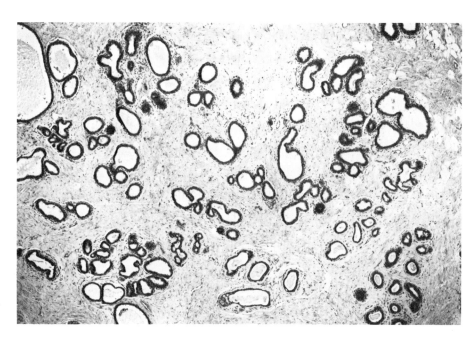

Fig. 7.**8** Blunt duct adenosis in mastopathy.

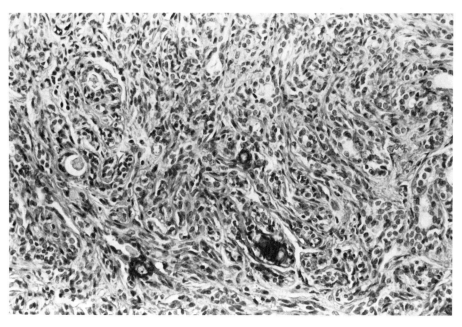

Fig. 7.**9** Microglandular and sclerosing adenosis with psammomatous calcifications.

are hypertrophic, the cell nucleus is round, and the cytoplasma is light (Fig. 7.9). Myoepithelial adenosis surrounds terminal, small, or medium-sized ducts (pericanalicular extension) as nodular foci. They may also form invaginations in ectatic ducts (intracanalicular extension). In most cases, myoepithelial hyperplasia causes a more or less prominent productive fibrosis.

Sclerosing adenosis arises by increase of collagen and reticular fibers. The accumulation of fibers causes a dissociation and compression of the proliferating myoepithelial cells. In ultramicroscopy, the myoepithelial cells are separated from the fibrous stroma by a clearly defined basement lamella (Fig. 7.10). Small, multicentric, often only microscopic calcifications are seen in the parenchyma of sclerosing adenosis. Confluence of florid foci form palpable diffuse thickening or multinodular tumors (Fig. 7.11). In frozen section, these changes might be mistaken for scirrhous carcinoma.

Ductal Papillomatosis

Papillomas are arborescent proliferations of the ductal system which have a fibrovascular core in the interior of their branches and which are covered by an epithelium of varying differentiation (Fig. 7.12). They differ basically in that respect from the pseudopapillary types of epitheliosis. There usually is a regular cylindrical epithelium. Apocrine metaplasia is not rare.

Small multicentric ductal papillomas (microscopic papillomatosis) might be part of mastopathy. It affects the medium-sized and smaller ducts more often than the main ducts and rarely produces pathologic secretions. The large solitary papilloma (gross papilloma) is, on the contrary, a specific condition localized to the distal subareolar part of the lactiferous ducts with the specific symptom of a serous or sanguinous nipple discharge.

Papilloma and Papillary Cystadenoma

The solitary papillomas of the lactiferous ducts are elongated, worm-like formations 1 to 2 cm in length. They usually completely obliterate the lumen causing an interruption of x-ray contrast in ductography. As they generally are of soft consistency, they cannot be palpated. A serous or sanguinous nipple discharge is present in about 80% of the cases. They may appear at any age with the average age about 40. Papillary cystadenomas are pathogenetically similar lesions located in preexisting cysts.

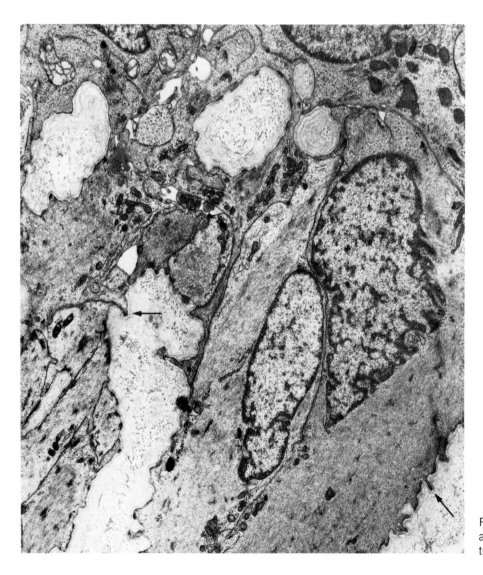

Fig. 7.**10** Myoepithelial cells in sclerosing adenosis. Distinct basement lamella. (Electron microscopy x 14,850.)

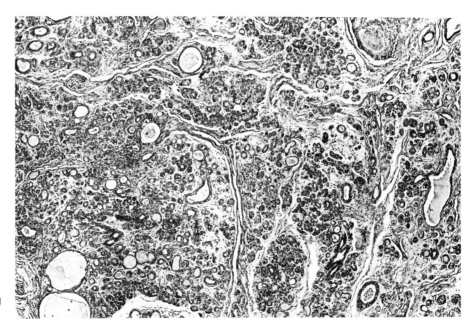

Fig. 7.**11** Diffuse multinodular sclerosing adenosis.

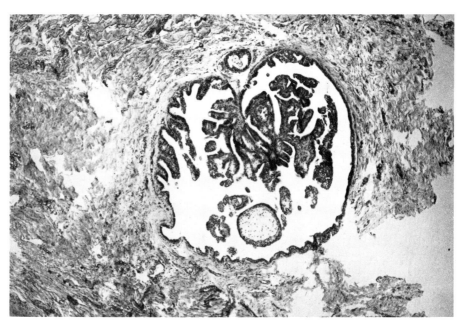

Fig. 7.**12** Ductal papillomatosis.

Histologically, the solitary papilloma consists of a ramified fibrous stroma covered by two or more layers of epithelium. Myoepithelial hyperplasia increases the abundance of cells in the papilloma (Fig. 7.**13**). The cells of the covering epithelium might show a foamy or apocrine transformation. Pronounced desquamation of cells is frequently present. The secretion retained within the ectatic ducts contains isolated cells or cells lying in pseudopapillary complexes. Sclerosis and hyalinosis of connective tissue stalk give rise to disturbances of vascularization in the larger papillomas leading to hemorrhage, necrosis, and degeneration. The walls of the affected ducts are almost always sclerotic and penetrated by cellular infiltrates (aseptic inflammatory reaction). Irregular tubular sproutings of the ductal epithelium in the pedicle of the papilloma might be mistaken for malignant stroma infiltration (tubular pseudoinfiltration) (Fig. 7.**13**). The complex cellular pattern and the pseudoinfiltration (infiltrating epitheliosis) might cause an overdiagnosis of malignancy in frozen sections. The most important histologic criteria to differentiate papillary cystadenoma from papillary carcinoma are seen in Table 7.**2**. The primary benign duct papilloma rarely becomes malignant. Contrary to diffuse microscopic papillomatosis, the general risk for malignant transformation of duct parenchyma in patients with solitary papilloma is not increased (Haagensen 1971). Segmental resection after exact preoperative localization with x-ray contrast technique is the therapeutic method of choice.

Table 7.2 Differential diagnosis of papilloma and papillary carcinoma

Papilloma	Papillary carcinoma
Well-developed, ramified fibrovascular core	Generally sparse connective tissue tumor rich of parenchyma
Often two types of epithelial cells	Uniform cell type
Complex glandular pattern apocrine and foam-cell transformation	Cribriform and trabecular pattern, no apocrine metaplasia
Different cell types but normochromic nuclei	Uniform cell type, but atypical hyperchromatic nuclei
Sclerosing adenosis as a concomitant finding	No sclerosing adenosis
Tubular pseudoinfiltration (infiltrating epitheliosis) at the base of the papilloma	When present, carcinomatous infitration of the stroma
Mitosis rare	Mitosis common

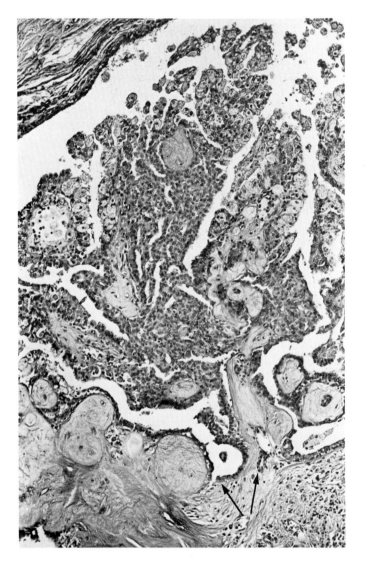

Fig. 7.13 Solitary cell-rich papilloma. Hyalinization of the central part of the stromal core, so-called tubular pseudoinfiltration in the papilloma stalk.

Relation of Cystic Mastopathy and Benign Hyperplasia to Carcinoma

Over decades, the relationship between mastopathy and mammary carcinoma has been a matter of controversy. In many cases, the hyperproliferative changes in different types of mastopathy were overemphasized as a predisposing factor in the histogenesis of carcinoma. The suspicion of a causal relationship was grounded on observations of questionable evidence:

1. The age distribution curve of breast carcinoma coincides closely to that of mastopathy
2. Patients with breast cancer have an increased frequency of mastopathy
3. Incidence of breast cancer is higher in patients which had previous operation for cystic disease than the expected incidence

The incidence peak of mastopathy lies in the perimenopausal age as does that of mammary carcinoma. The age peak of mastopathy is between 46 and 50 years (Sattelmacher and Jürgens 1955; Wiechern 1977), and according to Haagensen at the age of 53.5. Mammary carcinoma is most frequent between the age of 45 and 49. According to Prechtel and Schmidt (1979), the age peak for mastopathy lies ten years earlier than that of carcinoma. The age distribution of mammary carcinoma shows a bimodal pattern with one peak premenopausal and one postmenopausal (DeWaard et al. 1964). It is possible that this bimodal pattern is caused by epidemiological and constitutional differences in the disease (DeWaard et al. 1964; Jacobsen 1946). The synchronous appearance of mastopathy and carcinoma indicates similar predisposing factors for both diseases, but does not allow any conclusions as to causal relationship.

A coincidence of mammary carcinoma and cystic mastopathy (carcinoma in mastopathy) is seen in about 25% of the cases (22.2%, Davis et al. 1964; 28.6%, Wiechern 1977). The relative frequency of mastopathy changes in clinical biopsy material is 40% (38.2%, Bässler 1978; 41.8% Wiechern 1977), and in unselected biopsy material, 32.4%. The combination of mammary carcinoma and mastopathy is thus more rare than would be expected from the average frequency of mastopathy changes.

The association of carcinoma as a sequel of fibrous cystic mastopathy has been investigated in numerous retrospective and prospective studies. According to a summary made by Bässler in 1978, the frequency of mammary carcinoma following mastopathy diagnosed in biopsy is 3.17%. Several prospective studies reached the conclusion that the incidence of breast cancer in patients who had previous operations for cystic disease is between 2.5 and 5 times the expected incidence.

The So-called Proliferative (hyperplastic) Mastopathy

The inclusion of all forms of mastopathy in a single group lead to a difficult evaluation of its prospective significance. Subdividing mastopathy according to the degree of epithelial proliferation brought progress in the prognostic evaluation. The basis for this subdivision was the experience that obviously a significant increase in the risk for malignancy was present only in cases of abnormal and atypical epithelial proliferation (Kiaer 1954; Böhmig 1964; Davis et al. 1964; Möbius and Nize 1966; Marx et al. 1969). Prechtel (1972) recommended a subclassification into three groups: grade 1, simple mastopathy without epithelial proliferation; grade 2, mastopathy with epitheliosis but without cell atypia; and grade 3, mastopathy with atypical epithelial hyperplasia.

Investigations have proved that only certain of the proliferative alterations mainly included in grade 3 mastopathy predispose to the development of carcinoma. In a prospective study of 629 of their cases, Prechtel and Schmidt (1979) found a subsequent carcinoma within six years after the primary biopsy in 0.5% (3/629) in mastopathy type 1, 1.9% (2/103) in mastopathy type 2, and 2.0% (1/51) in type 3.

An improvement of the prognostic assessment of mastopathy with epithelial hyperplasia is to be expected in investigations based on histologically well-defined components. This presupposes dividing up the mastopathy syndrome in a spectrum of typical constituents. Page et al. (1978) have correlated the different tissue components of mastopathy found in 925 biopsies to the clinical course. They compared the carcinoma rate with a standard morbidity rate for each histologically well-defined category. Significant increase in the incidence rate was found in ductal hyperplasia (1.8), papillary apocrine changes (1.8), and atypical lobular hyperplasia (4.2). No increase of risk was seen in simple and sclerosing adenosis or in cystic mastopathy.

Investigations show that distinct hyperplastic components should be looked on more seriously in the prognostic evaluation of mastopathy than the degree of the general mastopathic transformation of the glandular tissue.

Atypical (Premalignant) Hyperplasias

The term atypical (premalignant) hyperplasia includes all pathologic proliferations of the ductal and lobular system that differ from the regular epithelial hyperplasias by having a higher degree of cell atypia but on the other hand not yet the degree of atypia as seen in intraductal or intralobular carcinoma.

This heterogenuous group is the borderline between benign and malignant lesions and is not clearly defined and thus open to very subjective interpretations. In the classification of mastopathy according to Prechtel (1972) it fits into the grade 3 mastopathy. The higher malignancy rate of mastopathy grade 3 leads to the conclusion that carcinoma gradually passes through different stages of epithelial hyperplasia (Fig. 7.**14**). This is not at all proved, although steps in a progression link could be hypothetically proposed. Wellings et al. (1975) have proposed development in five steps starting with simple adenosis (types 1 and 2) followed by transitional stages (types 3 and 4) to intraductal carcinoma (type 5). In this progression, the atypical lobule constitutes the link between benign epithelial hyperplasia and carcinoma in situ.

Atypical hyperplasia could be seen in ductal as well as in lobular compartments. It could be seen as isolated changes but was more frequent in combination with regular hyperplasia and/or preinvasive carcinoma.

Intraductal Atypical Hyperplasia

In slight degrees of atypical intraductal epithelial hyperplasia, the ductal epithelium is multilayered and nuclei in the secretory cells are pleomorphic and hyperchromatic (Fig. 7.**15**). With increasing proliferation, the epithelium

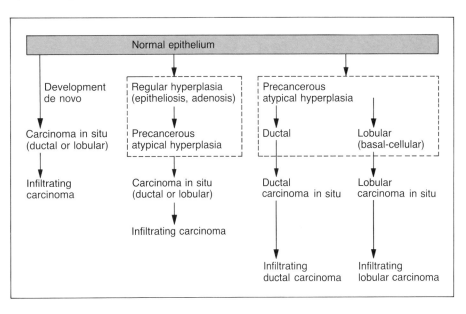

Fig. 7.**14** Hypothesis of the histogenesis of mammary carcinoma.

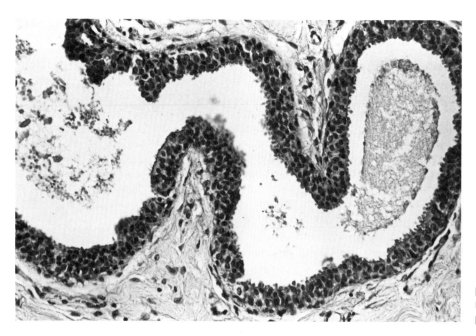

Fig. 7.**15** Atypical intraductal epithelial hyperplasia. Multilayered epithelium, enlarged nucleoli, pseudopapillary sprouting, and hyperchromatic nuclei.

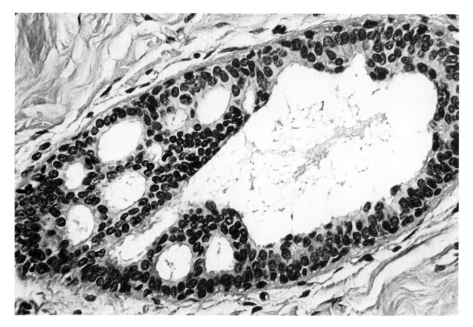

Fig. 7.**16** Intraductal carcinoma of cribriform type. Multilayered epithelium with hyperchromatic and irregular nuclei. The epithelium forms trabecula and arches (so-called Roman bridges). Rigid epithelial pattern.

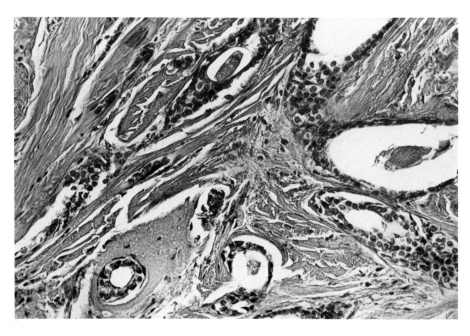

Fig. 7.**17** So-called tubular pseudoinfiltration (infiltrating epitheliosis). Irregular extraductal sprouting into sclerotic connective tissue.

forms thin pseudopapillary sprouts and epithelial bridges. The myoepithelial layer is usually preserved. Single mitoses can be seen. The cells might show apical secretion.

Differential diagnoses of intraductal carcinoma. Distinction from intraductal carcinoma especially of the clinging type might be difficult. According to Azzopardi, (1979), conclusive histologic criteria of clinging carcinoma are more pronounced nuclear pleomorphism, rigidity of the cellular pattern with the cells forming trabecular bars and curved epithelial bridges (roman bridges) (Fig. 7.**16**).

Extraductal Atypical Hyperplasia (Tubular Pseudoinfiltration)

Tubular pseudoinfiltration is a condition with extraductal sprouting that looks similar to, and might be mistaken for, a true carcinomatous infiltration. Azzopardi (1979) talks about infiltrating epitheliosis. The concept of infiltration is, however, so strongly connected with malignant proliferation that the description of the lesion could be misunderstood by the clinician.

Tubular pseudoinfiltration could often be seen around the bases of ductal papillomas with irregular sprouting tubules of different caliber and elongated strands within a sclerotic and hyalinized connective tissue (Fig. 7.**17**). The epithelium is cubical or flat. Myoepithelial cells could usually be demonstrated. Typically there is a triangular shape or acute narrowing of the tubules. Central components are tubular pseudoinfiltrations in a so-called radial scars (Hamperl 1975). This focal or multicentric lesion consists of an elastoid-hyaline core of connective tissue with radiating ectatic ducts showing different degrees of epithelial hyperplasia. Through the local transformation of the glandular architecture, a stellate lesion arises that both clinically and mammographically might be mistaken for a scirrhous carcinoma (Fig. 7.**18**). The prognostic significance of radial scars is a matter of question. Their

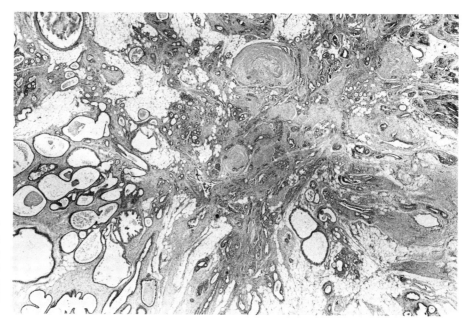

Fig. 7.**18** So-called radial scar. The center consists of elastoid-hyalin connective tissue with irregular proliferation of angular tubules (so-called tubular pseudoinfiltration). The periphery of the lesion consists of radiating ducts showing different degrees of epithelial hyperplasia.

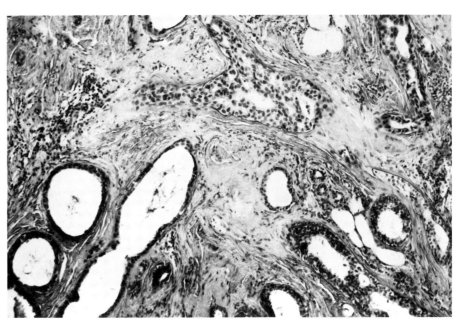

Fig. 7.**19** Section of radial scar with secondary malignant transformation of the epithelium.

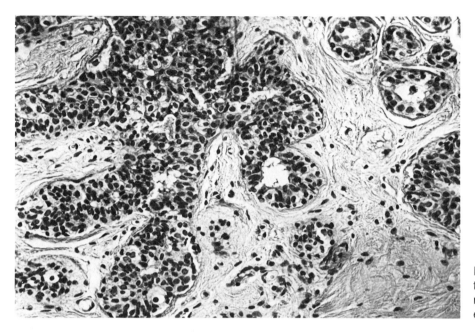

Fig. 7.**20** Atypical lobular hyperplasia of the epithelium. There is ectasia of the terminal ducts by multilayered and pleomorphic epithelium.

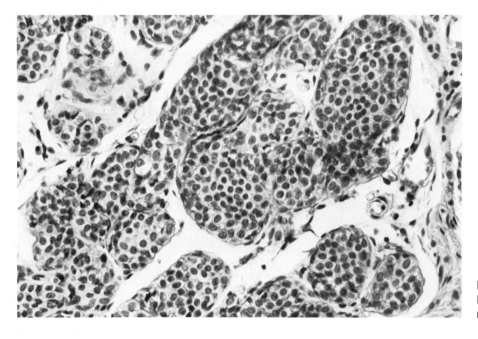

Fig. 7.**21** Lobular carcinoma in situ. Distension of the lobules by proliferation of monomorphic small cells.

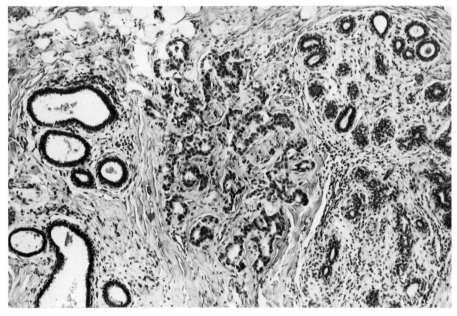

Fig. 7.**22** Cancerization of the lobules with extension of intraductal carcinoma into the lobules.

hitogenesis is also controversial (Fenoglio and Lattes 1974; Fisher et al. 1979; Linell 1980; Stegner et al. 1980). They could be seen in 4% to 16% of mammary biopsies. According to Linell et al. (1980) most, if not all, tubular carcinomas develop from radial scars. Sometimes they were found in combination with tubular carcinoma as well as with transitional stages between the two lesions (Fig. 7.**19**). Such observations point to the possibility of secondary malignant transformation of radial scars. In cytophotometric investigations, most radial scars are seen as benign lesions with normoploid distribution of the nuclear DNA (Stegner et al. 1980). Wide excision is accepted as adequate and sufficient therapy.

Intralobular Atypical Hyperplasia

In atypical hyperplasia in the lobular areas, the structure of the lobule is preserved and the number of terminal ducts is not generally increased. The epithelium of the terminal ducts is multilayered and the basal cells dominate (Fig. 7.**20**). Nuclei are hyperchromatic and irregularly placed. The cells lining the lumen are usually cylindrical. The differential diagnoses between lobular carinoma in situ and so-called lobular cancerization in conjunction with intraductal cancer has to be made. Criteria of lobular carcinoma in situ are the dilatation of the lobules filled by monomorphic cells (Fig. 7.**21**). Generally the cylindric secretory cells are missing.

Lobular cancerization is the centrifugal extension of an intraductal carcinoma into the lobular system. Typical are the large pleomorphic cells of ductal character (Fig. 7.**22**).

The different forms of atypical ductal and lobular epithelial hyperplasia are not specifically defined nor uniformly evaluated by pathologists. The question is open whether they are forms of florid benign hyperplasia or, in certain cases, a preneoplastic lesion.

A focal, doubtful finding at biopsy should always lead to careful sectioning of the entire specimen. In multifocal lesions, the increase or decrease in degrees of atypia seen in complementary sections could be helpful for diagnosis. Even for the most experienced there will be a gray zone of doubtful findings. The special technique of cell analysis, particularly DNA cytophotometry and immunocytology could be expected to offer further possibilities for diagnosis of borderline lesions and for evaluation of their prospective significance.

References

Azzopardi, J. G.: Problems in breast pathology. In Major Problems of Pathology, Vol. 11. W. B. Saunders Ltd., Philadelphia 1979

Bässler, R.: Pathologie der Brustdrüse. In Doerr, W., G. Seifert, E. Uehlinger: Spezielle Pathologische Anatomie Springer, Berlin, Heidelberg, New York 1978

Böhmig, R.: Mastopathia fibrosa cystica, ihre Epithelproliferationen und deren Beziehungen zum Carcinom. Erg. Allg. Pathol. 45: 39–116, 1964

Bonser, G. M., J. A. Dossett, J. W. Jull: Human and experimental breast cancer. Pitman Medical, London 1961

Davies, J. C.: Human colostrum cells: Their relation to periductal mononuclear inflammation. J. Pathol. 112: 153–160, 1974

Davis, H. H., M. Simons, J. B. Davis: Cystic disease of the breast: Relationship to carcinoma. Cancer 17: 957–978, 1964

DeWaard, F., E. A. Baanders-Van Halewijn, J. Huizinga: The bimodal age distribution of patients with mammary carcinoma: Evidence for the existence of two types of human breast cancer. Cancer 17: 141–151, 1964

Fenoglio, C., R. Lattes: Sclerosing papillary proliferations in the female breast. A benign lesion often mistaken for carcinoma. Cancer 33: 691–700, 1974

Fisher, E. R., A. S. Palekar, N. Kotwal, N. Lipana: A nonencapsulated sclerosing lesion of the breast. Am. J. Clin. Pathol. 71: 240–245, 1979

Haagensen, C. D.: Diseases of the Breast. W. B. Saunders, Philadelphia 1971

Hamperl, H.: Über fluoreszierende Mesenchymzellen (Fluorocyten). Leitz-Mitt. Wissensch. u. Technik 4: 243–246, 1960

Hamperl, H.: The myothelia (myoepithelial cells) normal state; regressive changes; hyperplasia; tumors. In Current Topics in Pathology. Springer, Berlin, Heidelberg, New York 1970

Hamperl, H.: Strahlige Narben und obliterierende Mastopathie, Beiträge zur pathologischen Histologie der Mamma. XI. Virchows Arch. Pathol. Anat. 369: 555–568, 1975

Jacobsen, O.: Heredity in breast cancer. A genetic and clinical study of two hundred probands. Nyt Nordisk Fortay Lewis Ltd., Copenhagen, London 1946

Kiaer, W.: Relation of fibroadenomatosis ("chronic mastitis") to cancer of the breast. Munksgaard, Copenhagen 1954

Linell, F., O. Ljungberg, I. Andersson: Breast carcinoma. Aspects of early stages, progression and related problems. Munksgaard, Copenhagen 1980

Marx, E., H. Schulz, R. Maecker: Klinische Bewertung der Epithelproliferationen in gutartigen Mammatumoren und Mastopathien. Bruns' Beitr. Klin. Chir. 217: 220–231, 1969

McFarland, J.: Residual lactation acini in the female breast. Their relation to chronic cystic mastitis and malignant disease. Arch. Surg. 5: 1–64, 1962

Möbius, G., H. Nizze: Mastopathia fibrosa cystica und Epithelproliferationen in weiblichen Brustdrüsen des Sectionsgutes. Frankfurter Z. Pathol. 75: 297–305, 1966

Page, D. L., R. V. Zwaag, L. W. Rogers, L. T. Williams, W. E. Walker, W. H. Hartmann: Relation between component parts of fibrocystic disease complex and breast cancer. J. Nat. Cancer Inst. 61: 1055–1063, 1978

Prechtel, K.: Beziehungen der Mastopathie zum Mammakarzinom. Fortschr. Med. 90: 43–45, 1972

Prechtel, K., H. Schmidt: Eine sechsjährige Verlaufsstudie bei Frauen mit bioptisch gesicherter Mastopathie. Verh. Dtsch. Ges. Pathol. 63: 609–612, 1979

Sattelmacher, P. G., G. Jürgens: Über die Altersabhängigkeit des Mammakarzinoms. Münch. Med. Wschr. 97: 1021–1023, 1955

Stegner, H.-E.: Screening beim Mammakarzinom? Dtsch. Med. Wschr. 104: 1655–1658, 1977

Stegner, H.-E., J. Bahnsen, B. Hinz: Cytophotometric analysis of nuclear DNA-content in so-called obliterating mastopathy with epithelial hyperproliferation. Pathol. Res. Pract. 170: 146–159, 1980

Theele, Ch., R. Bässler: Über Größenordnung, Formen und Varianten der Drüsenläppchen der Mamma. Pathologe 2: 208–219, 1981

Wellings, S. R., H. M. Jensen, R. G. Marcum: An atlas of subgross pathology of the human breast with special reference to possible precancerous lesions. J. Natl. Cancer Inst. 55: 231–273, 1975

Wiechern, E.: Matrixstrukturen beim Mammakarzinom. Eine korrelationspathologische Analyse von 2582 Mammabiopsien. Inaugural Dissertation Hamburg 1977

Chapter 8

Pathology of Malignant Diseases of the Breast

H.-E. Stegner

Pathogenesis of Breast Cancer

Development of breast cancer is biphasic in nature and progresses from intraepithelial stages to infiltrating carcinoma after various periods of latency.

Areas of predilection for developing cancers are the extralobular and intralobular terminal ducts (Fig. 8.1). On stimulation of the normal breast with mammotropic hormones, these parts of the ducts yield the most proliferative activity (Van Bogaert 1979). They are the roots for neogenesis of normal lobular structures. Most breast cancers are ductal or ductular in nature, with only a small fraction originating primarily in the acini. Opinions are contradictory concerning the initial stages in cancer formation. Histogenetically proposed possibilities are as follows: (1) the continuous development through primarily benign epithelial hyperplasia; (2) the development from atypical (pre-malignant) epithelial hyperplasia; and (3) the development de novo from a normal ductolobular epithelium.

According to Wellings et al. (1975), cancer formation is accomplished by gradual dedifferentiation of hyperplastic changes, but the authors fall short in their theory by failure to convincingly demonstrate any real continuity between the different stages of development. Similarly, Gallager and Martin (1969) are of the opinion that epithelial hyperplasias are the initial morphologically recognizable step in cancer development. Although lacking a precise or uniform definition, the preneoplastic hyperplasia can nonetheless be described as a "borderline lesion" falling somewhere between a benign, regularly proliferating hyperplasia of the diseased breast and a noninfiltrating carcinoma (ductal and lobular carcinoma in situ). The literature describes it as an atypical hyperplasia (Ashikari et al. 1974; Azzopardi 1979), or in some instances it falls within the melange of hyperplastic mastophathy (mastopathy grade 3: Prechtel 1971). Its rate of transformation to cancer is estimated to be 2% to 4%.

When comparing the total number of breast cancers, the development through pre-existent atypical hyperplasias becomes of secondary importance, but approximately one third of the manifest cancers show a coincidence with proliferative hyperplastic changes in breast tissue (Fig. 8.2). It is therefore likely that most breast cancers develop not by focal degeneration of hyperplastic lesions, but rather arise de novo from normal or morphologically "near normal" structures of the ductolobular unit whereby cells are made carcinogenic by some initiating factor. In keeping with this idea, it appears that the terminal duct segment demonstrates a hypersensitivity to certain carcinogens.

Carcinoma In Situ

Intraductal Carcinoma (DCIS)

Intraductal cancers are in situ growing cancers with solid, papillary, or cribriform differentiations. Due to segmental spreading or by synchronous dedifferentation, the lobules can be involved (so-called lobular cancerization). Should these tumors be in proximity of the nipple, cells can penetrate the epidermis of the nipple, a symptom of Paget's disease, which in most cases is the epidermal manifestation of a cancer localized deeper within the duct system.

Intraductal cancer mostly appears as a solid obstructively growing cancer that exhibits considerable degrees of both cellular and nuclear pleomorphism. It is the central portion of the tumor that undergoes necrosis and later degenerative calcification. These necrotic plugs become recognizable on the cut surface and have given the disease its name, comedocarcinoma (Fig. 8.3). The calcium precipitates, which can reach sizes greater than 1 mm (Hamperl 1968; Stegner et al. 1972; Stegner and Pape 1972), are not only a key mammographic indicator of the malignant process, but in the case of comedocarcinoma enhance the radiologic discovery of preinvasive cancer

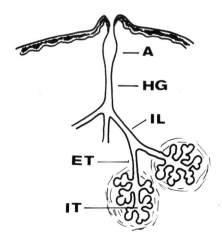

Fig. 8.1 Organization of the ductal-lobular system; HG, main duct; A, ampulla of main duct; IL, interlobular duct; ET, extralobular terminal duct; IT, intralobular terminal duct.

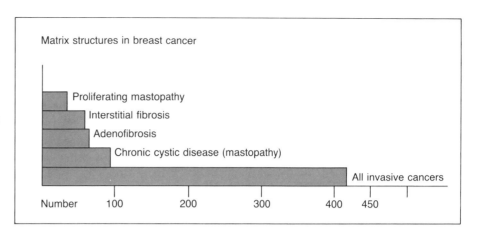

Fig. 8.**2**   Matrix structures in breast cancer. Of 416 investigated carcinomas 94 (22.6%) were observed in combination with chronic cystic disease (mastopathy) and 54 (13%) with adenofibrosis. Those with interstitial fibrosis composed 51 (12.3%) of all cases, and there were 25 (6%) cases combined with proliferating mastopathy. In the remaining cases, the parenchyma showed normal age-dependent structures.

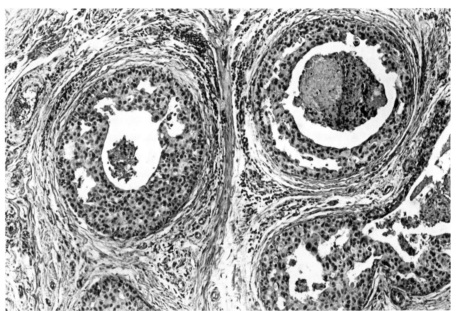

Fig. 8.**3**   Intraductal carcinoma of comedo type with accumulation of detritus in the lumen of the ducts, intact basement membrane, and periductal lymphoid cell infiltration.

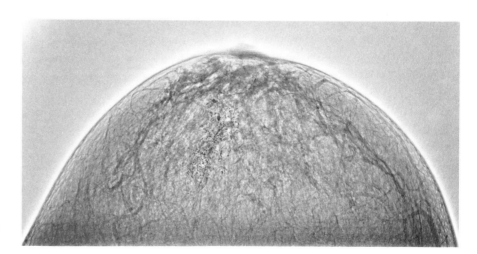

Fig. 8.**4**   Typical microcalcifications in the mammogram by intraductal carcinoma.

stages (Fig. 8.**4**) and are of greatest importance in early cancer diagnosis.

A variant of the intraductal comedocarcinoma is the clinging type described by Azzopardi (1971). In this type, the atypical epithelium forms only a peripheral layer of cancer cells, which form irregular, pseudopapillary processes and epithelial bars (so-called Roman bridges) (Fig. 8.**5**). Little or no detritus is found in the affected ducts. In intraductal carcinomas of a highly differentiated cribri-

form type, the degree of necrosis is small (Fig. 8.**6**). In the case of a classical comedocarcinoma, periductal lymphoid cell infiltration is frequently observed.

On ultramicroscopic investigation of the intraductal comedocarcinoma, a great variety in shape of the cancer cells is evident (Fig. 8.**7**). Polymorphic and coarsely heterochromatic nuclei with large nucleoli and cytoplasm rich with mitochondria, ergastoplasm, and Golgi structures are found. Striking characteristics of intraductal

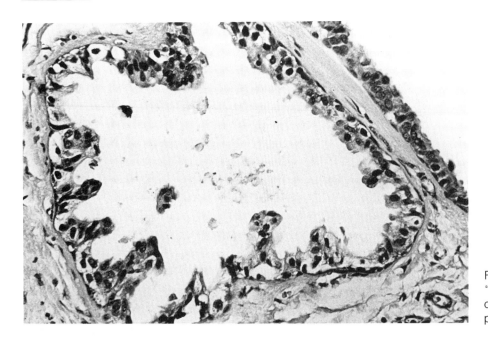

Fig. 8.**5** Intraductal carcinoma of the "clinging type." Ducts are lined with a layer of atypical cells that form stroma-free, pseudopapillary sprouts.

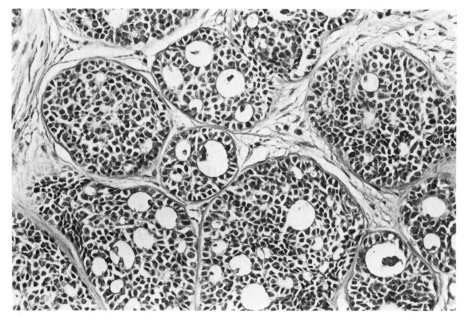

Fig. 8.**6** Intraductal carcinomas of the cribriform type. Intact basement membrane, and no evidence of necrosis.

carcinomas include dark and light cells (arising from the different amounts of organelles not unlike those found in invasive ductal cancer) and in highly differentiated types, secretory granules. Displaced myoepithelial cells can usually be found within the neoplastic epithelium and the unit of malignant cells can include non-neoplastic foam cells. The ducts are enclosed within a continuous or discontinuous basement membrane (Ozello 1971).

Intraductal carcinomas in situ (DCIS) constitute 3.3% to 5.6% of all breast cancers (Wulsin and Schreiber 1961; Kouchoukos et al. 1967; Farrow 1970; Silverberg and Chitale 1973; Westbrook and Gallager 1975; Carter and Smith 1977). Moreover, bilateral development is found in 10% to 31.9%. Contrary to earlier opinions, bilateral development of intraductal carcinoma is thus not less common than in lobular carcinoma in situ (CLIS).

The histological diagnosis of intraductal carcinoma requires serial sections of the biopsy material. However, it has to be kept in mind that it is always a tentative diagnosis since (1) the complete excision of the lesion is not guaranteed and (2) even with serial sections occult infiltration of the stroma cannot be ruled out. In 50 intraductal cancers, Gillis et al. (1960) were able to detect 14 cases of previously unrecognized stromal invasion after sectioning additional paraffin specimens. These findings explain that lymph node metastases were found in 1% to 4% of intraductal carcinomas without observed invasion. It is a theoretical speculation whether single tumor cells can penetrate a discontinuous basement membrane and ultimately cause lymphatic metastasis.

To refrain from radical therapy for intraductal carcinomas is justified because of the relatively low possibility of lymphatic and hematogenous spread. Gallager (1975) looks at intraductal carcinoma with no demonstrable stromal infiltration as "minimal" breast cancer. Simple mastectomy and removal of the proximal axillary lymph nodes is, however, the most common and adequate therapy. According to Fisher et al. (1978) and Lagios et

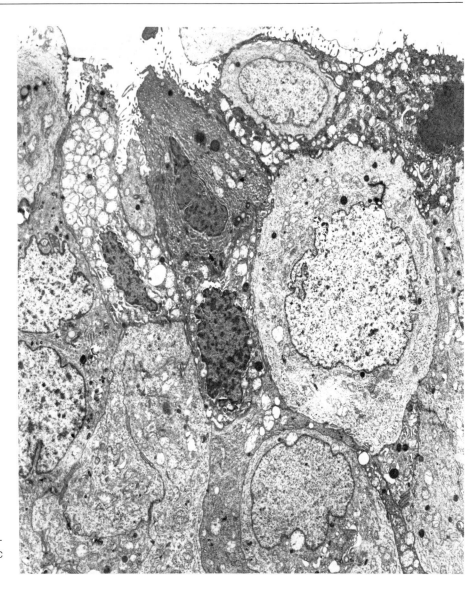

Fig. 8.**7** "Light" and "dark" cells of intraductal carcinoma. Electron microscopic magnification x 6500.

al. (1982), segmental resection under controlled clinical conditions may be justified in intraductal processes of less than 25 mm in extension. The responsiveness to radiation therapy of noninfiltrating ductal carcinomas has not yet been tested sufficiently.

Intralobular Carcinoma (LCIS)

Histologically, the LCIS is a proliferation of monomorphic cells within the lobules and the intralobular terminal ducts with distension of the acini (Fig. 8.**8**). These cells are small with relatively good contour. The round nuclei contain fine nucleoli. The incidence of mitosis is low. Haagensen (1971) divides the cases on the basis of cell types so that those with stronger cell polymorphy and less intensive cell cohesiveness are type B variety and those more uniform in nature are type A (Fig. 8.**9**A, B). Cytophotometric analysis of the nuclear DNA reveals that the monomorphic type generally displays a normal diploid distribution of DNA, whereas the histograms of the polymorphic type B exhibit the unimodal DNA pattern often found in infiltrating carcinomas (Sachs et al. 1976; Stegner 1977; Zippel and Citoler 1977). These cytophotometric differences might indicate possible variations in malignant potential. Ultramicroscopically,

the cells of the LCIS of type A correspond to indeterminate basal cells (Fig. 8.**10**). They contain only a sparse assortment of organelles, but also more highly differentiated types with intracytoplasmic vacuoles and fine cytoplasmic filaments could be seen. The cell complexes of the LCIS are surrounded by a continuous, electron microscopic basement lamella. The myothelium is retained (Fig. 8.**11**). In approximately 80% of all cases, the extralobular ducts are involved in the cell proliferation (Wheeler and Enterline 1976; Andersen 1977). In the classic case, the extralobular ducts are obliterated by the same uniform cell population as are the acini, but also mural, cribriform, and papillary variants of intraductal cell proliferates could be observed (Fechner 1972). Clover-leaf-like pattern is typical of the ducts involved (Fig. 8.**12**).

Unlike Bässler (1969) and Hamperl (1971), who assumed that a segmental spread of the LCIS occurred via appositional growth, Azzopardi (1979) proposed that the typical spread of the LCIS occurs by pagetoid spread; that is, via active penetration of the tumor cells between preexisting normal epithelial cells.

Clinically the LCIS is an asymptomatic, nonpalpable, and frequently multicentric neoplasia with a high specificity

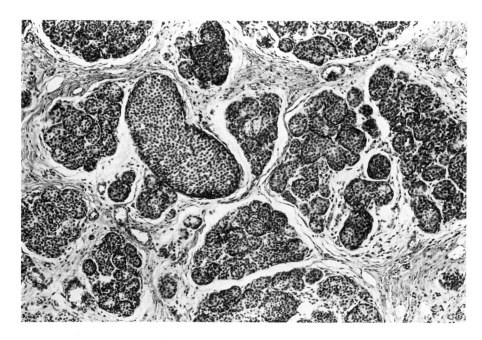

Fig. 8.**8** Lobular carcinoma in situ (LCIS), monomorphic type.

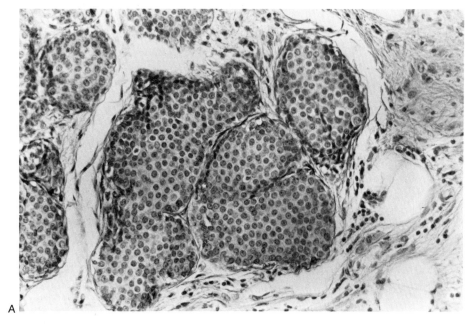

A

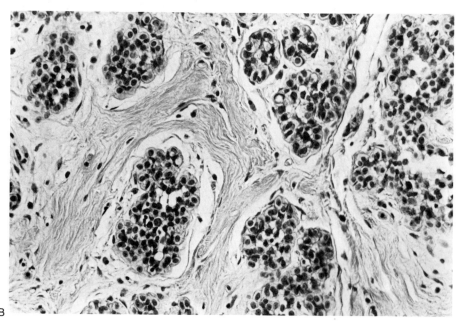

B

Fig. 8.**9** A: Lobular carcinoma in situ (LCIS), monomorphic type (Type A).
B: Polymorphic type (Type B); poor cell cohesiveness. Intact lumina of the terminal ducts, partly pagetoid cellular character.

for women of premenopausal age. Since it is nonpalpable in nature, it is almost always detected incidentally in biopsy material taken for some other reason. Microcalcifications in adjacent areas of proliferating mastopathy may serve as indirect criteria. Actual calcifications within the LCIS foci are seldom seen. Although statistics pertaining to the incidence of the LCIS in the normal population are unavailable, it is known that approximately 70% of all cases are multicentric in the same breast, 30% occur bilaterally (Table 8.1), and the incidence in breast biopsy material is 0.8% to 1.5%.

From circumstantial evidence, it is clear that the LCIS plays an important role in the development of breast cancer. It is found as an accompanying component of most types of infiltrating breast cancers but mostly in combination with small cell carcinomas (Fig. 8.13). A histogenetic connection could be drawn between the LCIS and these solid carcinomas, which were previously referred to as carcinoma solidum simplex, but are currently classified as infiltrating lobular carcinoma. Direct transformation of the LCIS into an infiltrating carcinoma has been seen occasionally in the form of microglandular extensions or through monocellular dispersions (Fig. 8.14). The time of latency for transformation into invasive carcinoma is rather long. More specifically, in approximately 25% of all cases of biopsy-identified LCIS not subjected to ablative therapy, breast cancer developed in the same breast within an observation period of 5 to 25 years (McDivitt et al. 1969). Moreover, of 172 patients observed by Andersen (1977), 26 (15%) developed an ipsilateral invasive carcinoma, whereas 19 (11%) developed contralateral invasive carcinoma over a median observation period of ten years. According to Wheeler and Enterline (1976), the likelihood for cancer formation in patients with LCIS is 2 to 4 times greater

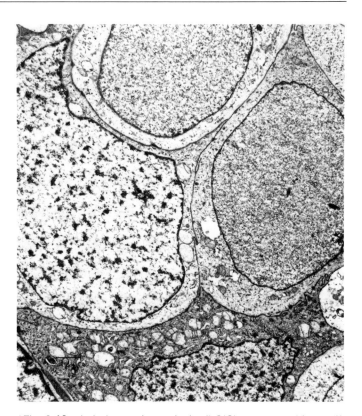

1Fig. 8.10   Lobular carcinoma it situ (LCIS) monomorphic, undifferentiated type. (Electron microscopic magnification x 10,000.)

Table 8.1   Frequency of multicentric and bilateral foci of LCIS

Reference	Multicentric (residual foci)	Bilateral
Antonius and Jones (1963)	83%	9%
Benfield et al. (1965)	80%	40%
Newmann (1966)	86%	23%
McDivitt et al. (1967)	70%	30%
Urban (1967)		35%
Farrow (1968)	63%	52%
Lewison and Finney (1968)	62%	46%
Hutter and Foote (1969)		29%
Warner (1969)	70%	15%
Haagensen (1971)		25%
Kaufmann et al. (1971)	66%	13%
Donegan and Perez-Mesa (1972)		26%
Andersen (1974)	59%	32%
Gaton and Czernobilsky (1974)		23%
Wheeler et al. (1974)	84%	
Dall'Olmmo et al. (1975)	58%	21%
Total	71%	28%

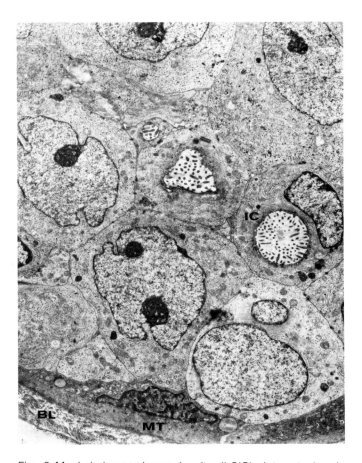

Fig. 8.11   Lobular carcinoma in situ (LCIS). Intracytoplasmic canaliculi (IC), myothelial cells (MT), and basement lamella (BL). Electron microscopic magnification x⁻7500.

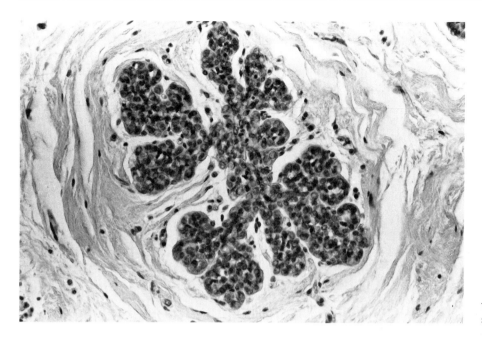

Fig. 8.**12** LCIS spreading to the ductal system. "Clover-leaf-like" figure of duct cross section.

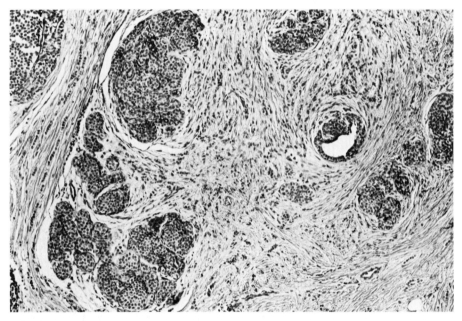

Fig. 8.**13** Lobular carcinoma in situ (LCIS) in combination with infiltrating lobular carcinoma.

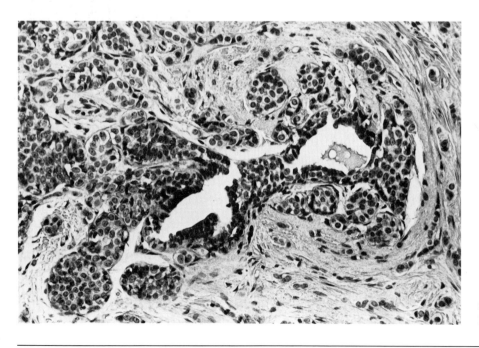

Fig. 8.**14** Lobular carcinoma. Pagetoid spreading to extralobular duct, with stromal infiltration.

than in the normal population. An accurate prognosis for the individual patient's cancer risk cannot possibly be made. Figures given are based on a group prognosis and that is why there is no standard therapy. The therapeutic spectrum ranges from diagnostic procedures only to bilateral mastectomy. Intense follow-up using all modern facilities should be chosen only after careful consideration has been given to the individual characteristics of the patients such as age, endocrine status, family cancer history, and possibility for consequent follow-up.

Early Carcinoma (Minimal Breast Cancer)

To the pathologist and the clinician, the term "early cancer" has different meanings. The pathologist, basically interested in the histogenesis of carcinoma, evaluates the histologically defined changes and distinguishes atypical hyperplasia of precancerous significance from cancerous epithelium without stromal infiltration (carcinoma in situ). He classifies cases with discrete microscopic signs of stromal infiltration as early invasive carcinoma.

The histogenetic concept, however, is purely theoretical and of limited value in the clinical area. One of the primary concerns of the clinician is to know whether the cancer has already started to spread or if the likelihood of spread is negligible. It was with this in mind that Westbrook and Gallager (1975) suggested the term "minimal cancer" to include all noninvasive ductal or lobular carcinomas and invasive carcinomas up to the size of 0.5 cm in diameter. Thus, the term "minimal cancer" deals not with cancers showing similarities in early developmental stages, but rather with nonmetastatic cancers. The size of 0.5 cm has proven to be the threshold to metastatic spread. Thirty four percent of tumors with a diameter of 0.6 to 1.0 cm can be expected to involve lymph node metastasis with the percentage increasing to 40% to 60% with tumors up to 2 cm in diameter (Huhn and Stock 1977; Zippel 1979).

Early stages of breast cancer represent so far only a small fraction of the average clinical material. In larger treatment centers, the relative number of stage I tumors is approximately 10% to 25%, and according to the American College of Surgeons, minimal carcinoma (as defined above) constitutes approximately 9.1% of primary breast cancer (Beduani et al. 1981). They are mostly clinically occult and have been diagnosed through mammography. The adequate therapy of minimal breast cancer is a subject for discussion. Different modalities for breast-preserving surgery in these cases are evaluated in controlled clinical trials. The pathologist is requested to refine his judgment to a degree that far exceeds the decision between benign and malignant. For selective therapy, many parameters have to be considered such as type of tumor, size, contour, histological grading, and degree of differentiation (Thomsen et al. 1980).

Tumor Growth

Tumor Border

The configuration of the tumor border often gives an indication of the histology of the carcinoma. The following main types can be distinguished:

1. Carcinomas with starlike extensions (scirrhous, irregular carcinoma, stellate carcinoma). This category includes the majority of fibrosing, infiltrating ductal carcinomas, as well as certain infiltrating lobular carcinomas. The cut surface macroscopically clearly reveals a fibrous, gray-yellow center and star-like extensions. They form distinct, isolated foci in the fat-rich, age-atrophic, mammographically "empty" breast. In the parenchyma-rich breast, they are often eccentrically located at the margin of the glandular parenchyma (Fig. 8.**15**).

2. Circumscribed multinodular carcinomas (convoluted type). These rare types of carcinomas are composed of several nodular subunits that together form a relatively smooth outer contour, except for some minor loss of clarity in mammograms due to fine, connective tissue extensions. Histologically they mostly are infiltrating ductal carcinomas, but also medullary carcinomas belong to this group.

3. Rounded nodular carcinomas. These carcinomas consist of a single nodular structure that contrasts sharply with the surrounding tissue (Fig. 8.**16**). The rare mucinous carcinomas and medullary cancers with lymphoid stroma also show this sharp demarcation.

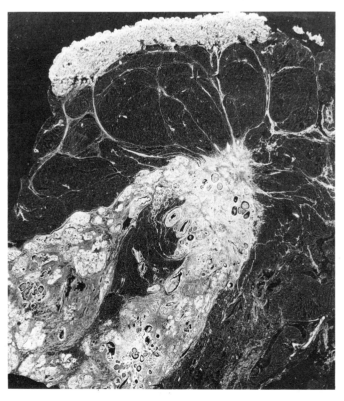

Fig. 8.**15** Scirrhous carcinoma occurring eccentrically in the parenchyma. Cooper's ligaments are easily distinguished. Contact copy of histological section.

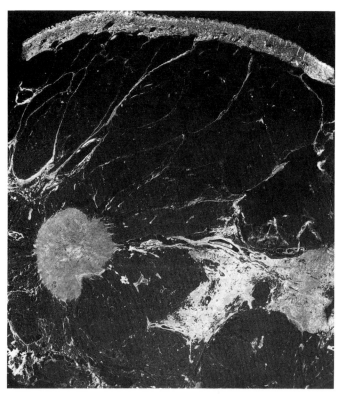

Fig. 8.**16** Round, nodular carcinoma. Contact copy of histological section.

Central necrosis and liquefaction of the parenchyma-rich medullary cancer could clinically and mammographically give the impression of a cyst.

4. Intracystic carcinomas. Although papillary carcinomas can cause multicystic tumors through secretion and bleeding, cancer development within pre-existing cysts is extremely rare (Fig. 8.**17**).

5. Diffuse carcinomas. Diffuse carcinomas cause the entire breast, or a large portion of it, to become indurated with no circumscribed tumor mass detectable either clinically or mammographically. Such diffuse propagation is seen in the inflammatory carcinomas and sometimes in the infiltrating lobular carcinomas. As a rule these are rapidly growing tumors with early dissemination. The rapid progression of intramammary metastasis covers the often small primary tumor.

In keeping with the previous clinical belief that both the shape of growth and outer demarcation of the carcinoma are accurate prognostic tools, Gallager (1974) found that tumors with a star-like structure up to a size of 5 cm were associated with a five-year survival rate of 71%, whereas similar-sized tumors of a nodular configuration yielded a five-year survival rate of 58%.

Reaction of Surrounding Tissue

As fibrous tissue is often the shape-giving component associated with breast cancer, it is not surprising that the term "scirrhous" cancer is often used as the prototype for all breast cancers, since the word scirrhous denotes tumor with overgrowth of fibrous tissue. These fibers develop from fibroblasts and myogenic cells, but there is both light and electron microscopic evidence that tumor cells are intimately involved in fiber formation (Hamperl 1970; Shivas and Douglas 1972; Stegner and Maass 1973; Douglas and Shivas 1974; Al-Adnani et al. 1975).

Elastic and collagen fibers are constituents of the ductal system. A significant increase in periductal collagen and elastic fibers is formed in the majority of infiltrating ductal carcinomas, although a similar increase is also reported in benign proliferative, hyperplastic processes. Several investigators view the periductal enhancement of elastoid hyalin as an indirect criterion for potential malignancy of the lesion (Jackson and Orr 1957; Fenoglio and Lattes 1974). Bernath (1952) as well as Sümegi and Rajka (1972) found that on staining with congo red, methylviolet and Lugol's solution, elastoid hyalin exhibited histochemically amyloid-like reactions. Since the classic amyloid contains immunoglobulins, these investigators link the amyloid-like substance in the breast tumors to local immune reactions. However, the positive staining reactions are probably due to tissue elastin.

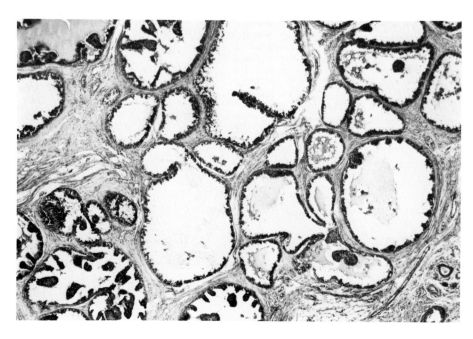

Fig. 8.**17** Intraductal, papillary carcinoma with cystic ectasia of the ducts.

Reactive fibroblastic proliferation and fibrosclerosis are a characteristic concurrent phenomenon seen in benign pseudoinfiltration. In cases of a preinvasive carcinoma of the breast, focal fibroelastosis may be a harbinger of malignant stromal infiltration. Bonser et al. (1961) and Azzopardi and Laurini (1974) suggest that fibroid elastosis is a nonspecific mesenchymal reaction occurring in both malignant and benign breast proliferative processes.

Cellular Infiltration

Infiltration from mononuclear cells in the periphery of the breast cancer is regarded as indicator of immunological defence (Moore and Foote 1949; Hamlin 1968; Berg 1971). Some invasion of the periphery of the tumor by lymphocytes and plasma cells is found in any type of tumor and in three fourths of all breast cancers. As a single parameter, lymphoid cell infiltration has no prognostic importance. Only the dense lymphoid infiltrates seen with the classic medullary carcinoma have any prognostic significance since in these tumors a significantly higher survival rate is found as compared with the ordinary ductal carcinomas. In clinical pathologic analysis, infiltration of lymphocytes did not demonstrate any positive correlation to survival time, but significant correlation was seen between the degree of lymphoid infiltration and the age of the patient, tumor size, and the degree of malignancy (Fisher et al. 1975).

Calcifications

As calcium deposits are commonly found in all types of tumors, it is not surprising that deposits of calcium crystaloids in the parenchyma and stroma are of great importance in mammographic diagnosis of breast cancer. Such calcium deposits are most frequently found in the cell detritus of both intraductal and infiltrating comedocarcinoma and more often in highly differentiated tubular and stroma-rich carcinomas than in poorly differentiated and stroma-poor carcinomas. Calcifications are never observed in medullary and rarely in lobular carcinomas. The size of these calcifications is 10 to 500 μm with aggregates reaching a size of more than 1500 μm. For the radiologist, irregular particle size, focal-shaped arrangement, and bizarre shapes arouse suspicion of possible malignancy. In benign lesions of the mammary parenchyma (particularly in fibrocystic disease and in scleradenosis), the calcium particles are usually even, relatively round (psammoma bodies), and more evenly distributed. In electron microscopy it is found that viable tumor cells excrete fine calcium particles (Stegner and Pape 1972) Fig. 8.18). Ahmed (1975) describes needle-like calcium crystals (hydroxyapatite) in intracytoplasmic vesicles. Following complete degeneration of these secretory cells, coarse cellular calcifications can be found free in the stroma. Extracellular calcification without connections to tumor cells are found in interstitial elastosis.

Lymphatic Spread

Histologic diagnosis of lymphatic spread can be made after identification of endothelium-lined lymphatic vessels (lacking elastic muscular wall structures) containing free cancer cells or cell complexes (tumor cell emboli) (Fig. 8.19). Although it appears that investigators have been unable to find significant correlations of prognostic value, Fisher et al. (1975) found lymphatic spread to be correlated to increased recurrence rate especially in large tumors with poor demarcation and a high degree of malignancy. Other authors were not able to find any significant correlation to the clinical course. The frequency in which lymphatic spread is found depends on the accuracy of the histologic interpretation. Misinterpretations are possible. Lymphatic dissemination of the tumor cell is dependent on the localization and aggressiveness of the tumor. The richly branched and ectatic subareolar lymphatic plexus offers good possibilities for spread. According to Citoler and Zippel (1974), 86% of all cases of breast cancer involving the subareolar region exhibit axillary lymph node metastasis regardless of tumor type and size.

Connections to the Skin

Parenchyma-rich, sharply contoured, nodular tumors, such as the mucinous carcinomas and medullary carcinomas, can bulge the cutis if in proximity to the skin. In contrast, the strongly fibrosing (scirrhous) cancers can cause retraction in the surrounding tissue through shrinkage of the stromal center, and even the smallest, subcu-

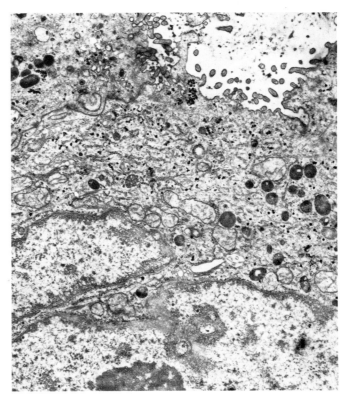

Fig. 8.**18** Intracytoplasmic and secreted calcium particles in cells of an intraductal comedo carcinoma. (Electron microscopic magnification x 10,800.)

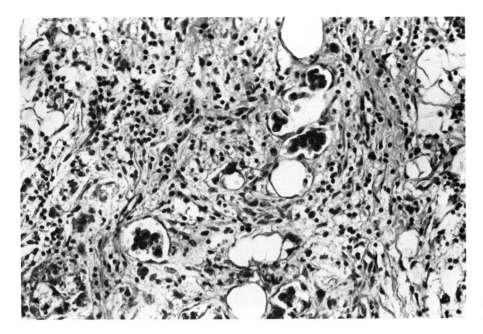

Fig. 8.**19** Lymphatic spread with tumor cell emboli in ectatic lymph vessels.

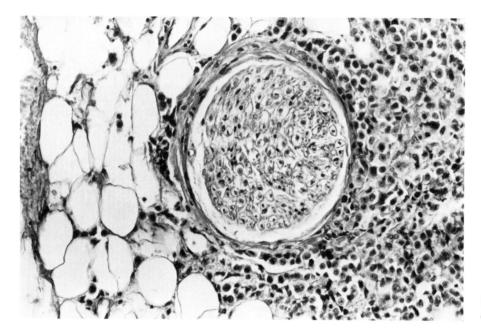

Fig. 8.**20** Perineural invasion of cancer cells.

taneously located scirrhous tumor can produce changes in the neighboring cutis through contraction of Cooper's ligaments (Fig. 8.**15**). When the breast skin contracts, the tension of the retinaculum increases thus causing the "plateau phenomenon" (Jackson and Severance 1944).

When deeply situated lymph vessels become blocked, the subsequent reduction of lymph flow causes localized skin edema in which the hair follicle openings appear like wide pores (peau d'orange). It is important to distinguish between the different subcuticular fixation phenomena of tumors growing close to the skin and the tumors that directly infiltrate the skin. Cancers massively infiltrating the corium initially cause an epidermal atrophy by pressure before penetrating the basement membrane and finally ulcerating. Tumor cells penetrating the epidermis from the stroma fail to show the pagetoid transformation characteristic of an intraepidermal spread.

Neural and Vascular Invasion

Neural infiltration was for a long time regarded as proof of the malignant nature of an epithelial growth (Fig. 8.**20**). Numerous investigations have, however, revealed infiltration of nerve sheets even from benign hyperplastic processes, as is certainly the case with infiltrating epitheliosis (Taylor and Norris 1967; Davies 1973; Azzopardi 1979).

Although neural invasion from malignant tumor is of little significance in prognosis, vascular invasion is a direct proof of hematogenic dissemination. Vascular infiltration is generally regarded as a bad sign even though as an indicator of poor prognosis it is more questionable. Moreover, with a frequency of 4.7% to 46%, vascular invasion lends itself to considerable misdiagnosis (Friedell et al. 1965; Fisher et al. 1975). Tumor cell complexes lying within tissue spaces are sometimes mistaken for vascular invasion. Additional staining (elastica-fibrin stain, phosphatase reaction) could be of diagnostic help. Fisher et al. (1975) did not find that vascular invasion influenced the clinical course. Teel and Sommers (1964) and Friedell et al. (1965) suggest a significantly poorer five-year survival rate in patients with vascular invasion independent of nodal status. Kister (1960), however, reported a significantly poorer ten-year survival rate only for patients who also had lymph node metastases.

Clinical Stages

The most widely accepted method for clinical staging has been developed by the Union Internationale Contre le Cancer (UICC), and is now used instead of previous staging systems (Table 8.2). Three parameters must be considered before surgery, namely, tumor (T), nodes (N), and metastases (M). Tumor size is determined through clinical examination or on the basis of mammographic image. The method used for measurement of tumor size must always be given. Not included in the TNM system are the location and the histologic degree of malignancy (grading). Regional lymph nodes are the palpable axillary, supraclavicular, and infraclavicular lymph nodes. Distant metastases are all the clinical and laboratory detected metastases including carcinomatous skin infiltration outside the breast area.

The merits of the TNM system include its simplicity, its clearness, and its adaptability to other neoplastic disease. The main disadvantage is the uncertainty in clinical diagnostic evaluation. The probability of error is 30% to 50% by palpation of regional lymph nodes. It appears that palpation is also not particularly dependable in determining the size of primary tumors. In contrast, mammographic measurement of tumor size coincides well with its histopathologically determined size.

The pretherapeutic clinical classification of the TNM system can be augmented by the postoperative histopathologic classification (pTNM) (Table 8.3). The exact size of the primary tumor can be measured on the histologic slides. In addition, lymph nodes are distinguished as micrometastases (less than 0.2 cm) and macrometastases (greater than 0.2 cm).

Table 8.2 Clinical staging of breast tumors (ICD-0 174), in accordance with TNM system

T — Primary tumor

Tis — Preinvasive carcinoma (carcinoma in situ), non infiltrating carcinoma or Paget's disease of the breast with no detectable tumor. Remarks: Paget's disease in combination with a detectable tumor is classified according to the size of the tumor

T0 — No evidence of a primary tumor

T1 — Tumor in its largest extension measures 2 cm or less
T1a, Without fixation to the underlying pectoral fascia and/or muscle
T1b, With fixation to the underlying pectoral fascia and/or muscle

T2 — Tumor in its largest extension measures more than 2 cm, but less than 5 cm
T2a, Without fixation to the underlying pectoral fascia and/or muscle
T2b, With fixation to the underlying pectoral fascia and/or muscle

T3 — Tumor measures more than 5 cm in its largest extension
T3a, Without fixation to the underlying pectoral fascia and/or muscle
T3b, With fixation to the underlying pectoral fascia and/or muscle
Remarks: Retractions of the skin or nipple or skin changes (other than those listed under T4b) can occur in T1, T2, or T3 without influence of the TNM classification

T4 — Tumors of all sizes with infiltration to the breast wall or skin
Remarks: Breast wall includes the ribs, intercostal muscles, and anterior seratus muscle, but not the pectoral musculature
T4a, Fixation to the breast wall
T4b, With arm edema, infiltration, or ulceration of the skin (including peau d'orange) or with skin nodes of the same breast
T4c, Both T4a and T4b

TX — The minimal requirements for the determination of mammary tumor do not exist
Remarks: Carcinomas with accompanying inflammation should be listed in a separate group

N — Regional lymph nodes

N0 — No palpable, homolateral, axillary lymph nodes

N1 — Movable, homolateral axillary lymph nodes
N1a, The lymph nodes are considered not affected
N1b, The lymph nodes are considered affected

N2 — Homolateral axillary lymph nodes with fixation internodulary or to the surroundings and considered affected

N3 — Homolateral, supraclavicular or infraclavicular lymph nodes that are considered affected, or an existing arm edema.
Remarks: The arm edema can be caused by interference of lymph drainage. Lymph nodes must not be palpable

NX — The requirement for classification of regional lymph nodes does not exist

M — Distant metastases

M0 — No evidence of distant metastases

M1 — Distant metastases are present

MX — The requirements for the detection of distant metastases do not exist

Classification

The classifications of breast cancers are based on a combination of morphologic, prognostic, and fine-structural parameters. With new findings come continuous changes and new definitions, although it is not an easy task to replace deeply ingrained definitions with current nomenclature. New information makes changes and new formulations necessary. Clarity and clinical applications are the goal of any classification, with the majority of most recent classifications resting on histogenetical principles (Table 8.**4**). Subclassification within the main categories of ductal and lobular carcinomas does not describe differences in topography, but rather differences in tumor differentiation. Although lobular carcinomas might be ductal in origin, the differentiation of cancer cells occurs within the functional-morphological specialization of the lobules.

Table 8.**3** Postsurgical histopathological staging (pTNM)

pT	Primary tumor
pTis	Preinvasive carcinoma (carcinoma in situ)
pT0	No evidence for primary tumor by histologic examination of resected material
pT1a,	Correspond to T1a, T1b, and are classified as: (1) tumor measures 0.5 cm or less (2) tumor measures more than 0.5 cm, but less than 1 cm (3) tumor measures more than 1 cm, but less than 2 cm
pT2a,	Correspond to T2a, T2b
pT3a,	Correspond to T3a, T3b
pT4a,	Correspond to T4a, T4b, T4c
pTx	The extent of the invasion cannot be determined
G	Histopathologic grading
G1	High degree of differentiation
G2	Moderate degree of differentiation
GX	Degree of differentiation cannot be determined
pN	Regional lymph nodes
pN0	No evidence of invasion of regional lymph nodes
pN1	Movable, homolateral axillary lymph nodes pN1a, Micrometastasis of 0.2 cm or less, in one or more nodes pN1b, Macrometastasis in one or more lymph nodes (1) Metastasis larger than 0.2 cm in one to three nodes (smaller than 2 cm) (2) Metastasis larger than 0.2 cm in four or more nodes (smaller than 2 cm) (3) Metastases with extracapsular growth (4) Positive lymph nodes, 2 cm or larger
pN2	Involvement of the homolateral axillary lymph nodes that are fixed among themselves or to neighboring structures
pN3	Involvement of the homolateral, supraclavicular, or infraclavicular lymph nodes Remarks: Homolateral nodes along the thoracic duct can be included in the pN3 category
pNX	Extent of invasion cannot be determined
pM	Distant metastases The pM category corresponds to the M categories

Table 8.**4** Histologic classification of breast tumours (WHO 1981)

I. Epithelial tumours

A. Benign
　1. Intraductal papilloma
　2. Adenoma of the nipple
　3. Adenoma
　　a. Tubular
　　b. Lacting
　4. Others

B. Malignant
　1. Noninvasive
　　a. Intraductal carcinoma
　　b. Lobular carcinoma in situ
　2. Invasive
　　a. Invasive ductal carcinoma
　　b. Invasive ductal carcinoma with a predominant intraductal component
　　c. Invasive lobular carcinoma
　　d. Mucinous carcinoma
　　e. Medullary carcinoma
　　f. Papillary carcinoma
　　g. Tubular carcinoma
　　h. Adenoid cystic carcinoma
　　i. Secretory [juvenile] carcinoma
　　j. Apocrine carcinoma
　　k. Carcinoma with metaplasia
　　　– squamous type
　　　– spindle-cell type
　　　– cartilaginous and osseous type
　　　– mixed type
　　l. Others
　3. Paget's disease of the nipple

II. Mixed connective tissue and epithelial tumours

A. Fibroadenoma

B. Phyllodes tumour [cystosarcoma phyllodes]

C. Carcinosarcoma

III. Miscellaneous tumours

a. Soft tissue tumours

B. Skin tumours

C. Tumours of haematopoietic and lymphoid tissues

IV. Unclassified tumours

V. Mammary dysplasia/fibrocystic disease

VI. Tumour-like lesions

A. Duct ectasia

B. Inflammatory pseudotumours

C. Hamartoma

D. Gynaecomastia

E. Others

Differentiation dictates the biological behavior of growth. Within certain limits, the endocrine regulatory system of the host becomes involved. Highly differentiated breast cancers develop specific hormonal receptors that make the tumors sensitive to endocrine therapy.

Thus, it appears that subclassification based on functionally specific structures (i. e., structural proteins, receptor proteins, specific secretions) will play an increasingly larger role in future modes of breast cancer therapy.

Histological Types

Infiltrating Ductal Carcinoma

Although the precursor of most infiltrating ductal carcinomas is probably intraductal in nature, the classification of breast cancer as an infiltrating, ductal carcinoma is independent of any concurrent intraductal component, although the latter could influence therapeutic modality and should be noted. Infiltrating ductal carcinoma with specific intraductal components are subclassified on the basis of these structural components (e. g., infiltrating comedocarcinoma, infiltrating papillary, or cribriform carcinoma).

Infiltrating ductal carcinomas without special differentiation (NOS, not otherwise specified) constitute approximately 80% of all breast cancers and histologically show a solid or glandular growth pattern with differing degrees of fibrosis (Fig. 8.**21**). Characteristic of the parenchyma-rich tumors is their relatively well-contoured, multinodular growth patterns, whereas the more fibrous (scirrhous) tumors exhibit irregular, star-like growth patterns with fine extensions of connective tissue (spicules). The center of the tumor may be composed completely of sclerotic collagen.

Medullary Carcinoma

Medullary carcinomas are parenchyma-rich tumors of "marrow-like" consistency with little stroma. Microscopically, these carcinomas appear as solid complexes or wide anastomotic cords of pleomorphic tumor cells. The tumor periphery is composed of dense infiltrates of mononuclear cells (lymphocytes and plasma cells). In larger tumors, necrosis and hemorrhage are often noted. Clinically and mammographically, centrally necrotic tumors can be mistaken for cysts. Medullary tumor cells are large and irregular, with hyperchromatic nuclei of bizarre shape and sometimes vesicular appearance (Fig. 8.**22**). Oddly enough, the high degree of wild cellular plemorphism and the great number of mitoses is in direct contrast to the low rate of metastasis and recurrences. Two thirds of the tumors fall within the group of grade III tumors, with the five-year survival rates ranging from 69% to 82.7% (Moore and Foote 1949; Richardson 1956; McDivitt et al. 1968). Such favorable survival rates differ greatly from those expected with common, infiltrating ductal carcinomas, although this difference becomes less pronounced after ten years (Schwartz 1969; Haagensen 1971; Flores et al. 1974). Ridolfi et al. (1977), adhering strictly to type-specific criteria, note a ten-year survival rate of 84%.

Infiltrating Lobular Carcinoma

The classic infiltrating, lobular carcinoma is a strongly fibrosing, small-cell tumor that growths in solid strings rather than clusters or with dispersion of cells. The overall small tumor cells of both primary tumor and metastasis may resemble the structure of a reticulum cell sarcoma (Fig. 8.**23**). The individual cell pleomorphism is insignificant. The tumor cells are mostly arranged in linear threads (Indian-file pattern) or surround the small ducts concentrically (target-pattern) (Fig. 8.**24**).

Variations of the infiltrating lobular carcinomas are the signet-ring type (Fig. 8.**25**), the tubuloalveolar type (Fisher 1973), and the alveolar type (Martinez and Azzopardi 1979) (Fig. 8.**26**).

Immunohistologic uncovering of function-specific structures results in an even larger variety of lobular cancers. Cytoplasmic vacuoles that give a positive reaction with Alcian blue PAS stain correspond ultramicroscopically with intracytoplasmic ductules (Eusebi et al. 1977; Steg-

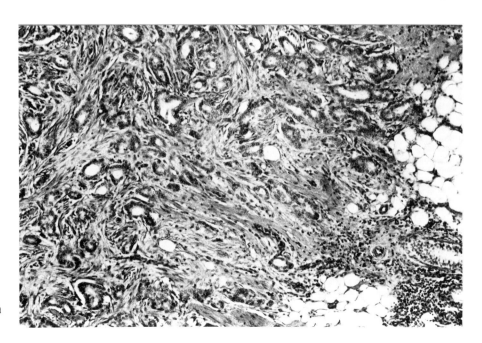

Fig. 8.**21** Infiltrating, ductal carcinoma (NOS) with solid and glandular formations.

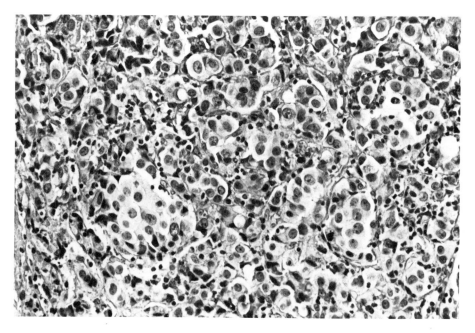

Fig. 8.22 Highly cellular pleomorphism in medullary carcinoma with lymphocytic infiltration).

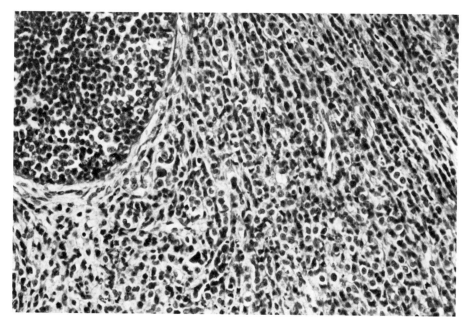

Fig. 8.23 Lobular carcinoma in situ (LCIS) in combination with infiltrating lobular carcinoma. Richness in cells and small cellular character could lead to a misdiagnosis of a lymphoreticular tumor.

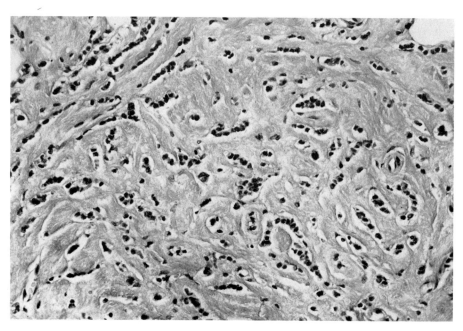

Fig. 8.24 Infiltrating lobular carcinoma. Relatively small tumor cells are arranged partially in an Indian-file pattern or dispersed in fibrous stroma.

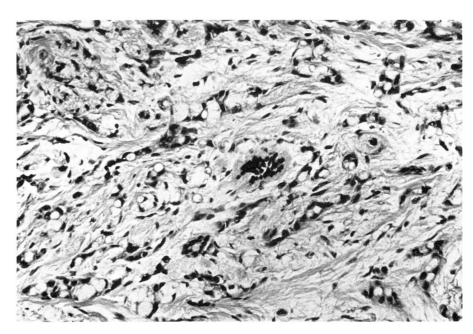

Fig. 8.**25** Signet ring cell type of an infiltrating, lobular carcinoma.

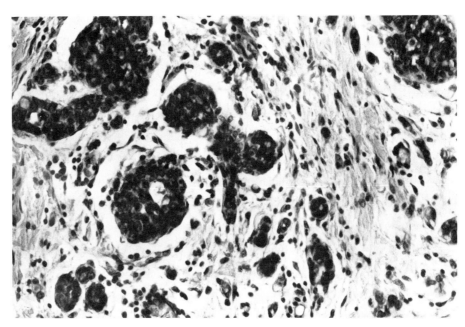

Fig. 8.**26** Infiltrating lobular carcinoma. Alveolar (microglandular) type.

ner et al. 1981) (Fig. 8.**27**). It is in this aspect that they differ from the mucous vacuoles present in colloid carcinomas. Casein, lectin receptors, and T-antigens can be detected on the membranes of the vacuoles via immunofluorescence and peroxidase-antiperoxidase technique (Klein et al. 1981; Stegner et al. 1981) (Fig. 8.**28**). Such data suggest the abortive synthesis of cell-specific secretions (milk proteins). Myoepithelial differentiation is suggested by the richness in cytofilaments, and unusually high activities of ATPase and ADPase (Scarpelli and Murat 1973).

Classification of an infiltrating, lobular carcinoma is independent of the absence or presence of an in situ component, and its frequency ranges from 3.7% to 5.8% (Bässler 1978).

Mucinous Carcinoma

Mucinous carcinomas (colloid carcinomas) are glandular-papillary or glandular-cystic growing tumors of a high degree of maturity. The mucinous secretion formed by the tumor is composed of neutral or weakly sulfated mucopolysaccharides and is retained within the glandular structures. Large "mucus lakes" often form that contain shed tumor cells as well as psammoma bodies (Fig. 8.**29**).

Examination of the ultrastructure reveals a well-ordered arrangement of tumor cells. The cytoplasm contains the structures necessary for mucin production (large Golgi apparatus, ergastoplasm, glycogen). Numerous desmosomes and membrane interdigitations form an impressive intercellular network (Fig. 8.**30**). The tumors have mostly a smooth border. The growth form is clinically mistaken for benign tumors (e. g., fibroadenoma). Mucinous carcinomas are regarded as prognostically favorable. They exhibit a long duration of symptoms and regional metas-

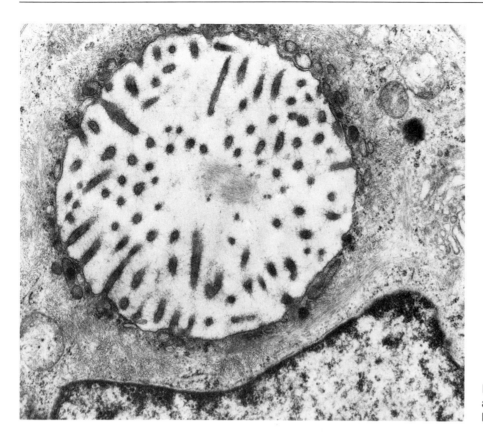

Fig. 8.**27** Intracytoplasmic vacuole – characteristic of breast cancer cells, especially in lobular carcinomas.

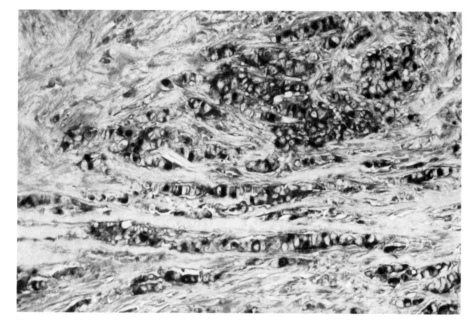

Fig. 8.**28** Demonstration of T-antigen (Thomsen-Friedenreich) in the cells of an infiltrating lobular carcinoma with the PAP method (from Stegner et al. 1981).

tases are seen less frequently than in other types of infiltrating breast cancers. The percentage of "pure" mucinous carcinomas is 1% to 2% of all breast cancers, and are usually found in older women (culmination at age 60). Mixed forms are common and prognostically less favorable, with recurrence and metastasis rates four times greater than for "pure" mucinous cancers (Haagensen 1971). For therapeutic and prognostic reasons, tumors with relatively small mucin-forming regions should be classified in accordance with the major structural components to which they are linked (Azzopardi 1979).

Tubular Carcinoma

The most highly differentiated of all the breast cancers are the tubular carcinomas. The irregularly extending tubules are embedded in fibrous stroma and formed by a one-layered epithelium. They have wide lumens (open glands). There is no myoepithelial layer. The cell polymorphism is poor. The cytoplasm is eosinophilic and mitosis is rare. Apocrine secretion can be seen. The stroma is rich in elastoid material. In two thirds of all cases of tubular carcinoma, concurrent components of intraductal carcinomas with papillary or cribriform patterns are observed (Fig. 8.**31**).

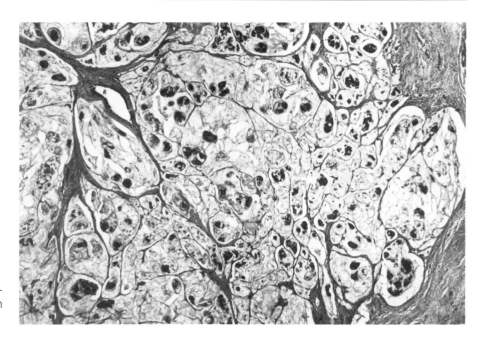

Fig. 8.**29** Mucinous carcinoma of the breast. Isolated tumor cell complexes within large "mucus lakes."

The tubular carcinoma is believed to have a favorable prognosis. Combinations with less differentiated growth components are not so rare (Fisher et al. 1975). Carstens et al. (1972) have found that such mixed forms are no more serious than the "pure" tubular carcinomas. Because of the high maturity of cells, it might be difficult to distinguish tubular carcinomas from benign lesions such as infiltrating epitheliosis (tubular pseudoinfiltration).

Tubular pseudoinfiltration is commonly found in so-called "radial scars" (Hamperl 1975). This pimarily benign lesion gives a focal radiating growth of the glandular structure with central sclerelastosis (Fig. 8.**32**). The most important differential criteria for pseudoinfiltration are listed in Table 8.**5**. Linell et al. (1980) believe that the majority, but not all, of tubular carcinomas originate from "radial scars." Egger (1981) finds a higher frequency of tubular forms occurring in small carcinomas rather than larger, more progressed tumors and concludes that perhaps a large number of carcinomas of different growth patterns originate as primary, tubular growing cancers.

Papillary Carcinomas

Infiltrating papillary carcinomas represent 0.3% to 1.5% of all breast cancers. Histology demonstrates branched papillary extensions within ectatic ducts and microcystic cavities. The papillae are usually lacking vascular stroma. The epithelium is single layered. Cells and nuclei are highly pleomorphic. Apocrine differentiation often seen in benign papillomas is absent (Fig. 8.**33**). McDivitt (1968) considers prognosis good whereas Kraus and Neubecker (1962) find no difference in prognosis as compared with the ordinary mammary carcinomas.

Adenoid-Cystic Carcinoma

With a frequency of approximately 1%, adenoid-cystic tumors of the breast exhibit patterns similar to those of the nasal pharyngeal area and the salivary glands and clinically show a favorable prognosis. These tumors are most prevalent in individuals in their 60s or 70s. Histology reveals island-like and trabecular cell complexes that contain slit-like or round cavities (Fig. 8.**34**). The lumina of these cavities are filled with an amorphous PAS-

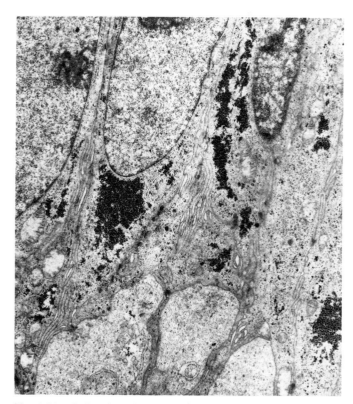

Fig. 8.**30** Cells of mucinous carcinoma. Good intracellular connections through membrane interdigitation and desmosomes. Large glycogen deposits in the infranuclear area of the cylindrical tumor cells. (Electron microscopic magnification x 10,000.)

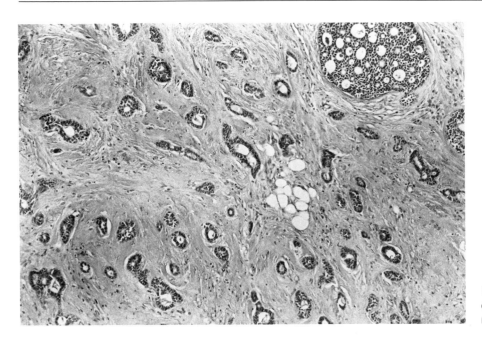

Fig. 8.**31** Highly differentiated tubular carcinoma with intraductal cribriform component

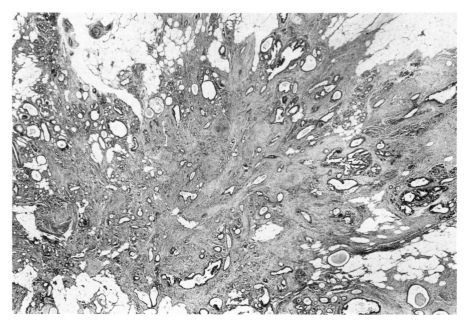

Fig. 8.**32** So-called radial scar (Hamperl). Radiation-like transformation of connective tissue with central sclerelastic core. Ectatic ducts in the periphery with hyperplasia of the ductal epithelium.

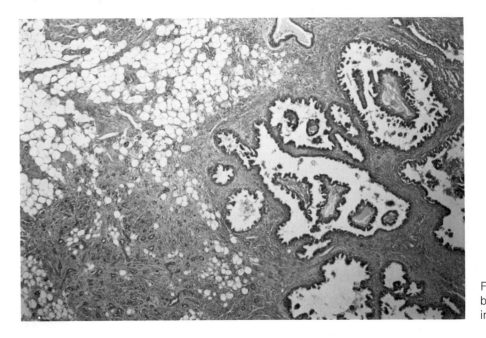

Fig. 8.**33** Papillary carcinoma: Papillary budding within highly ectatic ducts. Adjacent infiltrating tubular formations.

Table 8.**5** Histologic differential diagnosis: Radial scar versus tubular carcinoma

Radial scar with pseudoinfiltration	Highly differentiated tubular cancer
Total picture	
Stellate lesion	Stellate lesion
Elastoid hyaline core with tubular pseudoinfiltration (infiltrating epitheliosis)	Highly differentiated ("ordered") glandular structure
Radial ectatic ducts	Intraductal component (solid, papillary, or cribriform intraductal carcinoma)
Intraductal epithelial proliferations	
Retraction of surrounding tissue	
Epithelial formations	
Elongated tubuli and solid strands	Tubular formations
Narrow or "closed" lumina	"Open" glands
Irregular, "angular" formations	Trabecular, epithelial bridges
No extensions into the surrounding fat tissue	Infiltration of the surrounding fat tissue
Basal membrane	
Intact, sometimes ill defined	Intact, sometimes ill defined
Cell morphology	
One- or two-layered epithelium	One cell layer of cubic or cylindric cells
Two different cell types	Pale coloration of the cytoplasm
Plump cells with vesicular nuclei	Apical secretion in highly differentiated forms
Elongated cells with myoepithelial differentiation	No myoepithelial cells
	No focal apocrine metaplasia
Mitoses	
Rare, regular	Rare or moderately frequent, sometimes atypical
Stromal changes	
Loose and dense, collagenous stroma	Loose and dense collagenous stroma
Lots of elastoid material periductal and in nodular arrangement	Central sclerosis with lots of elastoid material

positive secretion and the cell complexes are separated by loose, edematous stroma. The tumor cells are cuboid or polygonal in shape and the nuclei slightly hyperchromatic. Mitoses are seldom seen. In addition to the ordered, cylindrical, sieve-like structures, undifferentiated solid or glandular areas are sometimes contained within these cell complexes.

Paget's Disease

Controversies concerning the histogenesis of Paget's disease still persist with the primary question remaining: Do Paget cells of the nipple epidermis originate in situ or are they tumor cells that secondarily have invaded the epidermis? Current findings suggest the derivation of these cells to be from intraepidermal metastasis.

Paget's disease is almost always found in conjunction with an intraductal or infiltrating carcinoma of the breast, and often a direct continuity between both lesions is evident (Fig. 8.**35**). Paget cells sometimes form glandular arrangements within the epidermis. This migration into the epidermis is not limited to intraductal carcinomas adjacent to the nipple (Fig. 8.**36**). Fisher et al. (1975) report that among 23 cases of Paget's disease, only two cases were associated with an intraductal carcinoma (DCIS). In 16 cases the accompanying carcinoma was an infiltrating ductal carcinoma (NOS). Of the remaining five cases, four were of type tubular and one a mucinous carcinoma.

On the basis of ultrastructural and/or histochemical comparisons, Neubecker and Bradshaw (1961), Sagebiel (1969), and Ozzello (1971) have substantiated the hypothesis that intraepidermal Paget cells are of metastatic cells driving from accompanying carcinomas. Bussolati and Pich (1975) lend further credence to support the histogenetic relationship between Paget cells and the parenchymal cells of the ductal-lobular system by demonstrating the presence of casein in Paget cells, although this finding does not fully substantiate the migration theory, since other epidermal structures (e. g., sebaceous glands) exhibit a positive casein reaction. Moreover, mammary carcinomas that invade the epidermis via the basal membrane do not lend themselves to Paget cell formation. Obviously, the intraepithelial spread of tumor cells is the prerequisite for pagetoid transformation.

Independent of the controversial theories surrounding the histogenesis of Paget's disease, the capacity for segmental and epidermal spreading is characteristic of all different types of breast cancer. Careful attention must be given to this property when considering breast-preserving surgical procedures (Fig. 8.**37**).

Inflammatory Carcinoma

Inflammatory carcinoma is a clinical term that refers to the accompanying symptoms of redness and warmth characteristic of this type of in general more advanced breast cancers. Clinically, inflammatory symptoms are experienced in 1% to 2% of all breast cancers (Robbins et al. 1974; Stocks and Simons-Patterson 1976).

Pathologists sometimes wrongly classify small cell carcinomas with extensive tumor cell dispersions as inflammatory carcinomas because they bear a striking resemblance to inflammatory mononuclear cell infiltration, but are histogenetically to be classified with the infiltrating lobular carcinomas.

The histologic substrate of the inflamed, reddened skin is the dermal lymphatic carcinomatosis, whose isolated tumor cell complexes (tumor cell emboli) within a mostly

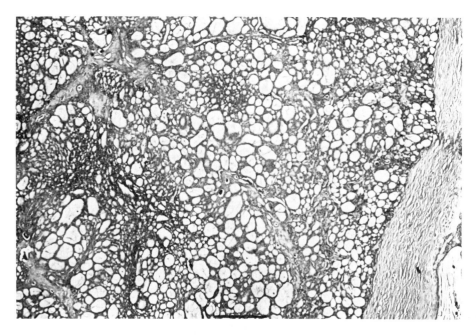

Fig. 8.**34** Low-power photo of adenoid cystic carcinoma of the breast.

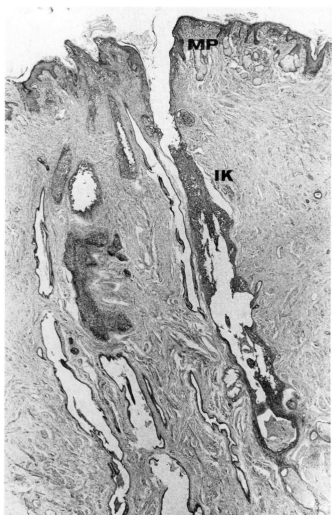

Fig. 8.**35** Intraductal carcinoma (IK) in association with Paget's disease (MP).

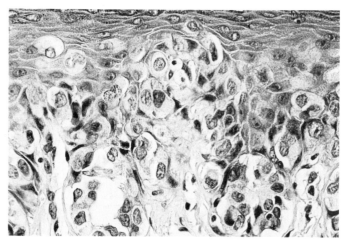

Fig. 8.**36** Paget's disease of the breast. Glandular arrangement of the Paget cells in the lower epidermal layers.

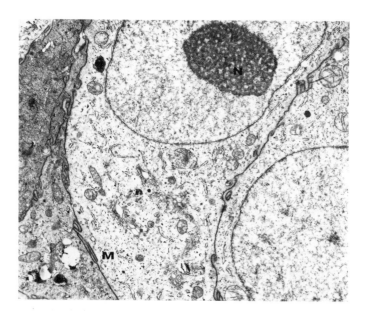

Fig. 8.**37** Intraepidermal Paget cell, "light" cytoplasm, large nucleus (N), basement membrane (M), and membrane interdigitation with neighbouring epidermal cells. (Electronmicroscopic magnification x 12,500.)

ectatic dermal lymph vessel system (Fig. 8.**38**). Lymphatic carcinomatosis does not, however, always lead to a clinical picture of an "inflammation," since edema and peau d'orange (cellulitis-like picture) are the clinical equivalents of a dermal lymphatic carcinoma. Lymphatic spread may also have a clinically occult course. In the case of clinically manifested as well as suspicious cases, a skin biopsy should be obtained before a choice of primary therapy is made, since radiation and systemic therapy are the preferred primary treatments for cancers where dermal lymphatic spread is present.

Other Rare Types

This heterogenous group of rare breast tumors is of interest to the pathologist mostly because of its histogenetic complexity. This group is only of clinical relevance if definitive differences of biological behaviour exist between these tumors and the more common types of carcinomas and if selective therapeutic procedures are indicated.

Squamous Carcinoma

The ontogenetic derivation of the breast as a dermal gland is directly reflected by the potency of epidermal differentiation. Although it is rare for squamous cancers to derive from the ductal-lobular system, they have been observed in pure form or in combination with cystosarcomas and carcinosarcomas. Light microscopy of large-cell ductal carcinomas sometimes reveals a structure resembling a squamous epithelial cancer. True cases of squamous cancer can be discerned ultramicroscopically through identification of cellular attributes associated with the squamous epithelium (tonofibrils in connection with desmosomes) (Fig. 8.**39**).

A favorable prognosis is usually expected for primary squamous cancer of the breast. The most effective treatment for these cancers is radical surgery. Adjuvant combination chemotherapy appears to be of little value.

Metaplastic Carcinoma

Epithelial metaplasia occurs in carcinomas with apocrine differentiation. These tumors exhibit the phylogenetic potency of the mammary glandular epithelium to form apocrine cells of the sweat glands type. The large tumor cells have an eosinophilic fine granular cytoplasm and arrange into papillary or acinar glandular formations. Apocrine carcinomas must be distinguished from primary sweat gland tumors that are sometimes located in the areolar region. Prognosis for apocrine carcinomas does not greatly differ from that expected for the common types of breast cancers (Frable and Kay 1968; Haagensen 1971).

Mesenchymal metaplasia appears to be the root of most osteosarcomas as well as chondrosarcomas. Both of these carcinomas are more rarely observed in a pure form than as mixed epithelial and mesenchymal tumors (carcinosarcomas). In metastases from mixed tumors, the different tissue components can appear alone or in combination.

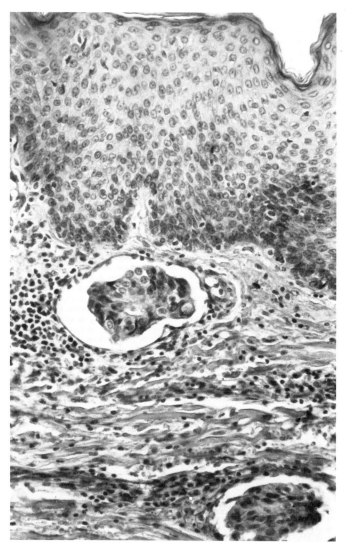

Fig. 8.**38** Dermal lymphatic carcinomatosis. Tumor emboli in ectatic lymph vessels of the corium.

Prognosis is unfavorable, with both cartilage- and bone-forming mixed tumors showing resistance to radiological and cytostatic treatments.

Lipid-Secreting Tumors

Carcinoma with secretion of specific products, particularly milk fat, form a special entity. Aboumrad et al. (1963) and Ramos and Taylor (1974) have described lipid-producing breast tumors. The tumor cells show mostly a solid growth pattern and contain a light, foamy cytoplasm, rich in neutral lipids. Nuclei are relatively uniform and eccentrically located in the cytoplasm with lipid droplets actively secreted from the tumor cells. Despite their high degree of maturity, these tumors are prognostically unfavorable, although the number of reported cases is far too small to allow for accurate prognosis.

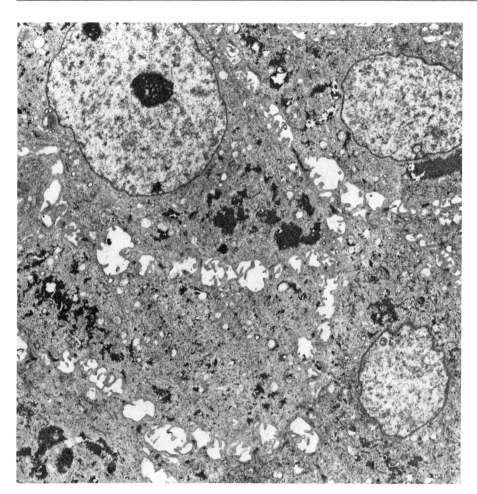

Fig. 8.**39** Electron microscopic picture of a squamous cell carcinoma of the breast. Characteristic desmosomal cell connections and abundance of glycogen in the cytoplasm of the polygonal tumor cells. (Electron microscopic magnification x 6500.)

Histological Grading

The process of tumor grading involves consideration of tumor histology and cytology and is based on three microscopic parameters, namely, tubular arrangement, nuclear pleomorphism, and the number of mitoses. The aim of tumor grading is to calculate the probability of treatment outcome. Viewed in conjunction with the clinical stages, histologic grading provides a clearer, more accurate picture of the individual prognosis. Histologic grading provides precise definitions in randomized therapeutic studies for comparison of collectives. This system is, however, not without its critics who claim that cytologic and histologic characteristics are subjective and therefore grading depends on the experience of the investigator. The reproducibility, as found through synchronous determinations by different investigators as well as repeated determinations by the same investigator, is mostly low but significant. Stenkvist et al. (1979) report values between 60% to 77%, which reflect the percentage of congruent determinations by investigators using the same histologic grading system. Also affecting the value of the grading system is the type of discriminants used. The grading recommended by the World Health Organization (WHO) (Scarff and Torloni 1968) is introduced by Bloom and Richardson (1957) and based on the following parameters:

1. Adenoid (tubular) differentiation
2. Hyperchromasia and number of mitoses
3. Nuclear pleomorphism (Table 8.**6**)

Partly through the modification of the original system, several investigators have demonstrated a significant correlation between the grade of the tumor and the survival time (Schiodt 1976; Bunting et al. 1976; Wallgren and Silfverswaerd 1976). Freedman et al. (1979) have gone on to suggest that histologic grading is more relevant to the course of the disease than clinical staging.

The integrating factor common to all grading systems is the degree of differentiation of the tumor cell, which is more exactly determined in ultramicroscopic cell analysis than by light microscopy. Ultramicroscopic grading of breast cancer was developed by Stegner et al. (1981), although its accuracy for predicting the course of the disease is not yet proved.

Hormone Receptors (Biochemical-Morphological Correlations)

The recognition of steroid receptors in the normal and neoplastic cell has improved insight regarding tumor growth, as well as given a logical basis for hormonal therapy in steroid-sensitive carcinomas. Estrogen receptor positive tumors compose 50% to 70% of primary breast cancers. This percentage drops for tumors where metastasis is present (Wittliff et al 1976). Moreover, in approximately 60% of all estrogen-receptor-positive cases, remission can be obtained through adjuvant endo-

Table 8.6 Grading of breast cancer (Scarff and Bloom)	Differentiation	Glandular	Mixed	Solid or disseminated
	Nuclear pleomorphy	Small	Moderate	High
Grade I: 3–5 points	Number of mitoses	Max. 1/HPF	2/HPF	3 and more/HPF
Grade II: 6–7 points	Total points	1	2	3
Grade III: 8 or 9 points				

crine therapy, whereas the remission probability is below 10% in patients without receptors (Maass et al. 1975; McGuire et al. 1975; Heuson et al. 1977).

It has been customary to differentiate between breast cancers on the basis of general topography, histogenetics, gross and fine structural morphology, and prognostic criteria, and the question is now where estrogen-receptor-positive and receptor-negative tumors fit in. Attempts to demonstrate a correlation between receptor contents and histologic type have proved unsuccessful (Terenius et al. 1974; McGuire et al. 1975; Rosen et al. 1975; Wittliff et al. 1976). It has been demonstrated, however, that the infiltrating lobular carcinomas and the group of highly differentiated tubular and papillary carcinomas exhibited more estrogen and progesterone receptors than did the less differentiated invasive ductal and medullary carcinomas (Rosen et al. 1975; Antoniades and Spector 1979; McCarty et al. 1980). Overall, it appears that receptor contents correlate better with the nuclear grading rather than with histologic type (Würz et al. 1979; McCarty et al. 1980; Stegner et al. 1981). Analyses where histologic type was not considered sought to correlate receptor contents with the ultrastructural differentiation of the cancer cell (Chabon et al. 1979; McCarty et al. 1980; Stegner et al. 1979, 1981); these investigations suggested a strong correlation between receptor contents and those ultrastructural parameters usually associated with a highly differentiated cell (e. g., gland formation, junctional complexes, secretory granules, and intracytoplasmic vacuoles).

To summarize the results obtained thus far concerning receptors, it has been demonstrated that tumors with a high, ultrastructural grade of differentiation (i. e., high intracellular organization, good intercellular connection, and specific products of synthesis) prove more often to be receptor-positive than less-differentiated tumors. Receptor-negative tumors are significantly more frequent with malignancy grade III. The formation of steroid receptors is strongly associated with the degree of differentiation of the tumor cell and is independent of established histologic classifications, and receptor formation is apparently not influenced by the histogenesis of the tumor, whether it derives from ductal or lobular origins.

Metastasis

Lymphatic Metastasis

As prognosis worsens with the number of lymph nodes involved, it is clear to see why nodal status has become an especially important prognostic parameter of breast cancer. Fisher (1978) reports that the rate of recurrence is doubled in cases where one to three axillary lymph nodes are metastatically involved; in cases where more than four lymph nodes are involved, the rate is five times as great when compared with cases where there is no lymph node involvement. Nodal status is the basis for any decision on adjuvant chemotherapy (Bonadonna 1980). It is obvious that careful histologic examination of axillary dissection material is essential. A rough investigation of sampled lymph nodes is no longer allowed, and the number of lymph nodes found depends on how extensively the surgeon performs the axillary dissection, as well as on the accuracy of the pathologist. The detection of lymph nodes within the dissected fat tissue is enhanced by staining with picric acid (Vogt-Hoerner and Gerard-Marchant 1958) or by the clearing technique (Haagensen et al. 1972). The probability of detecting nodal metastasis increases with the number of nodes examined and the number of histologic sections. The importance of careful examination of biopsied material is perhaps best illustrated in reports by Saphir and Amromin (1948), Pickren (1961), and Fisher et al. (1978), who show through systematic re-examination of previously examined lymph nodes that metastasis remained undetected in approximately 25% of all routinely examined cases.

The achievement in search for metastasis is determined by the capacity of the laboratory and the clinical relevance of the findings. According to the investigations of Fisher and Slack (1970), Huvos et al. (1971), Attiyeh et al. (1977), and Fisher et al. (1978), micrometastasis (less than 2 mm in diameter) have little bearing on prognosis. Of importance are only the larger metastatic infiltrations. Schremmer (1975) has recorded the size range of normal and metastatically infiltrated lymph nodes and found the average diameter of tumor-free lymph nodes to be 6.5 mm, whereas the metastatically infiltrated nodes showed an average diameter of 9.7 mm (1.8 to 40.6 mm).

Lymphatic metastasis occurs dependent on the site of the primary tumor and sequentially to the different groups of regional lymph nodes. Certain bypass mechanisms, however, allow for the omission of some lymph nodes groups. Reports by Haagensen et al. (1969, 1972) suggest that the central axillary lymph nodes are generally involved first and most frequently. Single metastasis is most often found in this group. The interpectoral lymph nodes (Rotter's nodes), the nodes along the axillary vein, the subscapular, and infraclavicular nodes are involved with decreasing frequency. Guided by practical surgical points of view, Berg (1955) proposed a classification of regional lymph nodes in three levels: level I, lymph nodes lateral and caudal of the minor pectoral muscle; level II, lymph nodes behind the minor pectoral muscle; and level III, lymph nodes medial and above the minor pectoral muscle.

Pathologic Aspects of the Regional Lymph Node Metastasis

Metastatic infiltrations of the lymph nodes in general show the same structure as the primary tumor. With ductal carcinomas, they may form island-like clusters with central necrosis similar to those found in the comedocarcinomas. Also the amount of fibrosis is repeated in the metastasis. In approximately 25% of all cases, however, the metastases have a histologic structure different from that of the primary tumor. This is possibly due to selection of heterogeneous (multiclonal) tumors (Schiodt 1966). The undifferentiated (anaplastic) components of mixed tumors possess a large metastasizing potential, but also an increase of differentiation may be found in nodal and distant metastases. Thus, a primary partially colloid cancer may show a pure mucinous structure in the metastasis. Through identification of type and structure of a metastatic node in occult carcinoma, type and location of the primary tumor may be deduced. Also of help is immunohistochemical detection via markers (e.g., lactoferrin, casein, T-antigen, and lectins) (Fig. 8.**40**).

The importance of non-specific reactions within the lymphoreticular tissue of a nodule is often debated. The so-called sinushistiocytosis is regarded as sign of a favorable immunologic defense situation by many investigators (Black and Speer 1958; Wartman 1959; Black et al. 1971). Other investigators did not find any correlation between sinushistiocytosis and survival rate (Berg 1956; Moore et al. 1960; Kister et al. 1969). A favorable prognosis was indicated, however, by T-cell hyperplasia (Tsakaklides et al. 1974).

Hematogenic Metastasis

Hematogenic metastasis is a sequential process that involves vascular invasion, transportation (embolization), and implantation (growth in other organs). The vascular invasion occurs through isolated cells or tumor cells that penetrate the vessel wall, thus reaching the free blood stream. Although embolization does not always lead to a manifest metastasis, the likelihood of metastasis does increase with the number of cell disseminated in the blood stream.

Currently appearing in the literature is the suggestion that spreading can occur through tumor biopsy. Although a blunt or sharp manipulation of a primary tumor can certainly result in an expulsion of cells, investigations have failed to correlate a decreased survival rate with tumor biopsy.

The process of metastasis begins with the accumulation of tumor cells within the inner walls of the endothelium. Shielded by thrombocytes and fibrin, the tumor cells are then ready to proceed with their destructive growth.

Diffusion of cancer cells usually emanates from a production center or multiplicator. For hematogenic spread, the lungs are of central importance. Following lymph node metastasis, invasion of the lungs occurs via the thoracic duct or through direct invasion to the thoracic venous system via the azygous vein and the internal mammary vein. Further pulmonary metastasis often involves the visceral pleura and the parietal pleura, and it is from the pulmonary area that other organs are affected. Although the intimate association between tumor cells and host tissue is not fully understood, it does appear that the specific environment of the host tissue is critical to the metastatic process. Moreover, it appears that local vascular activity has little bearing on the site of metastasis. Each hematogenically spreading neoplasm has its own unique pattern of metastasis. Table 8.**7** illustrates the frequency and distribution of hematogen metastasis in breast cancer. The site of organ metastasis is apparently unassociated with the duration of the illness and early- and late-metastasizing breast tumors do not exhibit different patterns of metastasis. The special pathology of organ metastasis is not discussed in this chapter.

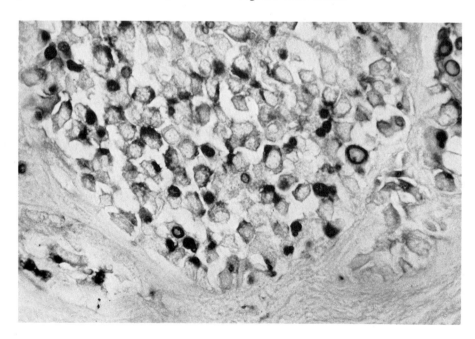

Fig. 8.**40** Identification of casein in cells of a ductal carcinoma of the breast. Immunoperoxidase technique.

Table 8.**7** Frequency and distribution of hematogenic metastases of breast cancers

Site	Percent
Lungs	63
Skeleton	58
Liver	51
Pleura	44
Adrenals	31
Skin	20
Peritoneum	17
Ovaries	13
Kidneys	13
Pancreas	10

Tumor Metastasis to the Breast

The breast is of little importance as a site of metastasis from tumors not originating in this area. Generally, metastasis from extramammary neoplasms represent 1% to 3% of malignant breast tumors (Baumgartner and Stamm 1966; Kleinert 1968). Infiltration of the breast can occur, however, with systemic diseases of the lymphoreticular apparatus, namely, leukemia and certain malignant lymphomas.

Lymphoma foci are often clinically and mammographically similar to sarcomas of the breast with diffuse, netlike manifestations seen only in the later stages (Fig. 8.**41**). Since they are histologically similar to diffusely growing lobular cancers with small anaplastic cells, careful differential diagnosis is critical. In such cases, the demonstration of cytochemical markers is particularly important (e. g., keratin, lectins and casein).

Among the most important extramammary epithelial tumors are malignant melanomas, uterine and ovarian carcinomas, and bronchial carcinomas. Metastases to the breast by extramammary tumors and mammary manifestations of lymphoblastomas and malignant lymphomas have an incidence peak at an earlier age than primary breast carcinoma.

Bilateral Breast Cancer

Since breast is a paired organ derived from genetically similar conditions and exposed to the same endocrine influences, it is not surprising that the probability of similar reactions in both breasts is high. The question of multicentric and bilateral cancer formation is of great importance in staged breast cancer therapy. Fisher et al. (1975) found in extended histology of 904 cases of breast cancer 121 cases (13.4%) with multicentric invasive and noninvasive foci. Multicentricity was most commonly noted in indistinctly contoured primary tumors, tumors larger than 5 cm, invasive comedocarcinomas, and growths within proximity of the nipple. In the case of the multicentric, noninvasive variety, the intraductal type occurred three times as frequently as the lobular type. Tellem et al. (1962) found in 64 mastectomy patients 26% of cancer involvement outside the primary tumor quadrant.

In 1 out of 100 cases of breast cancer, synchronously manifested, bilateral tumors are found. Histology, however, reveals a much higher percentage of multicentric foci in clinically manifest cases of carcinoma. This multicentricity may be the result of multicentric origin or might be contralateral metastasis (Table 8.**8**). By combining the cases of noninfiltrating and infiltrating tumors, Sandison (1962), Urban (1969), Slack et al. (1973), and Shah et al. (1973) found the percentage of cases with bilateral foci to be 14% to 25%.

Clinically, a subsequent manifestation of a latent, second carcinoma occurs in approximately 2% within the course of six years and in 6% within 20 years (Robbins and Berg 1964; Slack et al. 1973). Moreover, the general risk of developing a second carcinoma is 5 to 7 times greater in women with a previous history of breast cancer than in

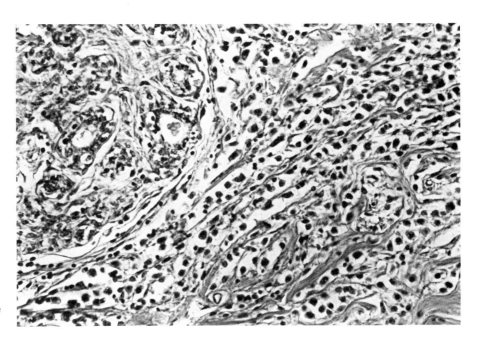

Fig. 8.**41** Malignant lymphoma of the breast.

Table 8.**8**   Bilateral breast cancer: Differential diagnosis, metastasis versus secondary carcinoma

Secondary tumor	Metastasis
Histological different type	Histological same type
Singular lesion	Multiple lesions
Simultaneous occurrence, no metastasis at other locations	Metachronic occurrence, further lymphogenic and/or hematogenic metastasis
Intraductal or intralobular accompanying component	Missing intraductal or intralobular accompanying component
Compact tumor core (central fibroelastosis)	Scant fibrosis
Prevalent upper outer quadrant	No predilection
No signs of lymphatic spread	Combined with lymphatic spread

the general female population (Leis 1970: Robbins and Berg 1964; Leis et al. 1965).

Dystopic (Paramammary) Carcinoma

In cases where the carcinoma originates within a peripheral glandular extension, an apparent dystopia can occur. For example, tongue-like, parenchymal extensions are often found in the upper lateral quadrant (axillary processus) and less frequently in the direction of the clavicle, sternum, or abdomen. Genuine dystopic cancers originate in accessory glandular tissue from the axilla caudally to the inguinal region corresponding to the embryonic milk-streak. It appears that aberrant glandular tissue is predisposed for malignant transformation, as well as for the formation of benign tumors.

Carcinomas of the axillary processus metastasize early into the neighboring pectoral lymph nodes. A nodular metastasis along the pectoral border may be the first clinical sign of an occult microcarcinoma of the dystopic glandular tissue.

Pathology of the Local and Regional Recurrence

Local recurrence following surgical treatment can occur in parenchymal residues in the thoracic region as well as the skin. A loco-regional recurrence is localized in the lymphatic drainage system. Causes of recurrence include incomplete removal of tumor tissue, latent lymphatic metastasis, and surgically caused spread (implantation metastasis). Approximately half of the cases of local recurrence occur before the end of the first year after primary treatment. The frequency depends on the stage of growth and on the thoroughness of the surgical procedure. Postsurgical radiation therapy appears to decrease the frequency of local recurrence when compared with

surgical therapy alone. Histopathology could disclose the cause of local recurrence. Local recurrence within scars often present small-celled, solid infiltrations between wide, collagen-containing scar fibers or a pronounced scattering of tumor cells. The cells have a discrete character and may be histologically mistaken for inflammatory infiltrations. Cutaneous aggregates occur as multiple tumor cell clusters that either arrange themselves in the collagen fibers of the corium or form larger, more compact nodes with central fibrous sclerosis. In the case of lymphatic spread, consolidated tumor cell clusters are not seen, although fine tumor emboli are found in ectatic lymph vessels. In cases of incomplete mastectomy, recurrence areas are surrounded by parenchymal residues. Multicentric tumor formation is to be considered in cases where foci are remotely situated from the original site of the primary tumor or when foci exhibit differing structural patterns.

Sarcoma of the Breast

Fibrosarcomas

Fibrosarcomas consist of spindle-shaped, fibroblast-like cells that are arranged in a fascicular, or twisted fashion. The intermediate tissue is rich in collagen and reticular fibers. Unlike the cystosarcomas, there is no epithelial component. The nuclei show varying degrees of pleomorphism ranging from uniform, spindle-like nuclei to bizarre, multinucleated cells. The stroma may be myxomatous. Fiber-rich tumors exhibiting little nuclear pleomorphism, sharp borders, and limited number of mitoses show local recurrence but rarely metastases in spite of extensive growth. Fiber-poor, mitosis-rich, highly nuclear pleomorphic tumors, however, exhibit rapid growth and a high tendency to metastasize. When making predictions regarding the prognosis, the most important histologic parameters are nuclear polymorphism, peripheral limitation, and the number of mitoses. Findings suggest that tumors with five or more mitoses per high power field are more likely to metastasize than those tumors with numbers of mitoses less than five (Norris and Taylor 1968; Barnes and Pietruszka 1977).

Cystosarcoma Phyllodes (Malignant Variety)

It was in 1838 that J. Müller described and named a group of mostly benign, although in some cases malignant tumors, whose structure and histogenetics appeared closely connected to fibroadenoma (Fig. 8.**42**). The most striking differences between cystosarcoma and typical fibroadenoma are the greater number of mesenchymal cells found in phyllodes tumors, and in the case of benign cystosarcoma, the high degree of cellular pleomorphism as compared with typical fibroadenoma (Fig. 8.**43**). Regardless of the differences, the similarities are strong enough for cystosarcoma growths to be given the names, giant fibroadenomas, juvenile fibroadenomas, or cellular intracanalicular fibroadenomas. As is the case with pure

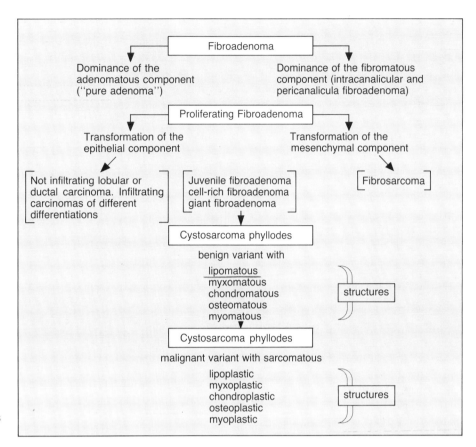

Fig. 8.**42** Classification of fibroadenomas and related tumors.

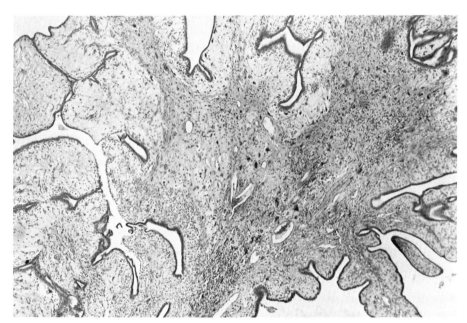

Fig. 8.**43** Cystosarcoma phyllodes. Benign type. In the stroma, multinucleated histiocytic cells.

mesenchymal tumors, genetically fixed differentiation potentials can be seen. Variations of cystosarcoma include a lipomyxomatous type, a chondromatous type, and on rare occasions, a myomatous type. The epithelial component consists of a two-layered epithelium, lining deep clefts. The deep split cavities produce the phyllodal structure of the tumor.

Macroscopically, cystosarcoma tumors are bulb-like or somewhat laminated tumors of gray-white, yellowish, or gray-red color. Unlike the firm fibroadenomas, the consistency of the cystosarcomas is much softer. Rapid tumor enlargement can be triggered by myxomatous changes

and by formation of cysts. Localization close to the skin of these bulb-like tumors can cause gross morphologic changes in the breast. The skin is freely movable over these pseudocapsulated tumors and enlargement of the venous pattern is seen. Skin fixation and retraction do not usually occur. Tumor sizes of 30 cm have been reported and where hemorrhagic necrosis and liquefaction are evident, the clinical impression of an advanced, incurable carcinoma arises (Fig. 8.**44**).

The features that distinguish the malignant cystosarcoma from the benign form include the presence of a sarcomatous stroma with enhanced cellular pleomorphism, an increase in mitoses, and overall aggressive growth pattern (Fig. 8.**45**). Degenerative changes in the myxomatous areas are often misdiagnosed as malignant cystosarcomas, as is histiocytic metaplasia. In the case of histiocytic metaplasia, it is the focal accumulations of highly pleomorphic, frequently multinucleated cells that resemble the cells of cutaneous histiocytomas. These cells can contain cytoplasmic inclusions of varying kinds, including hemosiderin. The sarcomatous matrix of the malignant cystosarcomas can contain metaplastic adipose, osseous, and chondroid foci (e. g., lipo-chondro-osteoplastic sarcomas). The malignant cystosarcoma differs, however, from pure sarcomas in that it contains an epithelial component. Findings report that distant metastases can be found in 30% to 50% of malignant cystosarcomas (Obermann 1965; Norris and Taylor 1967; Halverson and Hori-Robaina 1974). The spread is mainly hematogenous mostly to the lungs and skeletal system. Axillary lymph node metastases are extremely rare.

Histologic parameters are of great importance when choosing a suitable therapeutic modality and include determination of cell pleomorphism, number of mitoses, and tumor border. All of these parameters are critical for determining malignancy (Obermann 1965; Treves and Sunderland 1951; Lester and Stout 1954). As previously mentioned, misdiagnosis is possible. The overestimation of cell atypia, degenerative cell changes, and histiocytotic metaplasis is more common than the underdiagnosis of malignancy.

Benign and small cystosarcomas are removed by wide tumor excision. Recurrence due to remaining peripheral tumor extensions is common. Larger growths should be treated by simple mastectomy. Malignant cystosarcomas require radical therapy depending on their clinical stage. These tumors are relatively insensitive to radiation therapy.

Hemangiosarcomas

Hemangiosarcoma (malignant hemangioendothelioma) of the breast is a rare but nonetheless a highly malignant tumor, usually occurring during the fertile years of a woman. It is a rapidly growing, diffuse tumor that causes discoloration of the skin when superficially located. The blood-rich, sponge-like tumor contains necrotic or sclerotic areas.

The histologic diagnosis of biopsied material can be difficult without detailed clinical information since most of these tumors appear in combination with mature, well differentiated, cavernous angiomatous and solid endothelial structures (Hamperl 1973). Histologic parameters of prognostic significance include the degree of nuclear hyperchromatism, number of mitoses, and solid endothelial growth pattern. Hematogenous metastases occur to the skeletal system, lungs, liver, and other parenchymatous organs, whereas metastases to regional lymph nodes is seldom seen.

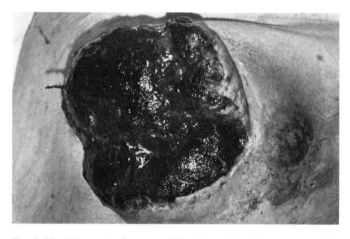

Fig. 8.**44** Hemorrhagic necrosis in ulcerated cystosarcoma phyllodes, benign type.

Liposarcomas

Liposarcomas exhibit an initially expansive pattern of growth and may later become ulcerated. Histology reveals in highly differentiated tumors many mature fat cells and lipoblasts. The more anaplastic types consist of round cellular elements, vacuolar lipoblasts, or multinucleated, pleomorphic giant cells (Fig. 8.**46**).

The stroma can become myxomatous. Lipoblastic sarcomas may be components of a malignant cystosarcoma phyllodes. Both lymphatic and hematogenous metastases have been observed with the metastatic potential dependent on histologic type (Breckenridge 1954; Jackson 1962)

Chondroplastic and Osteoplastic Mixed Tumors (Carcinochondroosteoid Sarcomas)

Extraosseous tumors with cartilage and bone-forming potential are oncologic rarities of particular interest to the histogenetically oriented pathologist. Both the general and comparative pathology deals with chondroid and osteoid metaplasias as possible differentiations of myoepithelial cells. Such chondroid-osteoplastic breast tumors are frequently observed among bitches and cats (Bomhard and Sandersleben 1973, 1974).

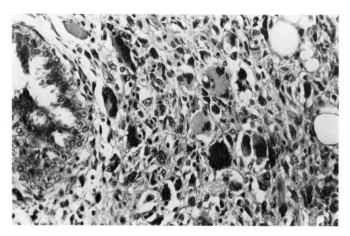

Fig. 8.**45** Malignant type of cystosarcoma phyllodes.

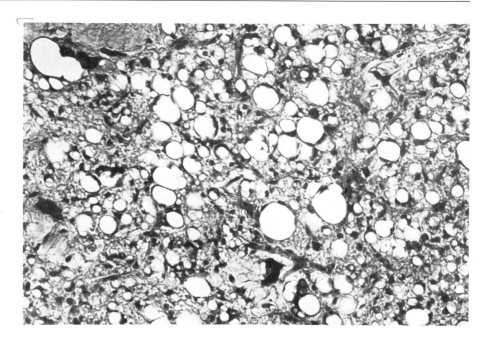

Fig. 8.**46**   Liposarcoma of the breast.

Hamperl (1970) considers the myoepithelial cell to be the link in the interpretation of mixed tumors as this cell can differentiate to epithelial as well as mesenchymal cells. Tumors that are histogenetically comparable are the mixed tumors or pleomorphic adenomas of the salivary gland (Seifert 1966). On histochemical and electronmicroscopic investigation, these tumors reveal an apparent cytogenetic connection to the myothelial cell (Azzopardi and Smith 1959; Mylius 1960; Hübner et al. 1969).

Both chondroid and osteoplastic mixed tumors occur as strikingly hard growths, are clinically fairly well demarcated, and show no preference for a particular age group. Depending on the composition of the tumor, the mammogram can show focal accumulation of bone. Descriptions of chondro-osteosarcomas of the female breast have been published by Kreibig (1925), Biggs (1947), Robb and McFarlane (1958), and Smith and Taylor (1969) have reported ten cases from the Armed Forces Institute of Pathology. Electronmicroscopic analyses have been performed by Gonzalez-Licea et al. (1966) and Llombart-Bosch and Peydro (1975).

Characteristics of these mixed tumors include a coarsely fibered stroma of a white-gray color, extensive hyalinization, liquefaction and necrosis, and focal accumulations of chondroid, osteoid, or bone tissue. Also characteristic is a cavernous system in which capillaries are usually found in abundance. Histology reveals strong cellular pleomorphism within cell-rich, sarcomatous tissue. The extracellular matrix is composed either of island-like chondroid areas or contains osteoid trabecular inclusions. The sarcomatous cells display many forms including undifferentiated connective tissue cells over fibro-chondro- and osteoblasts, as well as multinucleated, giant cells of the osteoblastic variety (Fig. 8.**47**).

The majority of these tumors contain carcinomatous tissue components in the form of solid or glandular structures. Generally, prognosis for the malignant mixed tumor is poor with survival times more than twelve months being rare, although cases with a better course

have been reported (Kennedy and Biggard 1967). These tumors are not sensitive to radiation therapy and little is known about the effect of cystostatic and endocrine treatment. In one case seen by the author, estrogen receptors were demonstrated.

Rare Types of Malignant Mesenchymal Tumors

Case reports are available regarding leiomyosarcoma, rhabdomyosarcoma, and neurogenic sarcomas of the breast, and they show the specific structural properties seen in other organ localizations. Alveolar rhabdomyosarcomas have been reported in children and adolescents as primary as well as secondary metastatic breast tumors (Fig. 8.**48**). Epidemiologic and therapeutic statements cannot be made on the basis of these occasional cases. Prognosis has proved due to effective chemotherapy.

Malignant Degeneration of Benign Tumors

In certain instances, both ductal and infiltrating lobular carcinomas can develop within fibroadenomas. The lobular type is the most common (Buzanowski-Konakry et al. 1975; Curran and Dodge 1962; McDivitt et al. 1967; Goldman and Friedman 1969). In half of these cases either non-invasive or invasive foci can be identified outside the fibroadenoma, which has to be considered when discussing therapy. In general, these malignancies developed from fibroadenomas show a more favorable prognosis than do the ordinary cancers, due to the strict demarcation of the tumors. The risk of a secondary malignancy of primary benign breast tumor is not greater than the risk of malignancy in normal breast parenchyma. A malignant transformation can only be determined microscopically.

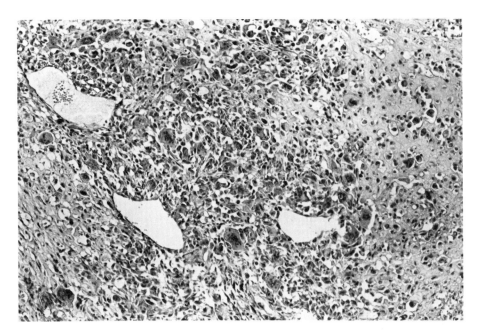

Fig. 8.**47** Carcino-chondro-osteoid sarcoma of the breast.

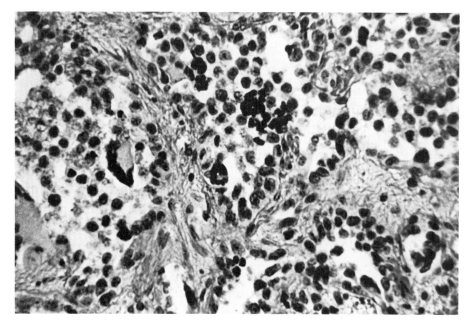

Fig. 8.**48** Alveolar rhabdomyosarcoma of the breast in a 14-years-old girl. The matrix of the tumor consists of undifferentiated, partially alveolarly arranged tumor cells. Characteristic are large, multinucleated rhabdomyoblasts.

In the case of malignant cystosarcoma phyllodes, this is most probably a primary malignant variety rather than a secondary transformation of an initially harmless fibro-adenoma.

Carcinomas of the Male Breast

Of all the cases of reported breast cancer, approximately 1% involve men with the average age of occurrence at 60 years (about five years later than that found in women) (Norris and Taylor 1969). According to Bässler (1978) most afflicted men are between the ages of 65 and 70.

These tumors originate most frequently in the central area of the breast. More often in men than in women, lymph node metastases are found at the time of initial examination. The histology is similar to that of the female carcinomas. The highly differentiated ductal types dominate; the infiltrating lobular carcinomas are found only occasionally (Giffler and Kay 1976; Yogore and Sahgal 1977). Similarly, the pattern of metastasis is not different from that found in female breast cancer with pleura, lung, and skeletal systems the preferred sites for spread. Scant information exists regarding the histogenesis of the carcinoma and its pathogenetic connections to benign hyperplasias of the male breast. Gynecomastia resulting from nonphysiologic, permanent hormonal stimulation appears to be predisposing for the formation of the carcinoma, and its appearance in conjunction with breast cancer is at a rate of 5% to 20%.

References

Aboumrad, M. H., R. C. Horn, G. Fine: Lipid-secreting mammary carcinoma. Report of a case associated with Paget's disease of the nipple. Cancer 16: 521–525, 1963

Ahmed, A.: Calcification in human breast carcinomas — Ultrastructural observations. J. Pathol. 117: 247–251, 1973

Al-Adnani, M. W., J. A. Kirrane, J. O'D. McGee: Inappropriate production of collagen and propyl hydroxylase by human breast cancer cells in vivo. Br. J. Cancer 31: 653–660, 1975

Andersen, J. A.: Lobular carcinoma in situ of the breast. An approach to rational treatment. Cancer 39: 597–2602, 1977

Antoniades, K., H. Spector: Correlation of estrogen receptor levels with histology and cytomorphology in human mammary cancer. Am. J. Clin. Pathol. 71: 497–503, 1979

Ashikari, R., A. G. Huvos, R. E. Snyder, J. C. Lucas, R. V. P. Hutter, R. W. McDivitt, D. Schottenfeld: A clinicopathologic study of atypical lesions of the breast. Cancer 33: 310–317, 1974

Attiyeh, F. F., M. Jensen, A. G. Huvos, A. Fracchia: Axillary micrometastasis and macrometastasis in carcinoma of the breast. Surg. Gynecol. Obstet. 144: 839–842, 1977

Azzopardi, J. G.: Problems in breast pathology. W. B. Saunders Ltd., Philadelphia 1979

Azzopardi, J. G., O. D. Smith: Salivary gland tumours and their mucins. J. Pathol. Bact. 77: 131–145, 1959

Azzopardi, J. G., R. N. Laurini: Elastosis in breast cancer. Cancer 33: 174–183, 1974

Barnes, L., M. Pietruszka: Sarcomas of the breast. A clinicopathologic analysis of the cases. Cancer 40: 1577–1585, 1977

Bässler, R.: Das sogenannte lobuläre Carcinom der Mamma. Dtsch. Med. Wschr. 94: 108–113, 1969

Bässler, R.: Pathologie der Brustdrüse. In W. Doerr, G. Seifert, E. Uehlinger: Spezielle pathologische Anatomie, Bd. 11. Springer, New York 1978

Baumgartner, H., H. Stamm: Das Problem der Mammatumoren. Fortschr. Geburtsh. Gynäk. 27: 60–111, 1966

Beduani, R., J. Vana, D. Rosner, R. Schmitz, G. P. Murphy: Management and survival of female patients with "minimal" breast cancer. Cancer 47: 2769–2778, 1981

Berg, J. W.: The significance of axillary node levels in the study of breast carcinoma. Cancer 8: 776–778, 1955

Berg, J. W.: Sinus histiocytosis: A fallacious measure of host resistance to cancer. Cancer 9: 935–939, 1956

Berg, J. W.: Morphological evidence for immune response to cancer. A historical review. Cancer 28: 1453–1456, 1971

Bernath, G.: Amyloidosis in malignant tumors. Acta Morph. Acad. Sci. Hungaricae 2: 137–144, 1952

Berndt, H., H. J. Gütz, K.-H. Jacobasch, B. Drahl, C.-N. Schremmer, R. Strohwig, G. P. Wildner, G. Wolff: Vorschlag zur pathologisch-anatomischen Klassifikation des Brustdrüsenkrebses nach dem TNM-System. Arch. Geschwulstforsch. 41: 146–163, 1973

Biggs, R.: The myoepithelium in certain tumors of the breast. J. Pathol. Bact. 59: 437, 1947

Black, M. M., F. D. Speer: Sinus histiocytosis of lymph nodes in cancer. Surg. Gynecol. Obstet. 106: 163–175, 1958

Black, M. M., A. J. Asire, H. P. Leis: Cellular responses to autologous breast cancer tissue. Correlation with stage and lymphoreticuloendothelial reaction. Cancer 28: 263–273, 1971

Bloom, H. J. G., W. W. Richardson: Histologic grading and prognosis in breast cancer. A study of 1409 cases in which 359 have been followed for 15 years. Br. J. Cancer 11: 359–377, 1957

Bomhard, D. V., J. v. Sandersleben: Über die Feinstruktur von Mammamischtumoren der Hündin. I. Das Vorkommen von Myoepithelzellen in myxoiden Arealen. Virchows Arch. Abt. A. 359: 87–96, 1973

Bomhard, D. V., J. v. Sandersleben: II. Das Vorkommen von Myoepithelzellen in chondroiden Arealen. Virchows Arch. Abt. A. 362: 157–167, 1974

Bonadonna, G.: Improved disease free and overall survival in operable breast cancer (N+) by surgical adjuvant chemotherapy. Vortr. Internat. Congress on Senology Hamburg 27.–31. 5. 1980

Bonadonna, G. P., P. Valagussa, A. Rossi, G. Tancini, C. Brambilla, S. Marchini, V. Veronesi: Multimodal therapy with CMF in resectable breast cancer with positive axillary nodes: The Milan Institute Experience. In: S. E. Salmon, S. E. Jones (eds.): Adjuvant therapy of Cancer III. Grune & Stratton, New York 1981, p. 435

Bonser, G. M., J. A. Dossett, J. W. Jull: Human and experimental breast cancer. Pitman Medical, London 1961

Breckenridge, R. L.: Liposarcoma of the breast. Am. J. Clin. Pathol. 24: 954–956, 1954

Bunting, J. S., E. H. Hemsted, J. K. Kremer: The pattern of spread and survival in 596 cases of breast cancer related to clinical staging and histological grade. Clin. Radiol. 27: 9–15, 1976

Bussolati, G., A. Pich: Mammary and extramammary Paget's disease. An immuno-cytochemical study. Am. J. Pathol. 80: 117–128, 1975

Buzanowski-Konakry, K., E. G. Harrison Jr., W. S. Payne: Lobular carcinoma arising in fibroadenoma of the breast. Cancer 35: 450–456, 1975

Carstens, H. B., A. G. Huvos, F. W. Foote, R. Ashikari: Tubular carcinoma of the breast. A clinicopathologic study of 35 cases. Am. J. Clin. Pathol. 58: 231–238, 1972

Carter, D., R. R. L. Smith: Carcinoma in situ of the breast. Cancer 40: 1189–1193, 1977

Chabon, A. B., R. J. Stenger, D. Tierstein, E. A. Johnson: Ultrastructural features of breast carcinomas in relation to their estrogen receptor activity. Vortr.: First Internat. Congr. on Hormones and Cancer, Rom 3.–6.10. 1979

Citoler, P., H.-H. Zippel: Carcinombefall der Mamille bei Mammacarcinomen. Gynäkologe 7: 186–189, 1974

Curran, R. C., O. G. Dodge: Sarcoma of the breast with particular reference to its origin in fibroadenoma. J. Clin. Pathol. 15: 1–16, 1962

Davies, J. D.: Hyperelastosis, obliteration and fibrous plaques in major ducts of the human breast. J. Pathol. 110: 13–26, 1973

Douglas, J. G., A. A. Shivas: The origin of elastica in breast carcinoma. J. Roy. Coll. Surg. Edinburgh 19: 89–93, 1974

Egger, H., A. H. Tulusan, M. L. Schneider: Surrounding lesions of small mammary cancers. Vortr. First Internat. Symp. on Minimal Invasive Cancer, Graz, 1.–4. Juli 1981

Eusebi, V., A. Pich, E. Macchiorlatti, G. Bussolati: Morpho-functional differentiation in lobular carcinoma of the breast. Histopathology 1: 301–314, 1977

Farrow, J. H.: Current concepts in the detection and treatment of the earliest of the early breast cancer. Cancer 25: 468–477, 1970

Fechner, R. E.: Infiltrating lobular carcinoma without lobular carcinoma in situ. Cancer 29: 1539–1545, 1972

Fenoglio, C., R. Lattes: Sclerosing papillary proliferations in the female breast. A benign lesion often mistaken for carcinoma. Cancer 33: 691–700, 1974

Fisher, B., N. H. Slack: Number of lymph nodes examined and the prognosis of breast carcinoma. Surg. Gynecol. Obstet. 131: 79–88, 1970

Fisher, B., E. A. Saffer, E. R. Fisher: Studies concerning the regional lymph node in cancer. IV. Tumor inhibition by regional lymph node cells. Cancer 33: 631–636, 1974

Fisher, E. R.: The pathologist's role in the diagnosis and treatment of invasive breast cancer. Surg. Clin. North Am. 58: 705–721, 1978

Fisher, E. R., R. M. Gregorio, B. Fisher: The pathology of invasive breast cancer. A syllabus derived from findings of the national surgical adjuvant breast project (protocol No. 4). Cancer 36: 1–263, 1975

Fisher, E. R., A. Paleka, H. Rockette, G. Redmond, B. Fisher: Pathologic findings from the national surgical adjuvant breast project (protocol No. 4). V. Significance of axillary node micro- and macrometastases. Cancer 42: 2032–2038, 1978

Fisher, E. R., S. Swamidoss, C. H. Lee, H. Rockette, C. Redmond, B. Fisher: Detection and Significance of occult axillary node metastases in patients with invasive breast cancer. Cancer 42 (1978) 2025–2031

Flores, L., M. Arlen, A. Elguezabal, S. F. Livingston, B. S. Levowitz: Host tumor relationships in medullary carcinoma of the breast. Surg. Gynecol. Obstet. 139: 683–688, 1974

Frable, W. J., S. Kay: Carcinoma of the breast. Histologic and clinical features of apocrine tumors. Cancer 21: 756–763, 1968

Freedman, L. S., D.-N. Eduards, E. M. McConnell, D. Y. Sownham: Histological grade and other prognostic factors in relation to survival of patients with breast cancer. Br. J. Cancer 40: 44–55, 1979

Friedell, G. H., A. Betts, S. C. Sommers: The prognostic value of blood vessel invasion and lymphocytic infiltrates in breast carcinoma. Cancer 18: 164–166, 1965

Gallager, H. S. (ed.): Early breast cancer. Detection and treatment. John Wiley & Sons, New York 1975

Gallager, H. S., J. E. Martin: Early phases in the development of breast cancer. Cancer .474: 1170–1178, 1969

Giffler, R. F., S. Kay: Small cell carcinoma of the male mammary gland. A tumor resembling infiltrating lobular carcinoma. Am. J. Clin. Pathol. 66: 715–722, 1976

Gillis, S. A., M. B. Dockerty, O. T. Glagett: Preinvasive intraductal carcinoma of the breast. Surg. Gynecol. Obstet. 110: 555–562, 1960

Goldman, R. L., N. B. Friedman: Carcinoma of the breast arising in fibroadenomas with emphasis on lobular carcinoma Cancer 23: 544–550, 1969

Gonzalez-Licea, A., J. H. Yardley, W. H. Hartmann: Malignant tumor of the breast with bone formation. Cancer 20: 1234–1247, 1966

Haagensen, C. D.: Diseases of the breast. W. B. Saunders, Philadelphia 1971

Haagensen, C. D., S. B. Bhonslay, R. J. Guttmann, D. T. Habif, S. J. Kister, A. M. Markowitz, G. Sanger, P. Tretter, P. D. Wiedel, E. Cooley: Metastasis of carcinoma of the breast to the periphery of the regional lymph node filter. Am. Surg. 169: 175–190, 1969

Haagensen, C. D., C. R. Feind, F. B. Herter, C. A. Slanetz, J. A. Weinberg: The lymphatics in cancer. Saunders, Philadelphia 1972

Halverson, J. D., J. M. Hori-Robaina: Cystosarcoma phyllodes of the breast. Am. Surg. 40: 295–301, 1974

Hamlin, J. M.: Possible host resistance in carcinoma of the breast: A histological study. Br. J. Cancer 22: 383–401, 1968

Hamperl, H.: Zur Frage der pathologisch-anatomischen Grundlagen der Mammographie. Geburtsh. Frauenheilk. 28: 901–917, 1968

Hamperl, H.: The myothelia (myoepithelial) cells. Normal state, regressive changes, hyperplasia, tumors. Clin. Trials Pathol. 53: 161–220, 1970

Hamperl, H.: Das lobuläre Carcinoma in situ der Mamma. Histogenese, Wachstum, Übergang in infiltrierendes Karzinom. Dtsch. Med. Wschr. 96: 1585–1588, 1971

Hamperl, H.: Beiträge zur pathologischen Histologie der Mamma. VI. Hämangiome der menschlichen Mamma. Geburtsh. Frauenheilk. 33: 13–17, 1973

Hamperl, H.: Beiträge zur pathologischen Histologie der Mamma. XI. Strahlige Narben und obliterierende Mastopathie. Virchows Arch. pathol. Anat. 369: 55, 1975

Heuson, J. C., E. Longeval, W. H. Mattheiem, M. C. Deboel, R. J. Sylvester, G. Leclercq: Significance of quantitative assessment of estrogen receptors for endocrine therapy in advanced breast cancer. Cancer 39: 1971–1977, 1977

Hübner, G., O. Kleinsasser, H. J. Klein: Zur Feinstruktur der Speichelgangcarcinome. Ein Beitrag zur Rolle der Myoepithelzellen in Speicheldrüsengeschwülsten. Virchows Arch. Pathol. Anat. 346: 1–14, 1969

Huhn, F. O., G. Stock: Zur Frage eingeschränkter sowie begrenzter Behandlungsmöglichkeiten von Mammakarzinomen. Befunddokumentation an 400 Operationspräparaten. Geburtsh. Frauenheilk. 37: 686–691, 1977

Huvos, A. G., R. V. P. Hutter, J. W. Berg: Significance of axillary macrometastases and micrometastases in mammary cancer. Ann. Surg. 173: 44–46, 1971

Jackson, D., A. O. Severance: The plateau test in breast carcinoma. Tex. State J. Med. 40: 328, 1944

Jackson, J. G., J. W. Orr: The ducts of carcinomatous breasts with particular reference to connective tissue changes. J. Pathol. Bact. 74: 265–273, 1957

Jackson, A. V.: Metastasizing liposarcoma of the breast arising in a fibroadenoma. J. Pathol. Bact. 83: 582–584, 1962

Kennedy, T., J. D. Biggard: Sarcoma of the breast. Br. J. Cancer 21: 635–644, 1967

Kister, S. J., S. C. Sommers, C. J. Haagensen, E. Cooley: Reevaluation of blood vessel invasion as a prognostic factor in carcinoma of the breast. Cancer 19: 1213–1216, 1960

Kister, S. J., S. C. Sommers, C. D. Haagensen: Nuclear grade and sinushistiocytosis in cancer of the breast. Cancer 23: 570–575, 1969

Klein, P. J., M. Vierbuchen, K.-D. Schulz, H. Würz, P. Citoler, G. Uhlenbruck, M. Ortmann, R. Fischer: Hormonabhängige Lektin-Bindungsstellen. II. Lektin-Rezeptoren als Indikator einer Hormonsensibilität vom Mammakarzinom. In G. Uhlenbruck, G. Wintzer: Symposium Carcinoembryonales Antigen (CEA) und andere Tumormarker. Tumor Diagnostik Verlag, Leonberg 1981

Kleinert, H.: Häufigkeit primärer doppelseitiger Mammakarzinome. Med. Klinik 63: 674–679, 1968

Kouchoukos, N. T., L. V. Ackerman, H. R. Butcher Jr.: Prediction of axillary nodal metastases from the morphology of primary mammary carcinomas. Cancer 20: 948–960, 1967

Kraus, F. T., R. D. Neubecker: The differential diagnosis of papillary tumors of the breast. Cancer 15: 444–455, 1962

Kreibig, W.: Zur Kenntnis seltener Geschwulstformen der weiblichen Brustdrüse. Virchows Arch. pathol. Anat. 256: 649–665, 1925

Lagios, M. D., P. R. Westdahl, F. R. Hargolin, M. K. Rose: Duct carcinoma in situ. Relationship of extent of non invasive disease to the frequency of occult invasion, multicentricity, lymph node metastases, and short-term treatment failures. Cancer 50 (1982) 1309–1314

Leis, H.P.: Diagnosis and treatment of breast lesions. Medical Examination Publ. Co. Inc., New York 1970

Leis, H. P. Jr., W. L. Mersheimer, M. M. Black, A. D. Chabon: The second breast. N. Y. State J. Med. 65: 2460–2468, 1965

Lester, J., A. P. Stout: Cystosarcoma phyllodes. Cancer 7: 335–353, 1954

Linell, F., O. Ljungberg, I. Andersson: Breast carcinoma. Aspects of early stages, progression and related problems. Munksgaard, Copenhagen 1980

Llombart-Bosch, A., A. Peydro: Malignant mixed osteogenic tumors of the breast. An ultrastructural study of two cases. Virchows Arch. Pathol. Anat. 366: 1–14, 1975

Maass, H., G. Trams, H. Nowakowski, G. Stolzenbach: Steroidhormone receptors in human breast cancer and the clinical significance. J. Steroid Biochem. 6: 743, 1975

Martinez u. Azzopardi 1979 zit. nach Azzopardi 1979

McCarty, K. Jr., Th. K. Barton, B. W. Fester, B. H. Woodard, J. A. Mossler, W. Reeves, J. Daly, W. E. Wilkinson, Sr. S. McCarty: Correlation of estrogen and progesterone receptors with histologic differentiation in mammary carcinoma. Cancer 46: 2851–2858, 1980

McDivitt, R. W., F. W. Stewart, J. H. Farrow: Breast carcinoma arising in solitary fibroadenomas. Surg. Gynecol. Obstet. 125: 572–576, 1967

McDivitt, R. W., F. W. Stewart, J. W. Berg: Tumors of the breast. Atlas of tumor pathology, 2nd series, Fasc. 2. Armed Forces Inst. of Pathology, Washington, D. C. 1968

McDivitt, R. W., R. V. P. Hutter, F. W. Foote, F. W. Stewart: In situ lobular carcinoma. A prospective follow-up study indicating cumulative patient risks. J. Am. Med. Assoc. 201: 82–86, 1969

McGuire, W. L., K. B. Horwitz, M. Delagaza: A biochemical basis for selecting endocrine therapy in human breast cancer. In: Breast Cancer: Trends in Research and Treatment. Raven Press, New York 1975

Moore, O. S., F. W. Foote Jr.: A relatively favorable prognosis of medullary carcinoma of the breast. Cancer 2: 635–642, 1949

Moore, R. D., R. Chapnick, M. D. Schoenberg: Lymph nodes associated with carcinoma of the breast. Cancer 13: 545–549, 1960

Müller, J.: Über den feineren Bau und die Formen der wechselhaften Geschwülste. Reimer, Berlin 1838

Mylius, E. A.: The identification and the role of the myoepithelial cell in salivary gland tumors. Acta Pathol. Microbiol. Scand. 139 (suppl.): 1–59, 1960

Neubecker, R. D., R. P. Bradshaw: Mucin, melanin, and glycogen in Paget's disease of the breast. Am. J. Clin. Pathol. 36: 49–53, 1961

Norris, H. J., H. B. Taylor: Relationship of histologic features to behavior of cystosarcoma phyllodes. Analysis of ninety-four cases. Cancer 20: 2090–2099, 1967

Norris, H. J., H. B. Taylor: Sarcomas and related mesenchymal tumors of the breast. Cancer 22: 22–28, 1968

Obermann, H. A.: Sarcomas of the breast. Cancer 18: 1233–1243, 1965

Ozzello, L.: Ultrastructure of intraepithelial carcinomas of the breast. Cancer 28: 1508–1515, 1971

Pickren, J. W.: Significance of occult metastases. A study of breast cancer. Cancer 14: 1260–1271, 1961

Prechtel, K.: Beziehungen der Mastopathien zum Mammakarzinom. Fortschr. Med. 89: 1312–1315, 1971

Ramos, C. V., H. B. Taylor: Lipid-rich carcinoma of the breast. A clinicopathologic analysis of 13 cases. Cancer 33: 812–819, 1974

Richardson, W. W.: Medullary carcinoma of the breast: A distinctive tumor type with a relatively good prognosis following radical mastectomy. Br. J. Cancer 10: 415–423, 1956

Ridolfi, R. V., P. P. Rosen, A. Port, D. Kinne, V. Mike: Medullary carcinoma of the breast. A clinicopathologic study with 10 years follow-up. Cancer 40: 1365–1385, 1977

Robb, D. M., A. McFarlane: Two rare breast tumours. J. Pathol. Bact. 75: 293–298, 1958

Robbins, G. F., J. W. Berg: Bilateral primary breast cancers. Cancer 17: 1501, 1964

Robbins, G. F., J. Shah, P. Rosen, F. Chu, J. Taylor: Inflammatory carcinoma of the breast. Surg. Clin. North Am. 54: 801–810, 1974

Rosen, P. P., C. J. Mendez-Botet, J. A. Urban, A. Fracchia, M. K. Schwartz: Estrogen receptor protein (ERP) in multiple tumor specimens from individual patients with breast cancer. Cancer 39: 2194–2200 (1977)

Sachs, H., B. Mayer, J. Bahnsen: Carcinoma lobulare in situ der Mamma. Med. Welt 27: 1819–1825, 1976

Sagebiel, R. W.: Ultrastructural observations on epidermal cells in Paget's disease of the breast. Am. J. Pathol. 57: 49–64, 1969

Sandison, A. T.: An autopsy study of the adult human breast. Nat. Cancer Inst. Monogr. No. 8 US Dept. of Health, Education, and Welfare, Washington, D. C. 1962

Saphir, O., G. B. Amromin: Obscure axillary lymph node metastases in carcinoma of the breast. Cancer 1: 238–247, 1948

Scarff, R. W., H. Torloni: Histological typing of breast tumors, International histological classification of tumours No. 2. WHO Genf 1968

Scarpelli, D. G., T. M. Murat: Recent contributions to our knowledge about the pathology of breast cancer. In M. L. Griem, E. V. Jensen, J. E. Ultmann, R. W. Wissler: Breast Cancer: A Challenging Problem. Springer, New York 1973

Schiodt, T.: Breast carcinoma. A histologic and prognostic study of 650 followed-up cases. Munksgaard, Copenhagen 1966

Schremmer, C.-N.: Die Größe der axillaren Lymphknoten beim Brustdrüsenkrebs der Frau nach präoperativer Bestrahlung mittels Telekobalt. Zbl. Chir. 100: 862–867, 1975

Schwartz, G. F.: Solid circumscribed carcinoma of the breast. Am. Surg. 169: 165–173, 1969

Seifert, G.: Mundhöhle, Mundspeicheldrüsen, Tonsillen und Rachen. In W. Doerr, E. Uehlinger: Spezielle pathologische Anatomie. Springer, New York 1966

Shah, J. P., P. P. Rosen, G. Robbins: Pitfalls of local excision in the treatment of carcinoma of the breast. Surg. Gynecol. Obstet. 136: 721–725, 1973

Shivas, A. A., J. G. Douglas: The prognostic significance of elastosis in breast carcinoma. J. Roy. Coll. Surg. Edinburgh 17: 315–320, 1972

Silverberg, S. G., A. R. Chitale: Assessment of significance of proportions of intraductal and infiltrating tumor growth in ductal carcinoma of the breast. Cancer 32: 830–837, 1973

Slack, N. H., T. Nemoto, B. Fisher: Experience with bilateral primary carcinoma of the breast. Surg. Gynecol. Obstet. 136: 433–440, 1973

Smith, B. H., H. B. Taylor: The occurrence of bone and cartilage in mammary tumors. Am. J. Clin. Pathol. 51: 610–618, 1969

Stegner, H.-E.- Morphologie prämaligner und maligner Veränderungen der Mamma. Gynäkologe 10: 129, 1977

Stegner, H.-E., C. Pape, B. Studt: Mikrocalcifikation bei Mammaerkrankungen. Histologische und ultrastrukturelle Aspekte. Arch. Gynäk. 212: 358–379, 1972

Stegner, H.-E., C. Pape: Beitrag zur Feinstruktur der sog. Mikrokalzifikation in Mammatumoren. Zbl. Allg. Pathol. Anat. 115: 106–112, 1972

Stegner, H.-E., H. Maass: Prognostische Kriterien aus der licht- und elektronenmikroskopischen Struktur der Mammakarzinome. Verh. Dtsch. Ges. Pathol. 57: 345–347, 1973

Stegner, H.-E., H. Maass, G. Trams, C. Pape: Estrogen receptors and ultrastructural pathology of mammary carcinoma. In G. Dallenbach: Functional morphologic changes in female sex organs induced by exogenous hormones. Springer, New York 1980

Stegner, H.-E., K. Fischer, A. Poschmann: Immunhistochemical localization of Thomsen-Friedreich antigen in normal and malignant breast tissue using peroxidase-antiperoxidase technique. Tumor Diagnostik 3: 127–130, 1981

Stegner, H.-E., J. Bahnsen, E. Fischer: Tumorgrading beim Mammakarzinom anhand licht- und elektronenmikroskopischer Kriterien. Pathol. Res. Pract. 173: 159–171 (1981)

Stenkvist, B., S. Westman-Naeser, J. Vegelius, J. Holmquist, B. Nordin, E. Bengtsson, O. Eriksson: Analysis of reproducibility of subjective grading systems for breast cancer. J. Clin. Pathol. 32: 979–985, 1979

Stocks, L. H., F. M. Simmons-Patterson: Inflammatory carcinoma of the breast. Surg. Gynecol. Obstet. 143: 885–889, 1976

Sümegi, I., G. Rajka: Amyloid-like substance surrounding mammary cancer and basal cell carcinoma. Acta Pathol. Microbiol. 80: 185–192, 1972

Taylor, H. B., H. J. Norris: Epithelial invasion of nerves in benign diseases of the breast. Cancer 20: 2245–2249, 1967

Teel, P., S. C. Sommers: Vascular invasion as a prognostic factor in breast carcinoma. Surg. Gynecol. Obstet. 118: 1006–1008, 1964

Tellem, M., L. Prive, D. R. Meranze: Four quadrant study of breast removed for carcinoma. Cancer 15: 10, 1962

Terenius, L., H. Johansson, A. Rimsten, L. Thosen: Malignant and benign human mammary disease: Estrogen binding in relation to clinical data. Cancer 33: 1364–1368, 1974

Thomsen, K., H.-E. Stegner, H.-J. Frischbier: Grundlagen und Grenzen der brusterhaltenden Therapie kleiner Mammakarzinome. Gynäkologe 13: 56–66, 1980

Treves, N., D. A. Sunderland: Cystosarcoma phyllodes of the breast: A malignant and a benign tumor. A clinicopathological study of 77 cases. Cancer 4: 1286–1332, 1951

Tsakaklides, V., P. Olson, J. H. Kersey: Prognostic significance of the regional lymph node histology in cancer of the breast. Cancer 34: 1259–1266, 1974

Urban, J. A.: Bilateral breast cancer. Cancer 24: 1310–1312, 1969

Van Bogaert, L.-J.: The proliferative behavior of the human adult mammary epithelium. Acta Cytol. 23: 252–257, 1979

Veronesi, U., R. Saccozzi, M. Delvecchio, A. Banfi, C. Clemente, M. De Lena, G. Gallus, M. Greco, A. Luini, E. Marubini, G. Muscolino, F. Bilke, B. Salvadori, A. Zecchini, R. Zucali: Comparing radical mastectomy with quadrantectomy, axillary dissection, and radiotherapy in patients with small cancers of the breast. N. Engl. J. Med. 305: 6–11, 1981

Vogt-Hoerner, G., R. Gerard-Marchant: Technique anatomo-pathologique de recherche et d'examen des ganglions lymphatiques. Bull. Cancer 45: 446, 1958

Wallgren, A., C. Silfverswaerd: Clinical and histological factors of prognostic importance in breast cancer. Int. J. Radiat. Oncol. Biol. Phys. 1: 611–617, 1976

Wartman, W. D.: Sinus cell hyperplasia of lymph nodes regional to adenocarcinoma of the breast and colon. Br. J. Cancer 13: 389–397, 1959

Wellings, S. R., H. M. Jensen, R. G. Marcum: An atlas of subgross pathology of the human breast with special reference to possible precancerous lesions. J. Natl. Cancer Inst. 55: 231–273, 1975

Westbrook, K. G., H. S. Gallager: Intraductal carcinoma in the breast. A comparative study. Am. J. Surg. 130: 667–670, 1975

Wheeler, J. E., H. T. Enterline: Lobular carcinoma of the breast in situ and infiltrating. In S. C. Sommers: Pathology Annual. Vol. 11. Appleton-Century-Corp., New York 1976

Wittliff, J. L., B. W. Beatty, E. D. Savlov, W. B. Patterson, L. A. Cooper: Estrogen receptors and hormone dependency in human breast cancer. In G. St. Arneault, P. Band, L. Israel: Breast cancer: A multidisciplinary approach. Springer, New York 1976

Wulsin, J. H., J. T. Schreiber: Improved prognosis in certain patterns of carcinoma of the breast. Arch. Surg. 85: 791–800, 1962

Würz, H., K. D. Schulz, P. Citoler, B. Sprenger, P. Weymar, R. Kaiser: Ergebnisse der Steroidrezeptor-Analyse beim Mammakarzinom. In H. Jung: Die Zusatz- und Nachbehandlung des Mammakarzinoms. Enke, Stuttgart 1979

Yogore, M. G., S. Sahgal: Small cell carcinoma of the male breast. Cancer 39: 748–1751, 1977

Zippel, H. H.: Das Mammakarzinom unter besonderer Berücksichtigung der Vor- und Frühstadien. Klinische, histologische, morphologische und zytophotometrische Untersuchungen am Krankengut der Universitäts-Frauenklinik Köln. Fortsch. Med. 97: 159–164, 1979

Zippel, H. H., P. Citoler: DNS-Messungen bei der lobulären Neoplasie der Mamma. Verh. Dtsch. Ges. Gynäkol. Geburtsh. 224: 519, 1977

Chapter 9

Epidemiology in Breast Cancer

H. P. Leis, Jr.

Introduction

Breast cancer is the most common cancer in women, accounting for 27% of all the cancers that develop in them. One out of every eleven women, or about 9%, will develop it during her lifetime. Every 15 minutes there are three new cases. In 1981, in the United States alone, about 110,000 new cases were found. There were over 1 million new cases in the world in 1980.

There is an increasing number of breast cancers in the United States. In 1969, there were 67,000 new cases with an incidence of 1 out of every 15 women, as compared with 110,000 in 1981, with an incidence of one out of every nine women. This is largely due to the fact that there are more women living longer into the cancer-prone years. In addition, there is also an increasing incidence per 100,000 women, predominately in those under the age of 55 and in blacks.

Breast cancer is also the leading cause of cancer death in women, accounting for 19% of these. It is also the leading cause of death due to all causes in women aged 40 to 44. Every 15 minutes, one women dies from it. In the United States alone, in 1981, approximately 36,800 deaths occurred (American Cancer Society 1981).

These facts emphasize the magnitude of the breast cancer problem and stress the importance of determining epidemiologic factors responsible for its development and of trying to isolate any preventive measures that might reduce its incidence (Leis 1970, 1975, 1977a, 1978a, 1979a, 1980a; Leis and Raciti 1976).

Breast cancer appears to be due to a constellation of epidemiologic factors rather than to a single one, including genetic predisposition, adverse hormonal milieu, immunologic incompetence, carcinogen exposure, and various adverse personal and demographic conditions. Therefore, it would seem highly improbable that any one epidemiologic factor of overwhelming importance in breast cancer will be determined, such as the single factor of smoking in the etiology of lung cancer. Although many etiologic factors in breast cancer are beyond the control of the physician and patient, there are a number of preventive measures that could be of importance.

After determining the etiology of breast cancer and defining preventive measures, the most important factor is early diagnosis (Leis 1977b, 1979b, 1980b; Pilnik and Leis 1978). Although one out of every 11 women, or 9%, will develop breast cancer during her lifetime, this is not a chance event that occurs randomly throughout the population. There is a group who has an increased risk for developing it. It is of paramount importance that the full armamentarium of diagnostic modalities be directed toward patients in this high-risk group so that if breast cancer develops in them, it will be detected in an early stage.

Beyond the obvious risk factors of a lump in the breast or of nipple discharge, the ones of major importance are sex, age, family history of breast cancer, previous benign breast disease, precancerous mastopathy, previous cancer in one breast, and adverse hormonal milieu as related to parity. Additional risk factors with a variable importance include other types of adverse hormonal milieu not related to pregnancy, reduced immunologic competence, carcinogenic exposure, adverse personal and demographic factors, certain parenchymal patterns seen on breast x-rays, and abnormal thermograms.

Early diagnosis offers better cure and long-term survival rates with less extensive surgery, less adjuvant therapy, and decreased local recurrence rates. With the use of less extensive procedures there is an improved cosmetic appearance (related to more effective breast reconstructions) and better arm and shoulder function (related to a decrease in arm edema) (Leis 1979c).

The importance of early diagnosis is emphasized in a series of 1,147 patients of ours treated until 1970 with potentially curable breast cancers, 82.9% of whom were treated with less than a radical mastectomy procedure. The ten year, absolute, disease-free survival rate was 64.8%, being 96.2% for those with stage 0 cancers, 73% for those with stage I cancers, and 43.1% for those with stage II cancers. The local recurrence rate was 7.3%, being 0% for those with stage 0 cancers, 5.7% for those with stage I cancers, and 11.9% for those with stage II cancers. Only 2.1% of the patients required skin grafts (Leis 1983a, b). (For definition of staging system, see p. 110, Chapter 10 „Prognosis in Breast Cancer".)

Sex

Obviously, the most significant risk factor is sex, with over 99% of breast cancers occurring in women (American Cancer Society 1981, Silverberg 1979). Short of arranging to have his patients reborn as men (transsexual operations would be to no avail), the physician can do nothing in this regard.

Age

Likewise, physicians have not been able to stop the process of aging and thus are also powerless against the next most important risk factor-age. Over 85% of breast cancers occur after age 45, and 67% after 50. The longer the patient lives the higher is her incidence chance for developing breast cancer (Schottenfeld 1976; Seidman 1972). Ironically, medicine's great accomplishment of dramatically increasing the life span has also brought about an increase in the number of breast cancer cases.

Genetic Predisposition

Response of the host organism to carcinogenic materials is controlled by its own intrinsic or genetic constitution, over which the physician has no control (Anderson 1976, 1977; Strong 1979). Female relatives of women with breast cancer have about a three times increased risk for developing such cancer (Lilienfeld 1963). This degree of risk is variable depending on the number and closeness of affected relatives, whether their cancers occurred in the premenopausal or postmenopausal years, and whether the cancers were unilateral or bilateral (Anderson 1974, 1976, 1977). Thus the risk could be as little as 1.5 times or lower if the relatives were distant with postmenopausal, unilateral cancers, or as much as nine times or higher if they were close relatives, that is mother or sister, and if the cancers were premenopausal and bilateral. Anderson (1977) has described four hereditary types in families with 50% risks.

Genetic predisposition is also underscored by a woman's genetically controlled type of earwax (wet or dry). There is a two times increased risk of breast cancer incidence in patients with the wet type (Matsunga 1962; Petrakis 1971).

There is a five times increased risk for whites compared with Orientals, but this difference in risk dramatically decreases when the latter move to Western nations such as the United States. The reported three times increased incidence in whites as compared with blacks is also diminishing (Thomas and Lilienfeld 1976).

Previous Breast Lesions

Patients who have had a biopsy for a benign breast disease have a tripled risk of breast cancer (Davis et al. 1969) and those with fibrocystic disease about a 2.5 times greater risk (Leis and Kwon 1979; Leis et al. 1978; Davis et al. 1969). Those with precancerous mastopathies, namely ductular or lobular epithelial hyperplasia with marked atypia, and apocrine metaplasia with marked atypia, have a five times increased risk, (Black and Kwon 1980; Black et al. 1972). In a 20-year follow up of 975 women who had benign breast biopsies, Rogers and Page (1979) noted that the risk for developing breast cancer was four to six times that of the general population if atypical lobular hyperplasia was present, and two to three times if atypical ductal hyperplasia was present in a patient over 45 years of age.

Haagenson (1971) reported a four times increased risk of breast cancer in patients with gross cystic disease after studying 1,693 such patients over a 20-year period. In a similar series of 1,720 patients studied by the author for the same period, the increased risk was 2.2 times, which is in keeping with the overall risk factor that has been determined for fibrocystic disease, and probably reflects the simultaneous occurrence of precancerous mastopathies with cystic changes. Today, cyst aspirations are routine (Leis 1980b:; Cammarata 1978), but serious consideration should be given to doing a formal biopsy of the first cyst with the removal of a surrounding wedge of breast tissue to determine whether there are any adverse changes in the tissue around the cyst, namely, precancerous mastopathy, a term coined by Black (Black and Kwon 1980; Black et al. 1972) to represent benign lesions with a high malignant transformation potential.

A radioimmunoassay for plasma levels of a protein isolated from human cyst fluid, called cystic disease protein (CDP), has been developed (Haagensen et al. 1977). In general, the plasma levels of this protein are low or absent in normal women, elevated moderately in a substantial number of women with gross cystic disease, and highly elevated in those with cancers with the levels increasing with disease progression.

Both CDP (Haagensen et al. 1977, 1978) plasma levels and carcinoembryonic antigen (CEA) (Haagensen et al. 1978; Tormey et al. 1977) plasma levels have been used to monitor responsiveness to breast cancer treatment and to indicate disease progression, alone and in combination. The interesting question is whether these markers might be of value in identifying women with preclinical (occult) cancers of the breast.

After removal of a breast for cancer, the risk of a patient's developing a second primary cancer in the remaining breast is five times the risk of initial breast cancer developing in women in the general population (Leis 1978b, 1980c).

There is a subgroup of patients who have an especially high risk for developing a second primary cancer in the other breast. This includes patients whose initial cancer in the first breast carried a good prognosis for extended survival, and whose age and constitutional status did not preclude at least a 20-year normal life expectancy. Thus patients under 50 years of age, in good health, with early cancers (stage 0 and I) that are either noninvasive, or if invasive, of a good prognostic type, are at high risk (Leis 1978b, 1980c; Leis and Urban 1978).

Also included are patients who have special features that indicate an increased risk for bilaterality, such as those with a close family history of breast cancer, especially if it was premenopausal and bilateral, those whose cancers in the first breast were multicentric and those who had evidence of precancerous mastopathy found by random biopsy of their other breast (Leis 1978b, 1980c; Leis and Urban 1978).

Finally those patients whose other breast shows a P2 (prominent duct pattern) or a DY (dense parenchymal pattern) on x-ray (Wolfe 1976), and those with an abnormal thermogram of the remaining breast must be considered to be a high risk (Byrne 1976; Gautherie and Gros 1980).

The physician has an obligation to follow his patients closely and to carefully instruct them in monthly self-breast examination when they have had biopsies for benign breast disease or are known to have fibrocystic disease. Furthermore, the surgeon should discuss with his patient the possibility of doing prophylactic bilateral mastectomies if they have evidence of precancerous mastopathy on their biopsy as well as other high risk factors. He should advise his patients who have undergone a unilateral mastectomy for cancer about prophylactic removal of their other breast, if they are in a high risk group for developing a second primary cancer. Nevertheless, this advice is seldom well received. Appropriate information about breast reconstruction should also be given in this context.

Parity

Nulliparous women have a three times increased risk for developing breast cancer (Thomas and Lilienfeld 1976; Dunn 1969), as attested to by the high incidence of breast cancer in Catholic nuns (Fraumeni et al. 1969). Some reports indicate that the association between breast cancer risk and parity relates to the age at which a woman first gives birth, and that parity exerts its protective influence predominantly against postmenopausal cancers (MacMahon et al. 1973; Henderson at al. 1974; Lilienfeld et al. 1975). Adami et al. (1978) reported, however, that age at birth of a first child did not seem to be an important factor as shown by a case-controlled study done in Sweden. Another finding is that breast feeding does not seem to influence the risk of breast cancer in a woman who has given birth (MacMahon et al. 1970).

There does seem to be about a four times lesser risk of breast cancer if first parity occurred before tha age of 18, and then a less pronounced but still decreased risk up to about the age of 28. After this age, parity shows little beneficial influence on risk. Indeed, if first parity occurs in the midthirties or later, it carries a four times increased risk, higher than that even for nulliparous women (MacMahon et al. 1973).

Parity seems to favorably affect not only the risk of breast cancer but also the subsequent course of the disease in women who do develop cancer. In an analysis of 608 women with operable breast cancer done by Papatestias et al. (1980), there was a five-year disease-free interval in 60% of parous women compared with 46% of nulliparous women.

Other Hormonal Factors

Prolonged menstrual activity increases the incident risk of breast cancer (Thomas and Lilienfeld 1976; Papaivannou 1974). Women whose menarche occurred before the age of 12, or who had 30 or more years of menstrual activity, have a 1.3 times increased risk (MacMahon and Cole 1972; Shapiro et al. 1968). Those whose menopause occurs after age 50 have a 1.5 times increased risk (MacMahon and Cole 1972; Shapiro et al. 1968; Trichopoulas et al. 1972). Artificial menopause (castration) before the age of 37 results in a three times decreased risk (Trichopoulos et al. 1972; Feinlieb 1968; Hirayama and Wynder 1962), but the recommendation of such castration would certainly not be well received.

Bulbrook et al. (1971) in their Guernsey Island studies of urinary androgen excretion, found subnormal levels of etiocholanolone and/or androsterone in women who later developed breast cancer as compared with controls who did not develop cancer, indicating that women with lower androgen urinary excretions are at risk for breast cancer.

The knowledge that some breast cancers are hormone dependent dates back more than 80 years (Leis 1976). There seem to be two types of hormone-dependent cancers. The first occurs in premenopausal women and is related to estradiol and estrone from the ovaries. The second occurs in postmenopausal women and is related to estrone produced through the metabolism of a steroidal precursor elaborated by the adrenal. It is postulated that the endocrine environment simply influences the susceptibility of the breast to carcinogens. It is suggested that when there are long periods of unopposed estrogen stimulation without progesterone antagonism, breast cancer may be induced by carcinogens. There are two open "estrogen windows." The first window opens between the ages of 8 and 10 and stays open until the onset of menses, or even longer if the cycles are anovulatory. The second window opens at about the age of 42 and can remain so for some 13 years. When menses are irregular, the long cycles may be luteally inadequate or anovulatory (Korenman 1980).

Consideration should be given by the physician to the administration of progesterone in selected patients to avoid these prolonged estrogen window phases and, of course, to the use of progesterone on a cyclic basis whenever exogenous estrogens are given (Leis 1976). Lafaye and Oubert (1979) have reported good results in the treatment of benign mastopathies by the local application of a progesterone cream to the breasts daily. Asch and Greenblatt (1977) recommend the use of an impeded androgen, danazol, in the management of benign breast disorders. Although the precise mechanism of danazol action is not known, it seems to blunt or inhibit the luteinizing hormone (LH) effect in the ovulatory woman and reduce gonadotropin levels in the menopausal woman. It suppresses ovarian function, resulting in a reduction of cyclic hormone stimulation of the breast. Recent studies indicate that it has a direct inhibitory effect on steroid receptors in target tissues.

Although not all studies agree, epidemiologic data suggest that women at increased risk for developing breast cancer excrete less estriol than estradiol and estrone. Estradiol is a stronger symptomatic estrogen and a weaker carcinogen than estrone, whereas estriol has a minimal, if any, symptomatic action and no carcinogenic potential (Leis 1976). Lemon (1970) postulates that estriol binds receptor sites and exerts an impeding or blocking action on the potential carcinogenic effects of estradiol and estrone. This could explain the protective influence of early parity. If a pure estriol fraction could be isolated, then one might consider its administration to young women who did not want to have a child at an early age, and it would seem logical to include it in any estrogen preparation for exogenous administration that contains estradiol or estrone.

A number of investigators have proposed a link between hypothyroidism and an increased risk for developing breast cancer (Blackwinkel and Jackson 1964; Edelstyn 1958), and others have claimed that thyroid hormones are even useful in the prevention and treatment of breast cancer (Lemon 1955; Loeser 1954). Although a report by Kapdi and Wolfe (1976) suggested that the prolonged intake of thyroid supplements might increase breast cancer risk, there seems to be general agreement that women with indications for taking thyroid supplements should continue to do so, and that hypothyroid patients should at least be maintained in a euthyroid state to avoid a possible increase in breast cancer risk (Gorman et al. 1977).

Shapiro et al. (1980) conducted a case-controlled study to determine whether the use of thyroid supplements increased the risk of breast cancer. Overall they found no grounds to suggest that the long-term use of thyroid supplements increased the risk of breast cancer.

Prolactin has been implicated in breast cancer epidemiology in some reports (Minton and Dickey 1973; McCallister and Welbourn 1962; Murray et al. 1972), but not in others (Lipsett and Bergenstal 1960; Wilson et al. 1974). Meites (1979) states that estrogen and progesterone cannot promote the growth and development of the breasts without the pituitary hormones and that prolactin is the most important of these hormones in the growth and development of the breast and in lactation.

Dopamine from the hypothalamus and dopamine-related drugs (reserpine, phenothiazines, chlorpromazine, dextroamphetamine, and others) inhibit the production of prolactin, whereas serotonin, also from the hypothalamus, as well as opiate peptides, thyrotropin, oral contraceptives, estrogens, and hormones from pituitary adenomas, increase its production. Both increased and decreased prolactin production and the agents causing them have been discussed in breast cancer epidemiology. At best the most that can be said is that the role of prolactin in breast cancer epidemiology is poorly understood (Leis 1976). Blichert-Toft et al. (1979) reported that bromocriptine, a prolactin-inhibiting drug, relieved mastalgia in fibrocystic breast disease. They hypothesized that it stopped breast pain by lowering serum prolactin concentrations, thereby decreasing the total stimulatory effect on the breast.

Despite all the evidence that estrogens are involved in the epidemiology of breast cancer, it is difficult to obtain any statistically valid evidence to indicate that the widespread use of estrogens for contraceptive purposes and menopausal symptoms is associated with an increased risk for developing breast cancer (Leis 1976). The report by Hoover et al. (1976) indicating that there might be a

relationship was based on a study of 1,891 women given conjugated estrogens for symptoms related to menopause for a mean period of 12 years. Forty-nine cases of breast cancer were observed as compared with an expected 39.1 cases, but the study did not indicate a definite cause and effect relationship between estrogen administration and breast cancer.

Black et al. (1980), in ongoing studies of their patients, have noted that although exogenous estrogen administration may have no observable impact on breast cancer incidence in the population as a whole, there may be subgroups that could be negatively affected. One group is that of premenopausal women, especially under the age of 35, with a family history of breast cancer who are taking oral contraceptives. Another group is that of menopausal women who are nulliparous or late parous who are taking estrogen replacement therapy. In these subgroups that have an already increased risk for developing breast cancer because of thier familial medical history and ther own nulliparity, there is a two times further risk from the use of exogenous estrogens. It is interesting to note that a recent report by Black et al. (1980) indicates that family history and oral contraceptive usage is especially important in women if their grandmothers or aunts were the ones who had breast cancer.

On the other hand, in premenopausal women under 40 with no familial history of breast cancer and in women aged 40 to 54 regardless of familial history, the use of oral contraceptives seems to reduce breast cancer development, as does estrogen replacement therapy in menopausal women with early first parity.

Paffenbarger et al. (1977) noted increases for women with prior history of benign breast disease who used oral contraceptives for six or more years. Brinton et al. (1979) found women to be at excess risk from birth control pills only if they had a history of previous breast biopsy, family history of breast cancer, or were older when their first child was born.

Greenwald et al. (1981) in discussing the relationship between breast cancer and menopausal exogenous estrogen administration, stated that there were six case-controlled studies as of January 1981 on this subject. Five showed no consistent relationship between menopausal estrogens and breast cancer. The one positive study by Ross et al. (1980) showed a moderately elevated risk that appeared to be limited to the subgroup of women who had intact ovaries and were exposed to high cumulative doses.

Immunologic Incompetence

There is an ever increasing body of evidence that suggests that immunologic mechanisms play an important role in the epidemiology of human breast cancer. Markers are being studied to measure the degree of immunocompetence of the host. Although still in the experimental stage, the entire field of immunology holds great promise for the future (Black 1977; Black and Zachrau 1978; Humphrey et al. 1980; Serrou et al. 1974).

At present, all that can be said is that there are certain patients with known immunologic deficiencies who have an increased risk for developing breast cancer, including older patients with thymic atrophy, other patients with decreased thymus-dependent lymphocytes, patients on chemotherapy, patients on immunosuppressant drugs, and patients exposed to heavy ionizing radiation (Leis 1978a, 1979a, 1980a; Leis and Raciti 1976).

Physicians must make an all-out effort to find ways of determining which patients are immunodeficient and to develop drugs or methods that could stimulate immunologic defense mechanisms. Of course, drugs known to reduce immunologic competence should be avoided whenever possible. Corticosteroids are often prescribed when they are not really needed, and only time can tell whether the use of adjuvant chemotherapy in breast cancer will result in benefits that reflect its theoretical advantages, or whether we will have actually done a disservice to our patients by reducing their immunologic competence.

Carcinogen Exposure

Several factors indicate that a viral agent, such as the mouse tumor virus (MTV), might be involved in the development of human breast cancer (Dmochowski et al. 1969; Spiegelman et al. 1980). Viral particles, similar to those found in the milk of mice with breast cancer that can be transmitted to the offspring causing mouse mammary carcinoma, have been found in the milk of women with breast cancer and in the milk of women with a familial history of breast cancer (Moore et al. 1969, 1971). This suggests the possibility that women who are asymptomatic, but carriers of such a B-type virus, are at increased risk for developing breast cancer, and that possibly it might be improper for women with a familial history of breast cancer to nurse their offspring.

Three case-controlled studies have reported a 2 to 3.5 times increased risk of breast cancer in women taking the rauwolfia alkaloid (reserpine) for hypertension (Armstrong et al. 1974; Boston CDSP 1971; Heinomen et al. 1974). However, Labarthe and O'Fallon (1980) in a community-based longitudinal study of 2,000 hypertensive women, found no evidence of such increased risk.

An association between alcohol consumption and increased breast cancer incidence has also been suggested (Williams 1976), and several common drugs have been implicated as possible cancer promoters, although there is no statistically, valid evidence to this effect, including methyldopa, phenothiazine, dextroamphetamine, some antidepressants, and some antihistamines. Certain chemicals, such as the polycyclic hydrocarbons as well as large doses of ionizing radiation, have potential carcinogenic effects (Williams 1976; Levin et al. 1974; Shubik and Hartwell 1957; Land 1980).

Recently, the question of whether methylzanthine, which is found in coffee, tea, cocoa, and cola or any product with caffeine, could be a carcinogen as well as a promoter of fibrocystic disease proliferation has been raised (Minton 1983).

The first recorded use of hair dyes was during the Egyptian third dynasty some 4,000 years ago (Heenan 1974). Some investigators have reported an increased risk of breast cancer in women exposed to hair dyes (Nasca et al. 1980; Shore et al. 1979), whereas others have not (Kinlen et al. 1977). A list of the ingredients in hair dyes that have caused cancer in laboratory animals may be obtained from the National Cancer Institute (Griesemar 1978. Although direct extrapolation of results from animals to humans is not possible, the Institute's test results do serve as a warning that these chemicals may be carcinogenic in humans (Griesemar 1978).

Ionizing Radiation

Although the carcinogenic effects of large doses of ionizing radiation may be delayed for 20 or more years (Land 1980; Advisory Committee 1972), there are certain patients, because of their past exposure, who have an increased risk for developing breast cancer including

1. Those who had multiple fluoroscopies for tuberculosis control (Mackenzie 1965; Boice and Monson 1977)

2. Those who had an excessive number of high dose diagnostic breast x-rays (Bailar 1976)

3. Those who had radiation treatments for mastitis (Mettler et al. 1969; Shore et al. 1977), gynecomastia (Lowell et al. 1968), and bleeding nipples, and now possibly in the ever increasing number of women who have chosen radiotherapy instead of surgery for the treatment of their breast cancers (Check 1981)

4. Those who received radiation treatment over the skin of the breast for acne and keloids (Baral et al. 1977)

5. Those exposed to ionizing radiation from atomic bombings such as at Hiroshima and Nagasaki (Wanebo et al. 1968; McGregor et al. 1977).

There is a considerable difference in radiation sensitivity in various ages (Upton 1977; Upton et al. 1977). The populations from which risk estimates have been made consisted largely of women under 30 years of age. Women exposed at over 30 years of age have an absolute risk less than half of that for younger women (Upton 1977; Upton et al. 1977).

Not only should physicians advise their patients about possible carcinogenic agents, but they should also use radiation carefully, both diagnostically and therapeutically, trying to keep the radiation dosage at a low level.

Regarding breast x-rays, it is important at the outset to differentiate between diagnostic and screening techniques. In the differential diagnosis of breast lesions, diagnostic mammography is an important aid, but it still should be used selectively and carefully with low-dose techniques. In diagnostic mammography, we do not advise it for patients under 25 years of age and for patients between 25 and 34 it is utilized as little as possible.

On the other hand, mammography for screening purposes on a yearly basis is a subject of considerable debate (Bailar 1976). Large doses of ionizing radiation produced an increased incidence of breast cancer as was seen from atomic exposures (Wanebo et al. 1968; McGregor et al. 1977), fluoroscoped patient (Mackenzie 1965; Boice and Monson 1977), and patients treated with radiation for mastitis (Mettler et al. 1969; Shore et al. 1977). Based on a linear hypothesis (Land 1980; Advisory Committee 1972) estimating risk from low doses by extrapolating from the observed risk from high doses, it was postulated that even relatively small doses of radiation could increase the risk for developing breast cancer when used routinely as a screening procedure over a period of years (Bailar 1976). Modern equipment has reduced radiation exposure to very low levels with better accuracy, especially in patients under 50 years of age.

The Consensus Development Meeting on Breast Cancer Screening (1977), held at the National Cancer Institute in September 1977, made certain recommendations for breast cancer screening with mammography, and the National Breast Cancer Task Force of the American Cancer Society in 1979, supported these recommendations which are as follows;

1. All women over the age of 50 may continue to have mammograms annually

2. Women 40 to 49 may have yearly mammography if they or their mothers or sisters have had breast cancer

3. Women from 35 on may have yearly mammography only if they have a personal history of breast cancer

4. A baseline mammogram for future reference should be done at the age of 35 to 40

In other patients, mammography is used at the judgment of the physician based on the difficulty of evaluating the breast clinically and the patient's number of risk factors as related to breast cancer development.

Personal and Demographic Factors

A 1.5 times increased risk for developing breast cancer has been reported for women living in a cold climate and in the western hemisphere (Stoll 1976). A two times increased risk has even been noted for affluent women, for Jewish women (Stoll 1976), and for those women with chronic psychologic stress, especially if they have and abnormal suppression of anger (Greer 1976).

The incidence of breast cancer varies markedly from one country to another. Rates tend to be higher in the developed countries, with populations of predominant European descent, and low in less-developed countries and in those with nonwhite populations. There is also a considerable variance of breast cancer rates in various sections of different countries (Thomas and Lilienfeld 1976; Stoll 1976).

Studies related to these variations in incidence by geographic area suggest that environmental, not racial or genetic factors, are responsible for these differences. This is emphasized by an increasing incidence of breast cancer when people from countries with a low incidence rate move to western countries and develop an increased incidence rate despite continuing to marry within their own race. This is well documented by the changing incidence from low to high of Japanese women who moved to Hawaii or mainland United States. The main factor that seemed to change was dietary with these patients assuming a western type of diet and becoming more obese (Thomas and Lilienfeld 1976; Stoll 1976).

There is a doubled risk of breast cancer for obese women, and a tripled risk for obese women with a wide body type and for those with the triad of obesity, diabetes, and hypertension (Leis 1978a; Thomas and Lilienfeld 1976; Stoll 1976; Miller 1981). There is a similar three times increased risk for those with a high dietary fat intake (Wynder 1980; Wynder et al. 1976, 1978). There is mounting evidence that the incidence of both breast and colon cancer might be reduced by a high fish and grain diet, and low beef and fat diet including milk products (Wynder 1980). Studies have indicated not only that selenium is essential for good nutrition, but that it appears to play a leading part in preventing cancer and may also be beneficial in its treatment (Uhlander 1980). Part of the benefit derived from a high fish diet may reflect its high selenium content.

Pauling (1979) believes that vitamin C may be effective in both the prophylaxis and treatment of cancer by making the immune mechanisms of the body more effective and by making normal tissue stronger by reinforcing its intercellular cement.

Knowing that there is a considerable daily dietary consumption of chemicals that may be carcinogenic, that the liver is the main detoxifying organ for the body, and that the water-soluble B-complex vitamins help liver function, then the advantage of taking supplemental B vitamins becomes obvious (Fredericks 1977).

Gonzalez (1980) in a review of the role of vitamin E in fibrocystic disease, discussed the contributions made by London and Abrams in this field. Vitamin E seems to be able to relieve breast tenderness and nodularity, cause cyst regression in many patients, and alterations in lipids and hormones. Its exact mechanism of action is not clearly understood, but it does seem to relieve most cystic breast disease. Since patients with fibrocystic disease are at increased risk for developing breast cancer there might be a resulting decreased incidence of breast cancer by causing a subsidence of fibrocystic disease.

It would seem to be advisable for a physician to recommend to his patients that they avoid obesity, that they use a diet that is high in fish and grains and low in beef and fats including milk products. They should avoid coffee, tea, cocoa, and cola to eliminate the methylzanthine in the caffeine occurring in these drinks, and they should take large doses of vitamin B complex and C, and a moderate dose of vitamin E daily.

Other Cancers of Organs

There is an increased risk of developing cancer of the breast as a second primary neoplasm in patients who have had either previous carcinoma of the ovary (Lynch et al. 1974), endometrium (MacMahon and Austin 1969), colon (Schoenberg et al. 1969), or of a major salivary gland (Dunn et al. 1972). MacMahon and Austin (1969), in a study of 869 women with endometrial cancer, reported a 30% increase in breast cancer over the expected number.

Trauma

There is no well-controlled scientific evidence to indicate that trauma as a single injury increased breast cancer incidence (Leis 1970, 1978a; Haagensen 1971; Donegan and Spratt 1979), but it is reasonable that it could aggravate a precancerous mastopathy causing a more rapid progression into carcinoma, or a pre-existing cancer causing a more rapid growth of the neoplasm (Pelner 1961). Trauma probably draws the patients attention to a pre-existing lesion, rather than serving as an etiologic agent (Donegan and Spratt 1979).

Breast X-Ray Patterns and Thermographic Abnormalities

Wolfe (1976) has reported on four parenchymal patterns seen on breast x-rays that have a statistically noteworthy difference in breast cancer incidence rates. By screening patients with P2 (prominent duct pattern) and those with a DY (dense parenchymal pattern), he estimated that one would be examining 27.4% of the population and finding 76% of the cancers. He estimated an increased risk of 17 times for the P2 pattern and 22 times for the DY pattern, with an average risk 20 times greater than that of patients with a normal pattern.

Other investigators, however, have estimated a much lower risk and recently these patterns have come under considerable question (Egan and Mosteller 1977; Krook et al. 1978; Mendel et al. 1977). Egan and Mosteller (1977) feel that the apparent increased risk of breast cancer in patients with DY patterns more realistically represents a delay in diagnosis due to the fact that early lesions may be hidden by the dense parenchyma. Check (1980) recently published a review article on this subject in which chellanges to the concept that breast parenchyma patterns can predict the development of breast cancer in healthy women were made by Moskowitz and Ernstr. Similar studies were reported by Cole, Wilkinson and Carlile. The question of the usefulness of these patterns is currently under investigation in studies sponsored by the American Cancer Society and the National Cancer Institute.

An abnormal thermogram appears to be a risk marker of significance. Byrne (1976) reported that a patient with an abnormal thermogram carried a 15 times increased risk for developing breast cancer compared with patients with a normal thermogram. Other reports, however, have indicated a lower risk factor associated with an abnormal thermogram (Isard 1972; Nyirjestym et al. 1977; Stark and Way 1974).

Gautherie and Gros (1980) have classified thermograms into five stages ranging from ThI to ThV, according to an increased probability of cancer. Stage ThIII represents indefinite situations in which the thermal signs are suspicious, but not conclusive. Approximately 90% of patients in their series presenting with the ThIV and V had a diagnosis of cancer established on first visit as contrasted with only 18% of the ThIII group.

One thousand two hundred forty-five women between the ages of 32 and 53 were followed during a 12-year period because they had a ThIII questionable thermogram. Sevenhundred eighty-four women were considered to have normal breasts and 461 benign mastopathies. Subsequently, malignancy was confirmed histologically in 38% of the normal group and 44% of the women with benign mastopathies.

Summary

"Medicine," said Lord Bryce, (1976) "is the only profession that labors incessantly to destroy the reason for its own existence." There is no better example than the physician's continuous search for factors related to the epidemiology of breast cancer.

With the knowledge of the major risk factors for developing breast cancer, it is possible to delineate a small group of women who have a substantially higher risk and another larger group with a moderately increased risk. Although the so-called "none group" cannot be forgotten, it is possible to direct the full armamentarium of diagnostic modalities toward those patients in the high-risk group so that if cancer develops, it can be detected in an early stage where the prognosis for cure is good with less extensive surgery, less adjuvant therapy, and better cosmetic and functional results.

Many factors that are associated with an increased risk for developing breast cancer are beyond the control of the physician, but there are a number over which he can exercise some control and he has an obligation to inform his patients about these.

The ultimate search for the woman with the highest risk for developing breast cancer would culminate in the finding of a 58-year-old, obese, wide body type, hypertensive, diabetic, hypothyroid, white, Jewish convert nun, on reserpine therapy for hypertension and estrogens for severe climacteric symptoms, living in a cold climate in the western hemisphere, whose mother and sister had bilateral premenopausal breast cancer, who has a wet type of earwax, a low estriol titer and subnormal levels of androgen excretion, who had a previous endometrial cancer, nursed from her mother, had B viral particles in her milk, whose menarche was at age 9, a DY parenchymal pattern on x-ray and an abnormal thermogram, who received multiple fluoroscopies for tuberculosis control when she was 19 years of age, had severe hepatitis and now has liver dysfunction, lives on a high fat, high beef, low fish and cereal diet that is deficient in vitamins, drinks an excessive amount of coffee, and dyes her hair. If she already has been treated for cancer of one breast, this further increases the risk of developing carcinoma of the other breast, especially if her remaining breast revealed precancerous mastopathy on random biopsy.

References

Adami, H. O., A. Rimstein, B. Stenkvist, et al.: Reproductive history and risk of breast cancer. Cancer 41: 747, 1978

Advisory Committee on the Biological Effects of Ionizing Radiations, National Academy of Sciences-National Research Council (BEIR Report): The effects of populations of exposure to low levels of ionizing radiation. Washington, D. C., U. S. Gov. Printing Office, 1972

American Cancer Society: Cancer Facts and Figures 1981: American Cancer Society, Inc., New York 1981

Anderson, D. E.: The role of genetics in human breast cancer. Cancer 24: 130, 1974

Anderson, D. E.: Familial and Genetic Predisposition for Breast Cancer. In B. S. Stoll: Risk Factors in Breast Cancer. William Heinemann Medical Books Ltd., London 1976

Anderson, D. E.: Genetics and the etiology of breast cancer. Breast 3: 37, 1977

Armstrong, B., N. Stevens, R. Doll: A retrospective study of the association between the use of rauwolfia and breast cancer. Lancet 2: 672, 1974

Asch, R. H., R. B. Greenblatt: The use of an impeded androgen-danazol in the management of benign breast disorders. Am. J. Obstet. Gynecol. 127: 130, 1977

Bailar, J. C.: Mammography: A contrary view. Ann. Intern. Med. 84: 77, 1976

Baral, E., L. E. Larsson, B. Mattson: Breast cancer following irradiation of the breast. Cancer 40: 2905, 1977

Black, M. M.: Immunopathology of breast cancer. In H. L. Ioachim: Pathology Annual. Appelton-Century-Crofts, New York 1977

Black, M. M., C. S. Kwon: Precancerous mastopathy: Structural and biological considerations. Path. Res. Pract. 166: 491, 1980

Black, M. M., R. E. Zachrau: Immunotherapy of breast cancer. In H. S. Gallager, H. P. Leis, Jr., R. K. Snyderman, J. A. Urban: The Breast. C. V. Mosby Co., St. Louis 1978

Black, M. M., J. H. C. Barcaly, S. J. Cutler et al: Association of atypical characteristics of benign breast lesions with subsequent risk of breast cancer. Cancer 29: 338, 1972

Black, M. M., C. S. Kwon, H. P. Leis, Jr., et al.: Family history and oral contraceptives: Unique relationships in breast cancer patients. Cancer 46: 2747, 1980

Blackwinkel, K., A. S. Jackson: Some features of breast cancer and thyroid deficiency. Cancer 17: 1174, 1964

Blichert-Toft, M., A. N. Andersen, O. B. Henriksen, et al.: Treatment of mastalgia with bromocriptine: A double-blind cross-over study. Br. Med. J. 1: 237, 1979

Boice, J. D., Jr., R. R. Monson: Breast cancer in women after repeated fluoroscopic examinations of the chest. J. Natl. Cancer Inst. 59: 823, 1977

Boston Collaborative Drug Surveillance Program: Relation between breast cancer and S blood-antigen system. Lancet 1: 301, 1971

Brinton, L. A., et al.: Breast cancer risk factors among screening program participants. J. Natl. Cancer Inst. 62: 37, 1979

Bulbrook, R. D., J. L. Hayward, C. C. Spicer: Relation between urinary androgen and corticoid excretion and subsequent breast cancer. Lancet 21: 395, 1971

Byrne, R.: Utilization of thermography as a risk indicator in breast cancer. Breast 2: 43, 1976

Cammarata, A., P. P. Rosen, H. P. Leis, Jr.: Breast biopsy: Surgical aspects, role of frozen section and specimen radiography. In H. S. Gallager, H. P. Leis, Jr., R. K. Snyderman, J. A. Urban: The Breast, C. V. Mosby Co., St. Louis 1978

Check, W. A.: Can mammographic parenchymal patterns foretell breast cancer? J. Am. Med. Assoc. 244: 221, 1980

Check, W. A.: Breast saving surgery: Radiation for early cancer gaining advocates. J. Am. Med. Assoc. 245: 661, 1981

Consensus Development Meeting on Breast Cancer Screening, National Cancer Institute, Bethesda, Maryland 1977

Coombs, L. J., A. M. Lilienfeld, I. D. Bross, et al.: A prospective study of the relationship between benign breast diseases and breast carcinoma. Prev. Med. 8: 40, 1979

Davis, H. H., M. Simons, J. B. Davis: Cystic disease and carcinoma of the breast: Relationship to carcinoma. Cancer 24: 1241, 1969

Dmochowski, L., G. Seman, H. S. Gallager: Viruses as possible etiologic factors in human breast cancer. Cancer 24: 1241, 1969

Donegan, W. L., J. S. Spratt: Cancer of the Breast. W. B. Saunders, Co., Philadelphia 1979

Dunn, J. E., Jr.: Epidemiology and possible identification of high-risk groups that could develop cancer of the breast. Cancer 23: 774, 1969

Dunn, J. E., Jr., K. O. Bragg, C. Sautter, et al.: Breast cancer risk following a major salivary gland carcinoma. Cancer 29: 1343, 1972

Edelstyn, G. A., A. R. Lyons, R. B. Webourn: Thyroid function in patients with mammary carcinoma. Lancet 1: 670, 1958

Egan, R. L., R. C. Mosteller: Breast cancer mammography patterns. Cancer 40: 2087, 1977

Feinlieb, M.: Breast cancer and artificial menopause: A cohort study. J. Natl. Cancer Inst. 41: 315, 1968

Fraumeni, J. F., Jr., J. W. Lloyd, E. M. Smith, et al.: Cancer mortality in nuns. J. Natl. Cancer Inst. 42: 455, 1969

Fredericks, C. F.: Breast Cancer: A Nutritional Approach. Grosset and Dunlap, New York 1977

Gautherie, M., C. M. Gros: Breast thermography and cancer risk prediction. Cancer 45: 51, 1980

Gonzalez, E. R.: Vitamin E relieves most cystic breast disease: May alter lipids, hormones. J. Am. Med. Assoc. 244: 1077, 1980

Gorman, C. A., D. V. Becker, F. S. Greenspan, et al.: Breast cancer and thyroid therapy: Statement by the American Thyroid Association. J. Am. Med. Assoc. 237: 1459, 1977

Greenwald, P., P. C. Nasca, W. S. Burnett, et al.: Breast cancer: Epidemiology and screening. N. Y. State J. Med. 81: 47, 1981

Greer, H. S.: Psychological Correlates of Breast Cancer. In B. A. Stoll: Risk Factors in Breast Cancer. William Heinemann Medical Books Ltd., London 1976

Griesemar, R. A.: Hair Dyes. National Cancer Institute Information Release. Bethesda, Maryland, February 10, 1978

Haagensen, C. D.: Diseases of the Breast. W. B. Saunders Co., Philadelphia 1971

Haagensen, D. E., Jr., G. Mazoujian, W. D. Holder, Jr., et al.: Evaluation of a breast cyst fluid protein detectable in the plasma of breast carcinoma patients. Ann. Surg. 185: 279, 1977

Haagensen, D. E., Jr., S. J. Kister, J. Panick, et al.: Comparative evaluation of carcinoembryonic antigen and gross cystic disease fluid protein as plasma markers for human breast carcinoma. Cancer 42: 1646, 1978

Heenan, J.: You're coloring your hair. FDA Consumer Publication No. 75–5005, U. S. Department of Health, Education and Welfare, National Institute of Health, Bethesda, Maryland 1974

Heinomen, O. P., S. Shapiro, J. Tuominen, et al.: Reserpine use in relation to breast cancer. Lancet 2: 672, 1974

Henderson, B. E., D. Powell, I. Rosario, et al.: An epidemiologic study of breast cancer. J. Natl. Cancer Inst. 53: 609, 1974

Hirayama, T., E. L. Wynder: A study of the epidemiology of breast cancer: The influence of hysterectomy. Cancer 15: 28, 1962

Hoover, R., L. A. Gray, Sr. P. Cole, et al.: Menopausal estrogens and breast cancer. N. Engl. J. Med. 295: 401, 1976

Humphrey, L. J., O. Singla, F. J. Volenec: Immunologic responsiveness of the breast cancer patient. Cancer 46: 893, 1980

Isard, H. J.: Breast thermography after four years and 10,000 studies. Am. J. Roentgenol. 115: 811, 1972

Kapdi, C. C., J. N. Wolfe: Breast cancer: Relationship to thyroid supplement for hypothyroidism. J. Am. Med. Assoc. 236: 1124, 1976

Kinlen, L. J., R. Harris, A. Garrod, et al.: Use of hair dyes by patients with breast cancer: A case-control study. Br. Med. J. 2: 366, 1977

Korenman, S. G.: The endocrinology of breast cancer. Cancer 46: 874, 1980

Krook, P. M., T. Carlile, W. Bush, et al.: Mammographic parenchymal patterns as a risk indicator for prevalent and incident cancer. Cancer 41: 1093, 1978

Labarthe, D. R., W. M. O'Fallon: Reserpine and breast cancer. J. Am. Med. Assoc. 243: 2304, 1980

Lafaye, C., B. Aubert: The action of local progesterone therapy on benign mastopathies: A study of 500 cases. Breast 5: 9, 1979

Land, C. E.: Low-dose radiation – A cause of breast cancer? Cancer 46: 868, 1980

Leis, H. P., Jr.: Diagnosis and Treatment of Breast Lesions. Medical Examinations Publishing Co., Flushing, New York 1970

Leis, H. P., Jr.: Risk factors in breast cancer. Am. Org. Reg. Nurse J. 22: 723, 1975

Leis, H. P., Jr.: Hormones in the epidemiology of breast cancer. Breast 2: 7, 1976

Leis, H. P., Jr.: Breast cancer – Patients at risk. In: Proceedings of the Third International Symposium on Detection and Prevention of Cancer. Marcel Dekker, Inc., New York 1977a

Leis, H. P., Jr.: The diagnosis of breast cancer. CA Cancer J. Clin. 27: 209, 1977b

Leis, H. P., Jr.: Epidemiology of breast cancer: Identification of the high-risk women. In H. S. Gallager, H. P. Leis, Jr., R. K. Snyderman, J. A. Urban: The Breast. C. V. Mosby Co., St. Louis 1978a

Leis, H. P., Jr.: Bilateral breast cancer. Surg. Clin. North Am. 58: 833, 1978b

Leis, H. P., Jr.: Breast cancer: Patients at risk. In P. Strax: Breast Cancer Screening. PSG Publishing Co., Littletown, Mass. 1979a

Leis, H. P., Jr.: Diagnosis of breast cancer: Clinical and preclinical. Compr. Ther. 5: 9, 1979b

Leis, H. P., Jr.: Selective and reconstructive surgical procedures for carcinoma of the breast. Surg. Gynecol. Obstet. 148: 17, 1979c

Leis, H. P., Jr.: Risk factors for breast cancer: An update. Breast 6: 21, 1980a

Leis, H. P., Jr.: Breast disease for the gynecologist. In H. S. Goldsmith: Practice of Surgery. Harper & Row Publishers, Inc., Hagerstown, Maryland 1980b

Leis, H. P., Jr.: Breast biopsy: Indications and techniques. Breast 6: 2, 1980c

Leis, H. P., Jr.: Managing the remaining breast. Cancer 46: 1026, 1980d

Leis, H. P., Jr.: The role of the modified radical mastectomy in breast cancer surgery. In I. Ariel: Progress in Clinical Cancer. Grune & Stratton, New York (in press) 1983a

Leis, H. P., Jr.: The surgeon's role in breast cancer: Changing concepts. Breast Cancer Res. Treat. 1: 5, 1981

Leis, H. P., Jr., C. S. Kwon: Fibrocystic disease of the breast. J. Reprod. Med. 22: 291, 1979

Leis, H. P., Jr., A. Raciti: The Search for the High Risk Patient for Breast Cancer. In B. A. Stoll: Risk Factors in Breast Cancer. William Heinemann Medical Books, Ltd., London 1976

Leis, H. P., Jr., J. A. Urban: The Other Breast. In H. S. Gallager, H. P. Leis, Jr., R. K. Snyderman, J. A. Urban: The Breast (Eds., C. V. Mosby Co., St. Louis 1978

Leis, H. P., Jr., J. A. Urban, R. K. Snyderman: Management of Potentially Malignant Lesions of the Breast. In H. S. Gallager, H. P. Leis, Jr., R. K. Snyderman and J. A. Urban: The Breast. C. V. Mosby Co., St. Louis 1978

Lemon, H. M.: Arrest of metastatic mammary carcinoma by cortisone and thyroid therapy. Forum 6: 414, 1955

Lemon, H. M.: Abnormal estrogen metabolism and tissue estrogen receptor proteins in breast cancer. Cancer 25: 423, 1970

Levin, D. L., S. S. Devesa, J. D. Goodwin, et al.: Cancer Rates and Risk. Publication No. 75-691, U.S. Department of Health Education and Welfare, Public Health Service, National Institute of Health, Bethesda, Maryland 1974

Lilienfeld, A. M.: The epidemiology of breast cancer. Cancer Res. 23: 1403, 1963

Lilienfeld, A. M., J. Coombs, I. D. J. Bross, et al.: Marital and reproductive experience in a community-wide epidemiological study of breast cancer. Johns Hopkins Med. J. 1975

Lipsett, M. B., D. M. Bergenstal: Lack of effect of human growth hormone and ovine prolactin on cancer in man. Cancer Res. 20: 1171, 1960

Loeser, A. A.: A new therapy for prevention of postoperative recurrence in genital and breast cancer: 6-year study of prophylactic thyroid treatment. Br. Med. J. 2: 1380, 1954

Lord Bryce: The Best of Sydney J. Harris, Houghton Mifflin Co., Boston 1976

Lowell, D. M., R. G. Martinean, S. B. Luria: Carcinoma of the male breast: Report of a case occurring 35 years after radiation therapy of unilateral prepubertal gynecomastia. Cancer 22: 585, 1968

Lynch, H. T., H. A. Guirgis, S. Albert, et al.: Familial association of carcinoma of the breast and ovary. Surg. Gynecol. Obstet. 138: 717, 1974

MacKenzie, I.: Breast cancer following multiple fluoroscopies. Br. J. Cancer 19: 1, 1965

MacMahon, B., J. H. Austin: Association of carcinomas of the breast and corpus uteri. Cancer 23: 275, 1969

MacMahon, B., P. Cole: The ovarian etiology of human breast cancer. In E. Grundman, H. Tulinius: Recent Results in Cancer Research. Springer-Verlag, New York 1971

MacMahon, B., T. M. Lin, C. R. Lowe, et al.: Lactation and cancer of the breast: A summary of an international study. Bull. WHO 42: 185, 1970

MacMahon, B., P. Cole, J. B. Brown: Etiology of human breast cancer: A review. J. Natl. Cancer Inst. 50: 21, 1973

Matsunaga, E.: The dimorphism in human normal cerumen. Ann. Genet. 25: 316, 1962

McCalister, A., R. B. Welbourn: Stimulation of mammary cancer by prolactin and the clinical response to hypophysectomy. Br. Med. J. 1: 1669, 1962

McGregor, D. H., C. E. Land, D. Choi, et al.: Breast cancer incidence among atomic bomb survivors, Hiroshima and Nagasaki, 1950–69. J. Natl. Cancer Inst., 59: 799, 1977

Meites, J.: Neuroendocrine control of the breast. Proceedings of Society for Study of Diseases of the Breast, Cambridge, Mass., June 8, 1979

Mendel, L., M. Rosenbloom, A. Naimark: Are breast patterns a risk index for breast cancer? A reappraisal. Am. J. Roentgenol. 128: 547, 1977

Mettler, F. A., Jr., L. H. Hempelmann, A. M. Dutton, et al.: Breast neoplasms in women treated with x-rays for acute postpartum mastitis. J. Natl. Cancer Inst. 43: 803, 1969

Miller, A. B.: Breast cancer. Cancer 47: 1109, 1981

Minton, J. P.: Methylxanthines and breast diseases. In: Proceedings of the Annual Meeting of the Society for the Study of Breast Diseases. Philadelphia, Pa., April 18–20, 1980 (in press) 1983

Minton, J. P., R. P. Dickey: Levodopa test to predict response of carcinoma of the breast to surgical ablation of endocrine glands. Surg. Gynecol. Obstet. 136: 871, 1973

Moore, D. H., N. H. Sarkar, C. E. Kelly: Type B virus particles in human milk. Tex. Rep. Biol. Med. 27: 1027, 1969

Moore, D. H., J. Charney, B. Kramaky: Search for a human breast cancer virus. Nature 229: 611, 1971

Murray, R. M. L., G. Mozaffarian, O. H. Pearson: In A. R. Boyns, K. Griffiths: Prolactin and Carcinogenesis. Alpha Omega Publishing Co., Cardiff, Wales 1972

Nasca, P. C., C. E. Lawrence, P. Greenwald, et al.: Relationship of hair dye use to benign breast disease and breast cancer. J. Natl. Cancer Inst. 64: 23, 1980

Nyirjestym, I., M. R. Abernathy, F. S. Billingsley, et al.: Thermography detection of breast carcinoma. A review and comments. J. Reprod. Med. 18: 165, 1977

Paffenbarger, R. S., et al.: Cancer risk as related to use of oral contraceptives during fertile years. Cancer 39: 1887, 1977

Papaioannou, A. N.: Etiologic factors in cancer of the breast. Surg. Gynecol. Obstet. 138: 257, 1974

Papatesias, A. E., M. Mulvihill, C. Josi, et al.: Parity and prognosis in breast cancer. Cancer 45: 191, 1980

Pauling, L.: Vitamin C and cancer. The Linus Pauling Institute of Science and Medicine Newsletter 1 (2), 1979

Pelner, L.: Host-tumor antagonism. XVLL. Trauma and Cancer. J. Am. Geriatr. Soc. 9: 58, 1961

Petrakis, N. L.: Cerumen genetics and human breast cancer. Science 173: 347, 1971

Pilnik, S., H. P. Leis, Jr.: Clinical diagnosis of breast lesions. In H. S. Gallager, H. P. Leis, Jr., R. K. Snyderman, J. A. Urban: The Breast. C. V. Mosby Co., St. Louis 1978

Rogers, L. W., D. L. Page: Epithelial proliferative disease of the breast: A marker of increased risk in certain age groups. Breast 5: 2, 1979

Ross, R. K., et al.: A case-control study of menopausal estrogen therapy and breast cancer. J. Am. Med. Assoc. 242: 1635, 1980

Schoenberg, B. S., R. A. Greenberg, A. Eisenberg: Occurence of certain multiple primary cancers in the female. J. Natl. Cancer Inst. 43: 15, 1969

Schottenfeld, D.: Epidemiology of breast cancer. Clin. Bull. Memorial Sloan-Kettering Cancer Center 76: 135, 1976

Seidman, H.: Statistical and Epidemiological Data on Cancer of the Breast. American Cancer Society, New York 1972

Serrou, B., J. B. Dubois, H. Pourquier, et al.: Immunodepression. In I. Severi: Multiple Primary Malignant Tumors. Perugia Univ. Med. School Press, Monteluce, Italy 1974

Shapiro, S., P. Strax, L. Venet, et al.: The search for risk factors in breast cancer. Am. J. Publ. Health 58: 820, 1968

Shapiro, S., D. Slone, D. W. Kaufman, et al.: Use of thyroid supplements in relation to the risk of breast cancer. J. Am. Med. Assoc. 244: 1685, 1980

Shore, R. E., L. H. Hemplemann, E. Kowalukm, et al.: Breast neoplasms in women treated with x-rays for acute postpartum mastitis. J. Natl. Cancer Inst. 59: 813, 1977

Shore, R. E., B. S. Pasternack, E. Thiessen, et al.: A case-control study of hair dye use and breast cancer. J. Natl. Cancer Inst. 62: 277, 1979

Shubik, P., J. L. Hartwell: Survey of compounds that have been tested for carcinogenic activity. Monography No. 6, National Cancer Institute, Bethesda, Maryland 1957

Silverberg, E.: Cancer statistics 1979. CA Cancer J. Clin. 29: 6, 1979

Spiegelman, S., I. Keydar, R. Mesa-Tejafa, et al.: Possible diagnostic implications of a mammary tumor virus related protein in human breast cancer. Cancer 46: 879, 1980

Stark, A. M., S. Way: The use of thermovision in the detection of early breast cancer. Cancer 33: 1664, 1974

Stoll, B. A.: Risk Factors in Breast Cancer. William Heinemann Medical Books Ltd., London 1976

Strong, L. C.: Establishment of the C H inbred strain of mice for the study of spontaneous carcinoma of the mammary gland. CA Cancer J. Clin. 29: 57, 1979

Thomas, D. P., A. M. Lilienfeld: Geographic reproductive and sociobiological factors in breast cancer. In B. A. Stoll: Risk Factors in Breast Cancer. William Heinemann Medical Books Ltd., London 1976

Tormey, D. C., T. P. Waalkes, J. J. Snyder, et al.: Biological markers in breast carcinoma: Clinical correlations with carcinoembryonic antigen. Cancer 39: 2397, 1977

Trichopoulas, D., B. MacMahon, P. Cole: Menopause and breast cancer. J. Natl. Cancer Inst. 48: 605, 1972

Uhlander, J.: Selenium. A mineral made to fight cancer. Prevention (Feb.) 128, 1980

Upton, A. C.: Radiobiological effects of low doses: Implications for radiobiological protection. Radiat. Res. 71: 51, 1977

Upton, A. C., G. W. Beebe, J. M. Brown, et al.: Report of the NCI ad hoc Working Group on the risks associated with mammography in mass screening for the detection of breast cancer. J. Natl. Cancer Inst. 59: 479, 1977

Wanebo, C. K., K. G. Johnson, K. Sato, et al.: Breast cancer after exposure to atomic bombings of Hiroshima and Nagasaki. N. Engl. J. Med. 279: 667, 1968

Williams, D.: Alcohol and cancer of the breast and thyroid. Lancet 24: 996, 1976

Wilson, R. G., R. Buchan, M. M. Roberts, et al.: Plasma prolactin in breast cancer. Cancer 33: 1325, 1974

Wolfe, J. N.: Risk for breast cancer development determined by mammographic parenchymal pattern. Cancer 37: 2486, 1976

Wynder, E. L.: Dietary factors related to breast cancer. Cancer 46: 899, 1980

Wynder, E. L., P. Chan, L. Cohen, et al.: Overview-Nutrition and breast cancer. Breast 2: 11, 1976

Wynder, E. L., F. A. MacCormack, S. D. Stellmen: The epidemiology of breast cancer in 785 United States Caucasian women. Cancer 41: 2341, 1978

Chapter 10

Prognosis in Breast Cancer

H. P. Leis, Jr.

Introduction

There are a number of gross and histologic parameters that have been used to predict prognosis and estimate survival in patients with breast cancer including the number of axillary nodes involved with tumor, histology of the nodes, size and/or contour of the primary lesion, growth rate (mitoses or doubling time), histologic type of the tumor, tumor differentiation (histologic grade and nuclear grade), extent of lymphocytic infiltration, mucin secretion, lipid contents, necrosis, and lymphatic and/or blood vessel invasion.

In general, prognosis seems to be based on a dynamic interplay between the anatomical extent of the cancer when it is first diagnosed and its growth potential (aggressiveness or virulence) on one side versus the degree of immunocompetence of the host (host-defense mechanism) and appropriate early treatment on the other side.

In 1980, the National Institute of Health re-emphasized the importance of prognostic factors by establishing research grants to stimulate retrospective studies to search for parameters based on histologic, histochemical, immunohistochemical, or other methods that would permit more precise predictions of the survival of patients with regional or local breast cancer.

Anatomical Extent of the Cancer

Stage

Cancer staging is representative of the anatomical extent or advancement of the cancer when diagnosed. It is based on the classical view that breast cancer was a singular lesion that grew progressively at the local site of origin, spread to the regional lymph nodes, and then disseminated distantly. The vast majority of patients with breast cancer show a direct relationship between the stage of the cancer when diagnosed and the length of survival. Although there are exceptions, in general, the earlier the cancer is diagnosed the better the prognosis.

There are many systems of breast cancer staging based on clinical, surgical, pathologic, and autopsy evaluations. The one that is in universal use is the TNM system. It offers details regarding T (tumor size), N (nodal status), and M (metastases). This system was developed by the International Union Against Cancer (1974) and a similar system developed by the American Joint Committee on Cancer Staging and End Results Reporting (1978).

For the general purpose of prognosis, however, a broad staging system can be used both clinically and pathologically; that is, stage 0 cancers (preclinical or occult cancers less than the 1-cm size that is usually needed for clinical palpation), stage I cancers (palpable tumors with negative homolateral nodes), stage II cancers (positive homolateral nodes), stage III cancers (locally advanced), and stage IV cancers (distant metastases).

The importance of staging as related to prognosis can be seen in a consecutive series of ours of 2,554 patients undergoing primary therapy for breast cancer at New York Medical College and affiliated hospitals, 1,174 of which have been followed for ten or more years. The absolute, ten-year survival rate based on pathologic staging was 96.2% for those with stage 0 cancers (98.8% for noninvasive and 93.1% for invasive), 73% for those with stage I cancers, 43.1% for those with stage II cancers, 11.3% for those with stage III cancers, and 0% for those with stage IV cancers.

Hutter (1980) has emphasized the fact that one of the most significant discriminators in staging and in predicting survival in breast cancer is the presence or absence of axillary lymph node metastases. The ten-year disease-free rate for patients with negative nodes according to Carbone (1981) is 75% and for those with positive nodes, 25%. Not only is the involvement of axillary nodes an important prognostic factor, but the number of nodes involved, the levels at which they are involved, whether there is extension through the lymph node capsule, and the determination of whether the involvement is microscopic or macroscopic is of great importance.

Clinical appraisal of axillary nodes is notoriously inaccurate, but it is mandatory at the onset in order to determine the most appropriate form of therapy. There is about a 33% difference in clinical and pathologic evaluation of nodes as to whether they are involved or not.

Cutler and Connelly (1969) found that among cases having clinically negative nodes, 38% were positive on pathologic examination and in cases with clinically positive nodes, 37% were pathologically negative. Fisher et al. (1976) reported that the false-positive and false-negative evaluation of the axilla was 24% and 39%, respectively, and the overall error in clinical staging was 32%. Smart et al. (1978), in their review of 8,587 cases of breast cancer, showed that 35% of clinically negative lymph nodes had metastases detected by pathologic examination, whereas those considered clinically positive contained metastases in 87%.

Cutler et al. (1969) emphasized the prognostic difference of clinical and pathologic staging. They reported a five- and ten-year survival rate for patients with pathologically negative nodes of 84% and 70%, and for the clinically negative nodes, 74% and 58%. In the pathologically positive group, the five- and ten-year survival rates were 52% and 33%, and in the clinically positive group, 58% and 38%. They also noted that patients with bilateral palpable axillary nodes had better survival rates than those with unilateral. Black and Asire (1969) correlated this as a host defense mechanism.

Berg (1955) has shown that the number of axillary nodes involved is inversely proportional to the patients survival. The more nodes involved, the worse the prognosis. The ten-year survival rate ranges from 38% to 54% when one to three nodes are involved, but it drops to 13% when four or more are involved according to Carbone (1981). Fisher et al. (1969) reported a five-year survival rate for patients with positive nodes of 49%. When only one to three nodes were involved, it was 62%, but when four or more nodes had metastases, then it was 35%. The American College of Surgeons (1979) reported on survival related to pathologically positive axillary lymph nodes in 8,248 patients. There was a progressive decline in five-year cure rate from 48% to 38% as the involvement increased from one to four lymph nodes, and then dropped more sharply to 29% when five lymph nodes were involved.

Not only is the number of nodes involved important, but the level of nodal metastases is of equal importance. Generally speaking, the spread is from the lowest level, or level 1, through the midlevel, or level 2, to the highest or apical level, level 3, with rare exceptions. Adair (1949) reported a five-year survival rate of 65.2% for level 1, 44.9% for level 2, and 28.4% for level 3 axillary node metastases.

Berg (1955) showed the distribution of lymph nodes at each level, from the lowest to the highest, was 45%, 35%, and 20%, respectively. The respective distribution of metastases, however, was 60%, 31%, and 9%. In general terms, the mortality for patients with level 3 involvement was twice that for level 2, which was in turn twice that for level 1. However, Smith et al. (1977) recently reported that survival seems to be more closely related to the total number of metastases than to the levels involved.

Lane et al. (1961) noted that if metastatic node involvement was only detected microscopically, the prognosis was much better than if the involvement was macroscopic. Pickren (1956) found that by doing multiple serial sections of axillary nodes initially judged to be free of metastases by routine pathologic examination, occult metastases were found, but that the survival rate was no different than in the patient with nodes free of cancer.

Huvos et al. (1971) defined micrometastases as smaller than 2 mm and macrometastases as larger than 2 mm and generally grossly visible. In a study of 227 patients treated for breast cancer at Memorial Hospital in New York, in 1960, they showed that the prognosis at level 1 was as good with micrometastases as though there were no nodes involved, and that for level 3 the eight-year survival

rate for patients with micrometastases was 59% compared with 29% for those with macrometastases. Attiyeh et al. (1977) have reconfirmed these findings on some of these same patients with ten and 14 year follow up. The 14-year survival for patients with metastases at only level 1 was 64%, those with micrometastases at any level was 67%, and for macrometastases at any level 36%. No patient who had only micrometastases had more than three lymph nodes involved.

Fisher et al. (1976) have reported that the extension of tumor through the capsule of the lymph node was associated with a 47% recurrence rate at 22 months compared with 30% for those with metastases restricted within the capsule. They further noted that involvement of extracapsular blood vessels was also a very serious sign.

Tsakraklides et al. (1974) have reported a difference in ten-year survival rates depending on lymph node morphology with the rates being 75% for those with lymphocyte predominance, 54% for germinal center predominance, 33% for lymphocyte depletion, and 39% for unstimulated.

Cancer Size and Contour

The size and configuration of the ordinary clinically invasive cancer can be used as an indicator of the probability of axillary metastases and survival. The 1979 American College of Surgeons Survey (1979) showed that as the size of the cancer increased, the frequency of axillary metastases increased, and the five-year survival rate decreased.

Tumor size is a determinant of importance in the prognosis of carcinoma of the breast. However, size estimated on clinical judgment is subject to a considerable amount of error. Because of this, pathologic size (i. e., the maximum diameter as measured in centimeters in the pathology laboratory) should be used.

As shown in studies by Fisher et al. (1969) there is an inverse relationship between tumor size and survival rate. Berg and Robbins (1966) in their long-term follow up of 1,458 breast cancer patients, noted that the smaller the cancer the better the survival. Goldenberg et al. (1961) reported a higher survival rate for breast cancer patients with small tumors regardless of the microscopic status of the axillary nodes. Eggers et al. (1941) reported a 75% five-year survival rate for patients with tumors less than 2 cm, 24% for those with tumors between 3 to 6 cm, and 16% when the tumor was larger than 7 cm.

Gallager and Martin (1969) defined minimal breast cancers as lobular carcinoma, in situ, non invasive intraductal carcinoma and invasive cancers up to 0.5 cm in maximum extent. They estimated a ten-year or more survival rate of over 90%. We (Leis 1975) as with Wanebo et al. (1974), include under minimal cancers those that measure up to 1.0 cm in size, and Hutter and Rickert (1976) as well as Wanebo et al. (1974) have also included favorable histologic types. Frazier et al. (1977), using the definition of minimal breast cancer of Gallager and Martin (1969) calculated a 20-year estimated survival rate of 93%. Wanebo et al. (1974) reported a ten-year survival rate of 95%. Our ten-year, absolute survival rate, as previously discussed for cancer less than 1 cm in size, was 96.2%, being 98.8% for noninvasive and 93.1% for invasive.

At the other extreme, the poor prognosis for cancers over 5 cm in size is emphasized by the fact that current TNM staging systems automatically place these tumors in stage III (International Union 1974; American Joint Committee 1978).

Fisher et al. (1969) calculated that, "if all tumors 2.0 cm or larger (70% of total) had been removed when they were 1.0 to 1.9 cm in size, at the end of five years the recurrence rate for all patients entered might have decreased by 10% to 18%, and the overall survival might have increased 11% to 20%." Nodal metastases, as well as the extent of involvement, is also related to cancer size. Johnstone (1975) noted that almost three quarters of patients with tumors larger than 5 cm already had nodal metastases when first seen. Berg (1955) reported that the larger the primary tumor, the higher the level of axillary metastases. Tumors larger than 6 cm had ten times the incidence of level 3 node metastases than cancers less than 2 cm. Pickren (1956) reported that tumors less than 1 cm had almost a 30% metastatic rate, whereas those over 4 cm had a rate of over 80%.

Another characteristic has been reported to be of prognostic significance, namely, the appearance of the tumor margin (contour or configuration). A relationship of the tumor contour to ten-year survival has been noted by Lane et al. (1961). Patients with an irregular contour, which composed 75% of the cases, had a 38% survival, whereas the patients with a rounded contour, composing the other 25%, had an 80% survival at ten years. Although there was no relationship of size to survival with rounded, contoured tumors, it was marked with those with irregular contours. Patients who had irregular contoured tumors smaller than 2.5 cm had a ten-year salvage of 52%, whereas those over 2.5 cm had a survival of only 25%. Silverberg et al. (1971a) also found that breast cancers with pushing margins were less likely to be associated with extensive lymph node metastases.

The same relationship of tumor conformation to axillary metastases was found by Gold et al. (1972) in the mammographic tumor images. The axillary metastatic rate was 56% for tumors with highly infiltrative margins compared with 21% for those with slightly infiltrative margins.

Tumor Location

Reports on the relationship between the location of the cancer in the breast and prognosis have not been uniform. Pack and Ariel (1960) state that most evidence indicates that a cancer in the lateral aspect of the breast carries a better prognosis than one occurring in the medial aspects. Reports by Cutler et al. (1963), Berkson et al. (1957), Hawkins (1944), Donegan (1967), Goldenberg et al. (1961), and Urban (1959) have all supported this. Berkson et al. (1957), in an analysis of 9,649 patients, found a five-year survival rate of 70.7% from medial lesions and 84.2% for lateral ones. Goldenberg et al. (1961) found a higher survival rate for lateral lesions regardless of whether there was axillary node metastases or not. Hawkins (1944) reported a five-year survival rate of 52.1% for medial-half cancers and 64.6% for outer-half ones. Urban (1959) noted that central and medial cancers have a worse prognosis than breast cancers in the outer aspect of the breast.

Handley and Thackray (1949) called attention to the occurrence and prognostic significance of metastases to the internal mammary lymph nodes. The worse prognosis for medial and central lesions is thought to be related to internal mammary node metastases. Spratt and Donegan (1967) collected a series of 2,742 cases from eight surgeons doing variable types of internal mammary node resection. Cancers in the central and medial quadrants metastasize to the internal mammary nodes in 28% of the cases, but in only 18% of lateral lesions. If there were axillary node metastases, then there were internal mammary node metastases in 25% of lateral lesions and 50% of medial or central ones. If axillary nodes were negative, then positive internal mammary nodes were found in 4% of lateral lesions and 13% of medial or central cancers.

Cutler et al. (1963) found that among breast cancers classified according to nuclear grade and sinus histocytosis, survival was not significantly influenced by location within the breast. Although Fisher et al. (1969) in a study of 1,063 breast cancers reported that the site of the primary cancer itself did not influence the prognosis when tumors were subareolar, survival rates were poorer, when tumors were in the middle vertical segment of the breast or diffuse.

Tumor Growth Potential (Aggressiveness or Virulence)

Screening studies, such as the one by HIP (New York Health Insurance Program), which was started in 1964 and ran for five years, and the BCDDP Study (Breast Cancer Detection Development Project), which was sponsored by the National Cancer Institute and the American Cancer Society and which was started in 1973 and also ran for five years, appear to have brought to light breast cancers at a frequency exceeding the expectation based on incidence figures (NIH 1980). This suggests that there may be different types of cancers with some lesions having little virulence and rarely making the transition to metastatic disease, whereas others are markedly virulent. Analysis of survival data by Bergson and Gage (1952), Cutler and Axtell (1963), and Fox (1979) also indicates two prominent breast cancer population groups with a striking difference in relative mortality. Based on the analysis of these studies, about 40% of accurately diagnosed patients with breast cancers would die at an exponential rate of 25% per year, whereas the remaining 60% would die at a rate of only 2.5% per year.

Patients with local breast cancers, that is, no lymph node involvement, generally exhibit a lower mortality rate than those with regional disease, that is, with lymph node involvement. However, one third of the patients in the analysis with regional disease also showed a low mortality emphasizing again the concept of a difference in tumor growth potential with some cancers being less virulent than others.

Invasive Quality

Smart et al. (1978) reported a rate of only 5% noninvasive cancers among 8,587 cancers registered in 1975. Beahrs et al. (1977), however, reporting on the NCI/ACS Breast Cancer Demonstration Detection Projects reported an incidence of 25% of noninvasive cancers by screening asymptomatic women.

Noninvasive cancers, which include lobular carcinoma in situ (sometimes called lobular neoplasia), and noninvasive intraductal carcinoma have a truly excellent prognosis (Leis 1978) approaching the 100% category for five-year survival. Farrow (1966) reported on 403 patients with noninvasive cancers of the breast collected over a 16-year period from Memorial Sloan-Kettering Cancer Center in New York City. No clinical evidence of recurrence was observed in any of the patients treated by simple mastectomy and partial axillary gland dissection.

Histologic Type

A number of reports, including those by Haagensen (1971), Wulsin and Schreiber (1962), and Fisher et al. (1976) have indicated that certain histologic types of cancer, even though they are invasive, carry a good prognosis. Black and Kwon (1978) have emphasized that such lesions account for only about one-fifth of the breast cancers seen in the United States and in most western countries. They stated that it should also be noted that the histological growth patterns commonly vary in different areas of the same primary tumor, and distinctive patterns are usually lacking in metastatic areas.

The following histologic types of invasive cancers have been credited as having a good prognosis by the indicated authors:

1. *Adenocystic* (Ackerman 1968; Cammoun et al. 1972; Cavanzo and Taylor 1969; Friedman and Oberman 1970; Schulenberg and Pepler 1969)
2. *Colloid* (gelatinous or mucinous) (Melamed et al. 1961; Norris and Taylor 1965; Silverberg et al. 1971b)
3. *Comedo with minimal stromal invasion* (Stapley et al. 1955)
4. *Medullary with lymphoid infiltrate* (Bloom et al. 1970; Hutter 1980; Moore and Foote 1949; Richardson 1956
5. *Papillary* (Dockerty 1964; Haagensen 1971; McDivitt et al. 1968; Tomcic et al. 1972)
6. *Tubular* (Carstens et al. 1972; McDivitt et al. 1968; Taylor and Norris 1970)

Histologic Grading

Grading is a measurement of the amount of neoplasia (the degree to which the tissue lacks normal histologic and cytologic differentiation) and may be recorded as a general or nuclear grade. Grading is recorded by numbers, but unfortunately general histologic grading is numbered in the opposite direction to nuclear grading. In general, the better the differentiation or grade (the closer the cancer is towards normal), the better the prognosis.

Haagensen (1971) credits von Hansemann in 1893 as being the first to call attention to a possible relationship between the behavior of malignant neoplasm and their degree of "anaplasia," but Tough et al. (1969) reported that a similar correlation was suggested even earlier by Dennis in 1891.

In 1925, Greenough (1925) developed a technique of grading mammary cancers that is the basis for the grading system used by most investigators today. He divided tumors into three grades based on structural differentiation such as the degree of tubule formation, the size and shape of cells and nuclei, and on the frequency of hyperchromasia and mitosis. On this basis, breast carcinomas were divided into 3 grades with grade 1 being well differentiated, grade 2, moderately differentiated, and grade 3, undifferentiated.

Greenough's method of grading was revived by Bloom in 1950, and in 1956 Bloom showed a close correlation between survival time and tumor grade. Other investigators who have confirmed the importance of the basic grading system of Greenough in relationship to survival time are: Barnett and Eisenberg (1964), Champion et al. (1972), Fisher et al. (1976), Hultborn and Tornberg (1960), and Tough et al. (1969). In the study by Fisher et al. (1976), grade 1, well-differentiated tumors were found to be correlated with older women, absence of nodal involvement, and good prognostic histological types of cancers.

On November 25th, 1919, Broders (1920) presented a paper before the Richmond Academy of Medicine and Surgery, which was published in the Journal of The American Medical Association in 1920. Although this classic paper was on squamous epithelioma of the lip, he was the first to emphasize the importance of the characteristics of the nuclei in estimating the degree of malignancy.

Black and Kwon (1978) and Black and Speer (1957) have emphasized the importance of nuclear rather than general grading in evaluating the degree of anaplasia of a breast carcinoma. They state that unlike general grading, with rare exceptions, the nuclear characterization of individual breast cancers are the same throughout the primary tumor and throughout the course of the disease. They reported a positive association between patient survival and the degree of nuclear differentiation of the primary tumor. Cutler et al. (1963), in a study of 1,067 women with proved cancers of the breast from the Yale-New Haven Medical Center, reported a definite correlation between patient survival and nuclear grade.

The essential features of the system of nuclear grade are nuclei showing marked variations in size and shape, prominent nucleoli, chromatin clumping, and numerous mitotic figures are considered to be undifferentiated and are designated as NG (nuclear grade) 1. At the other extremes, nuclei that are quite similar in size and appearance to those of the homologous noncancerous cells are considered to be well differentiated and are designated as NG 3. Nuclei whose appearance is intermediate between the two extremes are considered to be moderately differentiated and are designated as NG 2.

Growth Rate or Pattern (Doubling Time)

Gershon-Cohen et al. (1967 in their classic paper on "Biologic Predeterminism," first reported on breast tumor doubling times. These doubling times range from 23 to 209 days, with an average of 100 days. A tumor with a doubling time of 23 days takes only two years to reach a 1 cm size, whereas one with a doubling time of 200 days takes 17 years to reach this size.

Despite the valid observation that postoperative survival tends to have an inverse relationship to the size of the primary tumor at the time of diagnosis, it has long been known that some patients having large tumors experience prolonged postoperative survival, whereas others with smaller lesions die from rapidly disseminating disease.

Clinical studies suggest that the rapidity of growth may be more biologically significant than the absolute size. Denoix (1970) has emphasized that "the important fact is how long a tumor takes to reach a certain size, not time or size alone." When breast cancers were divided into stationary, slow growing, and fast growing, it was found that the slow growing had favorable survival characteristics, whereas the fast growing had unfavorable survival.

Breast cancers having a history of rapid growth and peritumor edema are designated as "evolving" cancers (PEV). These lesions have been subdivided according to the severity of the clinical characteristics. The five-year survival without recurrences for PEV 1 lesions is 36%, for PEV 2 lesions 11%, and for PEV 3 lesions 0%. Mourali et al. (1974) reported that PEV lesions make up a significant proportion (55%) of the breast cancers seen in Tunisia. It would seem that the growth rate rather than the size of the primary tumor when first noted may be the most important factor in relationship to survival. Small, slow-growing tumors should have a low precentage of nodal involvement and favorable survival rates (Black and Kwon 1978).

Necrosis

Carter et al. (1978) noted that tumor necrosis was associated with a greater rate of axillary metastases and mortality, and that tumors with necrosis and an infiltrative border were clinically even more aggressive. Patients with tumors that had an infiltrating border and necrosis had a 75% rate of axillary metastases and 29% ten-year survival. Those with smoothly circumscribed borders and no necrosis had a 30% rate of axillary metastases and 61% ten-year survival. Fisher et al. (1976), reporting on the pathologic findings from the National Surgical Adjuvant Breast Project, concluded that tumor necrosis was an ominous independent variable predicting treatment failure.

Blood Vessel Invasion

Blood vessel invasion is noted most frequently in veins and venules adjacent to uninvolved arteries. Its incidence has been reported as ranging from a low of 4.7% by Fisher et al. (1976) to a high of 46% by Friedell et al. (1965).

A number of other authors have also reported that blood vessel invasion has a negative effect on survival time (Delbert and Mendaro 1927; Teel and Sommers 1964; Kister et al. 1966; Bell et al. 1969; Ruiz et al. 1973; and Sampat et al. 1977). In the report by Friedell et al. (1965), they indicated that blood vessel invasion was prognostically significant only in the presence of nodal metastases. Fisher et al. (1976) noted that blood vessel invasion was more likely to be associated with a severe cell reaction in the tumor, lymphatic invasion, metastases in four or more axillary nodes, necrosis, and nuclear grade of 1.

Lymphatic Invasion

Hutter (1980) states that lymphatic invasion may be limited to the area of the primary cancer, diffuse throughout the breast substance and/or in dermal lymphatics, as in inflammatory carcinoma. Fisher et al. (1976) reported that their studies indicated a strong implication that lmyphatic invasion was an unfavorable pathologic finding in relationship to patients survival. They found it to be more likely associated with noncircumscribed large tumors of poor histologic grade and of no special histologic type, with blood vessel and perineural space invasion and nipple involvement. When present, there was an association with early tumor recurrence at 6 to 18 months.

Perineural Space Invasion

Fisher et al. (1976) reported that perineural space involvement was present in 104 of 378 cases in which such structures were recognized representing an incidence of 27.8%. Tumors with perineural space invasion were more likely to be associated with lymphatic invasion, nipple involvement, and the presence of metastases in axillary lymph nodes. Early tumor recurrence was also noted more frequently at the 18-month period of observation in its presence.

Miscellaneous Factors

The biologic significance and histogenesis of elastosis in mammary carcinoma are uncertain. Martinez-Hernandez et al. (1977) and then Van Bogaert et al. (1977) have indicated that elastosis in the tumor bed may indicate a more favorable five-year survival and possibly be a sign of slow growth, but this is open to question.

As previously indicated, there is a favorable prognosis in the mucinous (colloid) type of mammary carcinoma. However, little attention has been directed to the possible significance of lesser degrees of mucin that may occur in tumors. The intracellular mucin in signet cell carcinomas does not indicate a favorable prognosis (Harris et al.

1978). Hamlin (1968) has indicated that the presence of mucin, a favorable sign, was correlated with the degree of differentiation of the breast cancers she studied.

Fisher (1978) and Ramos and Taylor (1974) have recently described tumors rich in lipid, most of which had a very poor prognosis.

Hutter (1980) states that a number of other factors have been described including fibrous reaction, ductal hyalinization, alkaline phosphatase in stromal fibroblasts, and elastic amyloid, which are still of unproven significance.

Host Reactivity (Cell Reaction)

The immunologic responses to breast cancer tissue are a function of the antigenicity of the target tissue and the immunocompetence of the patient. Good host defensive response to cancer is indicative of a good prognosis.

Although not all authorities agree on the methods to measure host resistance, or on the reliability, value, and interpretation of such methods, there are definite tests that can be measured and used as a guideline for host response.

Lymphoreticuloendothelial Response

It has long been recognized that mammary carcinomas may have a lymphoid infiltrate at their periphery or among their cellular elements that has a prognostic significance. Sistrunk and MacCarty (1922) and Moore and Foote (1949) emphasized the importance of a lymphoid infiltrate. Subsequently, Black and his associates (Black 1965; Black and Kwon 1978; Black et al. 1975; Black and Speer 1958) indicated that the lethality of mammary carcinoma may be determined by the interaction of two factors, that is, one relating to the growth potential of the tumor as determined by nuclear grade and the other relating to host inhibitory or resistance factors that represent an immunologic response of the lymphoreticuloendothelial system. These include the degree of lymphoid infiltrate around the tumor, the degree of perivenous infiltrate in sections cut through the tumor, and the number of histocytes in the sinusoids of the regional lymph node (sinus histocytosis). These tests can be graded from 0 to 4, with the prognosis improving with the increase in grade.

The findings of the importance of lymphoid infiltrate in relationship to patient survival with breast cancer has been substantiated by Berg (1959), Fisher et al. (1976), and Hamlin (1968), but not by Champion et al. (1972). Support of the importance of sinus histocytosis has come from Wartman (1959), Masse et al. (1960), Anastassiades and Pryce (1966), Hamlin (1968), Silverberg et al. (1970), and Fisher et al. (1976), but not from Berg (1956) and Kister et al. (1969).

Cell-Mediated Immunity

These tests allow for the measurement of the amount of host resistance at the time of surgery, but there are other tests that can be done after surgery that offer an ongoing method of measuring the relative immunocompetence of the host. Black and Leis (1971, 1973) have reported on a test to measure the cellular response to autologous breast cancer tissue by a skin window technique, and Black et al. (1974) have reported on another method based on the leukocyte migration index. Black et al. (1976) have just completed a study related to the importance of a purified glycoprotein (Gp-55) in breast cancer regarding prognosis.

Other Prognostic Parameters

Hormone Receptors

The knowledge that some breast cancers are hormone dependent dates back 85 years ago to the time that Sir George Beatson (1896), a Scottish surgeon, first reported that inoperable mammary carcinoma in women could be induced to regress by excision of the ovaries. Since then, hormonal manipulations of various types, both additive and ablative, have been advocated for the prevention and treatment of breast cancer.

Jensen et al. (1967) reported the presence of a specific estrogen receptor (ER) that correlated well with the response to endocrine therapy. In 1974, at an International workshop chaired by McGuire (1975), data were reviewed that definitely demonstrated the predictive value of ER determination.

However, only recently have the prognostic implications of ER in breast cancer been brought to light. Bishop et al. (1979), Cooke et al. (1979) and Samaan et al. (1981) have all reported that ER-positive tumors have a better prognosis with the survival of ER-positive patients being statistically longer than that of ER-negative patients.

Biologic Markers

Much work is being done to identify biologic markers that could be used as prognostic parameters in breast cancer. The ideal marker would have to be sensitive, specific, easy to measure and related to cell replication rate. To date, no such ideal marker or combination of markers has been found.

Among the many markers being studied are carcinoembryonic antigen (CEA), a specific glycoprotein in gross cystic disease fluid called gross cystic disease fluid protein (GCDFP), or just cystic disease protein (CDP), human chorionic-gonadotrophin (HCG), serum ferritin, serum prolactin, placenta-like alkaline phosphatase, calcitonin, urinary steroids, serum zinc and copper, and lactic dehydrogenase (LDH) (Woo et al. 1978).

Since Gold et al. (1965) first described CEA, and Thompson et al. (1969) developed a radio immunoassay for it, it has become the marker most frequently referred to in breast cancer, but it has definite limitaions of sensitivity and specificity.

Abnormal levels have been reported in approximately 35% to 70% of breast cancer patients with metastatic disease, and Chu and Nemoto (1973) and Steward et al.

(1974) have reported changes in CEA levels during therapy correlating with the clinical course of the disease. Tormey et al. (1977a) state that CEA levels appeared to be elevated in the majority of patients with metastatic disease and that they were of prognostic importance in patients with metastatic breast cancer. Tormey et al. (1977b) also found human chorionic gonadotropin measurements to be of prognostic value.

Haagensen et al. (1977, 1978) have also found CEA to be a useful plasma marker. He also reported on the value of GCDFP, or which can be measured by a radioimmunoassay from plasma and which seems to be more specific than CEA. He found elevated plasma levels in 30% to 35% of patients with metastatic breast cancer and felt that serial measurements were useful in monitoring the effectiveness of therapy. Recently he reported that the two plasma protein markers, CEA and GCDFP, in combination seemed to be better than either alone for the diagnosis of metastatic breast cancer and for assessing the effectiveness of therapy in metastatic disease.

Woo et al. (1978) have emphasized the importance of the search for an optimum combination of biologic markers to evaluate prognosis in patients with breast cancer and to monitor treatment effects. He reported on an evaluation of seven combined blood and urine markers namely, plasma, CEA, three urinary polyamines, and three urinary nucleosides that seem to be of value in prognosis.

Thermography

Thermography is a safe, noninvasive procedure for evaluating the breast, but unlike mammography it is not able to detect any appreciable number of preclinical occult cancers and does not give an exact location for biopsy and histologic examination. However, an abnormal thermogram is a risk marker of significance (Byrne 1976) and recently it would seem to be a marker indicating prognosis as well (Gautherie and Gros 1980).

In a study by Gautherie and Gros (1980), a group of 1,245 women between the ages of 32 and 53 years were selected from 58,000 patients because they had the same abnormal thermograms of Th III, based on the thermogram staging of Gautherie of Th I to Th V according to an increased probability of cancer. These patients were carefully followed over a 12-year period. Among 784 women who were considered to have normal breasts by physical examination, mammography, and sonography, 38% subsequently developed cancers and 44% developed cancers among 461 patients who were considered to have benign mastopathy indicating the importance of thermography as a risk marker.

As to prognosis, there is a definite relationship between growth rate and metabolic heat production. The heat production is very high in patients with cancers that have a rapid growth rate or short doubling time and as previously stated, these are the cancers that carry a poor prognosis. Lesions, even though small, with an abnormal thermogram are indicative of cancers with a rapid growth rate and therefore thermography is of obvious importance in evaluating prognosis prior to surgery.

Length of Disease-Free Interval

Cutler (1968), reporting on findings of the End Result Section of the National Cancer Institute, noted that the time-free interval from primary treatment to recurrence and the number and location of recurrences are excellent prognostic factors. The shorter the time of the free interval and the greater the number of sites of recurrence, the poorer is the survival. In addition, recurrences in liver and brain have an extremely poor prognosis, whereas recurrences in the bones carry a much better prognosis.

Therapy

The importance of therapy is emphasized by the low survival rates in patients with untreated breast cancers. Vermund (1964) assembled the data from six studies on untreated breast cancer. The survival rate in this collected series of 1,308 patients, dated from the beginning of their disease, was 19% for five years and 5% for ten years. Bloom et al. (1962) found a survival rate for untreated patients with breast cancer to be 18% for five years and 4% for ten years.

Everson and Cole (1966), in a unique book entitled "Spontaneous Regression of Cancer," reviewed the world literature from 1900 to 1965 and studied cases described in personal communications. They were able to find only 176 cases that they considered to be adequately documented for consideration as spontaneous cancer regressions. Six of these were breast cancers. In the tumor-host relationship, it seems that there can be a biologic control of cancer without therapy, although this is very rare.

Almost any form of therapy can improve the survival rates just referred to, but no one form of therapy is applicable to or best for every patient with breast cancer. Therapy should be on a multidisciplinary approach basis utilizing the modalities of surgery, radiotherapy, hormone therapy, chemotherapy, and immunotherapy carefully and selectively and tailoring them to fit the needs of each individual patient (Leis 1980).

It must be emphasized that the primary aim in breast cancer must be cure and although cosmetic appearance and function results are of grave concern, lesser procedures must not be chosen if they jeopardize the cure of the patient. Appropriate therapy should be able to obtain ten-year, absolute, no evidence of disease survival rates in the range of 90% to 95% for patients with stage 0 cancers, 70% to 75% for those with stage I cancers, and 40% to 45% for those with stage II cancers.

The magnitude of the breast cancer problem was emphasized in the discussion on epidemiology. It was also pointed out that the epidemiology of breast cancer seems to be multifactorial, and therefore the likelihood of finding a realistic preventative approach in the near future is quite remote.

Early diagnosis, however, is possible and although there are some exceptions, in general, the earlier the diagnosis is made the better is the cure and/or long-term survival rates. Although the so-called "nonrisk" group cannot be ignored, by identifying women at increased risk for developing breast cancer, the full armamentarium of diagnostic aids can be directed toward them, so that if they develop cancer it can be diagnosed in an early stage. Not only does early diagnosis offer better cure rates, but it allows for less extensive surgical procedures, less adjuvant therapy, and better cosmetic and functional results.

Summary

Prognosis is based on a dynamic interplay between the anatomical extent of the cancer at the time of its diagnosis and its growth potential (aggressiveness or virulence) on one side and on the degree of immunocompetence of the host (host defense mechanism) and appropriate early therapy on the other side.

Of the many gross and histologic parameters that have been used to predict breast cancer prognosis, early diagnosis is of outstanding importance with special emphasis on nodal involvement including the type of metastases (microscopic or macroscopic) as well as the number and level of nodes involved and the size of the cancer.

Although early diagnosis is of great importance, there seem to be two prominent breast cancer population groups with a striking difference in their mortality rates. This suggests that there may be two different types of breast cancers with some lesions having little virulence and rarely making the transition to metastatic disease, whereas others are markedly virulent.

As to prognostic parameters related to a tumor growth potential (aggressiveness or virulence), the ones of major importance are the invasive quality of the cancer, its histologic type, grade, and growth pattern. Central necrosis, blood vessel invasion, and lymphatic invasion also seem to be of importance.

In general, patients who manifest good immunologic defense (host resistance) have a better prognosis. Measurements of the degree of immunocompetence of the host can be done by determining the lymphoreticuloendothelial response and the cell-mediated immunity of the host by a number of tests at the time of initial therapy and following it.

Other prognostic parameters including hormone receptor assay, biologic markers, and thermography may be of value and are under investigative studies.

There is a vast difference between the survival rates of treated versus untreated breast cancer patients. Therapy should be based on a selective, multidisciplinary approach, tailored to fit each individual patient, but never losing sight of the fact that cure rate is of primary importance, and that whereas cosmetic and functional results are of grave importance, they must be subservient to this.

References

Ackerman, L. V.: Surgical Pathology, 4th Ed. C. V. Mosby Co., St. Louis, 1968

Adair, F. E.: Surgical problems involved in breast cancer. Ann. R. Coll. Surg. Engl. 4: 360, 1949

American College of Surgeons Commission on Cancer. Final Report on Long-Term Patient Care Evaluation Study for Carcinoma of the Female Breast. 1979

American Joint Committee Handbook on Classification and Staging of Cancer by Site: Staging of Breast Cancer. American Joint Committee. Chicago 1978

Anastassiades, O. T., D. M. Pryce: Immunological significance of the morphological changes in lymph nodes draining breast cancer. Br. J. Cancer 20: 239, 1966

Attiyeh, F. F., M. Jensen, A. G. Huvos et al.: Axillary micrometastases and macrometastases in carcinoma of the breast. Surg. Gynecol. Obstet. 144: 839, 1977

Barnette, R. N., H. Eisenberg: Histologic grading in breast cancer. Conn. Med. 28: 123, 1964

Beahrs, O. H., S. Shapiro, S. Smart: Report of the working group to review NCI/ACS Breast Cancer Demonstration Detection Projects. September, 1977

Beatson, G. T.: On the treatment of inoperable cases of carcinoma of the mamma: Suggestion of a new method of treatment with illustrative cases. Lancet 2: 104, 1896

Bell, J. R., G. M. Friedell, I. S. Goldenberg: Prognostic significance of pathologic findings in human breast carcinoma. Surg. Gynecol. Obstet. 129: 258, 1969

Bergson, J., R. P. Gage: Survival curve for breast cancer patients following treatment. J. Am. Stat. Assoc. 47: 501, 1952

Berg, J. W.: The significance of axillary node levels in the study of breast cancer. Cancer 8: 776, 1955

Berg, J. W.: Sinus histiocytosis: A fallacious measure of host resistance to cancer. Cancer 9: 935, 1956

Berg, J. W.: Inflammation and prognosis in breast cancer. A search for host resistance. Cancer 12: 714, 1959

Berg, J. W., G. F. Robbins: Factors influencing short and long-term survival of breast cancer patients. Surg. Gynecol. Obstet. 122: 1311, 1966

Berkson, J. S., W. Harrington, O. T. Clagett et al.: Mortality and survival in surgically treated cancer of the breast. Proc. Mayo Clinic 32: 645, 1957

Bishop, H. M., R. W. Blamey, C. W. Elston et al.: Relationship of oestrogen-receptor status to survival in breast cancer. Lancet 2: 283, 1979

Black, M. M.: Reactivity of the lymphoreticuloendothelial system in human cancer. In I. Ariel: Progress in Clinical Cancer. Grune & Stratton, New York 1965

Black, M. M., A. J. Asire: Palpable axillary lymph nodes in cancer of the breast. Cancer 23: 251, 1969

Black, M. M., C. S. Kwon: Prognostic Factors in Breast Cancer. In H. S. Gallager, H. P. Leis, Jr., R. K. Snyderman, J. A. Urban: The Breast. C. V. Mosby Co., St. Louis 1978

Black, M. M., H. P. Leis, Jr.: Cellular responses to autologous breast cancer tissue. Correlation with stage and lymphoreticuloendothelial reaction. Cancer 28: 263, 1971

Black, M. M., H. P. Leis, Jr.: Cellular responses to autologous breast cancer tissue. Subsequent observations. Cancer 32: 384, 1973

Black, M. M., F. D. Speer: Nuclear structure in cancer tissues. Surg. Gynecol. Obstet. 105: 97, 1957

Black, M. M., F. D. Speer: Sinus histiocytosis of lymph nodes in cancer. Surg. Gynecol. Obstet. 106: 163, 1958

Black, M. M., H. P. Leis, Jr., B. Shore, et al.: Cellular hypersensitivity to breast cancer. Assessment by a leukocyte migration procedure. Cancer 33: 952, 1974

Black, M. M., T. H. C. Barclay, B. F. Hankey: Prognosis in breast cancer utilizing histologic characteristics of the primary tumor. Cancer 36: 2048, 1975

Black, M. M., R. E. Zachrau, A. S. Dion et al.: Cellular hypersensitivity to gp55 of RIII-MuMTV and gp55-like protein of human breast cancers. Cancer Res. 36: 4137, 1976

Bloom, H. J. G.: Prognosis in cancer of the breast. Br. J. Cancer 4: 259, 1950

Prognosis in Breast Cancer

Bloom, H. J. G.: The role of histology in the treatment of breast cancer. Br. J. Radiol. 29: 488, 1956

Bloom, H. J. G., W. W. Richardson, E. J. Harris: Natural history of untreated breast cancer. Comparison of untreated and treated cases according to histological grade of malignancy. Br. Med. J. 2: 213, 1962

Bloom, H. J. G., W. W. Richardson, J. R. Field: Host resistance and survival in carcinoma of the breast: Study of 104 cases of medullary carcinoma in a series of 1411 cases of breast cancer followed for 20 years. Br. Med. J. 3: 181, 1970

Broders, A. C.: Squamous-cell epithelioma of the lip. A study of 537 cases. J. Am. Med. Assoc. 74: 656, 1920

Byrne, R.: Utilization of thermography as a risk indicator in breast cancer. Breast 2: 43, 1976

Cammoun, H., G. Contesso, J. Rouesse: Les adenocarcinomes cyclindromateaux du sein. Ann. Anat. Pathol. 17: 143, 1972

Carbone, P. P.: Options in breast cancer therapy. Hospital Practice.: 53, 1981

Carstens, P. H. B., A. G. Huvos, F. W. Foote, Jr., et al.: Tubular carcinoma of the breast: A clinicopathologic study of 35 cases. Am. J. Clin. Pathol. 48: 231, 1972

Carter, D., R. D. Pipkin, R. H. Shepard, et al.: Relationship of necrosis and tumor border to lymph node metastases and 10 year survival in carcinoma of the breast. Am. J. Surg. Pathol. 2: 39, 1978

Cavanzo, R. J., H. B. Taylor: Adenoid cystic carcinoma of the breast. Cancer 24: 740, 1969

Champion, H. R., I. W. Wallace, R. J. Prescott: Histology in breast cancer prognosis. Br. J. Cancer 26: 129, 1972

Chu, T., T. Nemoto: Evaluation of CEA in human mammary carcinoma. J. Natl. Cancer Inst. 51: 1119, 1973

Cooke, T., D. George, R. Shields, et al.: Oestrogen receptors and prognosis in early breast cancer. Lancet 1: 995, 1979

Cutler, S. J.: End results in cancer. Report No. 3, NIH Publication No. 30, U. S. Government Printing Office, 1968

Cutler, S. J., L. M. Axtell: Partitioning of a patient population with respect to different mortality risks. J. Am. Stat. Assoc. 58: 701, 1963

Cutler, S. J., R. E. Connelly: Mammary cancer trends. Cancer 23: 767, 1969

Cutler, S. J., M. M. Black, L. S. Goldenberg: Prognostic factors in cancer of the female breast. Cancer 16: 1589, 1963

Cutler, S. J., C. Zippin, A. J. Asire: The prognostic significance of palpable lymph nodes in cancer of the breast. Cancer 23: 243, 1969

Delbert, P., A. Mendaro: Less cancers du sein. Masson, Paris 1927

Dockerty, M. B.: The grading and typing of carcinoma of the breast. J. Iowa Med. Soc. 54: 289, 1964

Donegan, W. L.: Staging and end results. In A. S. Spratt, Jr., W. L. Donegan: Cancer of the Breast. W. B. Saunders Co., Philadelphia 1967

Denoix, P.: Treatment of Malignant Breast Tumors. Springer-Verlag, New York 1970

Eggers, C., T. de Cholnoky, D. S. Jesup: Cancer of the breast. Ann. Surg. 113: 321, 1941

Everson, T. C., W. H. Cole: Spontaneous Regression of Cancer. W. B. Saunders Co., Philadelphia 1966

Farrow, J. H.: Late recurrence of breast cancer, J. Am. Med. Assoc. 195: 157, 1966

Fisher, B., N. H. Slack, I. D. J. Bross: Cancer of the breast: Size of neoplasm and prognosis. Cancer 24: 1071, 1969

Fisher, E.: The pathologist's role in the diagnosis and treatment of invasive breast cancer. Surg. Clin. North Am. 58: 705, 1978

Fisher, E. R., R. Gregorio, B. Fisher: Prognostic significance of histopathology. In B. A. Stoll: Risk Factors in Breast Cancer, Wm. Heinemann Medical Books Ltd., London 1976

Fisher, E. R., R. M. Gregorio, C. Redmond, et al.: Pathologic findings from the National Surgical Adjuvant Breast Project (Protocol No. 4) II. The significance of extra nodal extension of axillary metastases. Am. J. Clin. Pathol. 65: 439, 1976

Fox, M. S.: On the diagnosis and treatment of breast cancer. J. Am. Med. Assoc. 241: 489, 1979

Frazier, T. G., E. M. Copeland, H. S. Gallager, et al.: Prognosis and treatment in minimal breast cancer. Am. J. Surg. 133: 697, 1977

Freidman, B., H. A. Oberman: Adenoid cystic carcinoma of the breast. Am. J. Clin. Pathol. 54: 1, 1970

Friedell, G. H., A. Betts, S. C. Sommers: The prognostic value of blood vessel invasion and lymphocyte infiltrates in breast carcinoma. Cancer 18: 164, 1965

Gallager, H. S., J. F. Martin: The study of mammary carcinoma by mammography and whole organ sectioning: Early observations. Cancer 23: 855, 1969

Gautherie, M., C. M. Gros: Breast thermography and cancer risk prediction. Cancer 45: 51, 1980

Gershon-Cohen, J., S. M. Berger, H. S. Klockstein: Roentgenography of breast cancer moderating concept of "biologic predeterminism." Cancer 16: 961, 1963

Gold, P., S. O. Freedman: Demonstration of tumor-specific antigens in human colonic carcinomata by immunological and absorption techniques. J. Exp. Med. 121: 439, 1965

Gold, R. H., G. Main, C. Zippin, et al.: Infiltration of mammary carcinomas an indicator of axillary metastases. Cancer 29: 35, 1972

Goldenberg, I. S., J. C. Bailar, III, M. A. Hays, et al.: Female breast cancer re-evaluation. Ann. Surg. 154: 397, 1961

Greenough, R. B.: Varying degrees of malignancy in cancer of the breast. J. Cancer Res. 9: 453, 1925

Haagensen, C. D.: Diseases of the Breast. W. B. Saunders, Philadelphia 1971

Haagensen, D. E., Jr., G. Mazoujian, W. D. Holder, et al.: Evaluation of a breast cyst fluid protein detectable in the plasma of breast carcinoma patients. Ann. Surg. 185: 279, 1977

Haagensen, D. E. Jr., S. J. Kister, J. Panick, et al.: Comparative evaluation of carcinoembryonic antigen and gross cystic disease fluid protein as plasma markers for human breast carcinoma. Cancer 42: 1646, 1978

Hamlin, I. M. E.: Possible host resistance in carcinomas of the breast. Br. J. Cancer 22: 383, 1968

Handley, R. S., A. C. Thackray: The internal mammary lymph node chain in carcinoma of the breast. Lancet 2: 276, 1949

Harris, M., S. Wells, K. S. Vasudev: Primary signet ring cell carcinomas of the breast. Histopathology 2: 171, 1978

Hawkins, J. W.: Evaluation of breast cancer therapy as a guide to control programs. J. Natl. Cancer Inst. 4: 445, 1944

Hultborn, K. A., B. Tornberg: Mammary carcinoma: The biologic character of mammary cancer studied in 517 cases by a new form of malignancy grading. Acta. Radiol. Supp. 196: 1, 1960

Hutter, R. V. P.: The influence of pathologic factors on breast cancer management. Cancer 46: 961, 1980

Hutter, R. V. P., R. R. Rickert: The pathologic basis for therapeutic considerations in minimal lesions of the breast. Breast 2: 26, 1976

Huvos, A. G., R. V. P. Hutter, J. Berg: Significance of axillary macrometastases and micrometastases in mammary cancer. Am. Surg. 173: 44, 1971

International Union Against Cancer (UICC): TNM (Classification of Malignant Tumors), Second Edition, Geneva, 1974

Jensen, E. V., E. R. DeSombre, P. W. Jungblut: Estrogen receptors in hormone-responsive tissues and tumors. In R. W. Wissler, T. L. Dao, S. Wood, Jr.: Endogenous Factors Influencing Host-Tumor Balance. University of Chicago Press, Chicago 1967

Johnstone, F. R.: Carcinoma of the breast. Influence of size of primary lesion and lymph node involvement based on selective biopsy. Am. J. Surg. 124: 158, 1972

Kister, S. J., S. C. Sommers, C. D. Haagensen, et al.: Re-evaluation of blood vessel invasion as a prognostic factor in carcinoma of the breast. Cancer 19: 1213, 1966

Kister, S. J., S. C. Sommers, C. D. Haagensen, et al.: Nuclear grade and sinus histiocytosis in cancer of the breast. Cancer 23: 570, 1969

Lane, N., H. Goskel, R. A. Salerno, et al.: Clinicopathologic analysis of the surgical curability of breast cancers: A minimal ten year study of personal cases. Ann. Surg. 153: 483, 1961

Leis, H. P., Jr.: How much surgery for minimal breast cancer? Mod. Med. 75: 58, 1975

Leis, H. P., Jr.: Criteria and standards for evaluation of treatment results. In H. S. Gallager, H. P. Leis, Jr., R. K. Snyderman, J. A. Urban: The Breast. C. V. Mosby Co., St. Louis 1978

Leis, H. P., Jr.: Breast disease for the gynecologist. In H. S. Goldsmith: Practice of Surgery. Harper & Row, Inc., Hagerstown, Maryland 1980

Martinez-Hernandez, A., D. J. Francis, S. G. Silverberg: Elastosis and other stromal reactions in benign and malignant breast tissue. Cancer 40: 700, 1977

Masse, L., C. Masse, J. P. Chassiagne: Le prognostic de cancers du sein en function de la surcharge en histiocytes des sinus des ganglions axillaires. Mem. Acad. Chir. 86: 940, 1960

McDivitt, R. W., F. W. Stewart, J. W. Berg: Tumors of the Breast. Armed Forces Inst. of Pathology, Washington, D. C. 1968

McGuire, W. L., P. P. Carbone, M. E. Sears, et al.: Estrogen receptors in human breast cancer. An overview. In W. L. McGuire, P. P. Carbone, E. P. Vollmer: Estrogen Receptors in Human Breast Cancer. Raven Press, New York 1975

Melamed, M. R., G. F. Robbins, F. W. Foote, Jr.: Prognostic significance of gelatinous mammary carcinoma. Cancer 14: 699, 1961

Moore, O. S., F. W. Foote, Jr.: The relatively favorable prognosis of medullary carcinoma of the breast. Cancer 2: 635, 1949

Mourali, N., F. Tabbane, G. V. Hoerner, et al.: Choice of treatment according to rate of growth. Int. Cong. 353: 5, 1974

NIH: Correlation Between Microscopic Characteristics of Primary Breast Tumors and Subsequent Patient Survival. NIH Guide for Grants and Contracts. Vol. 9, No. 8. Bethesda, Maryland June 6, 1980

Norris, H. J., H. B. Taylor: Prognosis of mucinous (gelatinous) carcinoma of the breast. Cancer 18: 879, 1965

Pack, G. T., I. M. Ariel: Treatment of Cancer and Allied Diseases. The Breast, Chest and Esophagus, Vol. 4. P. B. Hoeber, Inc., New York 1960

Pickren, J. W.: Lymph node metastases in carcinoma of the female mammary gland. Bull. Roswell Park Memorial Inst. 1: 79, 1956

Ramos, C. V., H. B. Taylor: Lipid rich carcinoma of the breast. A clinicopathologic analysis of 13 examples. Cancer 33: 812, 1974

Richardson, W. W.: Medullary carcinoma of the breast. Br. J. Cancer 10: 415, 1956

Ruiz, U., S. Babeu, M. S. Schwartz, et al.: Blood vessel invasion and lymph node metastases: Two factors affecting survival in breast cancer. Surgery 73: 185, 1973

Samaan, N. A., A. U. Buzdar, K. A. Aldinger et al.: Estrogen receptor: A prognostic factor in breast cancer. Cancer 47: 554, 1981

Sampat, M. B., M. V. Sirsat, P. Gangadharan: Prognostic significance of blood vessel invasion in carcinoma of the breast in women. J. Surg. Oncol. 8: 623, 1977

Schulenberg, C. A., W. J. Pepler: Adenoid cystic carcinoma of the breast. Br. J. Surg. 56: 395, 1969

Silverberg, S. G., A. R. Chitale, A. D. Hind, et al.: Sinus histiocytosis and mammary carcinoma. Study of 366 radical mastectomies and a historical review. Cancer 26: 1177, 1970

Silverberg, S. G., A. R. Chitale, S. H. Levitt: Prognostic significance of tumor margins in mammary carcinoma. Arch. Surg. 102: 450, 1971a

Silverberg, S. G., S. Kay, A. R. Chitale, et al.: Colloid carcinoma of the breast. Am. J. Clin. Pathol. 55: 355, 1971b

Sistrunk, W. E., W. C. MacCarty: Life expectancy following radical amputation for carcinoma of the breast. Ann. Surg. 75: 61, 1922

Smart, C. R., M. H. Myers, L. A. Gloeckler: Implications from SEER data on breast cancer management. Cancer 41: 787, 1978

Smith, J. A., J. J. Gamez-Araujo, H. S. Gallager, et al.: Carcinoma of the breast: Analyses of total lymph node involvement versus level of metastases. Cancer 39: 527, 1977

Spratt, J. S., Jr., W. L. Donegan: Cancer of the Breast. W. B. Saunders Co., Philadelphia, 1967

Stapley, L. A., M. B. Dockerty, S. W. Harrington: Comedo carcinoma of the breast. Surg. Gynecol. Obstet. 100: 707, 1955

Steward, D. M., D. Nixon, N. Zamcheck et al.: Carcinoembryonic antigen in breast carcinoma patients. Cancer 33: 1246, 1974

Taylor, H. B., H. J. Norris: Well-differentiated carcinoma of the breast. Cancer 26: 687, 1970

Teel, P., S. C. Sommers: Vascular invasion as a prognostic factor in breast cancer. Surg. Gynecol. Obstet. 118: 1006, 1964

Thompson, D. M. P., J. Krupey, S. O. Freedman, et al.: The radioimmunoassay of circulating carcinoembryonic antigen of the human digestive system. Proc. Natl. Acad. Sci. U.S.A. 64: 161, 1969

Tomcic, S., S. Vulkcevic, Z. Vidovic: Histolskii drugi faktori u prognozi raka dojke i histoloski tip raka dojke i prognoza. Med. Arh. 26: 3, 1972

Tormey, D. C., T. P. Waalkes, J. J. Snyder, et al.: Biological markers in breast carcinoma: Clinical correlations with carcinoembryonic antigen. Cancer 39: 2397, 1977a

Tormey, D. C., T. P. Waalkes, R. M. Simon: Biological markers in breast carcinoma: Clinical correlations with human chorionic gonadotrophin. Cancer 39: 2391, 1977b

Tough, J. C., D. D. Carter, J. Fraser, et al.: Histological grading in breast cancer. Br. J. Cancer 23: 294, 1969

Tsakraklides, V., P. Olson, J. H. Kersey, et al.: Prognostic significance of the regional lymph node histology in cancer of the breast. Cancer 20: 1259, 1974

Urban, J. A.: Clinical experience and results of excision of the internal mammary lymph node chain in primary operable breast cancer. Cancer 12: 14, 1959

Van Bogaert, L. J., P. Maldague: Histologic variants of lipid secreting carcinoma of the breast. Virchows Arch. Abt. Pathol. Anat. 375: 345, 1977

Vermund, L.: Trends in radiotherapy of breast cancer. In: Proceedings of the Fifth National Cancer Conference. J. B. Lippincott Co., Philadelphia 1964

Wanebo, H. J., A. G. Huvos, J. A. Urban: Treatment of minimal breast cancer. Cancer 33: 349, 1974

Wartman, W. B.: Sinus cell hyperplasia of lymph nodes regional to adenocarcinoma of the breast and colon. Br. J. Cancer 13: 389, 1959

Woo, K. B., P. Waalkes, D. L. Ahmann, et al.: A quantitative approach to determining disease response during therapy using multiple biologic markers. Cancer 41: 1685, 1978

Wulsin, J. H., J. T. Schreiber: Improved prognosis in certain patterns of breast cancer. Arch. Surg. 85: 111, 1962

Chapter 11

Pregnancy and Carcinoma of the Breast

G. P. Rosemond and W. P. Maier

Introduction

Historical Notes

In 1896, Halsted performed his classic radical mastectomy on a lactating female with breast cancer who was reported to be alive and well more than 30 years later. In 1929, Kilgore reported a 70% five-year survival rate in lactating females with breast cancer with no involved axillary node and 11.5% five-year survival with nodal involvement. Bloodgood (Kilgore 1929) reported in 1929 a thirty-year follow-up on Halsted's case and dispelled the prevalent concept since the time of Billroth (1880) that a pregnant woman with breast cancer was incurable. He rejected the idea that milk fistula would result from biopsy. Bloodgood also mentioned in his writings the lack of harmful effect on the fetus from general anesthesia and suggested treating breast cancer occurring during pregnancy fundamentally in the same fashion as in a nonpregnant counterpart. Despite more optimistic previous evidence, Haagensen and Stout in 1943 included breast cancer during pregnancy in their categorically inoperable grouping. Although this was later canceled, the impact of their 1943 article was evident for years.

Cancer of the Breast in Young Women

Cancer of the breast is the most common malignant tumor to befall women. Experience has shown that it never occurs before mature development of the breast and rarely before the age of 20. Unusual before the age of 30, cancer of the breast becomes increasingly likely with advancing years and is the most common cause of death in women 40 to 44 years of age. Forty percent of breast cancers appear before the age of 50, the approximate age of menopause.

Cancer of the Breast in Pregnant Women

Less than 3% of breast cancers occur in women under the age of 30, whereas this age group has the highest pregnancy rate. After 35, pregnancy becomes less common. Incidence of breast cancer shows a real increase past the age of 35 with about 40% of all breast cancer occurring by the age of 50. In the 40 to 50 age group, pregnancy becomes increasingly infrequent. The average age of women with breast cancer associated with pregnancy or lactation is about 35. Odds are, therefore, such that coincidental pregnancy and breast cancer turn out to be less than 1 to 1,000.

The Philadelphia County Medical Society Experience

Incidence

The experience of the Philadelphia County Medical Society, (Maier and Rosemond 1977), seems to be a reasonably typical series. Between 1950 and 1963, 9023 breast cancers were identified. Eighty-five of these occurred during pregnancy or within six months of the termination of pregnancy. Six hundred and forty-nine cancers occurred in nonpregnant women under the age of 40. The age range of the pregnancy group was 21 to 49 years, 20 of whom were less than age 30 and 19 were 40 or over with an average age of 34. Fifty-seven were white and 28 black. This number of blacks, 33% was much higher than the expected approximate 20% and may be the result of a higher birth rate among blacks. Of the 85 patients, only 79 seemed acceptable for consideration as potential absolute five-year survivors. All were followed until death or five-year survival.

Treatment

Twenty-eight were treated during pregnancy and 57 during the six months postpartum. Thirty-four had no nodal involvement and 37 had axillary node involvement. The remaining six were unclassified or had widespread disease. Seventy-six had definitive treatment for possibly curable disease, usually radical mastectomy. Simple mastectomy or biopsy alone was performed in nine patients with advanced disease. Nine had therapeutic abortion and 29 ovariectomy. Radiation therapy, abortion, and ovariectomy were as a rule reserved for those with more extensive disease. Chemotherapy was not being used at the time this series was compiled. It can be speculated that modified radical mastectomy, including the interpectoral as well as all axillary nodes and total removal of the breast, might be preferred at present. The modified radical allows for more satisfactory rehabilitation and, in addition, reconstructive surgery, which often is so important to younger women. The lack of supporting evidence for the need of ovariectomy must always be considered when future pregnancy may be desirable.

Survival

The five-year survival rate of the 76 patients in this series was 49%, only slightly more unfavorable than one would expect in an overall all-age group. Seventy-one patients who unterwent radical mastectomy had a 53% five-year survival rate. Thirty-four patients with no axillary node involvement had a 76.5% five-year survival rate. The thirty-seven with involved nodes (the degree not stated) survived five years at a 30% rate. From the five patients with „widespread" disease, there were no five-year survivors. Two of three listed as unclassified survived at five years, one of whom refused surgery and was treated by radiation therapy alone, whereas the other had a total mastectomy and ovariectomy. Of the 20 treated while pregnant, the noninvolved node group (9) had a 78% five-year survival rate; the involved node group (11 patients) produced a drop in rate to 36%. Fifty-one fell in the six-month postpartum group. Five-year survival in the no-node group was 76%, and the node-positive group fell to 27%. The extent of nodal involvement was not clearly available.

Race

Blacks with nodal involvement had only an 8% five-year survival, whereas in whites with node involvement it was 40%. Without involved nodes the data were comparable between the two groups, but the difference between the two node-involved groups appears unexplainable from this material.

Pregnant vs Nonpregnant

Sex hundred an forty-nine nonpregnant women under the age of 40 (average age of 35) were compared. With no axillary node involvement, five-year survival nonpregnant was 80%; five-year survival pregnant was 76%; five-year survival with nodal involvement: nonpregnant 48%; pregnant 30%. There appeared to be little or no difference in the two groups when axillary nodes were not involved, but a striking difference was found in favor of the nonpregnant women when nodes were involved. This difference was influenced by the race dissimilarity previously mentioned. Once lymph nodes are involved, this study indicates that some unknown and unfortunate factor operates in an exaggerated pattern in the pregnant female. Consequently, the importance of diagnosis and treatment prior to lymph node extension is apparent.

Signs and Symptoms

Mass in the breast is by far the most common indicator of breast cancer in the female whether pregnant or not. Although the ratio of benign to malignant mass favors benign by at least a ratio of five to one, no real disagreement is found with Leis (1970) who has stated that "all true, three-dimensional dominant lumps should be biopsied, furthermore all areas of dominant thickening should be carefully studied". Needle aspiration preceding open biopsy is a proper sequence and should the mass be eliminated by aspiration or should a *positive* specimen be obtained by needle biopsy, the diagnosis is confirmed. This applies to both the pregnant and the nonpregnant female.

Erosion of the nipple indicating Paget's disease is rare in the pregnant female; nevertheless, it has been reported and the possibility of its presence must be taken into account. The nipple lends itself well to biopsy should cytology be inconclusive.

Discharge from the nipple as an indicator of malignancy is an uncommon and sometimes confusing sign. Milky discharge is physiological and should cause no concern. Occasionally, as the ductal structure of the breast rapidly expands, a spot of blood may accompany the milky discharge. In the writers' experience, this has always been momentary and of no consequence, but persistent serosanguinous discharge should be evaluated. Some have reported a so-called milk rejection sign, the baby refusing to nurse on the involved side during the postpartum period when cancer is present.

Common during pregnancy, tenderness alone is no indicator of malignancy. But when specifically associated with a mass, tenderness in no way rules out malignancy.

Diagnosis

Early diagnosis should be encouraged and identification from signs and symptoms is the responsibility of anyone who has the opportunity to make the diagnosis. Since most pregnant women are routinely evaluated by their obstetricians and since physiologic changes in the breast are so commonly observed in the developing pregnancy, there is an unusual opportunity to discover abnormalities. This is especially true should they appear early in the pregnancy before increasing enlargement complicates evaluation.

The prognosis of the mother with breast cancer depends on the same factors as in the nonpregnant woman with early diagnosis as the one controllable factor. The opportunity for early diagnosis is clear. Since prenatal examinations are routine, Hubay (1979) reasons that the former pessimistic attitude seems unjustified. Leavitt (1978) stresses the responsibility of the obstetrician and gynecologist.

The primary physician and the patient have a shared responsibility. Self-breast examination should be practiced regularly whether pregnant or not. There is no present trustworthy marker denoting the presence of breast malignancy in either the pregnant or nonpregnant female, but efforts continue toward this goal.

Lactation appears to have no protective effect as far as the mother is concerned. Suckling a cancerous breast prior to diagnosis seems to have no momentary or subsequent adverse effect on the infant.

Nursing the offspring may be beneficial to the baby, but MacMahon et al. (1970) concluded that prolonged lactation offered no protection to the mother against breast cancer.

The breast that is physiologically enlarged may present a confusing diagnostic problem, and a sign or symptom implying possible cancer should not be overlooked during lactation. Breast cancer appearing during the third trimester has a comparatively worse prognosis. It is suspected this is due to delay in diagnosis.

Because of the relatively poor prognosis of tumors discovered in the last trimester and presumably attributable to physiologic changes making diagnosis difficult, Peters and Meakin (1965) offer delaying definitive treatment until after delivery. Many believe that a few weeks delay near term is reasonable, but disregarding the stage of pregnancy, Clark and Reid (1978) support managing breast cancer in a similar mode as the nonpregnant woman.

Dexeus and Fernandez-Cid (1978) report a poor prognosis and suspect delay in diagnosis as a cause.

Diagnostic or therapeutic radiation must be particularly viewed with caution in the first three to four months of pregnancy, but not necessarily discarded.

Low-dose mammography with the abdomen properly shielded can be used as a diagnostic tool. Rickert (1971) reported a series of 368 pregnant women who had mammography with no adverse effect on mother or fetus. To avoid blame in the event of any coincidental genetic defect, specific patient consent should be obtained for mammography. The diagnostic radiologist should act as a consultant. Thermography is probably of scant value during pregnancy.

Chemotherapy is teratogenic and therefore contraindicated with a viable fetus.

Delay in diagnosis is not justified when a positive sign or symptom appears. Physiologic engorgement in the third trimester may present a problem, but delay can be minimized when attention is properly focused. There should be especial suspicion when there is strong family history of breast cancer and a special alert observed if the family history includes young victims and virgule or bilateral disease. The premenopausal daughter, a descendant of a family with premenopausal breast cancer history, is specifically suspect.

During pregnancy, close attention should be focused on the breast throughout the period of essential total patient evaluation. Complications of unusual enlargement can be bothersome if overlooked and both benign and malignant tumors can appear. Some of these tend to be stimulated to rapid growth and whether benign or malignant, they must be adequately managed. The expected favorable conclusion is proportionately lessened when an obvious complication is neglected.

Pathology and Biopsy

As has been pointed out by Anderson (1979) and others, the pathologic features of breast cancer in the pregnant female are comparable to cancer in the nonpregnant. Inflammatory carcinoma, thought by some to be synonymous with breast cancer while pregnant, fortunately is as uncommon in the pregnant as in the nonpregnant. Cancer can grow slowly or rapidly in the pregnant female.

Pathology is comparable in the pregnant and nonpregnant. Inflammatory cancer has been reported, but none was found in the study of 85 patients (Philadelphia series) Previously referred to in this chapter.

There is no contraindication to biopsy of the breast or nipple during pregnancy. A milk fistula does not occur and both breast and nipple heal readily. Either local or general anesthesia may be used. The important objective is to obtain an adequate biopsy.

The mistaken notion that certain simple diagnostic procedures such as needle aspiration and biopsy should be postponed until after delivery can also cause unnecessary delay.

Treatment

As far as the cancer is concerned, treatment is basically the same for the pregnant as for the nonpregnant. Consideration of the fetus must of course be kept in mind and ample consultation between parties concerned with therapy and protection of the fetus is vital. Unless treatment is unnecessarily extensive, there is no immediate effect on the fetus (Muxi et al. 1976, 1978).

Abortion with or without ovariectomy has not proved beneficial as part of the primary treatment and should be reserved for widespread disease. Although provoked abortion has been advised by the overly enthusiastic therapist, therapeutic abortion does not influence the prospective mother's prognosis.

Surgery and/or radiation therapy should be given the same careful consideration for the pregnant as for the nonpregnant. General anesthesia does not disturb the fetus if properly used, but the use of radiation therapy is questionable until after delivery.

Surgical procedures to be contemplated for the pregnant are the same as for any young woman of similar age. The recent trend is toward a more conservative management program. Modified radical mastectomy, leaving the pectoralis major muscle intact and innervated, affords reasonable protection and excellent rehabilitation with possibly effective plastic surgery when desired. Any procedure including axillary node removal has both a therapeutic and staging advantage, and rehabilitation is extremely important to the young victim. Radiation therapy and chemotherapy should be used only after termination of pregnancy, as either can adversely effect the fetus.

Bilateral disease in the pregnant should be treated as in the nonpregnant.

Prognosis

Prognosis for the mother increasingly worsens as pregnancy progresses. As previously stated, this is probably the result of delay in diagnosis. Prognosis depends on early diagnosis, a controllable factor, and tumor biology, which to date is not controllable.

Axillary lymph node involvement, always a serious prognostic factor, seems to be particularly important during pregnancy. Such poor prognosis may be exaggerated in blacks.

Schweppe et al. (1979) believe pregnancy has a favorable influence on prognosis unless there is axillary lymph node involvement. Gogas and Skalkeas (1975) agree that axillary node metastasis is a poor prognosis factor and ascertain from case records that early age of onset of pregnancy has but trivial prognostic importance. Juret (1976) states that sometimes pregnancy seems to aggravate and at other times protect.

It has been said that breast cancer prognosis in the very young and the very old is equally poor, although Pienkowski (1977) believes that prognosis is worse in the young.

Pregnancy at an early age does afford a measure of protection, and there is no physiologic reason to discourage subsequent pregnancy in the successfully treated female. One such patient is known by the authors to have favorably survived a subsequent pregnancy only to develop metastatic disease six years after this pregnancy. Palliation was achieved for a time by oophorectomy in this case.

There is no contraindication to future pregnancy except the possibility of the motherless child. The prognosis of either the mother or child is unaffected.

The pattern is not any more predictable in the pregnant than in the nonpregnant. Vorherr (1979) refers to the potential hormonal influence, but concludes that the role of pregnancy and lactation in the development and prognosis of breast cancer is not determined.

Breast cancer cells do not appear to cross the placental barrier and produce immediate breast cancer in the fetus. The long-term genetic effect is probably not influenced in a different than expected manner.

General Discussion

Although adequately controlled studies are so far lacking, there is no present firm evidence except for consideration of the fetus to show that the pregnant and the nonpregnant should be managed in a dissimilar manner. Even though there are many diagnostic, therapeutic, and psychologic variables associated with pregnancy and the presence of a fetus, the principles of diagnosis and treatment apply similarly to the pregnant and the nonpregnant. Diekemp et al. (1976) has discussed incidence and management, and Zinns (1979) wrote an excellent review article on the subject that embraced numerous references. Of late there has been a large number of printed reviews on this matter. General credit has been given in the references; however, variations in management are few.

In spite of the fact that there are no circumstances characteristic of breast cancer occurring during pregnancy, the age of the mother at first pregnancy effects incidence, but certainly does not provide protection.

Janerich (1979) suspects that pregnancy decreases immunity in the short run and increases it in the long run. When the first full-term pregnancy takes place at a very early age (18 or younger), it appears to decrease the incidence of future breast cancer. Lactation seemingly has no analogous influence.

Previous pregnancy or future pregnancy are not harmful and may afford some measure of protection. Lactation appears to have no measurable effect. Endocrine factors associated with pregnancy do not seem to adversely effect prognosis.

Endocrine influences appear to be variably manifest. Byrd et al. (1962) have postulated that estrogen given to the healthy female may diminish the future incidence of breast cancer or may at least postpone its appearance. Gambrell et al. (1979) reason that oral contraception simulating pregnancy is protective. There is some indication that the incidence of breast cancer in the pregnancy and lactation time period is less than would be expected. Leo (1980) suggests that the blood of pregnant women may contain a chemotherapeutic substance.

At present there are no firm data signifying a direct cause-and-effect relationship between the "pill" and breast cancer.

Pike et al. (1979) point out high levels of estrogen, prolactin, and progesterone in high-risk girls. Stoll and Dexeus (1976) agree that breast cancer associated with pregnancy is coincidental, but propose that a slightly worse prognosis may be linked with immunosuppression associated with pregnancy as well as with delay in diagnosis and treatment.

If there is such a thing as an environmental factor related to causation of breast cancer, it would seem to apply principally, if not entirely, to postmenopausal cancer. MacMahon (1979) cites high fat diet as a causal factor. Hormone patterns are influenced by diet, and genetic influences are most likely primarily premenopausal. Environmental factors are probably unimportant in the premenopausal female.

Psychosocial Considerations and Conclusion

Cancer involving the young female is invariably a special problem. The younger the patient, the longer the life potential. Because of the potential loss of productive life years, breast cancer in the young always affords an exceptional problem. Present and future hub of the family, the young pregnant female with breast cancer should be regarded as unique.

The psychological effect of the diagnosis of cancer is often profound and may lead to radical and ill-timed decisions from abortion to removal of reproductive organs. Cancer of the breast during pregnancy may be an excuse for abortion, although observably it does not appear to be a reason.

Emotional factors may impair judgment. The serious problem of the motherless child must be considered.

Rehabilitation programs have reduced but not eliminated the fear of the potentially physically unattractive and therefore unwanted wife. Observation has shown that ablative breast surgery strengthens a strong marriage but may be used as an excuse to dissolve a weak one.

Emotional upset is so common as to be quite impossible to comparatively evaluate. It is important that the patient be managed as pragmatically as possible, but with concern for her individuality. Strong family support is fundamental to the psyche of the young female, especially if associated with pregnancy, but necessary whether pregnant or not.

Direction should be toward early diagnosis, adequate treatment of the disease, and as brief a disruption as possible of normal life. Donegan (1977) supports management similar to treatment of breast cancer occurring at any other time. Ribeiro and Palmer (1977) have discussed this subject advocating a similar approach.

Donegan and Spratt (1979) believe consultations are useful, and there is general accord that adequate deliberation is indicated when the possibility of breast cancer develops during pregnancy. The expertise of the obstetrician, diagnostic and sometimes therapeutic radiologist and occasional chemotherapist should be regarded and utilized.

Team management approach, markedly important in the management of any breast cancer, must be expanded to include not only the patient, the primary physician, the diagnostic and therapeutic radiologist, the anesthesiologist, the surgeon, and sometimes the chemotherapist, but the obstetrician and occasionally the pediatrician as well. One central fact should be kept in mind: The cancer must be treated.

References

Anderson, J. M.: Mammary cancers and pregnancy. Br. Med. J. I: 1124–1127, 1979

Billroth, Th.: Die Krankheiten der Brustdrüsen. In: Surgical Pathology. Charles E. Hackley, Stuttgart, Enke 1880

Byrd, B. F., Jr., D. S. Bayer, J. C. Robertson, S. E., Jr. Stephenson: Treatment of breast tumors associated with pregnancy and lactation. Ann. Surg. 155 (6):940, 1962

Clark, R. M., J. Reid: Carcinoma of the breast in pregnancy and lactation. Int. J. Radiat. Oncol. Biol. Phys. 4:693–698, 1978

Dexeus, S., A. Fernandez-Cid: The effects of pregnancy and lactation on the prognosis of mammary carcinoma. Tokoginecol Pract. 36(405): 551–566, 1977 and Rev. Mex. Cir. Ginecol. Cancer 46(2): 44–61, 1978

Diekemp, U., J. Bitran, D. J. Ferguson- Breast cancer in young women. J. Reprod. Med. 17(5): 255–278, 1976

Donegan, W. L.: Breast cancer and pregnancy. Obstet. Gynecol. 50(2): 244–252, 1977

Donegan, W. L., J. Spratt: Cancer of the breast: Mammary carcinoma and pregnancy. Major Probl. Clin. Surg. 5: 448–63, 1979

Gambrell, R. D., F. M. Massey, T. A. Castaneda, A. W. Boddie: Breast cancer and oral contraception therapy in premenopausal women. J. Reprod. Med. 23(6): 265–271, 1979

Gogas, J., G. Skalkeas: Prognosis of mammary carcinoma in young women. Surgery 78(3): 399–342, 1975

Haagensen, C. D., A. P. Stout: Carcinoma of the breast: Criteria for operability. Ann. Surg. 118: 859–870, 1943

Haagensen, C. D.: Diseases of the Breast. Saunders, Philadelphia 1956

Halsted, W. S.: Surgical Papers. Vol. 2.The Johns Hopkins Press, Baltimore, Maryland

Harrington, S. W.: Cancer of breast: Results of surgical treatment when the cancer occurred in the course of pregnancy or lactation and when pregnancy occurred subsequent to operation, 1910–1933. Ann. Surg. 106: 690–700, 1937

Hubay, A. A., F. M. Barry, C. C. Marr: Pregnancy and breast cancer. Surg. Clin. North Am. 58(4): 819–831, 1979

Janerich, D. T.: Pregnancy, breast-cancer risk and maternal-fetal genetics. Lancet 1(8128): 1240–1241, 1979

Juret, P.: Pregnancy and breast cancer: Two entities with complex interferences. Critical study of the dossier. J. Chir. 2: 211–30, 1976

Kilgore, A. R.: Tumors and tumor-like lesions of breast in association with pregnancy and lactation (with a note by Bloodgood, J. C.: The treatment of tumors of the breast during pregnancy and lactation). Arch. Surg. 18: 2079–2098, 1929

Leavitt, T.: The role of the obstetrician-gynecologist in the diagnosis and treatment of breast cancer. Breast 4(3): 19–22, 1978

Leis, H. P., Jr.: Diagnosis and Treatment of Breast Lesions. Medical Examination Publishing Co., New York 1970

Leo, S.: A physiological approach to the treatment of cancer. Curr. Ther. Res. 27(1): 132–136, 1980

MacMahon, B.: Lactation and cancer of the breast: A summary of an international study. Bull. W. H. O. 42: 185–194, 1970

MacMahon, B.: Dietary hypotheses concerning the etiology of human breast cancer. Nutr. Cancer I(2): 28–41, 1979

Maier, W. P., G. P. Rosemond: Cancer of the breast in pregnancy. Gynec. Obst. I Chapter 67, 1977

Mausner, J. S., M. S. Shimkin, N. H. Moss, G. R. Rosemond: Breast cancer in philadelphia hospitals, 1951–1964. Cancer 23: 260–274, 1969

Muxi, M.: Breast cancer and pregnancy. Acta Obstet. Ginecol. Hisp. Lusitana 24(5): 289–308, 1976

Muxi, M.: Breast cancer and pregnancy: Results of a survey conducted by the social security administration of Barcelona, Spain. Toko-Ginecol. Pract. 37(419): 307–312, 1978

Peters, M. V., J. W. Meakin: The influence of pregnancy in carcinoma of the breast (prognostic factors in breast-cancer). Prog. Clin. Cancer 1: 471–506, 1965

Pienkowski, F.: The course of breast cancer in women less than 35 years of age. Nowotwory 27(3): 197–204, 1977

Pike, M. C.: The hormonal basis of breast cancer. Natl. Cancer Inst. Monogr. (53): 187–93, 1979

Ribeiro, G. G., M. K. Palmer: Breast carcinoma associated with pregnancy: A clinician's dilemma. Br. Med. J. 2: 1524–1527, 1977

Rickert, R. M.: Nuclear DNA content in hyperplastic lesions of cystic disease of the breast with special reference to malignant alteration. Cancer 28(3): 620–7, 1971

Schweppe, K. W.: Carcinoma of the breast and pregnancy (author's translation). Geburtshilfe Frauenheilkd. 39(12): 1083–8, 1979

Stoll, B. A., S. Dexeus: Effect of pregnancy and lactation on prognosis (risk factors in breast cancer). In: B. A. Stoll: New aspects in Breast Cancer, Vol. 2. William Heinemann Medical Books, Chicago 1976

Vorherr, H.: Pregnancy and lactation in relation to breast cancer risk. Semin. Perinatol. 3(3): 299–311, 1979

Zinns, J. S.: The association of pregnancy and breast cancer. J. Reprod. Med. 22:297–301, 1979

Chapter 12

Schematic Survey of Treatment of Breast Cancer

F. E. Rosato and J. O. Strömbeck

For clearness in the survey the TNM class is regarded as equal to the pTNM class. This means that N1a includes cases of micrometastasis of the axillary nodes (pN1a), N1b includes cases of periglandular growth pN1b (III), and N3 cases of metastasis of the internal mammary lymph nodes pN3.

The purpose of this survey is to be a guide to the possible treatment regimens of the various stages of breast cancer, as well as to provide the location in this book where these different treatments can be found. The survey is not meant to be a rigid how-to-do-it treatment guide. The evaluation is based on the TNM classification. A more detailed description of the TNM and pTNM classification is found on page 77, and only a summary is presented here.

T1	≤ 2 cm	a. without fixation fascia/muscle
T2	> 2–5 cm	b. with fixation fascia/muscle
T3	> 5 cm	
T4	Extension to chest wall/skin	
		a. chest wall
		b. skin edema/infiltration or ulceration
		c. both
N1	Mobile axillary	
		a. not considered metastatic
		b. considered metastatic
N2	Fixed axillary	
N3	Supraclavicular / edema of the arm	

Schematic Survey of Treatment of Breast Cancer

Table 12.**1**

Stage	TNM classification			Possible Therapy			
				Surgery	Radiation	Chemo-therapy	Hormonal Therapy
I	T1a	N0	M0	Modified radical mastectomy, page 132.	0	0	0
	T1b	N1a	M0	Lumpectomy and axillary node dissection, page 132. Quadrantectomy and axillary node dissection, page 127.	Postoperative irradiation, page 188.	0	0
II	T0	N1b	M0	Modified radical mastectomy, page 132. Radical mastectomy, page 136.	None or alternatively post-operative, radiation, page 190.	None or alternatively depending on receptor status and age, page 202.	
	T1a	N1b	M0				
	T1b	N1b	M0				
	T2a	N0	M0				
	T2a	N1a	M0				
	T2a	N1b	M0				
	T2b	N0	M0				
	T2b	N1a	M0				
	T2b	N1b	M0				
IIIa	T3a	N0	M0	Lumpectomy alternatively mastectomy to reduce tumor burden, page 132. Modified radical, radical mastectomy, page 132, 136. Extended radical mastectomy, page 138.	Alternatively preoperative ir-radiation or chemotherapy, page 187.	Alternatively postoperative chemotherapy or hormonal therapy according to receptor status and age, page 202, 218.	
	T3b	N0	M0				
	T3a	N1	M0				
	T3b	N1	M0				
	T1a	N2	M0				
	T1b	N2	M0				
	T2a	N2	M0				
	T2b	N2	M0				
	T3a	N2	M0				
	T3b	N2	M0				
IIIb	T1a	N3	M0				
	T1b	N3	M0				
	T2a	N3	M0				
	T2b	N3	M0				
	T3a	N3	M0				
	T3b	N3	M0				
	T4a T4b T4c	any N	M0				
IV	Any T	Any N	M1	Biopsy for diagnosis and re-ceptor status, page 41.	For local control, page 194.	According to receptor status and age, page 203, 218.	

Chapter 13

Surgical Technique of Breast Quadrantectomy and Axillary Dissection

U. Veronesi, A. Costa and R. Saccozzi

Indications for the Breast Quadrantectomy Plus Axillary Dissection

Quadrantectomy is a term coined by one of us (U. V.) in 1973 to define an operation consisting of the complete removal of the quadrant of the breast harboring a primary cancer. This operation was devised as a result of a number of factors all pushing toward a more extensive use of conservative procedures. The first factor is a better understanding of the natural history of breast cancer and of the fact that the results of treatment are influenced more by distant spread, when it occurs, than by local or regional control of the disease. The second is the discovery of increasing numbers of cancers of minimal dimensions by means of new diagnostic techniques, especially mammography. The third is the more pressing demand for less mutilating procedures and the increasing requests from patients to be informed of the various possible treatments, including conservative techniques. Finally, there is a widespread belief that if a conservative treatment could be offered to women with early breast cancer, it would represent a tremendous tool for popularizing self breast examination and alertness in seeking medical advice at the first appearance of a lump in the breast.

The indications for quadrantectomy plus axillary dissection are for the moment limited to small primary carcinomas, located not too closely to the areola. What should be the size limit for such an operation is still uncertain. For the time being, there is evidence that for tumors 2 cm or less in diameter, quadrantectomy plus axillary dissection supplemented by postoperative radiotherapy give long-term results not different from the classic Halsted mastectomy.

Positioning of the patient and preparation of the skin

The patient is placed in the supine position with the arm stretched out at a right angle on an operating table that can be tilted along the longitudinal and transverse axes. Braces are placed on the opposite side of the table so that when it is tilted the patient will not slip or fall down. During the axillary dissection, the table should be tilted away from the operator about 25 degrees so that the side of the thorax and the axillary fossa are more accessible.

The skin of the chest wall is prepared and scrubbed with an appropriate antibacterial solution from the neck to the epigastrium including the medial half of the opposite breast just to the contralateral nipple. The ipsilateral arm is scrubbed down to the lower third of the arm.

Procedure of the Biopsy

No definitive treatment for suspicious breast cancer should be adopted until diagnosis is established by a satisfactory pathologic examination. The biopsy is then an essential step in the operative procedure for the surgical treatment of breast cancer. Since cancer cells are easily transplantable, the surgeon must take special care not to implant them in the operative field. Finally, in the removal of the involved quadrant, the surgeon should avoid re-entering the biopsy site.

In taking an adequate biopsy the following objectives must be considered:

1. To remove an adequate quantity of cancer tissue for an accurate pathologic diagnosis at frozen section examination and to allow an accurate measurement of the lesion
2. To limit the disruption of the anatomic integrity of the breast to a minimum
3. To avoid implantation of cancer cells

If a fine needle biopsy has previously unequivocally proved the diagnosis of malignancy and there are clear clinical and mammographic findings of carcinoma, the biopsy with frozen section examination may be avoided and the quadrantectomy directly performed.

The incision must be made just over the site of the suspicious lump in a radial direction. The tumor nodule must be carefully dissected and totally removed with a very limited margin of normal tissue in all directions (Fig. 13.1A). The surgeon should then cut the tumor in two parts and observe the cutting surface. In most cases the diagnosis is easy to assess at this macroscopic examination. If the mass is less than 2 cm in maximum diameter, the patient is considered to be a candidate for quadrantectomy. While the specimen is being processed in the pathology department to obtain the final histologic diagnosis, the mammary gland is carefully reconstructed with one layer of interrupted suture with a 0 silk (Fig. 13.1B). As the wound may obviously contain free-floating cancer cells, it is filled with a gauze soaked in a solution apt to destroy free cancer cells. Then the skin is

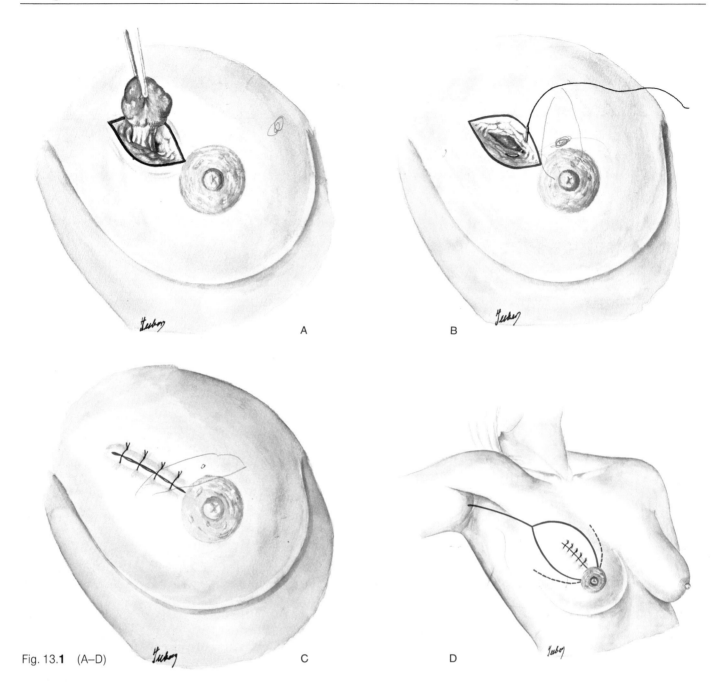

Fig. 13.**1**　(A–D)

closed with a continuous or interrupted suture. This suture must be tight and no fluid should spill from the wound (Fig. 13.**1**C). If this should happen, there is a risk of implantation of cancer cells during the subsequent quadrantectomy.

The Quadrantectomy

It was already said that the quadrantectomy technique aims to remove an entire quadrant of the breast, including the skin and the superficial pectoralis fascia. In this connection the quadrant does not refer to the usual anatomic quadrants (e. g., upper-outer), but to a quadrant of the breast with the tumor centrally independent of its clockwise orientation. The objective is therefore to obtain a complete and radical removal of the primary tumor and its potential surrounding infiltrations through

an excision of a good fourth of the entire breast. To perform such a radical operation it is obviously necessary that the primary cancer be of limited size and we believe that it is difficult to do an appropriate quadrantectomy for tumors whose diameter is larger than 2 cm.

Once the small operation for the biopsy is terminated, the malignant nature of the lesion confirmed, and the tumor itself measured and proved smaller than 2 cm, then all the instruments, gloves, and drapes must be changed and the skin rewashed.

The incision in the skin is first outlined with a sterile marking pencil (Fig. 13.**1**D). The shape of the incision is elliptical with the major axis radial from the nipple. A margin of at least 3 cm must be kept from the biopsy incision. If the axillary dissection is performed in continuity, a peripheral extension of the incision is made to give adequate exposure of the axilla. The en bloc operation is generally possible when the primary tumor is situated in the upper external quadrants or at the borders of it. In all other situations, the quadrantectomy must be carried out separately from the axillary dissection. The skin flaps are prepared with great accuracy to expose a portion of the mammary gland, which would extend on both sides for another 2 cm so that the lines of incision in the mammary gland will be 4 or 5 cm from the biopsy incision. The extent of normal skin and breast tissue removed laterally and superficially is therefore large. The deep plane of the excision is the superficial fascia of the pectoralis major muscle (Fig. 13.2). This plane of dissection may be many centimeters from the primary cancer if this is superficial and the breast is large and thick, but in other cases, when the cancer is deeply situated, only a few millimeters may divide the border of the tumor from the pectoralis muscle so that the plane of dissection is very close to the edge of the tumor or to the biopsy focus. In this case we suggest that the corresponding superficial portion of the pectoralis major muscle be dissected en bloc with the breast quadrant.

Once the dissection along the deep plane is terminated, the entire quadrant is totally removed.

Since a good cosmetic result is one of the major objectives of the quadrantectomy technique, it is important that the breast and the nipple be reconstructed with great care. This step will require time. The edges of the mammary gland must be sutured in one or two planes according to the thickness of the breast. However, the extent of reconstruction of the mammary tissue must be carefully evaluated in each case, since it is often advisable to limit the reconstruction to a minimum to avoid possible subsequent skin retractions or to produce a bulky and excessively prominent breast.

Great care is needed for the reconstruction of the nipple. One of the consequences of the quadrantectomy is the excessive protrusion of the nipple and sometimes its distortion. The protruded nipple tends in fact to bend in the direction of the removed quadrant. To avoid the nipple distortion, it is advisable to get it free from the mammary gland through an extensive dissection of the skin and by cutting the major ducts. Sometimes, when a portion of the areola has been removed, tiny skin flaps can be rotated to increase the amount of skin around the nipple.

The Axillary Dissection

As previously mentioned, the axillary dissection may be perfomed in continuity with the quadrantectomy or in discontinuity through a separate incision. In the latter case the incision that we recommend is a posterioanterior one that crosses the axillary fossa in an upward direction. The incision follows the cutaneous lines of Langer, 3 to 4 cm down the axillary fold and has a length of 12 to 15 cm. It gives excellent access to the axillary vein, but needs to be retracted downward to obtain access to the thoracodorsal vessels and nodes.

The first step of the axillary dissection, after the preparation of the skin flaps, is the exposure of the latissimus

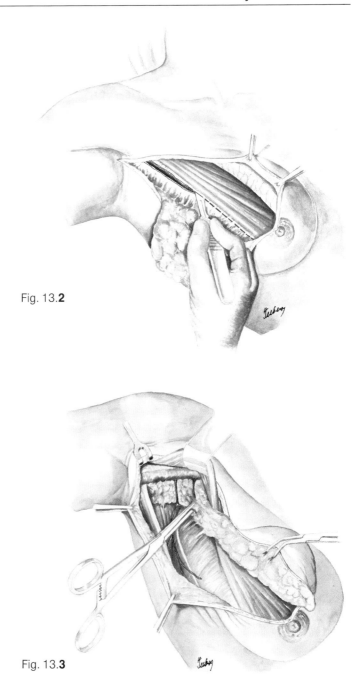

Fig. 13.2

Fig. 13.3

dorsi muscle. This muscle is a key point and once identified must be carefully followed upward to its white tendinous portion. After the latissimus dorsi muscle has been isolated, the axillary vein must be identified. The vein lies on the white tendon of the latissimus dorsi and may be reached superiorly after division of the small intercostobrachial nerves and vessels that cross over the white tendon. The vein may also be safely exposed by approaching it from its cranial side, once the fascia of the coracobrachialis muscle has been reached.

After the vein has been isolated in its lateral portion, it is advisable to expose the thoracodorsal vessels and nerve (Fig. 13.3). This may easily be done by cutting as laterally as possible the deep pectoralis fascia. Once the thoracodorsal vessels and nerve are exposed, the surgeon should free the lateral margin of the pectoralis major muscle from its fascial connections. The muscle is then retracted

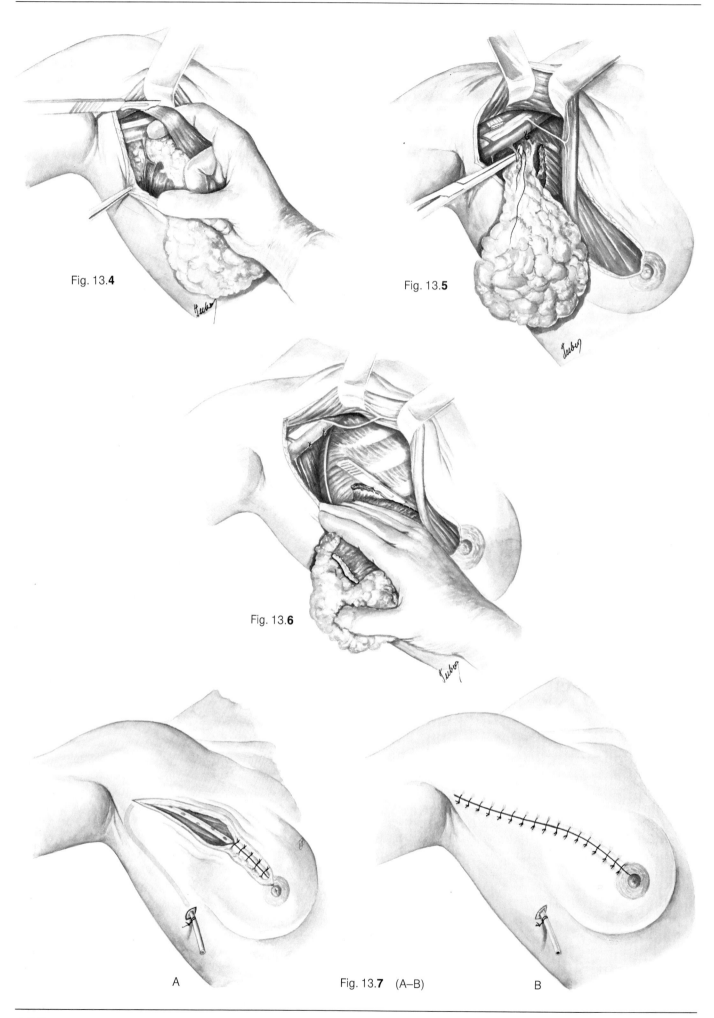

Fig. 13.4

Fig. 13.5

Fig. 13.6

A   Fig. 13.7 (A–B)   B

upward to give access to the structures situated deeply in the axilla. Great care must be paid not to injure the thoracoacromial vessels and the nerve to the pectoralis major. Other small nerves that reach the deep aspect of the pectoralis major muscle after crossing the pectoralis minor muscle may be found and cut. However, it may happen that one or two of them are of considerable size, if so, it is advisable to preserve them. The pectoralis minor muscle is divided 2 or 3 cm from its insertion on the coracoid process (Fig. 13.**4**).

The next step is the dissection of the apex of the axilla, which may easily be obtained with the incision of the costocoracoid fascia at the point of its reflection into the chest wall. The fat and areolar tissue in the area between the chest wall and the medial portion of the axillary vein contains the highest axillary lymph nodes. In order to help the pathologist to orient the specimen, it is advisable to put a silk marking tie on the tissue excised from the apex of the axilla.

Once the apex of the axilla has been cleared, the operation continues by dissecting all the axillary vein and artery, with isolation and ligation of all their branches directed toward the breast and the pectoralis minor muscle (Fig. 13.**5**). Finally, the costal insertions of the pectoralis minor muscle are dissected and the long thoracic nerve is identified and isolated. All the axillary fatty and areolar tissue containing the axillary lymph nodes and vessels is then set free and removed (Fig. 13.**6**).

Suction drain is employed and the wound closed. (Fig. 13.**7**A, B).

Postoperative radiotherapy is started two to three weeks after surgery and given with high-energy technique to a total dose of 50 Gy.

If positive nodes are found, adjuvant chemotherapy is given with cyclophosphamide-methotrexate-fluorouracil (CMF).

Editors note: In the USA as in many other countries the quadrant resection is combined with *only* a level I axillary dissection, not dissection of the entire lymph chain.

Reference

Veronesi, U., R. Saccozi, M. Del Vecchio, A. Banfi, C. Clemente, M. De Lena, G. Gallus, M. Greco, A. Luini, E. Marubini, G. Muscolino, F. Rilke, B. Salvadori, A. Zecchini, R. Zucali: Comparing radical mastectomy with quadrantectomy, axillary dissection and radiotherapy in patients with small cancers of the breast. N. Engl. J. Med. 305: 6, 1981

Surgical Technique of Lumpectomy, Breast Amputation, Modified Radical and Radical Mastectomy

F. E. Rosato

Lumpectomy (Tylectomy)

This simplest approach essentially removes an entire tumor with a surrounding margin of normal breast as well as the overlying skin and usually includes the underlying pectoral fascia. Presently its use is confined to smaller lesions, less than 2 cm in diameter, particularly in old or very ill patients who are judged to be poor anesthetic risks. In most instances, it can be performed with local anesthesia. Recently it has assumed greater importance in combination with axillary nodal sampling and radiation therapy as definitive treatment for some breast cancers. In this setting, it is an alternative to quadrantectomy and is preferred in many centers.

An elliptical skin incision is made. If this incision is radially oriented, it might be more conspicuous than a curvilinear incision placed in Langer's lines. The mass is marked by insertion of a fine gauge needle to provide a constant reference point ensuring an adequate margin in all directions from the mass.

Electrocautary for hemostasis is applied only after the mass has been removed to prevent heat-induced destruction of estrogen receptor protein content. The skin is then closed and the wound drained.

Amputation (Total Mastectomy, Simple Mastectomy)

Definition and Technique

All surgeons are familiar with the initial McWhirter procedure (1949) which involves total mastectomy (also termed breast amputation or simple mastectomy) in combination with radiation therapy as a proposed modality for the control of breast cancer. In this approach, the entire breast with a margin of skin at least 4 cm on either side of the limits of a tumor is removed with the underlying pectoral fascia. Less extensive skin margins are acceptable when the procedure is done for early breast cancer (lesions less than 1 cm diameter) or for in situ or premalignant lesions. Also, if it is palliative in the situation where disseminated disease in known to be present, less skin is resected. The axillary tail of Spence is included in the en bloc specimen. Superior and inferior skin flaps are developed. In general, no axillary dissection is employed. Since most of the details of this procedure will be covered in the description of both the modified and radical procedures to follow, any further technical description is abbreviated.

Indications

This approach, total mastectomy combined with radiation therapy, was tested in a prospective randomized stratified study under the direction of Dr. Bernard Fisher (1977), which compared radical mastectomy, modified radical mastectomy, or total mastectomy combined with radiation therapy. He concluded that all these operations produced similar results when applied to a large population of critically analyzed patients (NSABP 1979). Nevertheless, the American Cancer Society and the National Cancer Institute subsequently published a summary paper recommending that either radical or modified radical mastectomy was the procedure of choice since an axillary dissection with careful analysis of the maximum number of nodes is important for prognosis as well as for decisions about adjuvant therapy. At this moment, therefore, the approach of breast amputation alone as a viable surgical alternative for the treatment of invasive breast carcinoma is not considered appropriate therapy. In carcinoma in situ, the procedure may be considered as an alternative to subcutaneous mastectomy, although others may still insist on obtaining some axillary nodal tissue.

In patients in the extremes of age, those in the eighth and ninth decades of life, in patients extremely ill for other reasons, in those in whom a breast cancer because of its size and breakdown produces local problems may all still be considered candidates for this procedure. In these situations, I personally prefer to at least perform a limited axillary sampling and remove a few of the level 1 nodes, those lateral to the pectoralis minor and medial to the latissimus dorsi muscle. This is usually simply accomplished without adding significant time or effort to the breast amputation.

Modified Radical Mastectomy

The modified mastectomy involves removal of the breast, overlying skin, and axillary nodes and spares the pectoralis major muscle. This has recently been established as an entirely satisfactory operation for breast cancer (Handley 1976). The work of Dahl-Iversen (1963) has documented a similar survival pattern with this approach compared with the classic radical mastectomy to be described. Nemoto and Dao (1975) have pointed out that as many

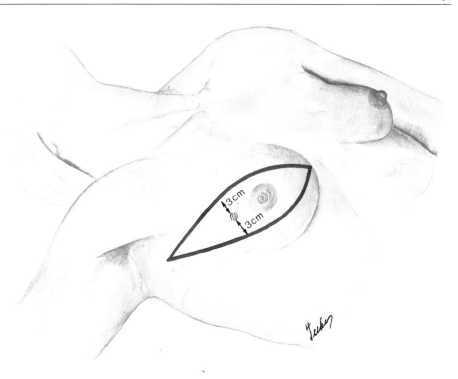

Fig. 14.**1** Patient positioned with arm at right angles supported but entirely movable on an arm board. Note elliptical incision with 3-cm margin of skin in all directions from tumor. The incision is oriented so that it slopes inferiorly as its progresses medially. Note that the nipple-areolar complex is included with the specimen since we make no attempt to preserve this complex.

nodes can be recovered with this operation as can be with the radical mastectomy. As previously indicated, the National Surgical Adjuvant Breast Project (NSABP 1979) found the modified mastectomy as effective as the radical mastectomy in a prospective carefully controlled study.

Skin Incision and Dissection of Skin Flaps

In general, I prefer incisions that are slightly oblique from the transverse line that extend more laterally than medially. Such an incision is more suited to dress and evening clothes style that predominate today (Fig. 14.**1**). There is less emphasis on excision of large amounts of skin with the breast specimen, and in general I believe that the en bloc breast resection should follow the usual precept and include at least 3 to 4 cm of skin in all directions from the margin of the tumor when palpable. I excise less skin when the lesions are small or deep-seated in the breast. After marking the limits of the necessary skin resection around the tumor, the ellipses are then continued in a medial and lateral direction conserving as much skin as possible.

Skin flaps are raised superiorly to the level of the clavicle and inferiorly to the fascia overlying the rectus abdominus muscle. Medially the dissection is carried over the opposite sternal midline and laterally to the latissimus dorsi muscle.

I do not feel that extremely thin flaps must be developed, but rather a plane found in the subcutaneous fat, which assures the removal of all underlying breast tissue. As much subcutaneous fat is preserved as is consistent with a total breast removal. In general, one can easily identify the plane between subcutaneous fat and breast tissue, and with careful attention there is little chance that breast

tissue will be retained in such flaps. Key to the development of flaps is the application of strong upward traction. I prefer to accomplish this with the use of towel clips rather than skin hooks with strong perpendicular upward traction balanced by countertraction on the underlying breast. One can apply a large number of such clips to afford a uniform degree of traction throughout the length of the flap and they are better handled by assistants than the finer more tenous skin hooks. I have not noted any problems with subsequent skin breakdown, scarring, or other complications with use of towel clips.

I prefer to develop the flaps with the use of a scalpel rather than scissors or electrocautery instruments (Fig. 14.**2**). Although there may be some diminished blood loss with the use of the electrocautery, in my experience this

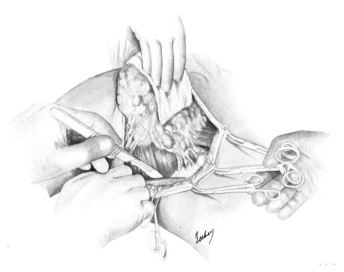

Fig. 14.**2** The technique of flap development is demonstrated. Here the lower breast flap is developed by knife dissection against the traction of upward pull on the skin and cranial elevation of the breast itself.

has not been significant. There is certainly a much reduced incidence of fluid accumulation beneath the flap when a knife is used as opposed to cautery. In addition, should residual breast tumor be required for hormone assay, this is easily done following a knife dissection; hormone receptor assay values after use of the cautery are sometimes falsely low due to heat-induced protein degeneration as a result of the heat developed by the instrument in the immediate neighborhood of the tumor.

Nipple-Areola

Under no circumstances do we attempt any conservation or preservation of the nipple-areolar complex as a part of the developed flaps. Should reconstruction be a consideration in the future, a nipple-areolar reconstruction could give such excellent results that preservation or banking of the original nipple areolar complex is no longer necessary. There have been several reports of tumor development at the site of an autotransplanted nipple-areolar complex (Allison and Howorth 1978; Tchendecker 1979). Anderson and Palleseu (1979) have shown that if careful multiple horizontal sectioning is done, there is about a 33% incidence of involvement of the nipple-areolar tissues with cancer. Therefore, the nipple-areolar complex is generally always included as part of the excised specimen.

Pectoralis Major and Minor Muscles

The overall results of cancer surgery using the modified mastectomy are comparable to those of standard radical mastectomy whether or not the pectoralis minor muscle has been removed. However, many surgeons feel that an adequate axillary dissection requires removal of the pectoralis minor muscle. I feel that if the nodes at all three levels, that is, those medial to the minor (level 3), beneath the minor (level 2), and between the minor and the latissimus muscles (level 1) are to be removed, the pectoralis minor muscle must in some way be mobilized (Fig. 14.**3**). I have in general accomplished this by disconnecting its attachment to the coracoid process, excising it from its medial rib and sternal attachments, and including it with the specimen. In so doing, the axillary artery and vein and underlying fibrofatty nodal tissue is clearly visualized allowing at least as complete an axillary dissection as would be possible with a radical mastectomy (Fig. 14.**4**). The average number of nodes removed has been 37. In mobilizing and excising the pectoralis minor, many of the nerves innervating the lower parts of the pectoralis major muscle are divided and that segment of muscle is denervated with unavoidable atrophy and thinning of the lower pectoralis major muscle. Whenever possible, therefore, an alternative approach preserving the pectoralis major innervation (lateral pectoral nerve) can be accomplished if the minor is mobilized by detaching its medial inferior origin from the sternun and ribs and performing the axillary dissection beneath the raised lower part of the muscle, leaving its insertion near the coracoid process intact. The innervation of the upper parts of both the pectoralis major and

minor muscle derives from medial branches of the intercostal nerves, which are generally left intact when such an approach is used.

Thoracodorsal Vessels and Nerves

Although surgeons generally do not hesitate to remove the thoracodorsal artery, vein, and nerve in order to assure wide margins around any tumor, nevertheless attention is always focused on preservation of these structures in order to maintain the function of the latissimus dorsi muscle. The thoracodorsal artery and vein run along with the nerve in the posterior axilla and have generally been sacrificed if clinically significant lymph nodes are seen in this area. If, on the other hand, no nodes are encountered and one considers selectively preserving the thoracodorsal nerve, one should also strive to preserve the thoracodorsal artery and vein. These vessels may be extremely important in later breast reconstruction if a latissimus dorsi myocutaneous flap is used. Since the edge of the latissimus muscle is the posterior extent of the axillary dissection, it is generally acceptable to preserve these structures without compromising the axillary dissection when there is no obvious disease present in this area (Fig. 14.**5**).

In performing the en bloc dissection, strong traction is applied to the pectoralis major muscle in an upward medial direction and the tissues between that muscle and the underlying pectoralis minor muscle (clavipectoral fasia) are included with the specimen.

Closure

For closure of this incision, I prefer a half dozen strategically placed 3-0 Vicryl sutures in order to line the incision properly and then skin staples. Soft drains, either 18 French red rubber, or similar-sized round polyurethene (Jackson-Pratt) drains are placed. One is put beneath the medial flap and the other beneath the lateral flap including the axilla. It is preferable to exit these drains through stab wounds in the axilla to further minimize skin scarring (Fig. 14.**6**). They are placed on continuous portable suction usually of the elastic bulb configuration where the suction can be replenished by both the nursing staff and the patients themselves. This is a closed drainage system. In general, blood and serum not exceeding 300 cc will be collected in the first three days after surgery and as soon as the 24-hour output falls below 35 to 50 cc the drains are removed usually over the course of the following three days.

I prefer the lightest dressing over the mastectomy incision for several reasons. Light dressings will promote the continued workings of the drains, whereas constrictive dressings will impede drain function. Light dressings have no adverse effect as do compressive dressings on flap circulation, and the incision can be more carefully observed and if necessary the drains manipulated into an area where some fluid might be seen accumulating.

Antibiotics are not used on a routine basis. The patients are ambulated on the day after operation and regular diet

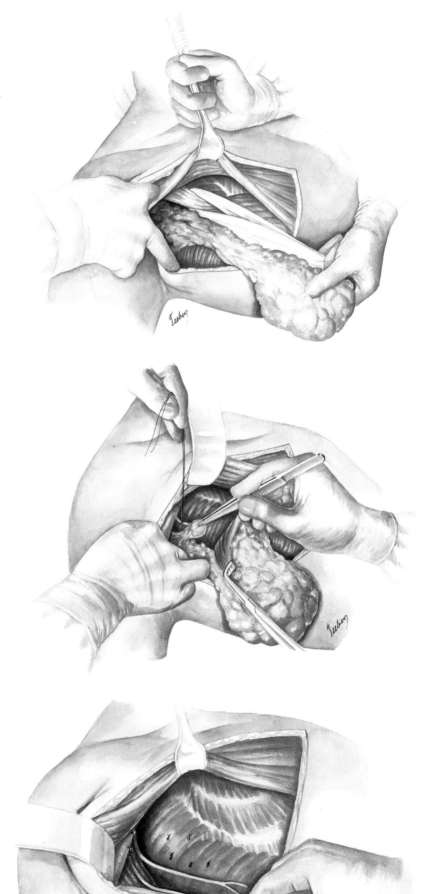

Fig. 14.**3** The pectoralis major muscle is being retracted medially while a Penrose drain that surrounds the pectoralis minor muscle defines it. The lateral pectoral nerves will likely be sacrificed if the pectoralis minor muscle is detached from the coracoid process.

Fig. 14.**4** The pectoralis minor muscle has been separated from the coracoid process and is being retracted inferiorly and laterally, its severed end held in a right-angle clamp. This exposes the neurovascular bundle, and the inferior axillary vein branches with nodal tissue are seen being dissected free from the vein. Continued medial traction on the pectoralis major muscle is necessary to allow such a view of the vein.

Fig. 14.**5** On completion of the dissection, the pectoralis major muscle, slightly retracted in this picture, is intact. The long thoracic nerve innervating the serratus anterior muscle can be seen medially and the thoracodorsal nerve, innervating the latissimus dorsi muscle can be seen slightly lateral in the diagram.

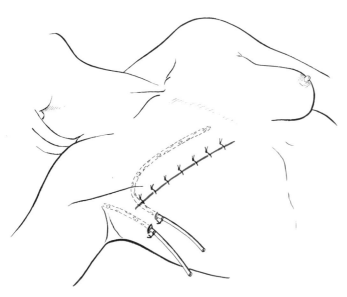

Fig. 14.**6** Diagrammatic representation of closed suction drainage of the mastectomy incision. Note that the two drains are exited through the axilla.

begun. Although earliest initiation of arm movement was formerly practiced, there have been increasing reports attesting to a decrease in flap seromas or mild edema when immobilization for a period of five to seven days is practiced. Therefore, we currently keep the arm on the operated side in a sling dressing and initiate movement from the fifth postoperative day.

Radical Mastectomy

The great contribution of William Stewart Halsted (1894, 1907) in the management of breast cancer remains evident to all practitioners today. His classically described radical mastectomy, which resulted in the removal of all breast tissue and an abundant overlying portion of skin, the entire pectoralis major and minor muscles, and all of the fibrous and fatty tissue beneath the axillary vein including nodes is still called a Halsted mastectomy. Breast cancer mortality before and after introduction of the Halsted mastectomy attests to the effectiveness of this treatment as the most definitive step in the management of breast cancer (Anglem and Leber 1971). Interestingly, until the advent of adjuvant chemotherapy, no further improvement in survival figures for patients with breast cancer had been documented. Within decades of the general acceptance of the Halsted radical mastectomy attempts were made to lessen the procedure in the hopes of still maintaining similar survival figures.

As previously mentioned (data from the American College of Surgeons' survey on the management of breast cancer), in the last decade there has been a definite decrease in the percentage of patients with breast cancer who are treated by a radical mastectomy, the great majority now being treated by a modified muscle-sparing mastectomy. In this survey conducted by the American College of Surgeons, whereas 70% of the operations for

breast cancer were radical mastectomy a decade ago, at the most recent reporting (1980) 70% were of the modified variety. Although one must be cautious and the follow-up period sufficiently long, it would appear at present that except in special circumstances the radical mastectomy has been replaced by the modified mastectomy without measurable changes in five-year cure rate or survival rates.

There are many studies also supporting the fact that the number of lymph nodes resected in a modified mastectomy is the same as in a radical mastectomy. It is my own belief that such a statement can only be made if the pectoralis minor muscle is detached and complete exposure of the axillary vein throughout its entire length from the superior surface of the first rib to the lateral margin of the latissimus dorsi muscle.

The performance of a modified mastectomy also makes subsequent reconstructive efforts considerably easier, although even after radical mastectomy they are possible since the advent of the myocutaneous flap. Even in the absence of reconstructive efforts, the cosmetic results with the modified mastectomy are certainly more acceptable than those following a radical mastectomy. The removal of both the pectoral muscles results in an acute angulation of the arm from the chest wall and a loss of infraclavicular fullness, neither of which occur following the modified mastectomy with conservation of the pectoral muscles. In addition, although difficult to document, in my own personal experience there is considerably less complaint of intermittent episodes of "chest tightness" following the modified mastectomy. There are no data suggesting less lymphedema with one procedure as opposed to the other and no changes in the "phantom breast phenomenon", which is pain interpreted as occurring in the previously excised breast.

Indications

Despite the obvious advantages of the modified over the classic Halsted mastectomy, there are still instances in which the Halsted radical mastectomy is clearly indicated. According to Sanders and Buchanan (1980), in some situations the incidence of recurrence is much higher when less than a Halsted mastectomy is done. Obviously when there is gross involvement of the pectoral muscles, nothing short of a Halsted mastectomy will be sufficient. In addition there is some evidence that tumors occurring in the periphery of the breast, those in the deeper third of the breast within 1 cm of the pectoral fascia, and any tumor larger than 4 cm might advantageously be treated by a Halsted mastectomy.

Technical Considerations

There are many basic articles outlining in detail the technique of Halsted mastectomy beginning with the papers of Halsted himself and additionally covered in detail in recent books such as Haagensen's text on surgery of the breast.

Several points are worth emphasis:

1. The same general principles that relate to the amount of skin removed can be applied to the technique of radical mastectomy and these were outlined in the previous section on modified mastectomy

2. In determining the sequence of steps in performing a mastectomy, it has always seemed more logical to commence with the axillary dissection, thus effectively sealing off lymphatic and vascular routes of spread and proceed from an axillary toward a medial thoracic direction. Once the pectoralis major insertion on the medial humerous has been detached, that muscle can be reflected medially and separated from its clavicular attachments (Fig. 14.7). Following division of the pectoralis minor muscle from the coracoid process, the axillary vein is fully exposed. I have not felt compelled to perform the vein dissection within the filmy adventitia layer preferring to leave this intact when dividing all the inferior branches. Irregular dilatation of the axillary vein sometimes results from such a dissection, and although unproved this may contribute to venous stasis problems and the development of subsequent arm edema

3. As previously stated, every attempt is made to preserve the thoracodorsal artery, vein, and nerve, although their sacrifice singularly or in any combination where tumor is present in the region is certainly in order

4. As the overlying breast, axillary content, and pectoralis major and minor muscles are swept medially, care must be exercised to secure the perforating branches supplying primarily the pectoralis major muscle along its medial margin. These perforators arise from the internal mammary and the medial anterior intercostal vessels and their identification from the medial underside of dissection prior to their division is worth every effort. If they are divided while on traction, they will often retract and their ligation frequently involves application of hemostats in an area where only intercostal muscles act as a barrier from the pleural cavity

5. Suction drainage catheters, as previously described, should again be used. Generally, the postoperative drainage is somewhat prolonged and slightly in excess of that following a modified mastectomy

References

Allison, A. B., M. B. Howorth: Carcinoma in a nipple preserved by heterotopic auto-implantation. N. Engl. J. Med. 298: 1132, 1978

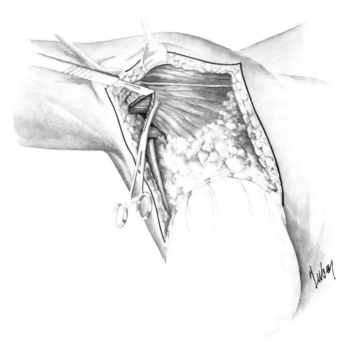

Fig. 14.7 Note the separation of the pectoralis major muscle from its lateral humeral attachments as one of the first steps in the performance of a radical mastectomy after the flaps have been developed.

Anderson, J., R. M. Palleseu: Spread to the nipple and areolar in carcinoma of the breast. Ann. Surg. 189: 367, 1979

Anglem, T. J., R. E. Leber: Characteristics of survivors after radical mastectomy. Am. J. Surg. 121: 363, 1971

Dahl-Iversen, E., T. Tobiassen: Radical mastectomy with parasternal and supraclavicular dissection for mammary carcinoma. Am. Surg. 157: 170, 1963

Fisher, B.: United States trials of conservative surgery. World J. Surg. 1: 327, 1977

Halsted, W. S.: The results of operations for the cure of cancer of the breast performed at Johns Hopkins Hospital from June 1889 to January 1894. Ann. Surg. 20: 497, 1894

Halsted, W. S.: The results of radical operations for the cure of carcinoma of the breast. Ann. Surg. 46: 1, 1907

Handley, R. S.: The conservative radical mastectomy of Patey: Ten year results in 425 patients' breasts. Dis. Breast 2:16, 1976

McWhirter, R.: Treatment of cancer of the breast by simple mastectomy and roentgenotherapy. Arch. Surg. 59: 830, 1949

Nemoto, T., T. L. Dao: Is modified mastectomy adequate for axillary lymph node dissection? Ann. Surg. 182: 722, 1975

NSABP: Progress report of the sixteenth semi-annual meeting of the National Surgical Adjuvant Project for breast and bowel cancers (NSABP), Spring meeting, Tuscon, Arizona, March 28–31, 1979

Sanders, G. B., J. B. Buchanan: Modified radical mastectomy: A word of caution. Breast 6: 2–6, 1980

Tchendekar, J. D.: Carcinoma in a heterotopically autoimplanted nipple. Cancer 42: 2502, 1979

Chapter 15

Extended Radical Mastectomy

J. A. Urban and R. A. Egli

Introduction

The extended radical mastectomy, which includes en bloc surgical excision of the internal mammary chain of nodes together with the radical mastectomy procedure (Urban 1951; Urban and Baker 1952), was devised to cope with the spread of breast cancer to the internal mammary lymph nodes (Sugarbaker 1953; Urban 1956; Wangenstein et al. 1956; Caceres 1958). Of necessity, its benefit is limited to patients who have internal mammary nodes containing metastatic breast cancer, but still do not have established systemic spread of disease. In the past, it was applied to patients with a relatively high risk of internal mammary spread of breast cancer, particularly those with central and medially located lesions (Urban and Castro 1971). Now we find that patients in this category show a lower incidence of internal mammary lymph node involvement because of the public awareness of the need for early diagnosis. It is necessary to select the proper patients more accurately in order to apply this procedure to those patients most likely to be benefited by it.

In 1976, Lacour published the results of an International Cooperative Study evaluating the effect of extended radical mastectomy. Patients were selected randomly for radical mastectomy or extended radical mastectomy. The study was carried out under the auspices of the Gustav Rousse Institute in Paris. One thousand five hundred eighty patients with infiltrating cancer were included; no adjuvant therapy was administered. An insignificant increase in five-year survival was noted in the patients undergoing the extended procedure. However, a subgroup of patients did show a distinct advantage following the extended operation. Patients whose lesions arose in the central and medial portion of the breast with proved positive axillary nodes and with primary lesions in the T1 or T2 category attained a five-year survival rate of only 52% following radical mastectomy, whereas the same group of patients achieved a 71% five-year survival rate with the extended procedure. One hundred ninety-two patients were included in this group and 32% of those undergoing the extended procedure had positive internal mammary nodes.

Currently, there is a great deal of disagreement regarding the significance of metastatic breast cancer in the internal mammary nodes. Donegan (1977) evaluated 113 patients following radical mastectomy in whom internal mammary nodes were biopsied extrapleurally at the time of initial surgery; 25 were shown to have metastatic cancer in the internal mammary nodes. No further treatment was administered to these nodes, and ten years later, only 1 of 20 or 5% of patients who had had positive internal mammary nodes survived. He concluded that the presence of metastatic cancer in the internal mammary nodes indicated an advanced stage of disease that was beyond control by local surgery or radiation therapy. Fisher (1969, 1979) who maintains that all breast cancers are systemic from their inception minimizes the significance of internal mammary node disease, which he believes is overshadowed by the presence of axillary node metastases as an indication of the presence of occult systemic disease. Veronesi, Bucalossi and Veronesi 1958; Veronesi and Valagussa 1981; Canellos et al. 1982, who originally advocated the extended operation, has reversed his attitude and now believes that resection of the internal mammary nodes has no effect on long-term survival. Several individuals now advocate extrapleural biopsy of the internal mammary nodes at the time of mastectomy (Morrow and Foster 1981) – not as a therapeutic procedure – but as an indication for the use of adjuvant multichemotherapy when internal mammary nodes are found to contain metastatic breast cancer, especially in patients whose axillary nodes are negative.

Despite Fisher's statement that any change in the local treatment of breast cancer will have no effect on the ultimate outcome of the disease, ten-year survival data on patients treated by different therapeutic regimens prove otherwise. When the presence of metastatic cancer is proved in internal mammary nodes by biopsy but no treatment is administered to these nodes, the ten-year survival rate obtained by Donegan (1977) was only 5%. Handley (1976), who performed extrapleural biopsy of the internal mammary nodes following the modified mastectomy procedure of Patey and then administered cobalt 60 therapy to the internal mammary area when the nodes were positive, obtained a ten-year survival rate of 22% in these patients. Radiation therapy, 4500 to 5000 rads, was administered to the nodal complex. When only internal mammary nodes were positive, 44% survived; when both axillary and internal mammary nodes were positive, 18% survived at ten years. Veronesi (1981), in his latest paper, reported that 45.8% of his patients with only positive internal mammary nodes survived ten years following the extended operation, and 20% of those who had involvement of both axilla and internal mammary nodes survived at ten years. His overall ten-year survival rate following the extended radical procedure for patients with positive internal mammary nodes was 26%. This is similar to the ten-year survival rate obtained by Koszarowski (1976) in Warsaw: 26.5% survival at ten years. Our own (Cody et al. 1982) personal ten-year survival rates in patients with positive internal mammary nodes following the extended radical operation with supplemental radiation therapy to the base of the neck when nodes were positive in the first internal mammary space or in the apex of the axilla was 46% overall. When only internal mammary nodes were positive, 45% were alive at ten years and 45% free of disease. When both axillary and internal mammary nodes were positive, 47% were alive, but only 35% free of disease. None of these patients received adjuvant multichemotherapy.

Patients whose involved internal mammary nodes were diagnosed by biopsy, but were not treated by surgical excision or radiation therapy, had essentially the same long-term survival as is noted in patients with untreated primary breast cancer (Donegan 1977). Even though the treated patients did better than those who were not treated, there is a great deal of room for improvement. Hopefully, the addition of adjuvant multichemotherapy to these patients will result in improved survival. At present, however, the effects of adjuvant multichemotherapy are not sufficiently encouraging to warrant the replacement of adequate primary therapy by inadequate local therapy plus multichemotherapy. Adjuvant multichemotherapy should be utilized as a supplement to adequate primary therapy. Local control achieved by adequate primary therapy diminishes the tumor load in the patient and should facilitate the effectiveness of adjuvant multichemotherapy.

Anatomy of the Internal Mammary Lymphatic-Vascular System

The internal mammary arteries arise from the undersurface of the subclavian artery opposite the thyrocervical trunk, descend behind the costal cartilages, and are separated from the underlying lung by a thin fascial layer and the parietal pleura. At the level of the third rib, the anterior transverse thoracic muscle appears behind the artery. The internal mammary veins lie between the artery and the sternal margin. Both vein and artery divide into two branches at the level of the third intercostal space, going inferiorly. Superiorly, the right internal mammary vein drains into the superior vena cava, whereas the left almost always drains into the left innominate vein. The right internal mammary lymphatics drain into the right lymphatic duct which empties into the right subclavian vein. The left lymphatic vessels draining the internal mammary nodal complex drain directly into the thoracic duct, or, rarely, by a separate pathway into the confluence of the internal mammary and subclavian veins. The internal mammary nodes are found most frequently in the first interspace, and then in diminishing frequency in the second, third, fourth, and fifth. In our own experience (Urban and Marjani 1971), 88% of patients had nodes in the first interspace, 84% in the second, 73% in the third, 46% in the fourth, and only 12% in the fifth. Nodes are found with equal frequency medial or lateral to the internal mammary vessels. The incidence of internal mammary nodes containing metastatic breast cancer shows a different distribution. The highest incidence occurs in the second interspace (17%) then in the first interspace (15%); 14% in the third, 5% in the fourth, and very rarely, 1% in the fifth interspace. Putti (1953), studying 47 cadavers, found internal mammary nodes present in 90% of the first interspaces, 89% in the second, 70% in the third, 46% in the fourth, 12% in the fifth, and 10% in the sixth. A total of 7.7 nodes were found in both internal mammary chains. We have found as many as ten nodes in one internal mammary chain, and as few as none in another at the time of surgery. Soerenson (1951) found an average of 3.5 nodes on each side. Ju (1957) had a similar experience in 100 autopsies. Abrao and Abrao (1954) found an average of 8.9 nodes on the right side and 7.3 on the left in 100 autopsies. In addition, they noticed retromanubrial lymphatic connection at the level of the first interspace in 20% of their cases. We (Urban and Marjani 1971) have never seen gross evidence of cross metastases from one internal mammary chain to the other in operable breast cancer patients (Abrao and Abrao 1954; Handlay and Thackray 1954).

We have applied the extended radical mastectomy to approximately 1000 patients at Memorial Sloan Kettering

Table 15.1 Node metastases in primary operable breast cancers undergoing combined procedure

Location		A	B	C	D	E	F	G	Total
Total No. of cases		224	321	80	81	75	26	8	815–100%
All nodes clear		127	156	29	35	12	5	2	366– 45%
Int. mammary only involved		28	18	12	7	1	1	0	67– 8.2%
Axillary only involved		27	79	11	15	36	11	4	183– 22.4%
Both int. mammary and axillary inv.		42	68	28	24	26	9	2	199– 24.4%
Overall group 55% positive nodes	815 cases	45% all nodes clear 33% positive int. mammary 47% positive axillary 15% cases with clear axilla had positive internal mammary nodes							

Cancer Institute in New York City, with only three postoperative deaths within 30 days of primary surgery. It has been applied mainly to patients with a high risk of internal mammary lymph node metastases from breast cancers arising in the central and medial portions of the breast. In the first 815 cases, 47% had positive axillary nodes, 29% positive internal mammary nodes (Table 15.1). In 8% only internal mammary nodes were involved. Fifteen percent of patients who had negative axillae had positive internal mammary nodes. This relatively high incidence of internal mammary node metastases reflects our selection of patients and is not typical of overall nodal involvement in the average patient.

Operative Procedure

After a positive biopsy has been obtained (Urban and Baker 1952), a wide skin incision is made about the breast extending at least 4 cm from the nearest palpable margin of the primary tumor (Fig. 15.1). Skin flaps are developed outside the superficial fascia which separates the subcutaneous fat from the underlying breast parenchyma. This fascia is transected at the base of the flap and the incision is beveled off to the underlying muscle fascia (Fig. 15.2). Flaps are developed to the clavicle above, the sternum medially, to the anterior margin of the latissimus laterally, and inferiorly to the sixth rib. The fascia overlying

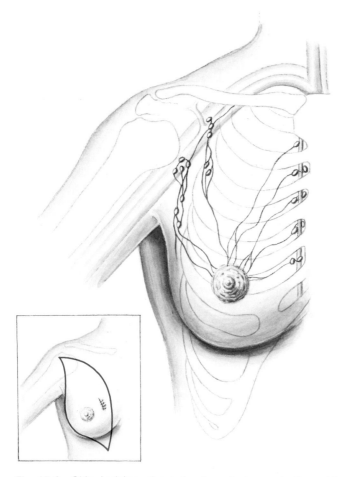

Fig. 15.1 Skin incision about the breast demonstrating wide margins about the tumor area.

the sternal head of the pectoral major muscle is dissected from this muscle downward to the plane that separates the sternal and clavicular heads. The major muscle is separated in this plane. Tissues overlying the first rib and the arch of the manubrium are dissected down to the bony structures and reflected downward exposing the lower margin of the first rib and the arch of the manubrium. Inferiorly, the rectus sheath is cleared to the level of the sixth rib where it is incised here or at the level of the fifth rib, and reflected upward exposing the lower portion of the fourth or fifth interspace. The pectoralis muscle is freed from the underlying chest wall by inserting a finger beneath this muscle just lateral to the second costal chondral junction elevating the muscle from the level of the first interspace above to the fifth interspace below (Fig. 15.3). Inferiorly, the major muscle is transected at its attachment to the costal chondral junction of the fifth rib and the tunnel beneath the muscle is completed (Fig. 15.4). The chest is entered through the first interspace just outside the costal chondral junctions of the first and second ribs. The internal mammary artery can now be palpated from within the chest lying just beneath the first rib. The artery usually extends upward and laterally, whereas the vein extends upward and medially at this level. The base of the neck can be explored by palpation from within the chest and the deeper mediastinal structures can also be examined before committing oneself to resecting the internal mammary area. If no gross evidence of metastatic disease is noted in these areas, the procedure is continued. The intercostal muscles of the first interspace are cut from the lower margin of the first rib and the arch of the manubrium exposing the areolar tissue that lies between the parietal pleura and the intercostal muscle and that contains the internal mammary vessels and nodes. This is reflected downward toward the operative specimen, the internal mammary vessels are doubly tied and cut, and the parietal pleura transected just below the lower margin of the first rib. In a similar fashion, dissection is carried through the lowermost portion of the fourth or fifth interspace, depending on the location of the primary tumor in the breast. With an upper inner quadrant lesion, dissection is usually carried down to the fourth interspace. If disease is found in the lower portion of the breast, dissection is usually carried down to the upper margin of the sixth rib to include this drainage area more thoroughly. Inferiorly, the internal mammary vessels lie between the intercostal muscles anteriorly and the anterior transverse thoracic muscle posteriorly. Dissection is carried through the entire thickness of the chest wall, the vessels are isolated, tied off, and cut just above the lower rib. Now the sternum is split vertically, just inside its ipsilateral margin, developing a trap door in the chest wall (Fig. 15.5). This portion of the chest wall, which contains the internal mammary vessels and lymph nodes, is now resected from the chest wall by cutting through the ribs and soft parts at the level of the costal chondral junctions of the second and third ribs with a scissors. The chest wall area containing the internal mammary lymph node complex is now reflected laterally still in continuity with the overlying breast and pectoral major muscle. The intercostal bleeders are tied off with 3–0 silk sutures, and bone wax is

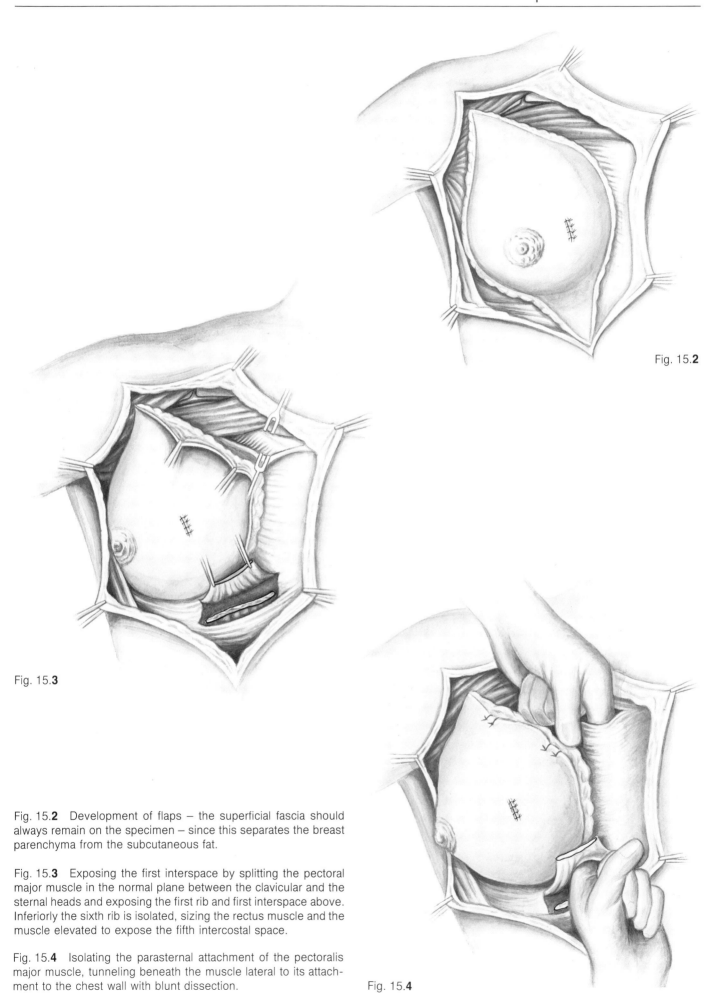

Fig. 15.**2**

Fig. 15.**3**

Fig. 15.**4**

Fig. 15.**2** Development of flaps – the superficial fascia should always remain on the specimen – since this separates the breast parenchyma from the subcutaneous fat.

Fig. 15.**3** Exposing the first interspace by splitting the pectoral major muscle in the normal plane between the clavicular and the sternal heads and exposing the first rib and first interspace above. Inferiorly the sixth rib is isolated, sizing the rectus muscle and the muscle elevated to expose the fifth intercostal space.

Fig. 15.**4** Isolating the parasternal attachment of the pectoralis major muscle, tunneling beneath the muscle lateral to its attachment to the chest wall with blunt dissection.

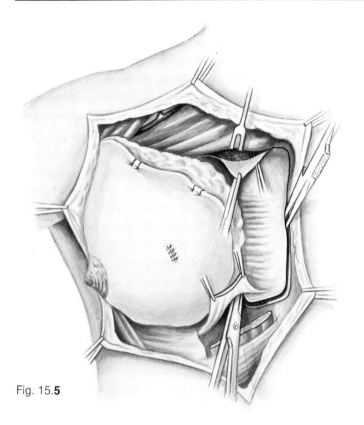

Fig. 15.**5**

Fig. 15.5 Resecting the parasternal portion of the chest wall en bloc with the perforating vessels and internal mammary vessels and the intact breast and pectoralis major muscle superficially.

Fig. 15.6 Demonstrating the defect in the chest wall following removal of the parasternal portion of the chest wall which contains the internal mammary nodes. The major and minor muscles have been stripped laterally from the chest wall and an underwater catheter has been inserted through the on interspace for drainage of the chest. Reconstruction of the defect is begun by suturing the mediastinal pleura to the periosteum on the anterior surface of the sternum.

Fig. 15.7 Final closure of the chest wall first utilizing heavy number two monafilament nylon sutures to over correct the defect in the chest wall by applying them through the ribs and opposing sternal margin under tension usually reducing the defect about one-third in size. This stabilizes the chest wall and avoids parado-xical motion. In B and C further completion of the closure by applying either the patient's own fascialata or sterile ox fascia, again under tension with interrupted stay sutures of No 3–0 monofilament nylon trimming the edges of the graft and tacking down the margins with continuous locked 3–0 chromic catgut suture.

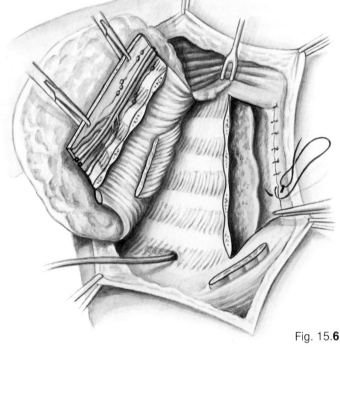

Fig. 15.**6**

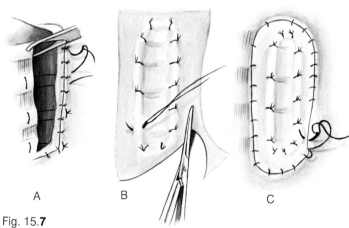

A   B   C

Fig. 15.**7**

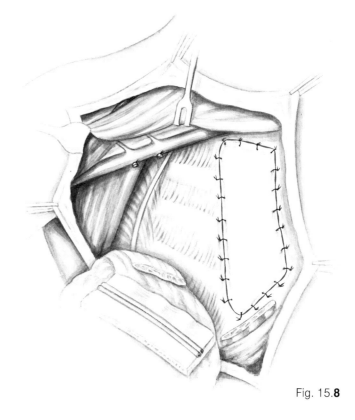

Fig. 15.**8**

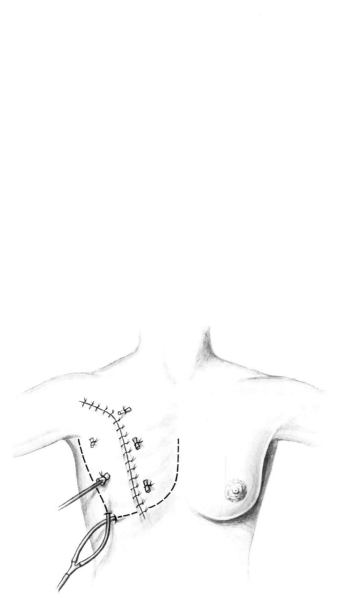

Fig. 15.**9**

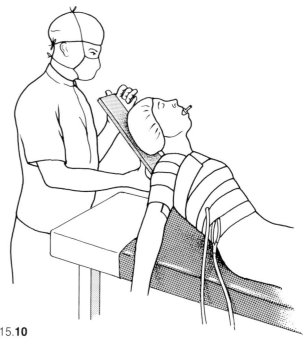

Fig. 15.**8** Appearance of the operative area following thorough axillary dissection – note all the tissues are being removed en bloc.

Fig. 15.**9** The complete closure of the operative defect by primary closure of the flaps using through and through stay sutures tied over gauge bolsters to distribute tension and closing the flap with interrupted 0000 nylon.

Fig. 15.**10** Supporting the patient with an aluminium arm board or similar support for application of wrap around dressing of gauze which is then reinforced with elastic tape in order to avoid dead space in the operative area.

Fig. 15.**10**

occasionally used to control oozing from the sternal marrow cavity. The pectoralis major and minor muscles are now reflected from the chest wall laterally and an underwater catheter is inserted into the chest cavity through the fifth or sixth interspace laterally. The defect in the chest wall is now reconstructed, first by suturing the free margin of the mediastinal pleura to the fascia overlying the sternum with a running suture of fine atranmatic catgut. The cut rib margins are then overapproximated to the sternal margin with four separate parallel heavy stay sutures of No. 2 dermalon (Fig. 15.**6**). These are applied through the anterior margin of the sternum first, carried across the space through the rib, over the rib, back through the rib, and through the anterior margin of the sternum. The sutures are all put in place and then snubbed up tightly to minimize the chest wall defect and also to stabilize the chest wall. The defect in the chest wall is usually diminished by approximately one third by this maneuver and the tense sutures serve as a stabilizing support (Fig. 15.**7**). Finally, sterile ox fascia or other tissue (autogenous fascia lata) is applied over the stabilized chest wall anchoring the fascia to the margins of the defect with interrupted double 0 dermalon, applied under tension. Excess fascia is trimmed off and the margins approximated to the underlying chest wall with a running atraumatic 00 chromic catgut suture. This type of closure results in a flexible support of the chest wall, which prevents paradoxical motion to a great extent. The radical mastectomy procedure is completed in the usual fashion (Fig. 15.**8**). Before closing the skin flaps, a stab wound is made in the lateral lower skin flap for exit of the underwater catheter. This is anchored in place with a silk suture, tied over a gauze bolster, which approximates the skin to the chest wall, and holds the underwater catheter in place. Two reliavac catheters are placed through the lower skin flap and the skin margins are closed. The underwater catheter is attached to a pleurovac and the reliovac drains to a suitable container (Fig. 15.**9**). The underwater catheter is usually removed two days follow-

ing surgery and the reliovacs are usually kept in place for five to six days (Fig. 15.**10**). The patients undergoing the extended procedure are usually hospitalized for eight days. We have performed 1000 extended radical procedures with only three postoperative deaths within one month of surgery. One death occurred from a coronary infarction, another from a cerebrovascular accident, and a third from an uncontrolled perforated peptic ulcer. This minimal mortality is only possible through careful postoperative care of the patients with particular reference to pulmonary ventilation and pleural drainage (Fig. 15.**11**).

Findings

Seven hundred eighty-four consecutive patients were operated on between 1951 and 1972. Only 3.5% had tumors presenting in the outer portion of the breast. All other tumors impinged on the vertical line extending from 12 to 6 o'clock, or were located medial to it. The average tumor measured 3.1 cm in diameter, as examined in the pathology laboratory. Forty-four percent had positive axillary nodes and 30% positive internal mammary nodes. Metastatic cancer was found in internal mammary nodes most often in the second interspace (17%); 15% in the first interspace; 14% in the third interspace; 5% in the fourth interspace; and 1% in the fifth interspace. Forty-eight percent of patients had all nodes negative, 22.5% only axillary involvement, 8% only internal mammary involvement. Twenty-one and one half percent had involvement of both axillary and internal mammary nodes 14% of patients with negative axillae had positive internal mammary nodes. Twenty-two percent of all patients received postoperative cobalt 60 radiation therapy to the base of the neck, usually receiving 4500 rads in air within a five-week period. Nine percent received radiation therapy to the chest wall – usually patients with very large primary tumors adjacent to the pectoral muscle. At 10 years post. op. local recurrence in the operative field occurred in 6.1% of all patients; it appeared as the first sign of recurrent cancer in only 18 (2.3%) patients. Local recurrence appeared in 30 (3.8%) patients coincident with or following the appearance of distant metastases.

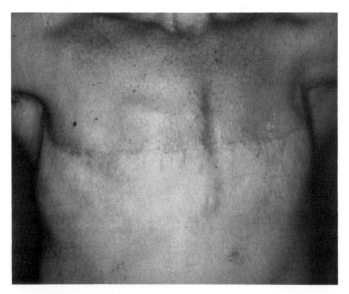

Fig. 15.**11** Modified mastectomy on right for intraductile carcinoma. Extended mastectomy on left for infiltrating lobular carcinoma with positive axilla and positive IM nodes.

Results

Seven hundred eighty-four patients were treated by the extended operative procedure between 1951 and 1972 at the Memorial Sloan Kettering Cancer Center in New York City. Overall crude ten-year survival is 54% free of disease, 59% alive. When only axillary nodes contained metastatic cancer, 49% are free of disease and 55% alive. When only internal mammary disease is present, 43% are free of disease and 51% alive. When both axillary and internal mammary nodal areas are involved with disease, 26% are free of disease and 36% are alive at ten years. When all nodes were negative, 71% were alive and free of disease; 73% were alive at ten years. Two percent of patients were lost to follow up and 5% died of other causes while free of evidence of disease. All included as though they had died of breast cancer.

After 25 years, 21% of patients with both axillary and internal mammary involvement are free of disease. However, at 25 years, 22% of patients were lost to other causes or lost to follow up without evidence of recurrent breast cancer. This high attrition rate from other causes indicates the difficulty of evaluating long-term results on a crude survival basis.

Almost all current trials of treatment for breast cancer use the life-table method for calculating survival. This shows the patients likelihood of death from breast cancer most accurately. Disease-free patients who are lost to follow up or die of other causes are eliminated from this study at that point and are not counted as dead of disease. However, in the life-table method, all deaths from cancer in patients dying of cancer, as well as patients with recurrent disease who die of other causes, are counted as deaths from cancer. Figs. 15.**12** to 15.**15** depict the survival rates based on life-table analysis. Fig. 15.**12** covers the overall group, and then each category of nodal involvement is covered separately regarding the presence or absence of adjuvant radiation therapy. No adjuvant chemotherapy was administered to any of these patients. The addition of radiation therapy did not significantly effect the survival rate. The drop off in survival rate appears to level off at 12 to 15 years in all categories. This would indicate that a 15-year follow up is probably the

ideal time interval for evaluating the effectiveness of any particular therapeutic regime for primary breast cancer.

Using the life-table method for calculating survival, at ten years 82% of all patients with all nodes negative survived; 63% with only axillary involvement; 56% with only internal mammary involvement; and 38% with both nodal areas involved with metastatic cancer survived at ten years. At 15 years, these figures dropped to 78%, 56%, 48%, and 30%. The survival rate at 25 years, using life-table analysis, is identical to that at 15 years. Seventy-seven percent with all nodes negative survived at 25 years, 55% when only axillary involvement was present, 47% with only internal mammary involvement, and 28% with both areas involved. These data would certainly indicate that adequate primary treatment succeeded in obtaining long term survival in a significant number of patients without the use of any systemic form of therapy.

During the last ten years, we have found a diminishing number of patients with positive internal mammary nodes, probably due to public awareness of the importance of early diagnosis. In addition, we have encountered an increasing number of patients who refuse permission for adequate primary surgery. Currently, the average tumor seen in our patients measures 1.8 cm. The average axillary involvement is 30% and involvement of internal mammary nodes has become exceedingly low less than 15% in the so-called high risk group of patients with inner and medial lesions. We now select patients for the extended radical procedure by preliminary extrapleu-

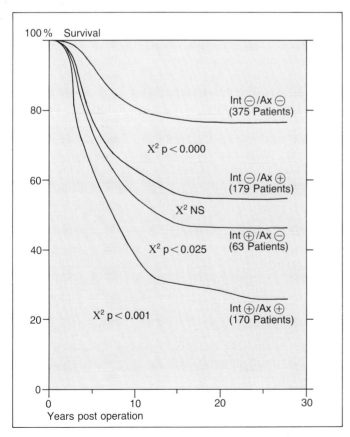

Fig. 15.**12** Life-table analysis of all patients undergoing extended radical mastectomy between 1951 and 1972 – in relation to nodal involvement.

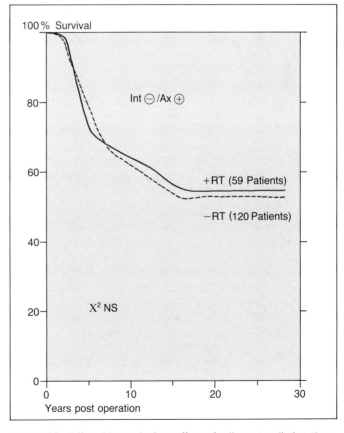

Fig. 15.**13** Life-table analysis – effect of adjuvant radiation therapy on survival of patients with only axillary node involvement.

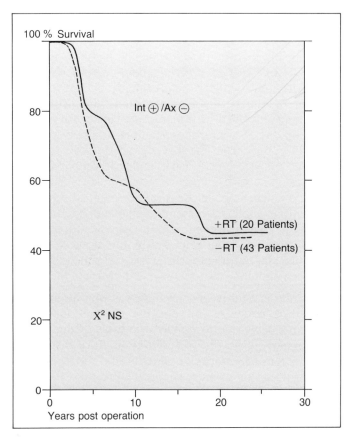

Fig. 15.**14** Life-table analysis showing the effect of adjuvant radiation therapy on patients with only internal mammary nodal disease.

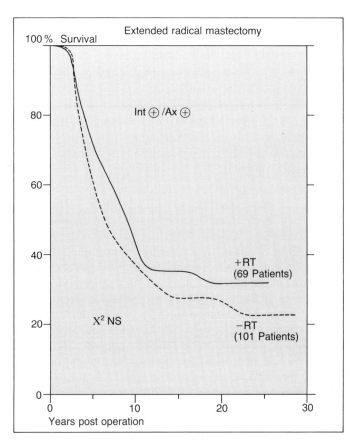

Fig. 15.**15** Life-table analysis showing the effect of adjuvant radiation therapy on the survival of patients with both internal mammary and axillary nodal disease.

ral biopsy of the internal mammary nodes at the time of mastectomy for a known breast cancer. This is applied primarily to patients with central and inner half lesions. Between 1973 and 1979, 72 extended radical procedures were performed as the initial primary operation. This was applied to patients with larger tumors. These proved to have 46% axillary involvement and 33% internal mammary involvement. During this same time interval, 89 other patients with central and inner half lesions were evaluated by extrapleural biopsy of the internal mammary nodes at the time of mastectomy. Forty-six underwent a radical mastectomy and 43 underwent the Patey type modified radical mastectomy. Only 14 of 89 (15%) patients had positive internal mammary nodes. We were unable to convince some patients of the potential benefit of the extended radical procedure. Only six of these 14 patients agreed to be converted to the extended procedure and eight were treated by application of supervoltage radiation therapy (5000 rads of cobalt 60 therapy in a five-week period). Early follow up of these patients at six years shows that one of those who underwent extended radical mastectomy died of liver metastases, or a failure rate of 17%. Two failures occurred in the eight patients treated by radiation therapy to the internal mammary nodes with a maximum follow up of five years (Table 15.**2**).

Several authors have maintained that lymphoscintigraphy represents an accurate means for evaluating the status of the internal mammary nodes. Ege (1982) has written on the use of radioactive antimony injected into the posterior rectus sheath with imaging done three hours later. She claims a high rate of accuracy in detecting metastatic disease in the internal mammary nodes. However, she has not correlated her findings with histopathologic examination of biopsied internal mammary nodes. Matsuo (1974), in Japan, used radioactive gold in a similar fashion and claimed a high rate of correct diagnoses – 90% correct in positive cases whose metastatic cancer was corroborated by biopsy and 44% correct when metastatic disease was suspected. We attempted to repeat Ege's study on 12 patients, but were unable to obtain any significant correlation between the radiographic findings and the histopathologic examination of the internal mammary nodes which were excised in regard to the presence or absence of metastatic breast cancer. However, this technique of radioactive imaging is an excellent one for localization of the internal mammary nodes for accurate positioning of radiation therapy portals (Osborne et al. 1983).

We believe that the extended radical procedure, when well performed and applied to selected patients with internal mammary node involvement who are still clinically free of disease, is an ideal operative procedure. It has yielded excellent local control: 2.3% local recurrence as the first sign of recurrent cancer and a moderately satisfactory long-term survival rate at 10 to 25 years. Supplementing this therapeutic approach with the addition of adjuvant multichemotherapy will hopefully add

Table 15.**2** Extrapleural biopsy of i.m. nodes 1973–1979

Number	Procedure	Findings
72	1° Ext. Rad Mast.	46% ax +, 33% IM +
46	Rad Mast. with I.M. Bx.	44% ax +⎫14/89–15%
43	Patey Mod. Mast. with I. M. Bx	25% ax +⎭IM + *

- *● 6 Converted to ERM
- ● 6 4 NED to 84 Mos.
- ● 1 DOC–NRD
- ● 1 Failure

- ● 8–Rx. with 5000 R Co60
- ● 6 NED to 61 Mos.
- ● 2 Failures

Cody-Urban

still further to the survival rate. This data should serve as a good bench mark for evaluating the curability of patients with breast cancer by a local primary attack on the breast and regional nodes. Adequate primary treatment of the breast and regional nodes of patients with primary operable breast cancer should be continued.

References

Abrao, A., A. Abrao: Estudo Anatomico da Cadeia Ganglionar mammaria interne em 100 cases. Rev. Paul. Med. 45: 317, 1954

Bucalossi, P., U. Veronesi: Long term results of radical mastectomy with removal of internal mammary chain. Acta Unio Int. Contra Cancrum 15: 1052, 1985

Caceres, E.: Radical mastectomy with resection of internal mammary chain. Acta Unio Int. Contra Cancrum 15:1061, 1958

Canellos, G. P., S. Hellman, U. Veronesi: The management of early breast cancer. N. Engl. J. Med. 1430–1432, 1982

Cody, H. S., III, S. S. Bretsky, J. A. Urban: The continuing importance of adequate surgery for operable breast cancer: Significant salvage of node-positive patients without adjuvant chemotherapy. Cancer 32: 242–256, 1982

Donegan, W. L.: The influence of untreated internal mammary metastases upon the course of mammary cancer. Cancer 39: 533–538, 1977

Ege, G. N.: Radiocolloid lymphoscintigraphy in the management of breast cancer. Contemp. Surg. 20: 33–43, 1982

Fisher, B.: Breast cancer management – alternative to radical mastectomy. N. Engl. J. Med. 301: 326–328, 1979

Fisher, B., N. H. Slack, R. K. Ausman, I. D. J. Bross: Location of breast carcinoma and prognosis. Surg. Gynecol. Obstet. 705–716, 1969

Handley, R. S.: The conservative mastectomy of Patey: 10 year results in 425 patients. Breast 3: 16–19, 1976

Handley, R. S., A. C. Thackray: Invasion of internal mammary lymph nodes in carcinoma of the breast. Br. Med. J. 1: 61, 1954

Ju, Cited by Haagensen – Diseases of the Breast; W. B. Saunders & Company, P. 38, 1957

Koszarowski, T.: Rational approach to the efficiency of internal mammary lymph node dissection in breast cancer. Breast 2: 44–47, 1976

Lacour, J., P. Bucalossi, E. Caceres, G. Jacobelli, T. Koszarowski, M. Le, C. Reuneau-Roquette, U. Veronesi: Radical mastectomy versus radical mastectomy plus internal mammary dissection. Cancer 37: 206–214, 1976

Margottini, M.: Arguments in favor of supra radical operations for cancer of the breast. Acta Unio Int. Contra Cancrum 15:1037, 1958

Matsuo, S.: Studies on the metastasis of breast cancer to lymph nodes. II Diagnosis of metastasis to internal mammary nodes using radiocolloid. Acta Med. Okayama 28: 361–371, 1974

Morrow, M., R. S. Foster: Staging of breast cancer. A new rationale for internal mammary node biopsy. Arch. Surg. 116:748–751, 1981

Osborne, M. P., W. S. Meijer, S. D. J. Yeh, J. J. DeCosse: Lymphoscintigraphy in the staging of solid tumors. Surg. Gynecol. Obstet. 136: 384–391, 1983

Putti, F.: Riciersche Anatomiche sue Linfonodi Mammari Interni. Chir. Ital. 7: 161, 1953

Sorensen, B.: Recherches-sur-localisation des ganglion lymphatiques Parasternaux par rapport aux espaces intercostaux. Int. J. Chir. 11: 501, 1951

Sugarbaker, E. D.: Radical mastectomy combined with incontinuity resection of the homolateral internal mammary node chain. Cancer 6: 969, 1953

Turner-Warwick, R. T.: Lymphatics of the breast. Br. J. Surg. 46: 574–582, 1959

Urban, J. A.: Radical excision of the chest wall for mammary cancer. Cancer 4: 1263–1285, 1951

Urban, J. A.: Radical mastectomy with en bloc incontinuity resection of the internal mammary lymph node chain. Surg. Clin. N. A. 36: 1065, 1956

Urban, J. A., H. W. Baker: Radical mastectomy with en bloc excision of the internal mammary lymph node chain. Cancer 5: 992–1008, 1952

Urban, J. A., E. B. Castro: Selecting variations in extent of surgical procedure for breast cancer. Cancer 28: 1615–1623, 1971

Urban, J. A., M. A. Marjani: Significance of internal mammary lymph node metastases in breast cancer. Am. J. Roentgenol. Radiother. Nucl. Med. 111: 1971

Veronesi, U., P. Valagussa: Inefficiency of internal mammary nodes dissection in breast cancer surgery. Cancer 47: 170–175, 1981

Wangenstein, O H., F. J. Lewis, S. W. Arhelgu: The extended or super radical mastectomy for carcinoma of the breast. Surg. Clin. N. Am. 36: 1951, 1956

Chapter 16

Nipple Discharge and Paget's Disease

F. E. Rosato and R. S. Boova

Nipple Discharge

Introduction

Nipple discharge is the second most common symptom in breast disease, the finding of a breast mass being the most common (Rimstein et al. 1976). Approximately 7% to 10% of all patients with breast disease will have abnormal breast secretions. Nipple discharge is at least twice as frequent in benign disease as it is with malignant breast lesions (Devitt 1977; Leis et al. 1967, 1973).

Physiologic Breast Secretions

Physiologic breast secretions are usually milky, whereas pathologic breast secretions may be serous, serosanguinous, or purulent.

Lactation results from prolactin stimulation of the mammary gland. Hyperprolactinemia in the nonpuerperal state may be the result of abnormal hypothalamic-pituitary interaction or a number of exogenous factors.

The hypothalamic-pituitary relationship may be upset in the postpartum period in the Chiari-Frommel or Sheehan's syndromes. Amenorrhea with galactorrhea also occurs in the Ahumada-del Castello and the Forbes-Albright syndromes, which are not associated with the postpartum period.

Other organic causes of abnormal lactation include primary hypothyroidism, Cushing's syndrome, chest wall trauma including thoracotomy, herpetic infection of thoracic nerves, hysterectomy, breast biopsy, and certain pituitary and hypothalamic lesions.

Several drugs can cause hyperprolactinemia and resultant breast discharge. These include phenothiazine derivatives (chlorpromazine and prochlorperazine), tricyclic antidepressants, and oral contraceptives both during usage and following discontinuance. Reserpine and methyldopa have also been associated with hyperprolactinemia (Archer 1977; Barnes 1966).

In addition, lactation may be the result of persistent mechanical stimulation. This may even occur during repeated breast self-examination (Leis et al. 1973). Nonlactiferous breast secretion may occur with vascular engorgement of the breasts as occurs in pregnancy, during the premenstrual phase, and with birth control pills (Rosemond and Maier 1975).

Galactorrhea secondary to hypothalamic-pituitary imbalances may be controlled medically with ergot derivates (Archer 1977). Lactiferous secretions caused by mechanical stimulation or medications will cease with termination of the inciting factor.

Pathologic Breast Secretions

The overall incidence of nipple discharge among patients with breast problems seen by physicians approximates 7% to 10% (Leis et al. 1967, 1972). Secretions are found in some 8% to 12% of patients with breast malignancy (Barnes 1966). However, among patients with nipple discharge, benign breast disease is causative in nearly 85%. The likelihood of cancer is related to the presence of a palpable mass (Atkins and Wolff 1964; Devitt 1977; Rosemond and Maier 1975). The incidence of carcinoma may be as high as 33% when nipple discharge is associated with a mass, whereas in the absence of a mass, nipple discharge will be caused by malignancy in 10% to 15% of cases (Rimsten et al. 1976). The occurrence of malignant disease increases in patients over age 60 with nipple discharges (Copeland and Higgens 1969; Seltzer et al. 1970). Some authors report a greater incidence of malignancy than benign breast disease in patients over age 60 with pathologic nipple discharge (Leis et al. 1967).

Discharges are described differently by many authors, including milky, cheesy, purulent, watery, serous, serosanguinous, or bloody. We prefer three categories: serous (milky, clear, yellowish, or greenish), bloody, or purulent. The type of discharge is not reliable in estimating the likelihood of malignancy. Carcinoma may occur with serous or sanguinous discharges. A bloody discharge is more likely due to benign disease. However, carcinoma is more likely to have bloody than serous discharge (Urban and Egeli 1978). Discharge of any type in a patient over age 60 is highly suspicious for cancer (Seltzer et al. 1970).

It is generally accepted that intraductal papilloma is the most frequent cause of nipple discharge (Funderburk and Syphax 1969, Haagensen 1971). However, many reports are found in which fibrocystic disease was a more frequent cause of abnormal breast secretion (Barnes 1966, Rimsten et al. 1976). Other causes include chronic subareolar abscess, mastitis, carcinoma, duct ectasia, and trauma.

Evaluation of a secreting breast is straightforward when a coincident mass exists. This may occur in 40% to 60% of cases (Madalin et al. 1957; Urban and Egeli 1978). In these instances, breast biopsy is certainly indicated.

In secreting breasts without a mass, a multitude of diagnostic techniques have been utilized. Cytology, contrast mammography, and transillumination have been employed with varying success. In the absence of a palpable mass, mammography is unlikely to identify a mass lesion. This mode should be utilized, however, in anyone with suspected breast disease. Cytology of the discharge has not had extensive application in the United States, but is used more in Europe. According to Franzen (see Chapter 1), there are many false-positive readings when malignant cells are found in such discharges and treatment should not be based exclusively on such positive findings. However, if no malignant or atypical cells are found, it is very rare for a cancer to be associated with such discharge.

If the offending duct can not be localized, the surgeon has several alternatives. If there is little suspicion of carcinoma, he may choose to observe the discharge for a short time until the pathologic duct can be identified.

Complete central duct excision has also been advocated when there is failure to localize the discharge (Shallow et al. 1950, 1953; Urban and Egeli 1978). This entails a large biopsy specimen that will include the pathologic duct and prevents recurrent discharge. This technique has been associated with minimal difficulty even in lactating and postpartum women.

The third alternative as advocated by Seltzer et al. (1970) is simple mastectomy, particularly if the patient is over age 60. In the patients reported by Seltzer, there was a 32% incidence of malignancy in patients over age 60 presenting with nipple discharge and no palpable mass. This aggressive approach has been challenged in that two thirds of patients in this age group would be treated by mastectomy for benign breast disease.

Chronic subareolar abscess with purulent discharge is treated by (wide) excison of the affected major duct, including a segment of the nipple which should be removed with the specimen, and the incision drained (compare Chapter 6). Our approach to the secreting breast is outlined in Fig. 16.**1.**

Nipple Discharge in the Male Breast

Carcinoma of the male breast is more frequently associated with discharge than is carcinoma of the female breast. Discharges present in 1% to 5% of women with breast caner whereas 10% to 15% of men with breast cancer will present with a discharge. Other causes for discharge in men are gynecomastia or hormonal treatment with estrogen or androgens. As in women, the diagnosis must be established by biopsy (Haagensen 1971, Leis et al. 1967, 1973).

Paget's Disease

Nipple discharge from the ductal system must be distinguished from changes seen with Paget's disease of the breast. The changes in Paget's disease consist of eczema, desquamation, crust formation, erosion or ulceration of the nipple and areola. The cutaneous manifestations originate on the nipple and extend to the areola and may result in symptomatic itching and burning. These characteristics may occur alone or in combination with a breast mass. Infrequently, a breast mass may be the only finding present; however, typical skin changes are seen in over 70% of cases.

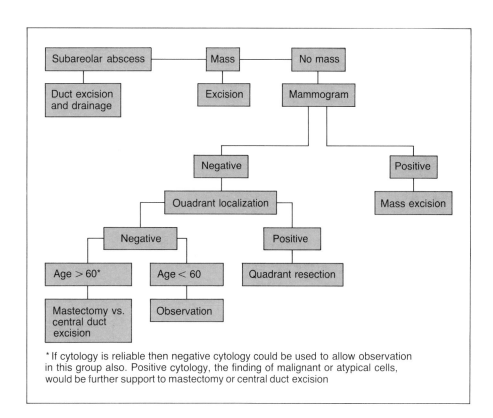

* If cytology is reliable then negative cytology could be used to allow observation in this group also. Positive cytology, the finding of malignant or atypical cells, would be further support to mastectomy or central duct excision

Fig. 16.**1** Nipple discharge

Although the skin changes with Paget's disease often manifest early, frequently the delay in diagnosis exceeds one year due to continued treatment for eczema (Ashikari et al. 1970; Kister and Haagensen 1970).

Histologically, Paget's disease is carcinoma arising in the nipple ducts. It can be infiltrating or noninfiltrating intraductal carcinoma. Tumor cells may spread up through the duct system to the nipple or down the ducts and disperse into the breast parenchyma. Paget's cells (relatively large, neoplastic epithelial cells with hyperchromatic nuclei and pale-staining cytoplasm), epidermal hypertrophy, and round cell infiltration of the skin constitute typical histologic findings in Paget's disease of the breast.

This entity is treated as any other breast cancer. Prognosis is determined by axillary lymph node status. Patients presenting with skin changes only infrequently have axillary lymph node metastasis (5% to 13%), whereas those patients presenting with breast mass with or without skin changes have axillary lymph node involvement in 50% to 66% of instance.

Patients with noninfiltrating intraductal carcinoma should have 100% salvage following mastectomy. Patients with cutaneous manifestation, no palpable mass, and no axillary lymph node metastasis have a minimum ten-year survival of 80%. Ten-year survival for patients with a palpable mass and negative axillary nodes approximates 70%, whereas those with positive axillary nodes have a ten-year survival ranging from 20% to 40% (Ashikari et al. 1970; Kister and Haagensen 1970).

Other dermatologic diseases that may mimic Paget's disease include eczema, eruptions associated with birth control pills, herpes simplex, and congenital nipple inversion (Rosemond and Maier 1975). It is imperative that any nipple-areolar lesion be regarded as Paget's disease on presentation. Immediate full thickness biopsy will avoid delay in diagnosis. With minimal eczematous lesions, a two-week trial with Kertatolytic or steroid creams may be employed, but biopsy should follow promptly if complete cure does not ensue.

References

Archer, D. F.: Current concepts of prolactin physiology in normal and abnormal conditions. Mod. Trends 28: 1977

Ashikari, R., K. Park, A. Huvos, J. Urban: Paget's disease of the breast. Cancer 26: 680–685, 1970

Atkins, H., B. Wolff: Discharges from the nipple. Br. J. Surg. 51: 602–606, 1964

Barnes, A.: Diagnosis and treatment of abnormal breast secretions. N. Engl. J. Med. 275: 1184–1187, 1966

Copeland, M., T. Higgins: Significance of discharge from the nipple in nonpuerperal mammary conditions. Ann. Surg. 151: 638–648, 1960

Devitt, J. E.: Value of the History in the office diagnosis of breast cancer. CMA Journal, 116: 1127–1131, 1977

Funderburk, W., B. Syphax: Evaluation of nipple discharge in benign and malignant disease. Cancer 24: 1290–1296, 1969

Gensen, H. A.: Diseases of the Breast – Revised Reprint

Kister, S., C. Haagensen: Paget's disease of the breast. Am. J. Surg. 119: 606–609, 1970

Leis, H., J. Dursi, W. Mersheimer: Nipple discharge – Significance and treatment. N. Y. State J. Med. 67: 3105–3110, 1967

Leis, H., S. Pilnik, J. Dursi, E. Santoro: Nipple discharge. Int. Surg. 58: 162–165, 1973

Madalin, H., O. Clagett, J. McDonald: Lesions of the breast associated with discharge from the nipple. Ann. Surg. 146: 751–763, 1957

Rimsten, A., V. Skoog, B. Stenkvist: On the significance of nipple discharge in the diagnosis of breast disease. Acta Chir Scand. 142: 513–518, 1976

Rosemond, G., W. Maier: Nonlactational Nipple Discharge. Diseases of the Breast, 1975

Seltzer, M., L. Perloff, R. Kelley, W. Fitts: The significance of age in patients with nipple discharge. S. G. O, 131: 519–522, 1970

Shallow, T., F. Wagner, R. Colcher: Adequate breast biopsy. Arch. Surg. 67: 526–536, 1953

Shallow, T., S. Eger, F. Wagner: Management of breast lesions. Postgrad. Med. 8: 499–505, 1950

Urban, J., R. Egeli: Non-lactational nipple discharge. CA–Cancer J. Clin. 28: 130–140, 1978

Chapter 17

Cystosarcoma Phyllodes

M. D. McDaniel and R. W. Crichlow

Introduction

Cystosarcoma phyllodes, the leaf-like cystic breast tumor first described by Johannes Mueller in 1868, is uncommon. It comprises only about 0.3% (Ariel 1961) to 0.9% (Dyer et al. 1966) of all breast tumors, or about 1% (Blumencranz and Gray 1978) to 2.9% (Lester and Stout 1954; Treves 1964) of all fibroadenomatous tumors, and there are only some 700 cases reported in series in the literature to date (Hart et al. 1978; Andersson and Bergdahl 1978; Blumencranz and Gray 1978; Browder et al. 1978; Lester and Stout 1954; Halverson and Hori-Rubaina 1974; McDivitt et al. 1967; Hajdu et al. 1976; Norris and Taylor 1967; Oberman 1965; Hafner 1962; Lee and Pack 1931; Blichert-Toft et al. 1975; Rosen and Urban 1975; Rao et al. 1964; Hill and Stout 1942; Lawrence 1972; Long et al. 1962). The unpredictable behavior of cystosarcoma phyllodes, poorly understood because of its rarity, demands treatment and follow-up different from that required with carcinoma or fibroadenoma, and it therefore merits separate discussion.

Clinical Features

History

The "average" Western patient with cystosarcoma phyllodes is best described as a menstruating woman (Tanphiphat et al. 1978; Blumencranz and Gray 1978; Treves and Sunderland 1951) about 45 years old (Pietruszka and Barnes 1978; Blumencranz and Gray 1978; Browder et al. 1978; Lester and Stout 1954; Treves 1964; West et al. 1971; Oberman 1965; Haagensen 1971; Hafner et al. 1962; McDivitt et al. 1967; Lee and Pack 1931; Rao et al. 1964; Hill and Stout 1942), but there is a wide range of characteristics in the population of afflicted patients, who could be of any age (Amerson 1970; Browder et al. 1978).

Although certain authors have thought that blacks (Lester and Stout 1954), nulliparous women (Tanphiphat et al. 1978; Blumencranz and Gray 1978), and those who had difficulty lactating (Lee and Pack 1931) were more common than their opposites among those with cystosarcoma phyllodes, subsequent examination has shown no clear predisposition among those groups (Stromberg and Golladay 1978; McDivitt et al. 1967; Norris and Taylor 1967). There is no genetic predisposition towards the tumor (Treves and Sunderland 1951), nor has it been recently reported in men in the absence of gynecomastia (Reingold and Ascher 1970; Pantoja et al. 1976).

The length of time over which a patient has been aware of a mass in the location of a cystosarcoma phyllodes gives little information concerning its malignant potential (Treves and Sunderland 1951). Pain is an uncommon complaint in cystosarcoma phyllodes, usually occurring only with large and/or ulcerated lesions (Treves and Sunderland 1951; McDivitt et al. 1967; Hafner et al. 1962; Lee and Pack 1931; Notley and Griffiths 1965; Maier et al. 1968).

Age at time of diagnosis is not an accurate predictor of malignancy in those with cystosarcoma phyllodes (Pietruszcka and Barnes 1978; Treves and Sunderland 1951; McDivitt et al. 1967). Nulliparity was felt to be associated with malignancy in those with cystosarcoma phyllodes by several authors (Treves and Sunderland 1951; McDivitt et al. 1967), but pregnancy has been associated in several instances with onset or rapid growth of both malignant (Ariel 1961; Lester and Stout 1954; Haagensen 1971; Reich and Solomon 1958) and benign (Pandya 1978; Treves and Sunderland 1951; West et al. 1971; Bader and Isaacson 1961; Lee and Pack 1931) tumors. One detailed report (Naryshkin and Redfield 1964) of pregnancy and lactation following excision of an apparently benign cystosarcoma phyllodes demonstrated no hormone imbalance associated with this diagnosis or recurrence of tumor associated with changing hormone levels.

In short, cystosarcoma phyllodes occurs in a wide range of patients without specific clinical or historical features that either indicate the diagnosis or distinguish benign from malignant behavior.

Physical Examination

A striking feature of this lesion is the large size that it may attain – up to 20 kg in the descriptions of Mueller (1838) and Lee and Park (1931). The overlying skin may be stretched and shiny, with enlarged subcutaneous veins (Browder et al. 1978; Hafner et al. 1962). Ulceration may result from pressure necrosis alone and not necessarily from invasion of the skin by tumor (Browder et al. 1978; Dyer et al. 1966; Treves and Sunderland 1951; Haagensen 1971; Lee and Pack 1931; Hill and Stout 1942). Decreased mobility of the tumor with respect to the pectoral muscle or fascia may be secondary to large size alone (Lawrence 1972; Haagensen 1971), or may be an indication of biologic malignancy with invasion of these underlying structures (Hafner et al. 1962; Maier et al. 1968).

More recently, when breast masses tend to be seen by physicians at earlier stages, described cystosarcoma phyllodes range in size from small masses (Salm 1978; Azzopardi 1979) to the enormous tumors of the earlier series (Treves 1964; Lee and Pack 1931). When a cystosarcoma phyllodes attains a large size, it usually does so rapidly after a long resting period (Norris and Taylor 1967; Lee and Pack 1931). This historical feature of rapid growth is not necessarily an indication of biologic malignancy (Lester and Stout 1954; Treves and Sunderland 1951; Long et al. 1962), but in several large series (Pietruszka and Barnes 1978; Browder et al. 1978; Treves and Sunderland 1951; Kessinger et al. 1972; McDivitt et al. 1967; Hajdu et al. 1976), the mean size of metastasizing (biologically malignant) tumors is larger than the size of biologically benign tumors. However, even small tumors can be malignant, since tumors as small as 2.5 cm have subsequently metastasized (Lester and Stout 1954).

Cystosarcoma phyllodes may range in shape and consistency from smooth and rubbery [in small tumors (McDivitt et al. 1967)] to multilobulated with cystic areas [more often in large tumors (Treves and Sunderland 1951)]. Nipple discharge is uncommon (Treves and Sunderland 1951; McDivitt et al. 1967; Lee and Pack 1931) and bloody discharge is rarely reported (Bader and Isaacson 1961; McCormick and Pillay 1977; Treves and Sunderland 1951; McDivitt et al. 1967). Bilateral cystosarcoma phyllodes (about 1% of reported cases) is rarer than bilateral fibroadenoma and occurs as often in biologically benign (Stromberg and Golladay 1978; Lester and Stout 1954; Bader and Isaacson 1961; Treves 1964) as in malignant lesions (Reich and Solomon 1958; Notley and Griffiths 1965).

Enlargement of axillary lymph nodes, although worrisome in carcinoma, seldom implies involvement of the nodes by cystosarcoma phyllodes. Hematogenous, not lymphatic, metastasis characterizes cystosarcoma phyllodes; reaction to local infection accounts for most axillary lymphadenopathy in this disease (Dyer et al. 1966; Treves and Sunderland 1951; West et al. 1971; Cooper and Ackerman 1943; Lee and Pack 1931; Hill and Stout 1942). Of those groups of axillary nodes reported to have been examined microscopically [particularly in the early experience with cystosarcoma phyllodes, when radical operations were more frequently undertaken (Norris and Taylor 1967)], only ten of 146 contained metastatic tumor (Treves and Sunderland 1951; Norris and Taylor 1967; Cooper and Ackerman 1943; Fernandez et al. 1976; Hoover et al. 1975; Minkowitz et al. 1968; Reich and Solomon 1958; Long et al. 1962) (Hart et al. 1978; Salm 1978; Pietruszka and Barnes 1978; Blumencranz and Gray 1978; Browder et al. 1978; Ariel 1961; Lester and Stout 1954; Treves 1964; West et al. 1971; McDivitt et al. 1967; Oberman 1965; Haagensen 1971; Hafner et al. 1962; Gibbs et al. 1968; Hill and Stout 1942; Geist 1964; Maier et al. 1968).

Clinical Course

Since at the time of diagnosis, one has no highly accurate clinical or histologic (see below) indication of the likely future behavior of a given cystosarcoma phyllodes, one can only project a statistically likely course based on retrospective study of the available data.

Cystosarcoma phyllodes does not usually kill its host. Typically, complete cure is effected by wide local excision or simple mastectomy. Lee and Pack, reviewing their own cases and the extant literature in 1931, reported only five recurrences among 91 cases, and only one death due to tumor metastasis. These authors were hesitant to classify cystosarcoma phyllodes as potentially malignant. However, subsequent series have demonstrated malignant recurrence or metastases in 3% to 12% of cases (Hart et al. 1978; Pietruszka and Barnes 1978; Tanphiphat et al. 1978; Browder et al. 1978; Lester and Stout 1954; Treves 1964; Treves and Sunderland 1951; West et al. 1971; Halverson and Hori-Rubaina 1974; Kessinger et al. 1972; McDivitt et al. 1967; Hajdu et al. 1976; Norris and Taylor 1967; Cooper and Ackerman 1943; Oberman 1965; Haagensen 1971; Rix et al. 1964; Long et al. 1962; Maier et al. 1968). Local recurrences have been excised as many as five times with apparent cure (McDivitt et al. 1967); however, in another instance local recurrence ten years after excision of the primary tumor foretold the death of the patient from metastasis (Treves and Sunderland 1951).

The 3% to 12% of patients who die of cystosarcoma phyllodes most commonly experience either local recurrence with extension into the chest (over 50%) or metastasis to lung and/or bone (about 40%). Occasional metastases have been found in nearly every organ (Wolfson et al. 1978; Rhodes et al. 1978; Ariel 1961; Lubin and Rywlin 1972; Hoover et al. 1975; Hines et al. 1976; Geist 1964; Aronson 1966). Kessinger et al. (1972) note that only 51% of those with distant metastases have local recurrence as well.

In those reports in which the time between initial therapy and malignant recurrence or metastasis is clearly documented, it is rare to find intervals of greater than 24 months; local recurrence or distant metastasis developing within one year of primary excision is a poor prognostic sign (Browder et al. 1978; Treves and Sunderland 1951; Hajdu et al. 1976; Norris and Taylor 1967; Haagensen 1971; Hoover et al. 1975; Hines et al. 1976). If death from cystosarcoma phyllodes is to ensue, this usually occurs within six years of initial therapy, although exceptionally long survivals of 7.5 (Rix et al. 1971) and 23 (Pietruszka and Barnes 1978) years have been reported. Only two patients with metastases from cystosarcoma phyllodes have apparently been cured; one with pulmonary metastasis, by pulmonary lobectomy (Hart et al. 1978), and one with axillary metastasis, by radical mastectomy (Long et al. 1962).

Pathology

Gross Appearance

Cystosarcoma phyllodes is often initially misinterpreted both grossly and microscopically. The skin changes of the in situ tumor have been discussed above, and may mimic the advanced stages of other malignant breast lesions. Similarly, at operation the tumor may appear to be well circumscribed (McDivitt et al. 1960) because it is surrounded by compressed breast tissue (Fig. 17.1); but there may actually be small invasive fingerlets of tumor advancing beyond the pseudocapsule (Haagensen 1971; McDivitt et al. 1960). Excision of a cystosarcoma phyllodes with too small a margin may amputate some of these projections and guarantee local recurrence (McDivitt et al. 1967; Oberman 1965). In the excised and divided specimen, the papillary intracanalicular projections of exuberant stroma, which gave this tumor its name, may not be evident or may be mimicked by intracanalicular fibroadenoma (Lee and Pack 1931). Although the cystic appearance, frond-like papillary projections, and intracystic hemorrhage of larger cystosarcoma phyllodes are nearly unique (Lee and Pack 1931; Blichert-Toft et al. 1975), the fibrous gray-white appearance of many smaller cystosarcoma phyllodes (McDivitt et al. 1960) is not. Even one so experienced in breast disease as Haagensen (1971) states emphatically that frozen sections should be studied at the time of all breast biopsies regardless of the clinical suspicion, because gross appearances are misleading and wider excision is appropriate for cystosarcoma phyllodes than for fibroadenoma.

Our experience with xeromammography in cystosarcoma phyllodes has been that these appear as well-circumscribed lesions (Fig. 17.2).

Histology

It is the microscopic appearance of cystosarcoma phyllodes, with distinct stromal and epithelial components, which is its defining characteristic. Although the cytologic appearance of a fine-needle aspirate is suggestive (Stawicki and Hsiu 1979), light microscopic sections remain the diagnostic means of choice.

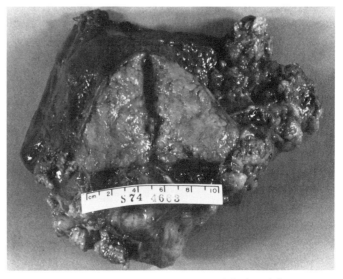

Fig. 17.**1** Gross appearance of excised lesion later proven microscopically to be cystosarcoma phyllodes.

In general, the stromal component consists of dense, hyperplastic connective tissue cells on a variably myxoid background (Fig. 17.**3**) (Azzopardi 1979). The stromal density and pleomorphism distinguish cystosarcoma phyllodes from fibroadenoma (Treves 1964; Treves and Sunderland 1951; Haagensen 1971; Rix et al. 1971; McDivitt et al. 1960). Overactive stromal growth, particularly seen adjacent to the epithelium-lined cystic, clefts (Azzopardi 1979; Oberman 1965), produces invagination (Fig. 17.**4**) into them and thereby papillae may be seen macroscopically. The stromal cells themselves usually differentiate along a fibrosarcomatous line (Azzopardi 1979), but less commonly liposarcoma (Pietruszka and Barnes 1978; Lester and Stout 1954; McDivitt et al. 1967; Haagensen 1971; Qizilbash 1976; McDivitt et al. 1960; Blichert-Toft et al. 1975; Aronson 1966), osteosarcoma (Lester and Stout 1954; Norris and Taylor 1967; Oberman 1965; Haagensen 1971; Fernandez 1976; Lubin and Rywlin 1972; Blichert-Toft et al. 1975; Kay 1971; Maier et al. 1968; Smith and Taylor 1969), chondrosarcoma (Pietruzska and Barnes 1978; Treves and Sunderland 1951; Norris and Taylor 1967; Oberman 1965; Haagensen 1971; Fernandez et al. 1976; Lubin und Rywlin 1972;

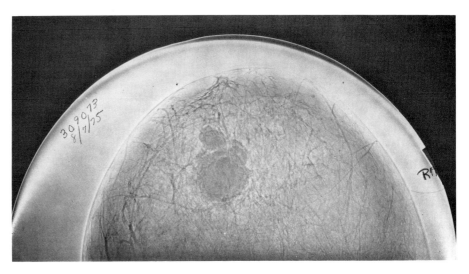

Fig. 17.**2** Xeromammogram of histologically proven cystosarcoma phyllodes.

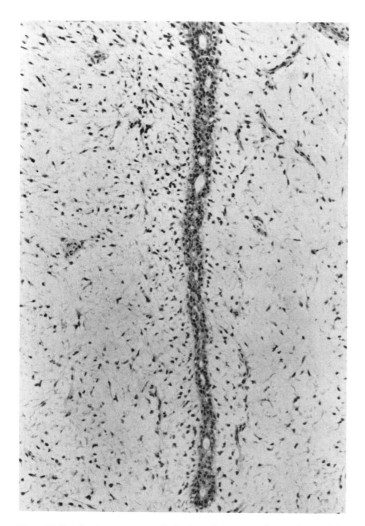

Fig. 17.**3** Cystosarcoma phyllodes (hematoxylin-eosin, x100). Dense stroma consists of pleomorphic cells.

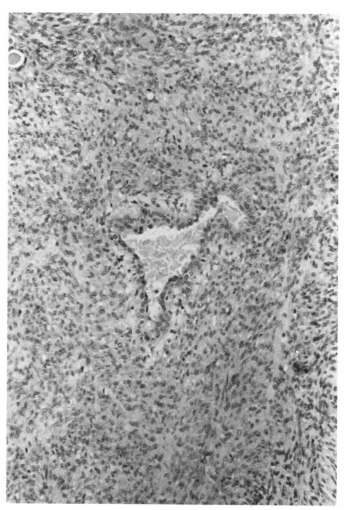

Fig. 17.**4** Cystosarcoma phyllodes (hematoxylin-eosin, x40). Note increased density of stromal cells adjacent to epithelium-lined cleft.

Blichert-Toft et al. 1975; Rao et al. 1964; Kay 1971; Hill and Stout 1942; Maier et al. 1968; Smith and Taylor 1969), rhabdomyosarcoma (Barnes and Pietruszka 1978; Pietruszka and Barnes 1978; Lester and Stout 1954), histiocytic metaplasia (Haagensen 1971), angiosarcoma (Lubin and Rywlin 1972), and hemangiopericytoma (Pietruska and Barnes 1978) have been described. The stromal cellular appearance varies widely with regard to atypia, mitotic activity, and the presence of tumor giant cells (Treves 1964; Fernandez et al. 1976), not only among different tumors, but within a given tumor (Lester and Stout 1954; Norris and Taylor 1967; Oberman 1965; Haagensen 1971; Rix et al. 1971; Blichert-Toft et al. 1975; Hill and Stout 1942). The fact that a small focus of anaplastic stroma might be missed on routine sampling could provide an explanation for the difficulty experienced in correlating histologic appearance with clinical behavior (Tanphiphat et al. 1978; Lester and Stout 1954).

The epithelial component is much more uniform. Although it is generally cuboidal, lining the cystic spaces in a single cell layer (McDivitt et al. 1960), hyperplasia (Pietruszka and Barnes 1978; Lester and Stout 1954; Treves 1964; Treves and Sunderland 1951; Norris and Taylor 1967; Haagensen 1971; Rix et al. 1971; McDivitt et al.

1960; Blichert-Toft et al. 1975; Hill and Stout 1942) has also been described. In rare instances (Pietruszka and Barnes 1978; Treves 1964; Norris and Taylor 1967; Haagensen 1971; Rix et al. 1971), malignant transformation of the epithelium occurs, but this is certainly not the rule. In one series (Pietruszka and Barnes 1978), the more benign-appearing epithelium tended to be associated with histologically more malignant stroma, but the significance of this is unclear.

The light microscopic appearance of recurrences and distant metastases of cystosarcoma phyllodes is most commonly the same as the stroma of the primary lesion (Azzopardi 1979; Lubin and Rywlin 1972). Two variations of this common pattern have been reported. First, the stroma of a recurrent lesion may appear far more malignant than the primary, and may foretell the clinical appearance of distant metastases (Lester and Stout 1954; Treves 1964; Treves and Sunderland 1951; Hajdu et al. 1976; Rix et al. 1971; Blichert-Toft et al. 1975; Long et al. 1962). Second, in only one reported instance (West et al. 1971), the epithelial component metastasized; it is usually the stromal component alone which metastasizes (Fernandez et al. 1976).

Clinicopathologic Correlation

Frustration with the unpredictable behavior of cystosarcoma phyllodes has prompted numerous retrospective attempts to correlate the gross and microscopic appearance of cystosarcoma phyllodes with the clinical course of afflicted patients.

Grossly, as we have seen, there is no close clinicopathologic correlation, except perhaps that benign lesions may tend more toward cystic growth patterns than malignant lesions (Treves and Sunderland 1951; McDivitt et al. 1967) and hemorrhage and necrosis may be more common in histologically malignant tumors (Pietruszka and Barnes 1978; Norris and Taylor 1967). Focal calcification occurs in both benign and malignant cystosarcoma phyllodes (McDivitt et al. 1967; McDivitt et al. 1960).

Microscopically also there is no clearcut clinicopathologic correlation. Stromal differentiation along lines other than fibrosarcoma is not correlated with malignant behavior (McDivitt et al. 1967; Haagensen 1971). Cellular pleomorphism and anaplasia, high mitotic activity, presence of tumor giant cells, extensive growth of stroma relative to epithelium, and infiltrating as opposed to "pushing" margins are all worrisome as predictors of malignant behavior (Hart et al. 1978; Pietruszka and Barnes 1978; Browder et al. 1978; Treves 1964; Treves and Sunderland 1951; Halverson and Hori-Rubaina 1974; Norris and Taylor 1967; Oberman 1965), but are not thoroughly reliable. A benign course may follow excision of a histologically quite malignant lesion (Blumencranz and Gray 1978), and metastasis and death have been reported following excision of histologically benign lesions (Lester and Stout 1954; West et al. 1971; Norris and Taylor 1967; Rix et al. 1971; Blichert-Toft et al. 1975).

Because of the histologic similarity between cystosarcoma and fibroadenoma, it is tempting to postulate that the former arises from the latter (Blumencranz and Gray 1978; Haagensen 1971; Lee and Pack 1931; Hill and Stout 1942; Notley and Griffiths 1965; Maier et al. 1968).

Circumstantial evidence supporting this theory includes:

1. The frequently noted history that a cystosarcoma phyllodes has been diagnosed following rapid growth of a longstanding breast mass that formerly was firm and rubbery, as a fibroadenoma (Maier et al. 1968)

2. That the mean age of patients with cystosarcoma phyllodes is slightly older than those with fibroadenoma, suggesting development of the former from the latter (Treves 1964; Azzopardi 1979)

3. Fibroadenomata are often found in adjacent breast tissue following mastectomy for cystosarcoma phyllodes (Lee and Pack 1931)

4. Areas of hyalinized stroma that appear to represent degenerating fibroadenoma are frequently found within a clearcut cystosarcoma (Pietruszka and Barnes 1978; Treves and Sunderland 1951; Lee and Pack 1931; Hill and Stout 1942).

Far more intriguing, however, is the hypothesis that the stromal change characteristic of cystosarcoma phyllodes is somehow induced by the duct epithelium. Although one seldom has the opportunity to examine early lesions, both Salm (1978) and Azzopardi (1979) describe satellite lesions with early sarcomatous change in a pericanalicular distribution, and note that it is the stroma directly adjacent to the epithelial canaliculi that shows the most marked hyperplasia and pleomorphism.

Treatment

The treatment of cystosarcoma phyllodes is primarily surgical. Because the rate of metastasis varies among different series, and each surgeon's approach depends on his experience with the aggressiveness of these tumors, precise recommendations vary regarding the appropriate operation.

It is generally agreed that wide local excision will cure most "benign" cystosarcomas (Blumencranz and Gray 1978; Treves and Sunderland 1951; McDivitt et al. 1967; Norris and Taylor 1967; Cooper and Ackermann 1943; Oberman 1965; Haagensen 1971). Treves and Sunderland (1951) recommended radical mastectomy for histologically malignant cystosarcoma phyllodes, based on their finding of a 25% metastatic rate for these tumors. However, as McDivitt et al. (1967) pointed out, that recommendation was not followed even at their own hospital. Simple mastectomy or wide local excision was subsequently substituted for radical mastectomy in 9 of 13 "malignant" cystosarcoma phyllodes with 100% apparent cure, indicating that achievement of local control is essential for cure. The choice between wide local excision and simple mastectomy will be determined by the size of the tumor (Tanphiphat et al. 1978; Treves and Sunderland 1951; Norris and Taylor 1967), radical mastectomy being reserved for those cases in which an adequate resection margin cannot be achieved by a less extensive procedure (Blumencranz and Gray 1978; McDivitt et al. 1967; Norris and Taylor 1967; Cooper and Ackerman 1943; Oberman 1965; Haagensen 1971; Long et al. 1962).

Axillary metastasis is rare, as discussed above. One could argue, however, as does Treves (1964), that "it would be regrettable to allow the rare case of metastatic axillary disease to slip by undetected by relying on simple mastectomy alone." Halverson and Hori-Rubaina (1974) agree; their only survivor with histologically malignant cystosarcoma phyllodes had a radical mastectomy as primary treatment. The contrary argument is offered by West et al. (1971) who stated that lymphatic dissemination of cystosarcoma phyllodes does not occur, that histologic appearance is of no prognostic value, and that cystosarcoma phyllodes is therefore best treated by simple mastectomy, with resection extended to other structures only if clearly involved.

Amerson (1970) stated that less aggressive therapy might be more appropriate in adolescents than in adults because cystosarcoma phyllodes appeared to be generally less virulent in this age group. However, review of cases reported from Western countries in those under 26 years of age (Andersson and Bergdahl 1978; Pietruszka and Barnes 1978; Tanphiphat et al. 1978; Blumencranz and Gray 1978; Browder et al. 1978; Stomberg and Golladay 1978; Lester and Stout 1954; Treves and Sunderland 1951; West et al. 1971; Halverson and Hori-Rubaina 1974; McDivitt et al. 1967; Azzopardi 1979; Hajdu et al. 1976; Norris and Tylor 1967; Oberman 1965; Haagensen 1971; Bader and Isaacson 1961; Hoover et al. 1975; Blichert-Toft et al. 1975; Naryshkin and Redfield 1964; Gibbs et al. 1968; Amerson 1970; Reich and Solomon 1958; Reed and Hiebert 1942; Simpson et al. 1969; Maier et al. 1968) reveals a mortality of 5.5% from cystosarcoma phyllodes. This is in the same range as the 3% to 12% mortality reported in the series noted earlier consisting mainly of adult patients, and would seem to indicate that the clinical course of cystosarcoma is the same in adolescents as in adults. No change in therapy would therefore be indicated for adolescents.

Nonsurgical modes of therapy have been less successfully attempted. From the few reported cases, it seems that there may be some response of primary cystosarcoma phyllodes to irradiation (Lee and Pack 1931), but that adjuvant irradiation does not necessarily improve the long-term outcome (Hart et al. 1978; Andersson and Bergdahl 1978; Blumencranz and Gray 1978; Treves and Sunderland 1951; West et al. 1971; Rix et al. 1971; Hafner et al. 1962; Bader and Isaacson 1961; Lubin and Rywlin 1972; Blichert-Toft et al. 1975). Variable response of metastases to irradiation is reported (Barnes and Pietruszka 1978; Hoover et al. 1975; Hines et al. 1976; Geist 1964; Aronson 1966) in terms of size reduction or pain relief.

Chemotherapy has most often been used in a desperate attempt to control metastatic disease. Response of metastases was reported with cyclophosphamide (Kessinger et al. 1972; Hoover et al. 1975) or thiotepa (Geist 1964), but other agents alone or in combination have not been useful (Tanphiphat et al. 1978; Blumencranz and Gray 1978; West et al. 1971; Kessinger et al. 1972; Hoover et al. 1975; Geist 1964).

Success of castration, estrogen, or testosterone administration has not been demonstrated in cases of cystosarcoma phyllodes (Tanphiphat et al. 1978; Treves and Sunderland 1951; McDivitt et al. 1967; Hoover et al. 1975; Geist 1964). Estrogen receptor activity has been identified in four out of ten cases assayed (Porton and Poortman 1981). Porton and Poortman indicate that relative scarcity of the epithelial component on histologic examination may be associated with significant estrogen receptor activity.

Follow-up

One's philosophy concerning the follow-up mandated by previous diagnosis of cystosarcoma phyllodes is strongly influenced by one's faith in the predictive value of the histologic appearance of the tumor. As discussed above, metastasis or malignant recurrence is almost always evident within six years of excision of the primary lesion,

more commonly appearing within the first two years of this period. Intensive surveillance (physical examination and chest x-ray) is necessary during this time period, keeping in mind that local "benign" recurrence has been reported at much longer intervals.

Summary

Cystosarcoma phyllodes is an uncommon tumor of uncertain etiology. Although its initial appearance may give rise to alarm, it is lethal to only 3% to 12% of afflicted patients; death usually occurs within six years of resection of the primary lesion, and follows extension of recurrent lesion into the chest or growth of metastases to the lung and/or bones. The histologic appearance of the primary tumor is a fair but not absolute prognosticator of biologic behavior. Cure is typically effected by wide excision of the primary lesion (not including routine axillary node dissection), but all afflicted patients should be suspected of having malignant disease and be followed appropriately.

References

Amerson, J. R.: Cystosarcoma phyllodes in adolescent females: A report of seven patients. Ann. Surg. 171: 849–858, 1970

Andersson, A., L. Bergdahl: Cystosarcoma phyllodes in young women. Arch. Surg. 113 (6): 742–744, 1978

Ariel, L.: Skeletal metastases in cystosarcoma phyllodes: A case report and review. Arch. Surg. 82: 275–280, 1961

Aronson, W.: Malignant cystosarcoma phyllodes with liposarcoma. Wisc. Med. J. 65: 184–187, 1966

Azzopardi, J. L.: Problems in Breast Pathology. WB Saunders Co., Philadelphia, pp. 346–365, 376–378, 1979

Bader, E., C. Isaacson: Bilateral malignant cystosarcoma phyllodes. Br. J. Surg. 48: 519–521, 1961

Barnes, L., M. Pietruszka: Rhabdomyosarcoma arising within a cystosarcoma phyllodes: Case report and review of the literature. Am. J. Surg. Pathol. 2: 423–429, 1978

Blichert-Toft, M., J. P. H. Hansen, O. H. Hansen, T. Schiodt: Clinical course of cystosarcoma phyllodes related to histologic appearance. Surg. Gynecol. Obstet. 140: 929–932, 1975

Blumencranz, P. W., G. F. Gray: Cystosarcoma phyllodes: Clinical and pathologic study. N. Y. State J. Med. 78: 623–627, 1978

Browder, W., J. T. Jr. McQuitty, J. C. McDonald: Malignant cystosarcoma phylloides: Treatment and prognosis. Am. J. Surg. 136: 239–241, 1978

Cooper, W. G., L. V. Ackerman: Cystosarcoma phylloides with a consideration of its more malignant variant. Surg. Gynecol. Obstet. 77: 279–283, 1943

Dyer, N. H., J. E. Bridger, R. S. Taylor: Cystosarcoma phylloides. Br. J. Surg. 53(5): 450–455, 1966

Fernandez, B. B., F. J. Hernandez, W. Spindler: Metastatic cystosarcoma phyllodes: A light and electron microscopic study. Cancer 37: 1737–1746, 1976

Geist, D.: Cystosarcoma phylloides of the female breast. Am. Surg. 30 (2): 105–108, 1964

Gibbs, B. F., R. D. Roe, D. F. Thomas: Malignant cystosarcoma phyllodes in a pre-pubertal female. Ann. Surg. 167: 229–231, 1968

Haagensen, C. D. Cystosarcoma phyllodes. In: Diseases of the Breast. 2nd ed. WB Saunders, Co., Philadelphia, pp. 227–249, 1971

Hafner, C. D., E. Mezger, J. H. Wylie, jr.: Cystosarcoma phyllodes of the breast. Surg. Gynecol. Obstet. 115: 29–34, 1962

Hajdu, S. I., M. H. Espinosa, G. F. Robbins: Recurrent cystosarcoma phyllodes: A clinicopathologic study of 32 cases. Cancer 38 (3): 1402–1406, 1976

Halverson, J. D., J. M. Hori-Rubaina: Cystosarcoma phyllodes of the breast. Am. Surg. 40: 295–301, 1974

Hart, W. R., R. C. Bauer, H. A. Oberman: Cystosarcoma phyllodes: A clinicopathologic study of twenty-six hypercellular periductal stromal tumors of the breast. Am. J. Clin. Pathol. 70: 211–216, 1978

Hill, R. P., A. P. Stout: Sarcoma of the breast. Arch. Surg. 44: 723–732, 1942

Hines, J. R., R. T. Gordon, C. Widger, T. Kolb: Cystosarcoma phyllodes metastatic to a Brenner tumor of the ovary. Arch. Surg. 111: 299–300, 1976

Hoover, H. C., A. Trestioreanu, A. S. Ketcham: Metastatic cystosarcoma phylloides in an adolescent girl: An unusually malignant tumor. Ann. Surg. 181: 279–282, 1975

Kay, S.: Light and electron microscopic studies of a malignant cystosarcoma phyllodes featuring stromal cartilage and bone. Am. J. Clin. Pathol. 55: 770–776, 1971

Kessinger, A., J. F. Foley, H. M. Lemon, D. M. Miller: Metastatic cystosarcoma phyllodes: A case report and review of the literature. J. Surg. Oncol. 4: 131–147, 1972

Lawrence, G. A.: Cystosarcoma phyllodes. Indian J. Cancer 9: 231–239, 1972

Lee, B. J., G. T. Pack: Giant intracanalicular myxoma of the breast. Ann. Surg. 93: 250–268, 1931

Lester, J., A. P. Stout: Cystosarcoma phyllodes. Cancer 7: 335–353, 1954

Long, R. T. L., A. E. Hesker, R. E. Johnson: Surgical management of cystosarcoma phyllodes: With a report of eight cases. Missouri Med. 59: 1179–1181, 1962

Lubin, J., A. M. Rywlin: Cystosarcoma phyllodes metastasizing as a mixed mesenchymal sarcoma. South. Med. J. 65: 636–637, 1972

Maier, W. P., G. P. Rosemond, P. Wittenberg, E. M. Tassoni: Cystosarcoma phyllodes mammae. Oncology 22: 145–158, 1968

McCormick, M. V., S. P. Pillay: Malignant cystosarcoma phyllodes associated with scirrhous carcinoma of the breast: A case report. S. Afr. Med. J. 52: 893–894, 1977

McDivitt, R. W., F. W. Stewart, J. W. Berg: Tumors of the Breast. Armed Forces Institute of Pathology, 2nd Series, Washington, D.C., pp. 117–123, 1968

McDivitt, R. W., J. A. Urban, J. H. Farrow: Cystosarcoma phyllodes. Johns Hopkins Med. J. 120: 33–45, 1967

Minkowitz, S., M. Zeichner, V. Di Maio, A. D. Nicastri: Cystosarcoma phyllodes: A unique case with multiple unilateral lesions and ipsilateral axillary metastasis. J. Pathol. Bacteriol. 96: 514–517, 1968

Müller, J.: Über den feineren Bau und die Formen der Krankhaften Geschwülste. G. Weiner, Berlin 1838

Naryshkin, G., E. S. Redfield: Malignant cystosarcoma phyllodes of the breast in adolescence, with subsequent pregnancy: Report of a case with endocrinologic studies. Obstet. Gynecol. 23: 140–142, 1964

Norris, H. J., H. B. Taylor: Relationship of histologic features to behavior of cystosarcoma phyllodes: Analysis of ninety-four cases. Cancer 20: 2090–2099, 1967

Notley, R. G., H. J. L. Griffiths: Bilateral malignant cystosarcoma phyllodes. Br. J. Surg. 52 (5): 360–362, 1965

Oberman, H. A.: Cystosarcoma phyllodes: A clinicopathologic study of hypercellular periductal stromal neoplasms of breast. Cancer 18: 697–710, 1965

Pandya, K. K.: Benign cystosarcoma phyllodes. J. Indian Med. Assoc. 70: 280, 1978

Pantoja, E., R. E. Llobet, E. Lopez: Gigantic cystosarcoma phyllodes in a man with gynecomastia. Arch. Surg. 111: 611, 1976

Pietruszka, M., L. Barnes: Cystosarcoma phyllodes: A clinicopathologic analysis of 42 cases. Cancer 41: 1974–1983, 1978

Porton, W. M., J. Poortman: Estrogen receptors in cystosarcoma phyllodes of the breast (letter to the editor). Eur. J. Cancer Clin. Oncol. 17 (10): 1147–1149, 1981

Qizilbash, A. H.: Cystosarcoma phyllodes with liposarcomatous stroma. Am. J. Clin. Pathol. 65: 321–327, 1976

Rao, R., J. Sanson, J. G. Gruhn: Cystosarcoma phyllodes: A clinicopathologic study of ten cases. Chicago Med. Sch. Q. 22: 24–29, 1964

Reed, H. L., A. E. Hiebert: Bilateral giant fibroadenoma simulating malignancy in pregnancy. J. Kans. Med. Soc. 43: 284–287, 1942

Reich, T., C. Solomon: Bilateral cystosarcoma phyllodes, malignant variant, with 14-year follow up: A case report. Ann. Surg. 147: 39–43, 1958

Reingold, I. M., G. S. Ascher: Cystosarcoma phyllodes in a man with gynecomastia. Am. J. Clin. Pathol. 53: 852–856, 1970

Rhodes, R. H., K. A. Frankel, R. L. Davis, D. Tatter: Metastatic cystosarcoma phyllodes: A report of two cases presenting with neurological symptoms. Cancer 41: 1179–1187, 1978

Rix, D. B., S. J. Tredwell, A. D. Forward: Cystosarcoma phylloides (cellular intracanalicular fibroadenoma): Clinical-pathological relationships. Can. J. Surg. 14 (1): 31–37, 1971

Rosen, P. P., J. A. Urban: Coexistent mammary carcinoma and cystosarcoma phyllodes. Breast 1: 9–15, 1975

Salm, R.: Multifocal histogenesis of a cystosarcoma phyllodes. J. Clin. Pathol. 31: 897–903, 1978

Simpson, T. E., R. L. Jr. Van Dervoort, H. B. Lynn: Giant fibroadenoma (benign cystosarcoma phylloides): Report of case in 13-year-old girl. Surgery 65: 341–342, 1969

Smith, B. H., H. B. Taylor: The occurrence of bone and cartilage in mammary tumors. Am. J. Clin. Pathol. 51: 610–618, 1969

Stawicki, M. E., J.–G. Hsiu: Malignant cystosarcoma phyllodes: A case report with cytologic presentation. Acta Cytol. 23: 61–64, 1979

Stromberg, B. V., E. S. Golladay: Cystosarcoma phylloides in the adolescent female. J. Pediatr. Surg. 13 (4): 423–425, 1978

Tanphiphat, C., S. Treesaranuvatana, C. Viratchai: Cystosarcoma phyllodes: A clinical and pathological study in Thai patients. J. Med. Assoc. Thai. 61 (3): 139–146, 1978

Toker, C.: Cystosarcoma phylloides: An ultrastructural study. Cancer 21: 1171–1179, 1968

Treves, N.: A study of cystosarcoma phyllodes. Ann. N. Y. Acad. Sci. 114: 922–936, 1964

Treves, N., D. Sunderland: Cystosarcoma phyllodes of the breast: A malignant and a benign tumor. Cancer 4: 1286–1332, 1951

West, T. L., L. H. Weiland, O. T. Clagett: Cystosarcoma phyllodes. Ann. Surg. 173: 520–528, 1971

Wolfson, P., B. J. Rybak, U. Kim: Cystosarcoma phyllodes metastatic to the pancreas. Am. J. Gastroenterol. 70: 184–187, 1978

Wulsin, J. H.: Large breast tumors in adolescent females. Ann. Surg. 152: 151–159, 1960

Chapter 18

The Postmastectomy Patient: Wound Care, Complications, and Follow up

K. I. Bland, L. S. Heuser, J. S. Spratt and H. C. Polk, Jr.

Introduction

The complex biologic behavior and growth characteristics of human mammary carcinoma requires a consideration of local and regional factors in its management. Current consensus would suggest that the majority of breast carcinomas have spread systemically at the time a primary tumor is diagnosed. These biologic observations have resulted in a trend to utilize more conservative surgical procedures for the breast and the axillary nodal areas, and, in many circumstances, provide the basis for application of adjuvant systemic therapy for the control of local, regional, and distant micrometastases. A continuing problem is the inability to recognize instances in which tumor progression and dissemination is beyond the ability of ablative operative procedures to control local disease.

Technological advances available through computerized tomography, radioscintigraphy, and xeromammography represent "state-of-the-art" procedures applicable in the pre-treatment staging of mammary carcinoma. Nonetheless, these diagnostic techniques need considerable refinement to identify regional and distant disease manifest at the time of primary therapy. Additionally, it is possible to assess the probability of dissemination of breast carcinoma by clinical and histopathological examination of the primary neoplasm. The identification of high-risk factors implicid for the recurrence of breast cancer in the postmastectomy patient is essential, and provides increasingly important data available to the clinician to plan the periodicity of followup.

The rehabilitation of the postmastectomy patient produces problems of varying complexity. The following chapter is organized to allow the clinician to have a more comprehensive approach to the physical, emotional, and social problems that accompany breast cancer in its post-treatment status.

Postmastectomy Wound Care

The various operative techniques employed in the treatment for breast carcinoma are described in detail in Chapters 13–15. We feel that the application of meticulous hemostasis and wound closure are paramount to ensure optimal wound healing. The application of the operative dressing is an essential part of the operative procedure and should not be left to surgical assistants or nurses who are unfamiliar with this detail. While we prefer closed-suction catheter drainage, commercially available as Hemovac®, Davol®, or Jackson-Pratt® tubing, each system should be appropriately placed to allow superomedial and inferolateral positioning of these apparati to ensure dependent and optimal aspiration. After the wound is closed the tubing is connected to continuous wall suction at 70 to 80 mm Hg pressure to ensure removal of all wound contents. An optional technique is wound irrigation with saline via the closed skin to flush and provide patency of the suction catheters. Thereafter, the skin is covered with strips of nonadherent, nonporous dressing (Telfa®), or a porous dressing (Adaptic®). Most important, thereafter, is the application by the operating surgeon of fluffs of 4×4 dressings of Kerlex®, inclusive of the entire operative site, to provide uniform compression within the limits of flap dissection. These compression dressings are then secured with an Elastoplast® elastic adherent dressing that is further secured by painting benzoine over the periphery of the dissected operative sites. This technique affords optimal dressing of the axilla with uniform compression, yet leaves the upper arm and forearm free of dressing application.

The patient will usually experience moderate pain in the operative site, shoulder, and arm in the immediate postoperative period. Due to the necessity of extensive flap development, the patient may experience hypesthesia and paraesthesia, as well as occasional "phantom" hyperesthesia. These sensations disappear gradually with wound healing (Schoenberg and Carr 1970). The patient should be assured that these abnormal sensations will subside within three to six months.

In the early postopertive period, the patient is encouraged to resume activity on the evening of her operative procedure. We regularly prescribe fluids by mouth within two to four hours postoperatively and often the patient is able to eat a normal or light meal before retiring. Early ambulation is encouraged. The current usage of portable suction units allows the patient to be up and about her room early postoperatively. We routinely encourage the patient to continue immobilization of the ipsilateral shoulder and upper arm, while mobility is permitted below the elbow in the forearm and hand. Application of closed-suction catheter techniques ensures wound evacuation in this circumstance. Isometric exercises, such as squeezing a ball, increase blood and lymph volume but do not facilitate lymph flow. First exercises should be graded active shoulder exercises.

While a moderate degree of bacterial contamination can be demonstrated in mastectomy procedures, we do not routinely administer preoperative, perioperative, or postoperative antibiotics unless other medical conditions (e. g., cardiac valves, prosthetic appliances, etc.) prevail. If postoperative erythema and cellulitis are evident, treatment with topical antibacterial creams such as Silvadene® are of particular value to prevent progressive epidermolysis and invasive soft tissue infections. Early debridement of obviously devascularized tissue is an important prophylactic adjunct to prevent progressive invasive infection. Stents applied over split-thickness skin grafts, which are necessary for large tissue defects, should be removed on the fifth or sixth postoperative day. Early and periodic wound care, including debridement with wet to dry saline dressings, affords optimal wound management to ensure adequate "take" of the graft application.

Suction catheter drainage, as a rule, is necessary for five to seven days postoperatively. The authors maintain a fetish with regard to the removal of the catheters and allow same only when the function of this closed system technique is terminated. Routinely, removal of the catheters is allowed only when less than 20 cc of serous or serosanguinous drainage is evident over a 24-hour interval. Thereafter, the wound is carefully inspected with regard to flap adherence and then the patient is encouraged to begin active range of motion of the ipsilateral arm and shoulder.

Complications of Mastectomy

Operative therapy for breast carcinoma can produce a variety of physical problems with regard to patient care. Rehabilitation for the postmastectomy patient has been greatly facilitated by the Reach to Recovery programs sponsored by the American Cancer Society. In most circumstances, a breast cancer patient is allowed to begin a gradual resumption of presurgical activities within two weeks after surgery. Young women usually regain full arm and shoulder range of motion before leaving the hospital, whereas older patients commonly may need intense exercise for several months before they can attain former levels of activity. Visits from volunteers of the American Cancer Society or the Visiting Nurse Association are particularly helpful for postmastectomy recovery.

Lymphedema

The pathogenesis of ipsilateral arm lymphedema following mastectomy is the ablation of the lymphatic system (nodes and channels) within the en bloc resection of the primary mammary tumor. The prevention of the subsequent increase in plasma hydrostatic pressure that follows the removal of these conduits may follow the surgical procedure, irradiation, or unchecked progression of neoplasm. Injury, capillary disruption, infection, or obstruction to lymphatic or venous outflow, hyperthermia, or exercise will accelerate protein leakage into these tissues. Previous attempts to evaluate the degree of arm lymphedema have been classified by Stillwell (1969) on the percentage of volume increase. This author grades an increase of less than 10% as insignificant, while an increase of greater than 80% is classified as severe. Lymphedema affects some 50% to 70% of all radical mastectomy patients but is severe and incapacitating in only approximately 10%, (Schottenfeld and Robbins 1970). Gilchrist (1971) stresses the importance of free and complete active range of motion of the arm and shoulder in the early postoperative period patient education with emphasis on the avoidance of excess sun exposure, injections, infections, or other potentially active or passive injury to the ipsilateral extremity and early recognition of incipient edema by the patient and its immediate therapy with compression massage of the edematous area. The early application of compression massage with the thumb, including stroking of the edematous extremity, often can alleviate and augment the prophylaxis of further edema. When it is severe, hospitalization for mechanical expression of tissue fluid, with application of an intermittent pneumatic compression device (Jobst® pump), may be helpful. The Jobst pump allows a progressive compression of the involved extremity in a proximal direction, thus allowing improvement to the obstructed flow of lymph. Additionally, the physician may wish to order antibiotic coverage, especially if there is evidence of supervening cellulitis, and may also prescribe diuretic therapy concomitant with a low salt diet. An elastic Ace bandage is applied when the patient is not treating herself with the pump, and the arm should be elevated at all times. We recommend daily measurements before and after Jobst therapy is used and the arm is elevated. The arm circumference is measured daily and recorded prior to therapy, which is on a repetitious cycle until optimal results have been achieved. At this point, the patient is measured for a Jobst Venous Pressure® sleeve, which is custom-tailored with a specific pressure at its distal surface. Daily application of treatment is necessary until the sleeve is received and therapy initiated.

Wound Infection

Although they occur rarely, infection and cellulitis of the postmastectomy wound or ipsilateral arm are serious complications. The majority of reported wound infections supervene as a result of primary tissue ischemia that occurs with flap dissection. Thereafter, progressive tissue necrosis allows wound bacterial proliferation with secondary infection. We do not administer prophylactic antibiotics routinely; however, topical irrigation of the wound with antibiotics is desirable for reduction of the bacterial flora. Infection produces an immediate disability that may progress to late postoperative edema of the arm. The compromised lymphatic flow, with resultant stasis produced with the standard technique of developing thin skin flaps, predisposes the wound to resultant infection. Early attempts at wound culture for aerobic and anaerobic organisms with immediate Gram stain are basic tenets for documenting the bacterial contaminant. Cellulitis uniformly responds to appropriate antibiotic therapy and elevation.

Seroma

The utilization of closed-system suction catheter drainage over the past decade has greatly facilitated a reduction in protracted serum collections. Seromas of the axillary dead space and the anterior chest wall are manifested in the first week postoperatively. In a retrospective analysis of 87 axillary regional lymph node dissections performed as isolated procedures discrete from en bloc breast resections, we (Bland et al. 1981a) observed seromas in 26% of patients treated for this operative site. Therapy consists of retention of the suction apparatus until drainage diminishes below 20 to 25 cc per day with the application of compression dressings after catheter removal for protracted circumstances.

Pneumothorax

This rare complication develops when the surgeon perforates the parietal pleura with tissue dissection or with attempts at hemostasis in the intercostal musculature. Pneumothoraces are more commonly recognized in the radical mastectomy procedure after removal of the pectoralis major musculature. Respiratory distress is recognized in the immediate postoperative period and pneumothorax is confirmed by chest x-ray. Early therapy, with closed thoracostomy drainage of the pleural space, is imperative.

Tissue Necrosis

The most commonly recognized complication of breast surgery is necrosis of the developed skin flaps or skin margins. Zintel and Nay (1964) observed major skin necrosis in 4% of their patients which is similar to that observed by other series. We (Bland et al. 1981a) observed an incidence of 21% for this complication with commonly associated wound infection for this operative site. Fitts et al. (1954) noted an incidence of marginal necrosis in 39% of patients in their series and demonstrated that patients with skin-edge necrosis were observed to have an increased incidence of postoperative arm edema.

Local debridement is usually not necessary in minor areas of necrosis (i. e., ≤ 2 cm^2 area). Larger areas of partial or full-thickness skin loss require debridement, and on occasion, the application of split-thickness skin grafts. Rotational composite skin flaps and subcutaneous skin tissue can be utilized from the lateral chest wall or the contralateral breast to cover the defect.

Hemorrhage

The utilization of closed suction catheter drainage allows early recognition of this rare complication. Hemorrhage is reported as a postoperative complication in 1 to 4% (Bland et al 1981; Zintel and Nay 1964) and is manifested with undue swelling at the operative site. Recognition of this complication is paramount and is treated by aspiration of the liquified hematoma and the establishment of patency of the suction catheters. The application of a light compression dressing reinforced with Elastoplast tape should diminish this occurrence.

Injury to Neurovascular Structures of the Axilla

Injury to the brachial plexus is also a rare complication of mastectomy. It is most commonly avoided by meticulous dissection in and about the neurovascular bundle and by staying parallel to the neurilemma and the wall of the axillary vein with en bloc resection of lymphatic structures and fatty tissues in this area. More commonly, one recognizes injuries to the thoracodorsal nerve and the long thoracic nerve of Bell in the postoperative period. The thoracodorsal, or subscapular, nerve innervates the latissimus dorsi muscle in its course with the subscapular vessels and is commonly sacrificed when lymph node tissue is discovered to be involved with metastasis in its dissection. Sacrifice of this nerve is a minimal physical disability with observed weakness of internal rotation and abduction noted with paralysis of the latissimus dorsi muscle.

Conversely, injury to the long thoracic nerve of Bell, which innervates the serratus anterior muscle, produces instability and unsightly prominence of the scapula, which is known as "winged scapula." The patient sustaining such an injury will often complain of shoulder pain at rest and motion for many months following the procedure. All attempts should be made to preserve this nerve, yet its involvement with invasive neoplasm or nodal disease may require that it be sacrificed to ensure adequate en bloc resection.

The lateral and medial anterior thoracic nerves to the pectoralis major muscles and the motor innervation to the pectoralis minor exit the brachial plexus and enter the posterior aspects of these muscles in the proximal portion of the axilla. Preservation of the pectoralis major and its functional integrity is the objective of the modified radical mastectomy. Thus, maintenance of the integrity of the anterior thoracic nerve is paramount to ensure subsequent function.

Technical precision must be exercised in dissection of the axillary vein and its tributaries. The surgeon should stay anterior and parallel to the vein surface with dissection of perivascular fat and lymphatics. The rare complication of injury to the vein with dissection is immediately controlled by use of vascular clamps and by suture repair with fine cardiovascular nylon. Tumor invasion of the axillary vein is best managed by vein resection and subsequent ligation of the proximal and distal ends. Ligation of the axillary vein for pre-existing venous tumor invasion has not been associated with an increased incidence of postoperative edema of the extremity (Zintel and Nay 1964).

Injuries to the axillary artery likewise must be carefully repaired with cardiovascular suture; however, such injuries are less likely to occur than venous injuries, as the axillary artery is located anterior and superior to the axillary vein. The axillary vein must be "skeletonized" in the performance of the axillary dissection, but there is no need to dissect the axillary artery. Lymphatics about the axillary artery serve an important prophylactic purpose in preventing postoperative arm edema, and rarely, except in extensive axillary involvement with neoplasm, are these perivascular lymphatics involved with disease.

Patient Education

The press and media exposure in the 1970s of the epidemiologic frequency and distribution of breast carcinoma has increased public awareness and has subsequently helped allay the cancerophobic fears that may delay early diagnosis. Much credit must be given to the early screening programs, notably the Health Insurance Plan of Greater New York (HIP), which preceded the American Cancer Society/National Cancer Institute-sponsored Breast Cancer Detection Demonstration programs (BCDDPs), that has as its primary motive the demonstration to the medical profession of the means by which earlier diagnosis of breast carcinoma to the lay and medical profession is feasible. While the ultimate impact on survival benefit would appear to allow detection and treatment in an earlier and more favorable stage of breast disease, the impact on disease-free interval and survival are unknown in this early phase of followup (Bland et al. 1981b). The first comprehensive study by the Gallup Organization (1973) was used to widely develop public information and education programs on breast carcinoma. This study commissioned by the American Cancer Society (ACS) in 1973 was undertaken to evaluate the effectiveness of the majority of public information and education programs with regard to breast carcinoma. This same survey organization was recommissioned by the ACS in 1976 and focused on breast self-examination as part of a larger survey of public perceptions of various practices for cancer detection (Gallup Organization 1977). This study implied that the total percentage of adult women regularly examining their breasts had increased 6% since 1973 from 18% to 24%. Lieberman Research Inc. prepared a third study in 1977 for the ACS with regard to the effectiveness of alternative breast cancer public education program. Researchers questioned over 5,500 women prior to, immediately after, and six months postparticipation in one of seven breast cancer public education programs, which varied in data content and the type of spokesperson. Results suggest that the level of a woman's knowledge about breast carcinoma not only increased as a result of exposure to these educational programs but, secondarily, reduced her anxieties about the disease process. All seven programs were effective in increasing the performance of breast self-examination (BSE) in women of all ages and also allowed an improvement in the confidence limits of the BSE. Additionally, this study also noted that former breast cancer patients, nurses, and trained laywomen were equally as successful as physicians in persuading women to examine their own breasts and in improving women's attitudes toward this practice. Most significant was the fact that former breast cancer patients were more successful than their health-allied colleagues in convincing women that BSE was easy to perform and in dispelling embarrassment or anxiety associated with the examination.

Because mastectomy is not a panacea for breast carcinoma, a patient's vulnerability to recurrence and mortality periodically requires women to reassess their life styles and future goals. A growing number of postmastectomy voluntary lay groups have been organized to dispel the fears and anxiety of mastectomy patients and to more appropriately allow the emotional problems to be resolved through such self-help groups. In most major institutions, a trained volunteer sponsored by the American Cancer Society's Reach to Recovery Program will visit the patient before and after surgery to provide her with emotional support and with literature on exercise programs, prostheses, clothing, and other aspects of the postmastectomy rehabilitation. All volunteers in the Reach to Recovery programs are mastectomy patients themselves and have become empathetic allies and role-models for successful rehabilitation after breast surgery.

The Impact of Breast Self-Examination (BSE) Practices on Breast Cancer Detection

Despite advances in the detection and therapy of many types of cancer, little improvement has been made in the cure rate for carcinoma of the breast in the past 35 years. As therapy of smaller- or earlier-stage cancers has generally allowed for improvement in survival rates compared to the larger-stage lesions, BSE has been widely recommended. Foster et al. (1978) studied 335 patients with breast carcinoma to determine the relation between BSE performance and the clinical and pathological stage of breast carcinoma at first diagnosis. Approximately one-fourth of the patients evaluated had practiced monthly BSE whereas one-half had never practiced the examination. The authors noted that a more frequent performance of BSE was associated with more favorable clinical stage and with fewer axillary lymph node metastases at pathological staging. Additionally, pathological examination disclosed an age-adjusted maximum tumor diameter, which was much less in those practicing monthly BSE (1.97 ± 0.22 cm as compared to 2.47 ± 0.20 cm for individuals performing BSE less than monthly). Mean tumor size was 3.59 ± 0.15 cm for women never performing BSE. These authors' data corroborated a more favorable clinical and pathological stage of breast cancer in patients practicing more frequent BSE.

Greenwell et al. (1978) examined the effects of BSE and breast examination by physicians on the stage of breast carcinoma in and about the time of diagnosis. Clinical and pathological staging information was compared to interview data on the method of initial detection for 293 patients. Tumors were detected in clinical stage I over one-half of the time when the detection modality was a routine physical examination, 38% in those in whom BSE was employed, and in only 27% of women if the detection was accidental. Over two-thirds of the patients practicing BSE at the time of diagnosis discovered their tumor by this method. These authors also confirm that routine examination of the breast allows detection of smaller tumors than by accidental discovery. It was projected that breast cancer mortality would be reduced by 18.8% to 24.4% through BSE or by routine physical examination, respectively. Feldman et al. (1983) estimated that the regular practice of BSE may result in a 10%, five-year mortality reduction for whites and a 17% reduction for non-whites. These findings have been recently disputed, however, since they have been retrospective and do not include an analysis of detection methods and actual survival patterns among breast cancer patients (Smith et al. 1980). Critics of BSE have expressed concern that some women could be deluded into a false sense of security by a false negative self-examination, and that they would substitute BSE for periodic clinical examination. Nasca (1981) notes that even the strongest supporters of BSE view this procedure as a complement to, rather than a substitute for, periodic clinical examinations and it is a point that continues to be emphasized in our educational programs. Reliable teaching models are needed to ensure acceptance of BSE through our educational measures and must include proficient teaching practices. Current research would also suggest that new communication approaches are necessary to reach women who do not respond to mass media techniques.

A recent national survey, funded by the National Cancer Institute, indicates that public awareness of BSE has increased. This study revealed that 96% of women surveyed were aware of BSE, representing a substantial increase from the 77% reported in 1973, using similar survey practices. Since 1973, the proportion of women acknowledging the monthly practice of BSE (40%) increased by 10%. Additionally, women who are taught BSE techniques by their personal physicians were more likely to continue the practice of this technique as compared to women who learned from other sources (Howe 1980).

Mammography

The application of current xeromammographic techniques should be appropriately credited as the only available methodology, other than physical examinations or BSE, to detect cancer of the breast at an earlier stage. The early studies by Egan (1960) and the subsequent reproducibility study by Clark et al. (1965) demonstrated the feasibility of applied radiography in diagnosing human mammary carcinoma by radiographic techniques. The HIP study originally demonstrated the usefulness of mammography in presumably asymptomatic women with a 40% reduction in breast cancer mortality being evident only in women over the age of 50. With the initiation of mass screening techniques by the BCDDP utilizing mammography, thermography, and physical examinations, as well as the teaching of BSE, the ACS and NCI were able to demonstrate in 27 national projects measures by which breast cancer screening would have national impact. All of these projects have now completed 60 months of operation time and the ultimate impact of breast cancer mortality is conjectural. A recent review by Bland et al. (1981b) would suggest a crude benefit to younger screenees employing the screening modalities of mammography and physical examination, with an applied benefit which was identical to the individual over the age of 50 years.

The increasing recognition of non-invasive carcinoma and minimal breast cancers has recently been reviewed by the BCDDP pathology review subcommittee, and they suggested the finding of more atypical epithelial hyperplasias and associated presumably pre-cancerous lesions. This report, which has recently been reviewed by Carlile (1981), recommended that the BCDDP should encourage concurrent review of multiple pathologic opinions in all borderline lesions to avoid overlooking cancer or over-diagnosing it. The National Cancer Institute Ad Hoc Working Groups on Mammography and Screening for Breast Cancer (1977) reported a similar interpretation of the HIP data. This group concluded that the HIP data justified the use of mammography as a screening device in individuals over the age of 50 if the radiation dosage can be implemented under one rad. Uncertainty continues to exist in assessing risk and benefit of mammography in doses greater than or equal to one rad.

A recent NCI population survey suggests there is an increase in public awareness of xeromammography since 1973. Sixty-one percent of the women surveyed were aware of xeromammography as compared with 43% in an earlier survey. However, a small percentage of women surveyed were aware of negative publicity concerning this technique, despite the fact that 19% reported having a mammographic examination (Nasca 1981).

Interval Clinical Examination

The HIP study suggested that periodic clinical examination and mammography contributed independently to a reduction in breast cancer mortality in individuals older than 50 years. While these early detection modalities were complementary in reducing breast cancer mortality, it was extrapolated that essentially one third of the lesions would have been missed had mammography not been performed and almost half would have been reported as false-negatives if clinical examination had omitted been done (NCI Ad Hoc 1977; Shapiro et al. 1973).

Previous screening results from the HIP study and the BCDDP were derived from projected data to detect breast cancer at its earliest and most favorable stage. Few data are able to refuter confirm the effectiveness of periodic physical examinations as conducted in a community setting on mortality. Greenwald et al. (1978) reported a higher percentage of stage I (T_1–T_2, N_0, M_0) tumors among women whose cancers were first detected through a routine physician examination than compared with cancers detected accidentally by the patient. As stated above, these authors estimate that routine physician examinations may reduce breast cancer mortality by 24% at five years followup. Physical examination of the breast, particularly when coupled with the knowledge of a patient's known risk factors, is accepted as a readily available, effective, and economic methodology of breast cancer detection.

The Relation of Dietary Factors to Breast Carcinoma

The exact relationship between breast carcinogenesis and fatty intake remains controversial. Evidence exists that suggests that hormonal imbalance and the utilization of metabolic substrate are altered by nutritional factors (Armstrong 1979; Hill et al. 1977, 1978). As early as 1942, Tannenbaum suggested that a high-fat diet increased the rate of carcinogen-induced and spontaneous breast carcinomas in laboratory animals, whereas other macronutrients did not enhance the effect of tumor incidence. Conversely, more current data (Fernandez et al. 1976) have demonstrated a retardation in the progression of breast cancer when fats were restricted in the diets of animals susceptible to this neoplasm. A recent report (Chan et al. 1977) also notes that in contrast to animals fed a low-fat diet, ovariectomized animals on a high-fat diet had a significant tumor yield before and after removal of the estrogenic effect of ovarian function.

The influence exerted by dietary factors in the etiology of breast carcinoma has recently been reviewed (Wynder 1980) and is generally supported by several epidemiologic approaches. A positive correlation is known to exist between dietary intake of fat in various populations and the mortality from breast carcinoma, although it is recognized that such correlation does not necessarily mean causation. The remarkable differences in the incidence of breast carcinoma and its mortality rate internationally, especially with alterations in rates with time as countries progress to "westernization," reflect the important etiologic environmental factors in this neoplasm. In the majority of population groups, total fat intake accurately reflects the risk of developing breast cancer, especially among postmenopausal women (Enig et al. 1978). Numerous tumorigenic agents are present in food-stuffs that would be expected to cause a higher incidence rate of cancer occurrence in certain geographic parts of the world. However, these neoplastic agents represent only one of the possible mechanisms involved in nutritional carcinogenesis. Rather than a specific food component appearing to enhance tumor carcinogenesis, it would appear that specific deficiencies or excesses of calories or macro/micronutrients are able to modify carcinogenesis by a number of currently unexplained mechanisms (Wynder 1980). This excessive consumption of dietary macromolecules and calories may cause them to act as cocarcinogens or other modifying factors, and in one study they have been linked to the development of approximately one third of the cancers in men and one-half of all cancers among women (Wynder 1978).

The relationships observed to date support the premise that obesity predisposes to a metabolic and endocrine hormonal milieu that promotes the occurrence of breast carcinoma. Donegan et al. (1978) previously demonstrated that breast cancer recurrence after radical mastectomy was evident in subjects with high preoperative body weight and suggested that the biologic mechanisms involved may promote growth of residual cancer after the original operative procedure. A more recent study (Donegan et al. 1978) correlates the preoperative obesity index (weight/height) to the recurrence of mammary cancer. A significant association was found between cancer recurrence and a high obesity index. Additionally, the disease-free survival rate of obese patients was half that of thinner women. This difference in recurrence rate was maintained regardless of the axillary lymph node

status and was unassociated with significant differences in menopausal status or mean duration of follow up.

Sohrabi et al. (1980), in a retrospective analysis, found no association between obesity per se and the time or frequency of recurrence of mammary carcinoma. Their sample did reaffirm that recurrence of breast carcinoma was related to tumor size and the pathologic status of axillary lymph node metastasis. Obesity was similarly related to tumor size and nodal status.

The Physician's Role in Follow up

Because of the propensity for breast carcinoma to recur and metastasize, a cost-effective lifetime followup plan is desirable. Guidelines for the extent of evaluation and followup have been based primarily on clinical impressions, but there are little factual data to support most of the proposed recommendations. There is a growing trend to perform extensive laboratory and radiographic studies at more frequent intervals. It would, therefore, seem quite desirable to look critically at our preconceived opinions and to allow physicians and nurses to evaluate more objectively their followup practices. The purpose of followup is not to generate and record costly laboratory and x-ray data, but to discover conditions that can be handled beneficially early in their evolution.

The difficulties involving attempts to define recurrence of neoplasm are legend. Kuzma and Dickson (1966) previously noted that the "diagnosis" of recurrent cancer depends upon a variable relationship of when that cure was attempted, co-existing illnesses, and physician prejudices. Polk and Spratt (1971), in a retrospective analysis of patients with carcinoma of the colon and rectum, analyzed the value of followup examinations in the detection and timely treatment of recurrences after resection for intended cure of colorectal cancers. Additionally, they evaluated the efficacy of the various methods of treatment for recurrent cancer. These authors emphasize that followup examinations are expensive and time-consuming and should be scheduled to permit discovery of neoplasms not controlled by primary therapy, with the intent of providing beneficial treatment for patients with recurrent disease where time makes a difference. Any additional therapy should provide control of recurrent disease in certain patients while allowing palliation in the remainder. Sixty-five percent of all recurrences had been detected by the end of the second postresection year whereas 88% of the recurrences were observed by the end of the fourth postoperative year. Peak interval recurrence rates corresponded precisely with the three- to six-month interval commonly scheduled for reexaminations. This study emphasized that an interval recurrence rate of 2% was sufficient to justify followup examinations every two months in the first postoperative year, every three months in the second year, every six months in the third and fourth years, and annually thereafter. Beyond the forty-eighth month postresection, patient education as to signs and symptoms of recurrent neoplasm is the major resource in the detection of late recurrence. An organized system of followup designed

for specific recurrent neoplasms, sufficiently early[
allow retreatment for cure, appears to be justified. [
appreciable salvage rate attending this early report m
be tempered with regard to locally recurrent colon c
cer. A more current analysis (Polk and Spratt 1979) nc
a disappointing disease-free survival for patients in wh
curative reexcision of the perineum was performed, v
or without associated resection of viscera as warranted
operative findings. This dismal survival rate, free
disease, underlies the palliative nature of this reopera
approach when the primary operation had been a sl
dard abdominoperineal procedure.

While we advise women to begin monthly BSE at age
the routine performance of this examination in a patient
with previously diagnosed and treated breast cancer is
paramount. Ideally, this procedure should be performed
one week after cessation of the menses in the premenopausal female at a time when there is less breast congestion and sensitivity. We routinely advise postmenopausal
women to examine the contralateral breast at the beginning of each month (Fig. 18.**1**). A convenient time for
BSE is while the skin is wet as with bathing, as this
optimizes the ability to palpate peripheral and deep
breast masses. The examinations should be performed in
sequence: first with the patient's arms at her side and then
extended over the head while *viewing* each breast in the
mirror. Thereafter, the hands should be pressed firmly
against the hips so that skin and nipple dimpling or
retraction is exaggerated. The second phase of the examination is *palpation,* which should be systematically performed with the fingers of the opposite hand with the
ipsilateral arm in a relaxed and hyperextended position.
Additionally, examination should include detailed
examination of skin contour, the areolar-nipple complex,
and finally palpation of the axilla for lymph node metastasis.

Abnormalities or evidence that metastases have developed have been the subject of previous reviews (Ackerman and del Regato 1970) and include: (1) pain in the
vertebral bodies, long bones, ribs, etc. (bone metastasis);
(2) persistent cough, hoarseness, or hemoptysis (metastasis to the mediastinum, the lungs or the pleura with or
without pleural effusion); (3) constipation, jaundice or
other digestive abnormalities (metastasis to the liver, or
gastrointestinal tract); and (4) alterations in mentation or
focal neurologic deficits (metastasis to the central nervous system). The above sites represent the more common sites of breast cancer metastases, but virtually any
part of the body represents a site for involvement.

The only mechanism for evaluating the benefits for the
treatment of the breast cancer patient is careful followup;
however, the value of the earliest possible detection of
recurrent lesions needs to be assessed. Tumors that recur
locally can theoretically still be treated for cure with the
present knowledge that there is little chance for cure of
distant metastases. Smaller tumor volumes can be palliat-
ed much longer than advanced disease, but a still unan-
swered question is the interval between the appearance of
detectable metastases and the occurrence of symptoms.
Uniform agreement suggests that routine testing should

II asymptomatic breast cancer, the possibility exists that
75% of the positive bone scans actually represent false-
positive studies.

Scanlon et al. (1980) noted that physicians who obtain an
accurate history, perform a physical examination, and
evaluate symptoms will identify most recurrences at a
relatively early stage, and that extensive routine testing
may not be of value. These authors evaluated two groups
of breast cancer patients to study the symptomatic versus
asymptomatic recurrences with regard to tumor size,
location of recurrence, extent of nodal involvement,
grave local signs, stage of tumor, menopausal status, and
treatment mode–chemotherapy versus no chemotherapy. In a comparison of patients with ≤ 3 nodes involved
compared to those with ≥ 4 nodes, there was a statistically significant difference between the two groups.
Patients with ≥ 4 nodes were more likely to have
symptomatic recurrences than those with fewer involved
nodes ($P < 0.0126$). Additionally, there was a significant
difference for distant metastases, which were more likely
to be symptomatic than those recurring locally. No
differences were noted in comparison of the symptomatic
versus the asymptomatic recurrence groups with regard
to size of the primary tumor, menopausal status, disease-
free interval, or the presence of grave local signs.

Although physicians' recommendations are variable with
regard to patient followup, the integration of known risk
factors (age, menopausal status, family or personal
history, tumor size, stage of disease, etc.) are important
criteria to be considered on an individual basis in follow-
up. Current recommendations by the National Cancer
Institute include visits that are generally scheduled every
three months in the first two years postmastectomy and at
least every six months for the next three years, with yearly
interval examination five years postmastectomy. The
importance of systematic monthly BSE of the
contralateral breast is emphasized. In the noncompliant
patient, careful scrutiny, with more frequent intervals of
followup is desirable. At each examination, the physician
should examine the patient's mastectomy site, regional
(supraclavicular and cervical) lymph nodes, both axillae,
lungs, abdomen, and the opposite breast. Additionally,
annual laboratory examinations should include a complete blood count (CBC), chest x-ray and SMA-18,
mammography of the contralateral breast, pelvic examination with Pap smear, and rectal examination. Any
woman who presents with *symptomatic* skeletal, gastroin-

How to examine your breast

Fig. 18.**1**

This figure is taken from a booklet published by the American Cancer Society.

1

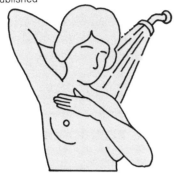

In the shower:

Examine your breasts during bath or shower; hands glide easier over wet skin. Fingers flat, move gently over every part of each breast. Use right hand to examine left breast, left hand for right breast. Check for any lump, hard knot or thickening.

2

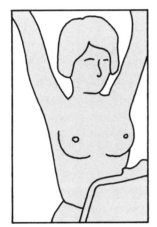

Before a mirror:

Inspect your breasts with arms at your sides. Next, raise your arms high overhead. Look for any changes in contour of each breast, a swelling, dimpling of skin or changes in the nipple.

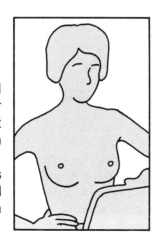

Then, rest palms on hips and press down firmly to flex your chest muscles. Left and right breast will not exactly match – few women's breasts do. Regular inspection shows what is normal for you and will give you confidence in your examination.

3

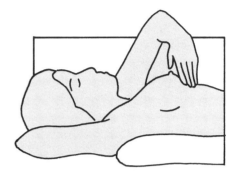

Lying down:

To examine your right breast, put a pillow or folded towel under your right shoulder. Place right hand behind your head – this distributes breast tissue more evenly on the chest. With left hand, fingers flat, press gently in small circular motions around an imaginary clock face.

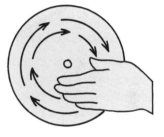

Begin at outermost top of your right breast for 12 o'clock, then move to 1 o'clock, and so on around the circle back to 12. A ridge of firm tissue in the lower curve of each breast is normal. Then move in an inch, toward the nipple, keep circling to examine *every part of your breast,* including nipple. This requires at least three more circles. Now slowly repeat procedure on your left breast with a pillow under your left shoulder and left hand behind head. Notice how your breast structure feels.

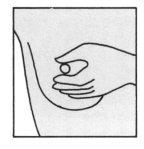

Finally, squeeze the nipple of each breast gently between thumb and index finger. Any discharge, clear or bloody, should be reported to your doctor immediately.

testinal, or central nervous system symptoms should have sequential evaluation by bone, liver-spleen, and brain radionuclide or computerized-axial-tomography (CAT) scans, respectively.

Recent studies (Scanlon et al. 1980) have suggested that annual examinations are too infrequent in the first four years postmastectomy; thus, there is scientific validity to the concept of examinations at three-month intervals because they are more likely to disclose recurrent tumor at a time when tumor burden is relatively small.

The Opposite Breast

Management of the contralateral breast most often refers to planned postoperative observations of the remaining breast following mastectomy for breast cancer. To formulate this treatment plan, however, several other clinical situations must be considered to encompass all women with bilateral breast cancer. These included: 1) synchronous breast cancers in one or both breast(s), 2) metastatic lesions to the remaining breast, and 3) non-simultaneous primary breast cancers in the remaining breast. Formulating a screening program for observing the remaining breast requires study of the incidence of occurrence of each of the previous possibilities.

Simultaneous Primary Breast Cancers

The reported incidence of simultaneous breast cancer ranges from 0.2% to 12% (Urban et al. 1977; Donegan and Spratt 1979). This broad range is probably due to two factors. The lowest incidence is reported in those series where the simultaneous cancers are both clinically evident, i.e., palpable lesions are present in both breasts. The highest incidence is reported from series where a contralateral breast biopsy is routinely done with each mastectomy or a sophisticated mammographic screening program scrutinizes both breasts.

The true incidence rate of simultaneous (synchronous) bilateral breast cancer is probably somewhere between these extremes. The number of minimal and in situ cancers found during biopsy and mammography that would grow on to invasive metastasizing breast cancers is as yet unknown. Pathologic interpretation of premalignant lesions is not uniform. These factors also affect reported incidence of bilateral cancers.

Metastases to the Opposite Breast

The dermal and subcutaneous lymphatics are routes for metastases from a primary cancer in one breast to the contralateral breast. Although this is not an uncommon occurrence, a contralateral breast lesion is more frequently observed as a second primary rather than a metastasis. Histologic criteria are helpful for differentiating primary and metastatic disease. A carcinoma in the contralateral breast should be considered a second primary cancer if it is of different histologic type, if the degree of nuclear differentiation of the second lesion is significantly greater than the original primary, or if there

is contiguous in situ carcinoma with the invasive lesion. Anatomical location favors metastases to occur in the fat at the periphery of the breast, near the midline or in the axillary tail. Metastases also tend to be multiple and show expansile growth rather than an infiltrative stellate pattern characteristic of primary cancer. Previous studies have shown that initial recurrence as a metastasis postmastectomy occurs in the opposite breast in 1.5% of cases–while 3% of all surgical cases developed new primary breast lesions. Followup periods ranged from one to ten years (Donegan and Spratt 1979).

Nonsimultaneous Breast Cancer

The last clinical situation is that of a second primary breast cancer occurring in an individual with a previous mastectomy for breast cancer. There is widespread belief that women at highest risk for the development of breast cancer are those having had a cancer in the opposite breast. Close scrutiny of the available data, however, would not allow such a sweeping statement. The actual incidence of second primary breast cancer varies according to the method(s) by which it is reported and the duration of observation. For example, one series reported an overall incidence rate of 3% of second primary cancers after mastectomy. What is not taken into consideration is the age of the women at risk and the length of time they are followed up. Calculated yet another way, when age and probable duration of life in which to develop a second cancer are considered, it is estimated that there is a 0.7% per year chance of developing a second cancer (Donegan and Spratt 1979).

Spratt and Hoag (1966a, b) reported 30 new breast cancers among 3643 person-years of observation, producing an age-specific incidence rate of non-simultaneous breast cancers no different than expected in the general population (P > 0.8). These data were updated and reaffirmed by Spratt (1977) and were earlier reported by Watson (1953). A more detailed breakdown of the Spratt and Hoag data suggests that if the first cancer occurs before age 55, there is a greater probability of non-simultaneous clinical cancer in the contralateral breast than is seen in the general population.

The clinician must consider the individual case. Two examples follow. The first is a 70-year-old woman with a large invasive lesion and axillary metastases at the time of mastectomy. Her chances of developing a second primary cancer of the opposite breast depend mainly on the number of years she lives to develop the second cancer. Most studies would indicate that her five-year survival rate from the first lesion is 30% and her ten-year survival rate is 15%. The probability of dying from her first cancer is much greater than her cumulative chances of developing a second primary tumor (Cancer Patient Survival 1976; Leis 1980).

The other extreme is a 40-year-old premenopausal woman with a minimal (≤ 1.0 cm, in situ) breast cancer of the first breast but with no tumor invasion or axillary metastases at mastectomy. Her five-year survival rate of this lesion is almost 90% and her life expectancy is nearly

30 years at age 40 (Cancer Patient Survival 1976). Her cumulative chances of developing a second primary breast cancer grow with each year she survives the first lesion. The clinician must then tailor the postoperative examinations of the remaining breast to each woman's individual situation.

Figure 18.2 is an algorithm which we currently utilize in the followup of the postmastectomy patient. The integration of the patient's menopausal status with the breast parenchymal pattern determined on xeromammogram allows one to categorize patients with regard to risk. Patient mammograms are assigned to a specific parenchymal pattern according to the Wolfe classification (Wolfe 1976). This system will allow sequential interpretation of breast parenchymal alterations according to the following classification:

N_1 = A breast composed mainly of fat.
P_1 = Prominent ducts in the subareolar area involving only a small portion of the breast.
P_2 = More severe involvement with a prominent duct pattern.
DY= Severe involvement with mammary dysplasia, with or without the presence of ducts.

The physician should be aware that utilizing this method of followup for the postmastectomy patient acknowledges that the P_2/DY parenchymal pattern represents a high risk with regard to the subsequent development of carcinoma, and that a time interval of observation after the baseline mammogram is necessary to allow the radiologist to observe any subsequent changes in breast parenchyma. This is a key concept in the mammographic interpretation of subtle alterations in breast parenchyma.

The Tumor-Host Relationship

The endocrine and biochemical heterogeneity of mammary carcinoma is adequately demonstrable in histological section or at morphometric analysis. Conversely, the functional heterogeneity of this neoplasm is inconsistent with regard to its clinical responsiveness. Experimental and clinical evidence suggests that a tumor may differ in terms of its karyotypes, biosynthetic activities, proliferative characteristics, hormone dependence, antigenicity, as well as varying reponsiveness to irradiation and cytotoxic chemotherapeutic agents. The varying heterogeneity of a particular mammary carcinoma cell type will determine the pattern of growth of a tumor and its proclivity to dissemination (Carter 1977). Atkins (1974) has suggested that the functional heterogeneity of human breast carcinoma presents a range of behavior. At one end there is a tendency to remain localized for long periods of time. Other breast cancers disseminate at an early stage and are quite acute. Evidence exists for the heterogeneous nature of breast carcinoma from extensive endocrinological investigations as well as the studies on cellular kinetics, and suggests a remarkable spectrum with regard to variations in doubling times of the mammary neoplasm (Stoll 1969; Slack et al. 1969). Controversy continues to pervade the literature with regard to evaluation of observations for the association between tumor doubling time and the degree and/or extent of metastatic spread (Tubiana and Malaise 1976). The time span between ablation of a primary tumor and the subsequent appearance of a local recurrence varies widely. Additionally, the interval between the development of a local recurrence and death is consistently short and rarely exceeds 24 months (Tough 1966). This earlier study indicates that the doubling rate for breast carcinoma is not constant and reflects growth of the heterogeneous cell population with sudden activation of growth that may occur at any stage of its disease. Further, it has been shown that a number of metastases – local, osseous, and visceral – often lead to demise of the host within 18

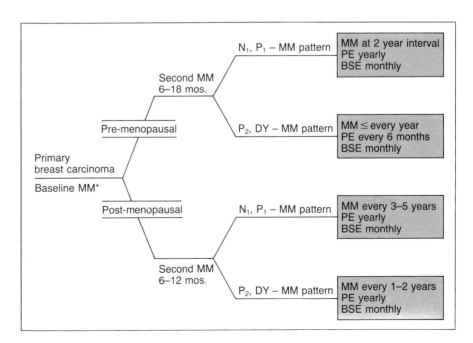

Fig. 18.2 Screening intervals for the postmastectomy contralateral breast
MM = mammogram; PE = physical exam (Physician); BSE = breast self-examination; N_1 = breast with mostly fat; P_1 = Prominent subareolar ducts; P_2 = More prominent duct pattern; DY = Severe mammary dysplasia

months of diagnosis and are thought to be more commonly associated in the younger woman in whom tumor doubling time is considerably shorter than for the elderly woman. This observation is noted to be compatible with alterations in the host immune-defense mechanism (Stoll 1976).

The growth rates for primary carcinoma of the breast remain a critical aspect of the natural history of the disease because optimal therapy is available only for "early" mammary lesions (Spratt and Spratt 1979). To establish strategy for the detection of early lesions, certain data must be known:

1. The time elapsing from inception of the cancer until it reaches a threshold size that is detectable.
2. The rate of growth in this predetectable stage.
3. The length of time between the threshold size and the time that it is no longer curable.
4. The percentage of cases in which metastases have occurred before the cancer reaches a detectable size.

We (Heuser et al. 1979a, b) have previously examined growth rates of carcinomas as a critical aspect of this natural history of the disease. The growth rates of 32 primary cancers were determined from serial mammographic views of tumor-nucleus shadows in a population of 109 cancers. These cancers were found on a screening population of over 10,000 women who received over 30,000 xeromammograms within a 36-month interval. The tumor volume doubling times ranged from 109 to 444 days (mean doubling time = 325 days, 9 tumors = no growth). Additional cancers, which were growing too fast to be measured by the radiographic techniques employed, were noted at subsequent evaluations. These cancers were determined to be more likely to metastasize, but because of the small sample size, the absolute percentage of tumors in this fast-growing group was not determinable but ranged between 17% and 77%. Additionally, the tumors classified as "fast-growing" had an incidence rate of 34% for positive nodes at surgery, while those classified as "slower-growing" had an incidence rate of 16% for positive nodes.

Local Recurrence of Mammary Carcinoma

Patients with more advanced primary tumors developed local recurrence earlier than patients with less advanced primary lesions. Haagensen (1971) points out the fact that local recurrence is a considerable threat following the usual types of mastectomies. He considers recurrence locally of three types: 1) the first (and least frequent) type is local recurrence in the axilla; 2) parasternal mound-like tumors which are the outward manifestation of metastases to the internal mammary chain of nodes and 3) the most frequent type of local recurrence, represented by nodules in the skin flaps of the chest wall. This author notes that chest wall recurrence is the most frequent type of local recurrence, and it has a significant correlation with the extent of axillary metastases. Chest wall recurrence is indeed rare when no axillary metastases are evident, but is distressingly frequent when ≥ 8 axillary

nodes are involved or when nodal size exceeds 2.5 cm in diameter.

Distinction between local and regional recurrence is important but not always possible. This distinction is inconsistent with regard to frequency and prognosis. Donegan (1979) notes that the mechanism of local recurrence is uncertain and suggests the etiology is related to several causes:

1. Retrograde embolization through transected lymphatics.
2. Incomplete local removal of neoplasm.
3. Transection of involved lymphatics and blood vessels with tumor implantation in the wound.
4. Implantation of hematogenous metastases in traumatized tissue of the thorax.
5. Lymphatic stasis, which follows regional lymph node dissections with secondary endolymphatic arrest and entrapment of neoplastic cells.

Thereafter, there is progressive growth of micro-metastases within regional nodes.

Untreated internal mammary nodes will produce biopsy-proven metastases and adenopathy in at least 10% (Donegan 1977). Additionally, nodes that remain untreated in any regional lymph node basin, which is demonstrated to be present in as many as 40% of clinically normal axillae, will have notable progression of micro-metastases to clinically palpable disease (Fisher et al. 1977). Local recurrences may occur essentially at any interval following mastectomy. However, wide agreement suggests that the *maximum* local recurrence rate occurs in the first two years after initial therapy and that nearly 90% of local recurrences have appeared by five years (Bruce et al. 1970; Donegan 1979; Donegan et al. 1966). Additionally, Donegan (1972, 1979) noted that the interval of observation is an important variable and must be uniform if comparisons of local recurrence are to be valid, as the incidence of recurrence postoperatively increases with length of observation.

As noted above, the majority of local recurrences at the site of primary breast cancer treatment represents tumors which were quite advanced at the time of curative surgery or, in part, reflects inadequate existing methods for clinical appraisal of the extent of tumor dissemination. Approximately 15% of all local recurrences developed ≥ 5 years after therapy of the primary breast neoplasm. The frequency of these local treatment failures depends to a great extent upon a number of clinical variables as well as on the interval from time of initial therapy. Deck and Kern (1976) observed a higher five-year relapse rate when axillary nodes were involved at the time of initial therapy than when axillary nodes were disease-free. These data have been substantiated by Donegan (1979) and, additionally, also correlate with primary tumor size, number of involved axillary nodes, histologic type of neoplasm, the presence of fascial fixation of the primary, and the presence of skin edema. Further, Haagensen (1971) reports an increasing incidence of local chest wall recurrence as a function of the number of nodes and stage (Columbia clinical classification) of disease. This author currently initiates prophylactic postoperative irradiation to the chest wall and the axilla in all patients found to have ≥ 8 axillary nodes at the time of mastectomy.

Locally recurrent tumor, while described above as the physiologic consequences of inadequate ablation with local tumor progression, remains a problematic circumstance for the surgeon and medical oncologist. Essentially no information is available with regard to the immunological reactivity of antitumor effect, and this basic relevant information is paramount in establishing disease control. Regrettably, locally recurrent tumor does identify that the patient has extremely poor host-tumor interrelationship, and it is this immunologic status, rather than the method of therapy, which will largely determine the outcome of disease. While we commonly consider locally recurrent disease the harbinger of systemic metastases, no evidence exists that the chest wall provides a reservoir of malignant cells that will eventually progress to distant metastases. Bruce et al. (1970) point out that this explains why postoperative irradiation may reduce (or control) local recurrence; however, such therapy has had no impact on patient survival.

Regional Recurrence of Mammary Carcinoma

The regional nodes may simply be considered traps for prevention of mammary tumor dissemination. The efficiency of endolymphatic entrapment is minimal (Fisher and Fisher 1967a, b). Indeed, the interval of lymph node arrest of labeled tumor cells is brief and cells have been observed to traverse lymph nodes to enter the efferent lymphatic or venous systems. Further, labeled tumor cells that initially lodge within the lymph nodes were observed to reside transiently within these lymphatic systems. Cancerous emboli usually enter the central portion of the axillary lymphatics initially. Haagensen (1971) suggests that the nodes of the central group are the most commonly involved nodal group, and that this group is also most often exclusively involved. The subclavicular (apical) nodes (level III) are usually the last lymphatic group involved by virtue of the sequential progressive dissemination in the five levels of axillary nodal groups. This latter group of nodes is, in essence, never exclusively involved with metastases.

Most pathologists distinguish between the levels of ipsilateral axillary lymph nodal metastases with mammary carcinoma. McDivitt et al. (1968) reported that crude and corrected five- and 20-year survival rates are inversely proportional to the level of nodal metastatic involvement. The generally defined levels include level I, the earliest order of nodal dissemination below the pectoralis minor muscle; level II, the nodal level within the borders of the pectoralis minor and beneath same; and level III, the highest nodal group (apical-subclavicular).

Many investigators currently consider that level III nodes should be functionally remote and not be considered "regional" lymph nodes despite their anatomical echelon for progression of disease. These observations are substantiated by a much improved survival rate when apical (subclavicular) nodes are enlarged, but microscopically uninvolved with tumor emboli. This observation of site-dependent heterogeneity of axillary nodes has been supported by Berg et al. (1973) and Fisher et al. (1974a, b) with regard to investigations of lymphocyte transformation in cells from nodes at various axillary levels in patients subjected to radical mastectomy. Metastases to the apical (level III) nodes is considered evidence of distant tumor spread and is supported by differences in survival rates for levels of nodal involvement (Haagensen 1971).

The grave prognostic significance of metastatic disease to the subclavicular (apical, level III) nodes has been emphasized above. It is interesting, however, that metastases to the other four axillary nodal groups have a similar prognostic significance (Haagensen 1971). Cutler et al. (1969) previously observed that the proportion (percentage) of nodal involvement was related to prognosis. This view differs from that of Fisher and Slack (1970), who failed to demonstrate that the discovery and examinations of a greater number of nodes in a specimen were more meaningful in determining prognosis than if only a few were recovered, and further, that anatomical variations accounted for the differences observed in the number of nodes recovered from the axillary portion of radical mastectomy specimens. The wide range in the number of nodes per specimen might be related to a combination of anatomical differences, errors in identification of nodes, and possible variations in the extent of surgical dissection. Specimens containing positive lymph nodal metastases were analyzed with regard to 1–3 or ≥ 4 nodes present. In patients having 1–3 positive nodes, there was no trend to indicate that when fewer nodes were examined, results were statistically different from those in which greater numbers were examined. It was similarly observed that when ≥ 4 nodes were positive, patients whose specimens contained 5–10 lymph nodes had recurrence rates almost identical to those in patients from whom more than 30 nodes were observed. Survival rates were lower when 1–3 positive nodes were observed than if none was present. The most unfavorable prognostic index was when ≥ 4 nodes were positive. A more recent prospective survey (Fisher et al. 1975) indicated there is a similar pathologic correlation between the number of involved axillary nodes and an early recurrence rate. Additionally, the presence of ≥ 4 nodes in this study was associated more commonly with a larger primary neoplasm, the presence of lymphatic, blood vessel or perineural extension, and greater tendency to more malignant histologic grade.

Metastatic disease rarely becomes clinically apparent in internal mammary nodal chains. Donegan (1979) and Handley (1927) have estimated that, from the findings of surgeons who have included this nodal group with mastectomy specimens, approximately one third of patients have metastases to the internal mammary nodal group at the time of mastectomy. Additionally, the proportion of subjects presenting with internal mammary nodal involvement escalates with the clinical stage of disease. Donegan (1977, 1979) attributes regional failure, in part, to extension of tumor beyond the boundaries of the classical-radical or modified-radical mastectomy performed for operable disease.

A clinically negative axilla contains nodal metastases in nearly 40% of patients with invasive mammary lesions. Regional failure of the axilla as the first site of recurrence is to be expected in an increasing number of patients in whom the metastases are left unresected. This represented the first site of regional failure after total (simple) mastectomy alone in one third of the patient population that Fisher et al. (1977) thought to have occult metastases.

The early studies of internal nodal metastases by Handley (1927) and Handley and Thackray (1949, 1954) were landmark contributions to our knowledge of the dissemination of mammary carcinoma in this regional area. These authors established three clinical dictums with regard to tumor emboli in this region:

1. Internal mammary metastases occur after involvement of the axillary nodes with an increasing proportion of regional metastases as a direct correlate of the number of axillary metastases.
2. Internal mammary metastases are more frequent than commonly suspected and are found in approximately one-quarter of all patients with operable breast cancer.
3. These regional metastases are more commonly observed with tumors of the medial one half and central zone of the breast than from lesions of the lateral half of the breast.

Additionally, the clinical stage of disease and the size of the primary tumor are important correlates for the likelihood of internal mammary metastases in that nodes are involved 3.5 times as frequently when the primary tumor is ≥ 8 cm compared with lesions ≤ 3 cm.

Halsted's early recognition of the propensity of the axillary-supraclavicular route of metastases was an important physiologic observation. Consequent to these observations, Halsted added excision of the supraclavicular nodes to his radical mastectomy procedures. Subsequently, the high morbidity and mortality rates led to the abandonment of the operation by Halsted's pupils. Dahl-Iversen (1963) observed that supraclavicular lymph node disease was commonly observed in patients developing recurrent disease after radical mastectomy. After an extensive experience with supraclavicular dissection, an incidence of metastases to this regional site was observed in 8.4% of subjects with known axillary metastases (Haagensen 1971; Dahl-Iversen 1963).

The reported incidence rate of isolated local-regional recurrence of breast cancer following modified or classical radical mastectomy is between 10% to 17% (Donegan et al. 1966; Bonadonna et al. 1978), and five-year survival from the time of recurrence is reported to be from 21% to 37% (Buzdar et al. 1979; Chu et al. 1976). Bedwinek et al. (1981) retrospectively analyzed seven clinical factors tested for prognostic significance in patients with isolated local-regional recurrence. This analysis was performed to characterize the natural history of patients with isolated recurrences and to identify those clinical factors that predict which subsets of patients have a good prognosis and those who do not. Only three clinical factors –

number of recurrences, size of the largest recurrence, and length of the interval from mastectomy to recurrence (disease-free interval) – were found to affect survival. Clinical stage of disease at initial diagnosis, number of histologically positive nodes at mastectomy, menopausal status, and location of recurrences (chest wall versus nodal) were noted to have no significant effect on survival or on disease-free survival. Eighty-one percent of patients ultimately developed distant metastases; the incidence of distant metastatic disease was similar for patients with factors predicting a good prognosis to those with factors predicting bad prognosis. The number of breast cancer recurrences and disease-free intervals have previously been shown to correlate with prognosis.

The Prognostic Value of Biochemical Markers

McGuire and associates (1977) have recently reported the prognostic significance of the estrogen-receptor (ER) levels in breast cancer patients having mastectomy and axillary node dissections. After analysis by stage of disease, type of radical mastectomy, adjuvant radiotherapy or chemotherapy, the recurrence rates were consistently lower in ER-positive patients than in the ER-negative individuals. These authors conclude that the absence of ER-protein in the primary breast cancer is a major prognostic determinant for patients undergoing mastectomy for stage I and II disease. Prognostically, a similar finding was supported by Fletcher et al. (1978) with regard to patients undergoing non-operative therapy for stage IV disease. The probability of response of metastases to chemotherapy or endocrine therapy appears to increase with concentration of ER. Estrogen receptor positivity is associated with a prolonged disease-free interval which appears to be independent of age, tumor size, menopausal and nodal status (Allegra et al. 1979). Lippman et al. (1978) reported a markedly higher responsiveness to cytotoxic chemotherapy by ER-negative (76%) than by ER-positive (12%) neoplasms. Other studies (Kiang et al. 1978; Gapinski and Donegan 1980) have contradicted this correlation between ER status and responsiveness to chemotherapy. These inconsistencies in reported results support attempts to individualize adjuvant endocrine and chemotherapy programs. If ER-positive cells respond to endocrine therapy and ER-negative cells primarily respond best to chemotherapy, and if most tumors are heterogeneous, then combined chemotherapeutic and endocrine approaches may be superior to sequential therapies (Mercer et al. 1978; Lippman and Allegra 1978).

The combination approach of additive endocrine therapy (tamoxifen) to L-phenylalanine mustard (L-PAM) combined with 5-fluorouracil has been reported recently by Fisher with other NSABP investigators (1981) for women with primary breast cancer and positive axillary nodes. Disease recurrence was reduced at two years for patients ≥ 50 years given the three-drug regimen whose tumor ER levels were ≥ 10 femtomole. Patients < 50 years were less responsive, with no benefit noted for those with 1–3 positive nodes, but a reduced treatment failure rate was observed for individuals with ≥ 4 nodes and high receptor levels.

Other combination chemo-hormonal therapy regimens have been reported to be effective for metastatic disease in phase II trials. Allegra and associates (1983) noted 50% complete remissions using additive, sequential tamoxifen and Premarin® with methotrexate and 5-fluorouracil. Future chemohormonal approaches appear justifiable to allow maximum antitumor effect, as the different mechanisms of action and of toxicity for the combination method may result in better response rates when compared to either therapy alone.

Patterns of Recurrent Disease for Operable Breast Carcinoma

Adjuvant chemotherapy for breast carcinoma must be recognized as a clinical experiment requiring a significant number of patients to ensure comparability for the many critical variables. Despite recent positive results as reported from the Milan Clinics with the use of cytoxan, methotrexate, fluorouracil (CMF) (Bonadonna et al. 1976), adjuvant chemotherapy has not been established as having absolute clinical value. Considering the prognosis for operable breast carcinoma, the rationale for cytotoxic drug combinations for women with positive nodes at mastectomy is based on the probability that in an adjuvant setting, intermediate analysis will also predict results for the long-term analysis. As most treatment failures appear to occur within the first 36 months following potentially curative surgery, current approaches utilize various forms of adjuvant systemic treatment as a rational attempt to improve prognosis when residual disease is regarded as a stage of micrometastases.

The early promising results of initial controlled trials with prolonged adjuvant chemotherapy (Bonadonna et al. 1976, 1977) have raised the possibility of the use of adjuvant therapy in patients with negative lymph nodes. Currently, factors obviating the use of adjuvant chemotherapy in individuals with uninvolved nodes include its followup and its potential long-term toxic side effects. A recent study by Nime et al. (1977) confirmed the development of visceral metastases in 43% of women with tumor cells demonstrated in intramammary lymphatic vessels, compared to 4% of women in a control group who had no intramammary tumor emboli. These findings could provide the basis for the selection of high-risk patients suitable for adjuvant chemotherapy.

Valagussa et al. (1978) reported patterns of primary treatment failures and their correlation with overall survival in patients with operable breast carcinoma. Relapse and survival rates were related to different patterns, with the intent to define on a clinical basis the high-risk groups in whom systemic adjuvant therapy was to be given. The ten-year relapse rate was 52.9% for this group treated with radical and extended radical mastectomy. Patients with negative axillary nodes and positive axillary nodes were noted to have a ten-year relapse rate of 27.9% and 75.5%, respectively. Relapse rates were affected by concomitant involvement of internal mammary nodes and were directly proportional to the size of the primary tumor in node-positive patients. Location of primary tumor as well as menopausal status revealed no direct effect on relapse and survival. Regardless of the nodal groups involved, sites of first relapse were documented to occur preferentially in distant organs and tissues.

The influence of adjuvant chemotherapy (CMF) on the patterns of first recurrence in operable breast cancer was evaluated by Valagussa et al. (1980). Clinical and laboratory reevaluations confirmed that surgery (radical mastectomy) with 12 CMF treatments allowed a higher probability for relapse as *single* bone or lung lesions (63%) compared to mastectomy alone or mastectomy with six CMF treatments (48% and 36%, respectively). *Mixed* osseous lesions were observed more commonly in the high-dose CMF group (38%) compared to the group treated with surgery alone or surgery with six cycles of CMF. The percentage of new disease manifestations was similar in the three treatment groups for cerebral metastases, lesions at other distant sites, and recurrence in the contralateral breast. Multiple organ involvement was least commonly observed in the group treated with both mastectomy and 12 cycles of CMF.

A current interim report from the National Surgical Adjuvant Breast Project (NSABP) analyzing the patterns of recurrence for breast carcinoma has been updated for patients with histologically positive axillary nodes treated with L-PAM following conventional radical or modified radical mastectomy (NSABP 1981). Overall results continue to indicate a significant difference in favor of patients receiving L-PAM (P = 0.03). The estimated survival rate was 55% for those who will be free of disease at six years among the L-PAM treated group, versus 45% of those in the placebo-treated group. Distributions by sites of first reported treatment failures indicate that patients on L-PAM have a lower percentage of regional recurrence than individuals receiving placebo. The sites of treatment failures for the subgroup of patients in which L-PAM was most effective were patients ≤ 49 years with one to three positive nodes. The incidence of local and regional treatment failures in each group were comparable; however, the L-PAM group revealed a much smaller percentage of distant recurrences (32.3% for placebo versus 12.5% for L-PAM). Detailed analysis of distant failure sites disclosed a statistically higher percentage rate of integumentary and skeletal recurrences in the placebo group as compared the L-PAM treated group.

References

Ackerman, L. V., J. A. del Regato: Cancer-Diagnosis, Treatment and Prognosis. Fourth Edition. C. V. Mosby Co., St. Louis 1970

Allegra, J. C., M. E. Lippman, R. Simon, E. B. Thompson, A. Barlock, L. Green, K. K. Huff, H. M. T. Do, S. C. Aitken, R. Warren: Association between steroid hormone receptor status and disease-free interval in breast cancer. Cancer Treat. Rep. 63: 1271, 1979

Allegra, J. C., T. M. Woodcock, S. P. Richman, K. I. Bland, J. L. Wittliff: A Phase II trial of tamoxifen, premarin, methotrexate and 5-fluorouracil in metastatic breast cancer. Breast Cancer Research and treatment 2: 93, 1982

Armstrong, B. K.: Diet and hormones in the epidemiology of breast and endometrial cancers. Nutr. Cancer 1: 90, 1979

Atkins, H. J. B.: The Treatment of Breast Cancer. Medical and Technical Publishing, Lancaster 1974

Bedwinek, J. M., J. L. Lee, B. Fineberg, M. Olwieza: Prognostic indicators in patients with isolated local-regional recurrence of breast cancer. Cancer 47: 2232, 1981

Berg, J. W., A. G. Huvos, L. M. Axtell, G. F. Robbins: A new sign of favorable prognosis in mammary cancer. Hyperplastic reactive lymph nodes in the apex of the axilla. Ann. Surg. 117: 8, 1973

Bland, K. I., T. W. Klamer, H. C. Polk Jr., C. O. Knutson: Isolated regional lymph node dissection: Morbidity, mortality, and economic considerations. Ann. Surg. 193: 372, 1981[a]

Bland, K. I., J. B. Buchanan, D. L. Mills, J. G. Kuhns, C. Moore, J. S. Spratt, H. C. Polk, Jr.: Analysis of breast cancer screening in women less than fifty years of age. J. Am. Med. Assoc. 245: 1037, 1981[b]

Bonadonna, G., E. Brusamolino, P. Valagussa: Combination chemotherapy as an adjuvant treatment in operable breast cancer. N. Engl. J. Med. 294: 405, 1976

Bonadonna, G., A. Rossi, P. Valagussa, A. Banfi, U. Veronesi: Adjuvant chemotherapy with CMF in breast cancer with positive axillary nodes. In S. E. Salmon, S. E. Jones: Adjuvant Therapy of Cancer. Elsevier/North-Holland Biochemical Press, Amsterdam 1977

Bonadonna, G., P. Valagussa, A. Rossi: Are surgical adjuvant trials altering the course of breast cancer? Semin. Oncol. 5: 450, 1978

Burce, J., D. C. Carter, J. Fraser: Pattern of recurrent disease in breast cancer. Lancet 433, 1970

Burkett, F. E., E. F. Scanlon, R. M. Garces, J. D. Khandekar: The value of bone scans in the management of breast cancer patients. Surg. Gynecol. Obstet. 149: 523, 1979

Buzdar, A. U., G. R. Blumenschein, T. L. Smith et al.: Adjuvant chemoimmunotherapy following regional therapy for isolated recurrences of breast cancer (Stage IV NED). J. Surg. Oncol. 12: 27, 1979

Cancer Patient Survival, Report Number 5, U. S. Dept. of Health, Education and Welfare. Public Health Service, NIH, Bethesda 1976

Carlile, T.: Breast cancer detection. Cancer 47: 1164, 1981

Carter, R. L.: Significance of local recurrence in secondary spread in breast cancer. In B. A. Stoll: New Aspects of Breast Cancer, Vol. 3. Heinemann Medical Books, Ltd London 1977

Chan, P. C., J. F. Head, L. A. Cohen, E. L. Wynder: Effect of high fat diet on serum prolactin levels and mammary cancer development in ovariectomized rats. Proc. Am. Assoc. Cancer. Res. 18: 189, 1977

Chu, F. C. H., F. Lin, J. H. Kim, S. H. Huh, C. J. Gormatis: Locally recurrent carcinoma of the breast: Results of radiation therapy. Cancer 37: 2677, 1976

Clark, R. L., M. M. Copeland, R. L. Egan: Reproducibility of the technique of mammography (Egan) for cancer of the breast. Am. J. Surg. 109: 127, 1965

Cutler, S. J., M. M. Black, M. Torbjom, S. Harvel, C. Freeman: Further observations on prognostic factors in cancer of the female breast. Cancer 24: 653, 1969

Dahl-Iversen, E.: An extended radical operation for carcinoma of the breast. J. R. Coll. Surg. (Edinburgh) 8: 81, 1963

Deck, K. B., W. H. Kern: Local recurrence of breast cancer. Arch. Surg. 111: 323, 1976

Donegan, W. L.: Mastectomy in the primary management of invasive mammary carcinoma. In J. D. Hardy: Advances in Surgery. Year Book Medical Publishers, Chicago 1972

Donegan, W. L.: The influence of untreated internal mammary metastases upon the course of mammary cancer. Cancer 39: 533, 1977

Donegan, W. L.: Local and regional recurrence. In W. L. Donegan, J. S. Spratt: Cancer of the Breast, 2nd Ed. W. B. Saunders Co., Philadelphia 1979

Donegan, W. L., J. S. Spratt: Cancer of the second breast. In W. L. Donegan, J. S. Spratt: Cancer of the Breast, 2nd Ed. W. B. Saunders Co., Philadelphia 1979

Donegan, W. L., C. M. Perez-Mesa, F. R. Watson: A biostatistical study of locally recurrent breast carcinoma. Surg. Gynecol. Obstet. 112: 529, 1966

Donegan, W. L., S. Jayich, M. R. Koehler, J. H. Donegan: The prognostic implications of obesity for surgical cure of breast cancer. Breast 4: 14, 1978

Donegan, W. L., A. J. Hartz, A. A. Rimm: The association of body weight with recurrent cancer of the breast. Cancer 41: 1590, 1978

Egan, R. L.: Experience with mammography in a tumor institution. Radiology 75: 894, 1960

Enig, M. G., R. J. Munn, M. Keeney: Dietary fat and cancer trends: A critique Fed. Proc. 37: 2115, 1978

Feldman, J. G., A. C. Carter, A. D. Nicastri et al.: Breast self-examination: Relationship to stage of breast cancer at diagnosis. Cancer (in press) 1985

Fernandez, G., E. G. Yunis, R. A. Good: Suppression of adenocarcinoma by the immunological consequences of caloric restriction. Nature 263: 504, 1976

Fisher, B., E. R. Fisher: The barrier function of the lymph node to tumor cells and erythrocytes. I. Normal nodes. Cancer 20: 1907, 1967a

Fisher, B., E. R. Fisher: The barrier function of the lymph node to tumor cells and erythrocytes. II. Effect of x-ray, inflammation, sensitization and tumor growth. Cancer 20: 1914, 1967b

Fisher, B., N. H. Slack: Number of lymph nodes examined and the prognosis of breast carcinoma. Surg. Gynecol. Obstet. 131: 79, 1970

Fisher, B., E. A. Saffer, E. R. Fisher: Studies concerning the regional lymph node in Cancer. VII. Thymidine uptake of cells from nodes of breast cancer patients relative to axillary location and histopathologic discriminants. Cancer 33: 271, 1974a

Fisher, B., E. A. Saffer, E. R. Fisher: Studies concerning the regional lymph node in cancer. IV. Tumor inhibition by regional lymph node cells. Cancer 33: 631, 1974b

Fisher, B., E. Montague, C. Redmond, B. Barton, D. Borland, E. R. Fisher, M. Deutsch, G. Schwarz, R. Margolese, W. Donegan, H. Volk, C. Konvolinka, B. Gardner: Comparison of radical mastectomy with alternative treatments for primary breast cancer. A first report of results from a prospective randomized clinical trial. Cancer 39: 2827, 1977

Fisher, B., C. Redmond, A. Brown et al.: Treatment of primary breast cancer with chemotherapy and tamoxifen. N. Engl. J. Med. 305: 1, 1981

Fisher, E. R., R. M. Gregorio, B. Fisher: The pathology of invasive breast cancer. A syllabus derived from findings of the National Surgical Adjuvant Breast Project (Protocol 4). Cancer 36: 1, 1975

Fitts, W. T., J. G. Keuhnelain, I. S. Ravdin, S. Schor: Swelling of the arm after radical mastectomy. A clinical study of its cause. Surgery 35: 460, 1954

Fletcher, W. S., B. S. Leung, C. E. Davenport: The prognostic significance of estrogen receptors in human breast cancer. Am. J. Surg. 135: 372, 1978

Foster, R. S., Jr., S. P. Lang, M. C. Costanza, J. K. Worden, C. R. Haines, J. W. Yates: Breast self-examination practices and breast cancer stage. N. Engl. J. Med. 299: 265, 1978

Gallup Organization, Inc. (prepared for the American Cancer Society.): Women's Attitudes Regarding Breast Cancer. Gallup Organization, Inc., New York November 1973

Gallup Organization, Inc. (prepared for the American Cancer Society): A Study Concerning Cigarette Smoking, Health Check-ups, Cancer Detection Tests. A Summary of Findings. Gallup Organization, Inc., Princeton, N. J. January 1977

Gapinski, P. V., W. L. Donegan: Estrogen receptors and breast cancer: Prognostic and therapeutic implications. Surgery 88: 386, 1980

Gilchrist, R. K.: The postmastectomy massive arm. A usually preventable catastrophy. Am. J. Surg. 122: 363, 1971

Greenwald, P., P. C. Nasca, C. E. Lawrence, J. Horton, R. P. McGarrah, T. Gabriele, K. Carlton: Estimated effect of breast self-examination and routine physicians examinations on breast cancer mortality. N. Engl. J. Med. 299: 271, 1978

Haagensen, C. D.: The surgical treatment of mammary carcinoma. In C. D. Haagensen: Diseases of the Breast. W. B. Saunders Co., Philadelphia 1971

Haagensen, C. D.: The natural history of breast carcinoma: The spread of breast cancer through lymphatics. In C. D. Haagensen. Diseases of the Breast, 2nd Edition. W. B. Saunders, Co., Philadelphia 1971

Handley, R. S.: Parasternal invasion of thorax in breast cancer and its suppression by use of radium tubes as operative precaution. Surg. Gynecol. Obstet. 45: 721, 1927

Handley, R. S., A. C. Thackray: The internal mammary lymph chain in carcinoma of the breast. Lancet 2: 276, 1949

Handley, R. S., A. C. Thackray: Invasion of internal mammary lymph nodes in carcinoma of the breast. Br. Med. J. 1: 61, 1954

Heuser, L., J. S. Spratt, H. C. Polk, Jr.: Growth rates of primary breast cancers. Cancer 43: 1888, 1979[a]

Heuser, L., J. S. Spratt, Jr., H. C. Polk, Jr., J. B. Buchanan: Relation between mammary cancer growth kinetics and the intervals between screening. Cancer 43: 857, 1979[b]

Hill, P., P. C. Chan, L. A. Cohen, E. L. Wynder, K. Kuno: Diet and endocrine-related cancer. Cancer 39: 1890, 1977

Hill, P., E. L. Wynder, P. Helman: Nutrition and hormone levels in relation to breast cancer and coronary heart disease. Clin. Oncol. 4: 35, 1978

Howe, H.: Proficiency in performing breast self-examination. Patient Counseling Health Education 2: 151, 1980

Khandekar, J. D., F. E. Burkett, E. F. Scanlon: Sensitivity, specificity, and predictive value of bone scans in breast cancer. Proc. Am. Assoc. Cancer Res. Proc. Am. Soc. Clin. Oncol. 19: 379, 1978

Kiang, D. T., D. H. Frenning, A. L. Goldman, V. F. Ascensao, B. J. Kennedy: Estrogen receptors and responses to chemotherapy and hormonal therapy in advanced breast cancer. N. Engl. J. Med. 299: 1330, 1978

Knight, W., III, R. B. Livingston, E. J. Gregory, W. L. McGuire: Absent estrogen receptor and increased recurrence rate in breast cancer. Proc. Am. Assoc. Cancer Res. Am. Soc. Clin. Oncol. 271, 1977

Kuzma, J. W., W. J. Dixon: Evaluation of recurrence in gastric adenocarcinoma patients. Cancer 19: 677, 1966

Leis, H. P., Jr.: Managing the remaining breast. Cancer 46: 1026, 1980

Lieberman Research, Inc. (prepared for the American Cancer Society): A Study of the Effectiveness of Alternative Breast Cancer PE Programs, Summary Report. Lieberman Research, Inc., New York 1977

Lippman, M. E., J. C. Allegra: Current concepts in cancer: Receptors in breast cancer. N. Engl. J. Med. 299: 930, 1978

Lippman, M. E., J. C. Allegra, E. B. Thompson, R. Simon, A. Barlock, L. Green, K. K. Huff, H. M. T. Do, S. C. Aitken, R. Warren: The relation between estrogen receptors and response rate to cytotoxic chemotherapy in metastatic breast cancer. N. Engl. J. Med. 298: 1233, 1978

Madoc-Jones, H., A. J. Nelson III, E. D. Montague: Evaluation of the effectiveness of radiotherapy in the management of early nodal recurrences from adenocarcinoma of the breast. Breast 2: 31, 1976

McDivitt, R. W., F. W. Stewart, J. W. Berg: Tumors of the Breast. Atlas of Tumor Pathology. Armed Forces Institute of Pathology, Washington D. C. 1968

Mercer, W. D., C. A. Carlson, T. M. Wahl: Identification of estrogen receptors in human breast cancer cells by immunofluorescence. Am. J. Clin. Pathol. 70: 330, 1978

Nasca, P. C.: Current status of breast cancer screening. Curr. Concepts Oncol. 3: 17, 1981

The National Cancer Institute Ad Hoc Working Groups on Mammography in Screening for Breast Cancer and a Summary Report of Their Joint Findings and Recommendations. Final Reports. J. Natl. Cancer Inst. 59: 466, 1977

Nime, F. A., P. P. Rosen, H. Thaler, R. Ashikary, J. A. Urban: Prognostic significance of tumor emboli in intramammary lymphatics in patients with mammary carcinoma. Ann. J. Surg. Pathol. 1: 25, 1977

NSABP progress report, Protocol No. B-05. A protocol for the evaluation of prolonged therapy of mammary carcinoma with L-phenylalanine mustard (L-PAM) as an adjuvant to surgery. Twentieth Semi-Annual Meeting of the National Surgical Adjuvant Project for Breast and Bowel Cancers. May 21–23, 1981

Polk, H. C., Jr., J. S. Spratt Jr.: Recurrent colorectal carcinoma: Detection, treatment and other considerations. Surgery 69: 9, 1971

Polk, H. C., Jr., J. S. Spratt Jr.: The results of treatment of perineal recurrence of cancer of the rectum. Cancer 43: 952, 1979

Scanlon, E. F., M. A. Oviedo, M. P. Cunningham, J. A. Caprini, J. D. Khandekar, E. Cohen, B. Robinson, E. Stein: Preoperative and followup procedures on patients with breast cancer. Cancer 46: 977, 1980

Schoenberg, B., A. C. Carr: Loss of external organs: Limb amputation, mastectomy, and disfiguration. In B. Schoenberg, A. C. Carr, D. Peretz, A. H. Kutscher: Loss and Grief: Psychological Management in Medical Practice. Columbia University Press, New York 1970

Schottenfeld, D., G. F. Robbins: Quality of survival among patients who have had radical mastectomy. Cancer 26: 650, 1970

Shapiro, S., P. Strax, L. Venet: Changes in 5-year breast cancer mortality in a breast cancer screening program. In Seventh National Cancer Conference Proceedings. JB Lippincott Co., Philadelphia 1973

Slack, N. G., L. E. Blumenson, I. D. J. Bross: Therapeutic implications from a mathematical model characterizing the course of breast cancer. Cancer 24: 960, 1969

Smith, E. M., A. M. Francis, L. Polissar: The effect of breast self-exam practices and physician examinations on extent of disease at diagnosis. Prev. Med. 9: 409, 1980

Sohrabi, A., J. Sandoz, J. S. Spratt, H. C. Polk Jr.: Recurrence of breast cancer: Obesity, tumor size and axillary lymph node metastases. J. Am. Med. Assoc. 244: 264, 1980

Spratt, J. S., Jr.: Multiple primary cancers, review of clinical studies from two Missouri hospitals. Cancer 40: 1806, 1977

Spratt, J. S., Jr., M. G. Hoag: Incidence of multiple primary cancers per man year of followup – 20 year review of the Ellis Fischel State Cancer Hospital patients with comparison to the general population. Ann. Surg. 164: 775, 1966[a]

Spratt, J. S., Jr., M. G. Hoag: Mortal diseases among 1,000 Ellis Fischel State Cancer Hospital Patients – With comparison to the general population. Mo Med. 63: 198, 1966[b]

Spratt, J. S., J. A. Spratt: Growth Rates. In W. Donegan, J. S. Spratt: Cancer of the Breast. Major Problems in Clinical Surgery. Second Edition. W. B. Saunders & Co., Philadelphia 1979

Stillwell, G. K.: Treatment of postmastectomy lymphedema. In Modern Treatment. Hoeber Medical Division, Harper and Row, New York 1969

Stoll, B. A.: Hormonal Management in Breast Cancer. Pitman Medical, London 1969

Stoll, B. A.: Effect of age on growth pattern. In B. A. Stoll: Risk Factors in Breast Cancer. New Aspects of Breast Cancer, Vol. 2. Year Book Medical Publishers, Inc., Chicago 1976

Tannenbaum, A.: The genesis and growth of tumors. III. Effect of a high fat diet. Cancer Res. 2: 468, 1942

Tough, I. C. K.: The significance of recurrence in breast cancer. Br. J. Surg. 53: 897, 1966

Tubiana, M., E. P. Malaise: Growth rate and cell kinetics in human tumors: Some prognostic and therapeutic implications. In T. Symington, R. L. Carter: Scientific Foundations of Oncology. Heinemann Medical Books, London 1976

Urban, J. A., D. Papachristou, J. Taylor: Bilateral breast cancer: Biopsy of the opposite breast. Cancer 40: 1698, 1977

Valagussa, P., G. Bonadonna, U. Veronesi: Patterns of relapse and survival following radical mastectomy: Analysis of 716 consecutive patients. Cancer 41: 1170, 1978

Valagussa, P., J. D. Tesoro-Tess, A. Rossi, G. Tancini, G. Bonadonna: Has adjuvant CMF altered the patterns of first recurrence in operable breast cancer with N+? Presented at Proceedings for Sixteenth Annual Meeting of the American Society of Clinical Oncology. San Diego, California, May 26–27, 1980

Watson, T. A.: Incidence of multiple primary cancer. Cancer 6: 365, 1953

Wolfe, J. N.: Risk for breast cancer development determined by mammographic parenchymal pattern. Cancer 37: 2486, 1976

Wynder, E. L.: Personal habits. Bull. N. Y. Acad. Med. 54: 397, 1978

Wynder, E. L.: Dietary factors related to breast cancer. Cancer 46: 899, 1980

Zintel, H. A., H. R. Nay: Postoperative complications of radical mastectomy. Surg. Clin. North Am. 44: 313, 1964

Chapter 19

Psychology of Breast Amputation

K. Gyllensköld

This chapter will deal with the psychology associated with breast amputation. For all patients the diagnosis of breast cancer will produce *an acute situational crisis*. The intensity and duration of this psychological crisis will vary but all patients will pass through some or all phases of such a crisis (Caplan and Grunebaum 1967; Parad 1969; Feigenberg 1970; Cullberg 1980; Gyllensköld 1976, 1981).

Situational Crisis

Definition of situational crisis: A situational crisis will be initiated when an external event, for example, a serious somatic illness, threatens a person's physical existence, social identity, personal security, or possibilities of basic satisfactions in life. A situational crisis follows a distinct pattern of initiation, development and completion and is accordingly divided into four phases (Table 19.1).

Table 19.1 Four phases of situational crisis

Name of phase	Duration	
1 Shock	From a few seconds to some days	The acute state
2 Reaction	One or several month after the shock	The state of psychologically working through
3 Reparation	Further months after the shock	
4 New-orientation	The time after all other phases have been passed through	

The different phases of the crisis overlap and the passing from one phase to another is gradual. Two phenomena are basic for our understanding of the situational crisis when dealing with breast cancer patients: the psychology of cancer illness and the psychology of the female breast.

Psychology of Cancer Illness

Feigenberg (1981) discusses two concepts of cancer illness: the medical or biological cancer concept (that of doctors) and the subjective cancer concept (that of laymen or of patients). *The medical cancer concept* is actually composed of many different objective concepts by which one is able to sort different types of cancer into diagnostic classes. With varying degrees of accuracy, one may predict the prognosis of a cancer illness. There are many different methods of treatments to be used that have been clinically studied and tested so that indications, contraindications, and secondary effects are known.

The subjective cancer concept comprises the individual patient's conception of cancer illness and is usually influenced by personal experiences, myths, and fantasies. There is no sharp border between fact and fiction. Patients and laymen often associate cancer directly with death. Cancer illness is regarded as being insidious, hard to control, and leading to horrible sufferings. The fact that, so far, no one has yet been able to fully explain the etiology of cancer gives rise to ideas that the patients themselves might be responsible. As one patient put it: "If you smoke too much, you get cancer of the lung. If you have had too many men, you get cancer of the uterus. What have I done to get cancer of the breast?"

Some patients and their families will read a lot on cancer and different treatments. They will want to know as much as possible, whereas others prefer not to.

The two here simplified concepts of cancer are well known to most hospital personnel dealing with cancer patients. The concepts are contradictory and yet an individual may harbor both of them. This goes for patients and their families as well as for medical personnel at times of hopelessness and despair, especially when caring for dying cancer patients or for instance when stricken with cancer themselves.

Psychology of the Female Breast

To both women and men, *the female breast* engenders all sorts of ideas and emotions, some being conscious, whereas others are totally unconscious. The range of a woman's experience of the breast is wide. It will start with her being nursed as an infant and pass through the development of her own breasts during puberty and adolescence, to her teenage and later grown-up sexual experiences, and then to her ability to nurse her own children. How a woman has experienced her breast development, her breasts in sexual relations, or when nursing seems to be of importance when she tries to cope with the situational crisis in connection to breast cancer illness (Bard and Sutherland 1955; Gold 1964; Rheingold 1964; Sutherland 1967; Gyllensköld 1976/1981).

In a psychological study (Gyllensköld 1976/1981), breast cancer patients associated the following to the meaning of the female breast: the breasts are visible signs of the female sex; the breasts are one of the most highly prized physical attributes of women; the breasts may give life and the milk production is exclusively female; the breasts are symbols of motherhood and fertility; the breasts are erotically sensitive and important in sexual relations (see also Bard 1952; Renneker and Cutler 1952; Vigman 1953; Bard and Sutherland 1955; Bressler et al. 1956; Lewinson 1956; Renneker 1956/1957; Gold 1964; Sutherland 1967; Hueston 1970; Peretz 1970; Schoenberg et al. 1970; Steiner and Aleksandrowicz 1970; Farrow 1971; Goldsmith 1971; Lewis 1971; Snyderman and Guthrie 1971).

A woman's breasts will have contributed to a high self-esteem if she has been content and pleased with them: their looks, how they feel, getting pleasure from having them caressed, having enjoyed nursing her babies. However, some women's identity may be exaggeratedly dependent on their physical outfit including their breasts. Such women "need" their breasts as concrete and visible evidence that they are real women and worthy of sexual relations and motherhood. When they have to face the loss of the breast, they will initially more or less unconsciously interpret the breast amputation as a violation of their personal integrity. They will equate the breast loss with loss of an indispensable part of their femininity. Such patients will need extra psychological support before any medical intervention. Before a mastectomy, they will show open or concealed aggression rather than direct signs of the underlying deep depression.

Sometimes women may unconsciously associate their breasts with emotions of guilt or shame because of unresolved neurotic conflicts. On a more conscious level, some women will complain of dissatisfaction with their breasts because of how they look or how they feel. Many women never seem to have had any pleasurable sexual experiences through their breasts (Kinsey et al. 1953; Gyllensköld 1976/1981). All this will contribute to a negative or uncertain self-esteem.

Whatever attitudes or experiences women have of their breasts, they inevitably constitute an important part of their personality. Therefore, many patients will experience a breast amputation as a loss of a significant part of their female identity, at the same time as they realize the loss to be a necessary condition for life to go on. Some patients will say: "It is all right if they take my breast away if only I may live." But there will be others to whom the loss of the breast will be comparable to loss of a loved one (c. f., Schoenberg et al. 1970; Parkes 1974).

Taking the above into account, it is obvious that to patients breast amputations will have psychological implications as well as surgical. A mastectomy because of cancer illness will be an event of vital psychological importance to the patient's future life.

The Shock Phase

When a patient gets a breast cancer diagnosis she will experience both a threat to her life and a threat to her identity as a female. In this situation she will be totally dependent on medical personnel in order to deal adequately and successfully with what has happened to her. Therefore, she will also experience emotions of great helplessness and dependency. At the time of diagnosis, the patient will be shocked and during *the shock phase* she will try to keep reality at a distance, since she will not yet be able to integrate what has actually happened. It is not uncommon to find a shocked patient quite calm on the surface while underneath there is chaos. Many patients will strive hard to keep their overtly calm behavior in front of doctors and nurses. But they will not hear or understand much of any information given. Although they seem to be listening, most of their psychological energy is used to somehow cope with the shock. At the time of diagnosis, one should give the patient psychological support rather than medical information that may be communicated later on when the shock phase is over.

During the shock phase, some patients will start unconsciously to use different psychological defense mechanisms to cope with the situation, such as denial, depersonalization, and suppression. *Denial:* "The doctors only told me that I am to have an operation. They never told me why or what kind of disease I have." (The author had actually been in the room overhearing the oncologist telling of the diagnosis to this patient who in a conversation later on that day expressed herself in the above cited way.) *Depersonalization:* "I felt it was not me sitting there – I was standing beside myself. And going home, I was sort of walking beside myself. It lasted the whole day." *Supression:* "Well, I don't know if I think about it at all. I have not had thoughts about it at all. I just feel empty." During the shock phase, a patient will mostly not be able to understand much of any medical information given to her. What she needs most is warmth and somebody who cares about how she is feeling.

The best help you can offer during the shock phase is, therefore, to be with the patient, to give physical contact, and to encourage her tell you what she is feeling and to listen. At some Swedish oncology centers patients will get a pamphlet at the time of diagnosis giving some necessary medical information and general advice. This pamphlet *does not* replace the dialogue between doctors and patients, but is an appreciated complement to this (Gyllensköld 1979). The pamphlet is meant to be taken home and read when the patient feels calmer and to show to her family so that they get informed as well. The information given are known facts of breast cancer etiology, the upcoming medical treatment, and the physiologic and psychologic reactions in connection with treatment. It also tells about necessary exercises that the patient will be taught by the physiotherapist to do after the mastectomy. A special paragraph gives information to the family, how they might help, and be supportive to the patient. Finally there is some information on the possibilities of having reconstructive breast surgery. The booklet is meant for patients with rather good prognosis. It is written in positive language, but not with the intention of giving false hopes. The text is the result of cooperation between two oncologists, a nurse, a physiotherapist, a psychologist, and two former breast cancer patients.

The Reaction Phase

Gradually and with support of what actually goes on in reality, the patient will pass into *the reaction phase* of the situational crisis. Now she will be able to more fully grasp the meaning of the diagnosis: that she is going to have a mutilating treatment and that she has a serious illness. Mostly this will mean that she will be occupied by thoughts of the illness and of accompanying emotions. To be concerned of very little else but the illness and its possible consequences is a psychologically normal and healthy way to react. Something extraordinary has happened and the patient is suddenly facing aspects of life and death that she perhaps never gave much thought to earlier.

At the surgical ward in connection with a breast amputation, a patient may experience:

1. Satisfaction and gratefulness on getting rid of the cancer tumor; getting help; being cared for.
2. Loss of femininity.
3. Feelings of being misshapen; mutilated; frightening for others to look at.
4. Reactivation of neurotic conflicts.

Parallel to the well-known feeling of relief at having the tumor removed, the patient may harbor feelings of having lost part of her womanhood. Every time she dresses or undresses she may notice that her body is misshapen: "I look mutilated." – "I feel like half a person." It is not unusual that patients express themselves like this and it is not surprising taking into account that the female body normally is equipped with two breasts, symmetrically placed, as with many other organs of the body. – "I feel like a deviate." – From a psychologic point of view, this is a normal reaction since a patient missing one breast as a matter of fact does not look like a "normal" woman. The patient's value as a person will not have changed, but her bodily look does deviate as far as the breasts are concerned. To obtain a well-functioning patient-doctor relationship, the doctor should not deny this fact but by his attitude show that he understands and respects the feelings of the patient.

The psychologically normal reaction to loss of the breast because of cancer is to grieve (Deutsch 1942; Bard and Sutherland 1955; Aronsson 1958; Jackson 1963; Feigenberg 1968; Francis 1969; Steiner and Aleksandrowicz 1970; Schoenberg et al. 1970; Harker 1972; Peretz 1972; Parkes 1974; Gyllensköld 1978/1981). In this context grieving means that the patient repeatedly goes over what has happened, reflects over the illness and the breast loss, feeling worried and sad. It is important that her sorrow is allowed to come to open expressions such as crying, since properly grieving will facilitate a healthy adaptation to reality. Within psychodynamic psychology, one speaks of psychologic health referring to an individual's ability to freely experience all kinds of emotions, from despair to happiness; to express these emotions in adequate ways, for instance to cry when sad as well as to smile and laugh when happy; to think flexibly, which will lead to an open and broad mind. A necessary condition to obtain this kind of health is to have free access to psychologic energy.

If, during a situational crisis, too much of this energy is bound by too heavy an unconscious use of defense mechanisms such as repression or denial, this will negatively affect the possibilities of regaining former psychologic health by finally reaching the phase of new orientation. Anyone being in a situational crisis will unconsciously use any kind of defense mechanism to be able to cope. Such mechanisms may be regarded as adaptive or maladaptive depending on how effectively they function as a shelter against anxiety in connection with the threat of the situational crisis and in what way they contribute or hinder the individual to ultimately pass through all the phases of the crisis (for a more lengthy discussion of this question of adaptivity versus maladaptivity see Gyllensköld 1976/1981).

Some patients will be more preoccupied by the threat of loosing their life than of loosing their breast. This goes for young as well as elderly patients. They will be able to adapt to their psychological situation by unconscious defenses like repression, suppression, denying, and/or reaction formation against emotions of anger, bitterness, hatred, or despair. For some this may be the best solution. Others may cope better, if given the opportunity to share their experiences with a caring other person. When confronted with the ultimate human fate – death – such emotions are as normal and frequent as feelings of humbleness, love, acceptance and integrity.

At times mastectomy patients who deny or repress anxiety, sorrow, or worries are characterized by family members or hospital staff as "fantastic" patients who never "complain." However, from a psychodynamic point of view, one does not regard it as very healthy when breast-amputated patients do not show any signs at all of grieving or being worried about the cancer illness. Sometimes patients as well as families, doctors, and other personnel seem to believe this to be the other way round. They will believe that one has a strong and good psychologic health if one never feels sad, worried, or anxious but always glad, satisfied, and happy.

Hospital staff will sometimes get feelings of panic when a patient, for instance, starts crying. They will tell the patient not to cry: "Everything is going to be all right." They might be afraid the patient otherwise will never stop crying or they may feel like crying themselves. But many have learned that just staying calmly and silently with the patient will eventually make her stop crying and will make her feel much better afterwards, because she has experienced the adequate and normal outlet for her sorrow. In order to regain psychologic well-being and to maintain it, the patient will benefit from being allowed to overtly express her emotions and to verbalize her thoughts and feelings and in this way share her psychologic situation with someone else. The grieving in the reaction phase may be regarded as a *"moratorium."* This word has originally been used in developmental psychology by the American psychologist, Erik Homburger Eriksson, standing for times of urgent changes in life when you are about to loose something important in order to gain something even more important (Eriksson 1968).

Incomplete grieving or repressed grieving will often lead

to unfinished crises, not seldom with added psychosomatic symptoms. Not only unresolved problems in this phase but also serious progression of the disease may hinder patients to reach the next two phases of the psychological crisis. The important subject of the psychology of terminal care is however not dealt with within this chapter.

The Reparation Phase

In *the reparation phase,* patients will be less occupied by thoughts of the loss of the breast and of cancer illness. They will be able to again take a more active part in what is going on in every day life and resume their work at home or their occupational work. They will begin to function more or less in the way they did prior to treatments. However, they will have spells of sadness and moments of worries that cancer might hit them again. But such moments will not be longlasting or of hindrance when it comes to being able to enjoy life.

The Phase of New Orientation

The *phase of new orientation* is characterized by a complete return to earlier activities and capabilities. Patients reaching this phase have no need to deny what has happened or the fact that they are different from before. They will have learned that you can cope with cancer sharing this knowledge with family and friends (see also Gyllensköld 1980).

The Family

Usually families are able to cope better when all members (including the patient) have the same amount and kind of information. Sometimes patients prefer the doctor to explain to the husband and/or to other family members what the illness and the surgery will mean. It might be of great importance to some patients that the doctor speaks to the family and underlines the importance of the patient doing recommended physiotherapy and not carrying heavy burdens or in any other way straining the arm on the operated side. In some families there may exist a belief that cancer is infectious and the doctor's explanation that this is not so might be beneficial. In some cases it may be good to inform the husband that the couple does not have to refrain from sexual life because of the breast amputation.

It might seem strange that it may be of immense value to family members to hear that it is *perfectly normal* for everyone in the family of a breast cancer patient to get emotionally upset, especially at the time of diagnosis, surgery, and other treatments. However, this is understandable bearing in mind that often hospital personnel as well as patients and laymen believe it to be a sign of good psychologic health not to experience, or at least not to show any kind of feelings of being worried, anxious, or sad.

Phantom Breast

Phantom Breast is a phenomenon that usually is not very well known, but a few authors have observed it (Kolb 1954; Löfgren 1968; Crone-Münzebrock 1950; Ackerly et al. 1955; Bressler et al. 1956; Gyllensköld 1976/1981), and one other author mentions the lack of it after breast amputation (Gallinek 1939). According to the literature, between 33% and 50% of mastectomy patients will, if they are asked, tell of phantom breast. In Gyllensköld 1976/1981, there is a discussion on the background of phantom breast experiences as well as lack of it.

Prosthesis

It is hardly necessary to say that the prosthesis is a very important matter in the rehabilitation of the breast-amputated patient. The use of the prosthesis is medically motivated since a one-sided breast loss will mean an oblique load to the back. But more important is its psychologic and social value.

Reconstruction of the Breast

The female breast to some women seems to be an invaluable part of their identity and therefore loss of the breast because of cancer illness will mean a serious blow to their personal integrity, resulting in states of deep depression. Modern surgical techniques are of great psychologic importance both when it comes to extended use of breast-saving surgery and to reconstructive surgery after mastectomy.

Usually mastectomy patients are offered the use of an external prosthesis. To some patients, however, the use of an external prosthesis will not be an adequate compensation. On the contrary, the external prosthesis may give rise to additional feelings of worthlessness and insecurity, thereby damaging an already lowered self-esteem. From a psychologic point of view, reconstruction of the breast is therefore of great importance to patients who are not content with an external prosthesis.

In a small scale pilot study undertaken by the author, all interviewed patients (8) were highly pleased with the result of the plastic surgery they had undergone in spite of some minor complaints of a certain asymetry and "hardness" of the reconstructed breast (2). Summarizing the results of that study, one may conclude that the reconstruction made it possible for the patients to regain their former level of psychologic well being with regard to occupational work as well as private life including an improved sex life. Looking at the results, one may speculate on the importance of reconstructive surgery for the patient's possibility of denying having had breast cancer. Here the denial serves as an adaptive defense or coping mechanism since the reconstructed breast, among other things, psychologically seems to serve as a shelter against otherwise unbearable conscious or unconscious notions of death and dying from breast cancer illness.

Although reconstruction of the female breast seems to be well known among women in general, some breast cancer patients seem to be somewhat reluctant to introduce this topic for discussion with their oncologist or with the surgeon who performed the mastectomy. Such patients will, for instance, believe that other people including the doctors will find them ungrateful, demanding, or peculiar, should they ask for a reconstruction. "When your life has been saved you should be grateful and stop complaining about having lost your breast." "If I'd admit missing my breast as much as I do, they might think I'm a sex maniac or something." Because of misunderstandings such as these, it is of great importance that the doctor takes initiative by introducing discussions of breast reconstruction.

From a psychological point of view, one would wish for the future that the psychology of the female breast will be even more widespread and well recognized so that breast-saving surgery will be more frequent and breast reconstruction will be an integrated part of breast cancer surgery.

"Reach to Recovery" organizations

Starting in the United States and now working in many European countries are organizations of former breast cancer patients who will send a volunteer to visit new patients at hospitals after the mastectomy (see "First European Conference on Reach to Recovery" 1980; Gyllensköld 1976/1981). Such organizations mostly work within national or local cancer societies. Their aim is to emotionally support the patient as well as to give her some advice on daily living as a "mastectomee." In different countries there are varying criteria for selection of volunteers. Before volunteers will start visiting patients, they will have gone through an instruction course (see First European Conference on "Reach to Recovery" 1980). To some patients the meeting with a Reach to Recovery volunteer seems to be like a turning point. Psychologically this has to do with the volunteer being a living and healthy proof of her own information.

References

Ackerly, W., W. Lhamon, W. T. Jr. Fitts: Phantom breast. J. Nerv. Ment. Dis. 121: 177–178, 1955

Aronson, M. J.: Emotional aspects of nursing the cancer patient. Ment. Hygiene (N. Y.) 42: 267–273, 1958

Bard, M.: The sequence of emotional reactions in radical mastectomy patients. Public Health Rep. 67: 1144–1148, 1952

Bard, M., A. M. Sutherland: Psychological impact of cancer and its treatment. IV: Adaptation to radical mastectomy. Cancer 8: 656–672, 1955

Bressler, B., S. I. Cohen, F. Magnussen: The problem of phantom breast and phantom pain. J. Nerv. Ment. Dis. 123: 181–187, 1956

Caplan, G., J. Grunebaum: Perspectives on primary prevention. Arch. Gen. Psychol. 17: 331–346, 1967

Crone-Münzebrock, A.: Phantomgefühl und Phantomschmerz nach Mammaamputation. Langenbecks Arch. Klin. Chir. 266: 569–575, 1950

Cullberg, J.: Keiner leidet ganz umsonst. Gütersloher Verlagshaus Gerd Mohn, Gütersloher 1980

Deutsch, H.: Some psychoanalytic observations in surgery. Psychosom. Med. 4: 105–115, 1942

Eriksson, E. H.: Youth and Crisis. W. W. Norton and Company, Inc., New York, 1968

Farrow, J. H., A. A. Fracchia, G. F. Robbins, E. Castro: Simple excision of biopsy plus radiation therapy as the primary treatment for potentially curable cancer of the breast. Cancer 28 (5): 1195–1201, 1971

Feigenberg, L.: Vad betyder cancer? Cancer 2: 1–5, 1968

Feigenberg, L.: Erfarenheter som psykiater vid en tumörklinik. Svenska Läkartidningen 67: 5641–5649, 1970

Feigenberg, L.: Psykosociala aspekter på cancer och cancervård. In R. Romanus, H. Høst, L.-G. Larsson, B. Rosengren, C.-M. Rudenstam: Klinisk onkologi. Esselte Studium, Stockholm 1981

First European Conference on "Reach to Recovery": A programme for mastectomees, Copenhagen, 19–20th May (International Union Against Cancer), 1980

Francis, G. M.: Cancer: The emotional component. Am. J. Nurs. 69: 1677–1981, 1969

Gallinek, A.: The phantom limb. Am. J. Psychiatr. 96: 413–422, 1939

Gold, M. A.: Causes of patients' delay in diseases of the breast. Cancer 17: 564–577, 1964

Goldsmith, H. S., E. S. Alday: Role of surgeon in the rehabilitation of the breast cancer patient. Cancer: 14–17, 1971

Gyllensköld, K.: Visst blir man rädd. . . Samtal med kvinnor som behandlats för bröstcancer. Forum, Lund 1976. Published in English by Tavistock Publications, Ltd., London, under the title Breast cancer. The psychological effect of the disease and its treatment 1981

Gyllensköld, K.: Psykologiska aspekter vid bröstcancerupplysning och diagnostik. Föredrag vid symposium arrangerat av Nordisk Cancerunion, September 1980, Stockholm 1979

Gyllensköld, K.: Underlag för vårdprogram för Tumör i bröstet. Socialstyrelsen, Utbildningsproduktion AB, Malmö, 1981

Harker, B. L.: Cancer and communication problems. Psychiatr. Med. 3: 163–171, 1972

Hueston, J. T.: Augmentation mammaplasty. Med. J. Aust. 7: 728–731, 1970

Jackson, C. L.: The grief process in physical illness. Smith Coll. Stud. Soc. Work 33: 2, 1963

Kinsey, A. C., W. B. Pomeroy, C. E. Martin, P. H. Gebhard: Sexual Behaviour in the Human Female. W. N. Saunders Co., London 1953

Kolb, L.: The painful phantom. American Lecture Series No. 235. C. C. Thomas, Springfield, Ill. 1954

Lewinson, E. F.: Psychological aspects of breast cancer. J. Gen. Psychol. 13: 99–115, 1956

Lewis, J. R.: Reconstruction of the breast. Surg. Clin. North Am. 51: 429–440, 1971

Löfgren, B.: Castration anxiety and the body ego. Int. Psychoanal. 49: 48–410, 1968

Parad, H. J. (ed.): Crisis Intervention. Family Service Association of America. New York, 1965

Parkes, C. M.: När den närmaste dör. Wahlström & Widstrand, Stockholm, 1974

Peretz, D.: Development, object – relationships and loss. In Schoenberg et al.: Loss and Grief: Psychological management in Medical Practice. Columbia University Press, New York/London 1970

Renneker, R. E.: Psychological impact of cancer. Yearbook of Cancer. Chicago, 1956/1957

Renneker, R. E., M. Cutler: Psychological problems of cancer of the breast. J. Am. Med. Assoc. 148: 833–838, 1952

Rheingold, J. L.: The Fear of Being a Woman. A Theory of Maternal Destructiveness. Grune & Stratton, Inc., New York, 1964

Schoenberg, B., A. C. Carr, D. Peretz, A. H. Kutscher (eds.): Loss and Grief: Psychological Management in Medical Practice. Columbia University Press, New York/London, 1970

Snyderman, R. K., R. H. Guthrie: Reconstruction of the female breast following radical mastectomy. Plast. Reconstr. Surg. 47: 565–567, 1971

Steiner, M., D. R. Aleksandrowicz: Psychiatric sequelae to gynaecological operations. Isr. Ann. Psychiatry Relat. Discip. 8: 186–192, 1970

Sutherland, A. M.: Psychological observation in cancer patients. Int. Psychiatr. Clin. 4: 75–92, 1967

Vigman, F. D.: The cult of the bust and its callypina counterpoint. Int. J. Sexol. 6: 210–213, 1953

Chapter 20

Radiation Treatment in Breast Cancer

A. Wallgren

Introduction

In the year after the discovery of the invisible and penetrating x-rays by Wilhelm Röntgen in 1895, Grubbe in America and Gocht in Europe used irradiation to treat cancer of the breast (Mansfield 1976). Since then, radiotherapy has been used instead of or as an adjunct to surgery in operable breast cancer, instead of or preceding surgery in locally advanced disease, and in the palliative treatment of metastatic disease.

The routines have varied. As in the surgical treatment of breast cancer, the role of radiotherapy in the treatment of primary breast cancer has been challenged during the last decade. There are several reasons for this. In the days of Halsted and Röntgen, most women only presented their breast cancers to the surgeons when the tumors were locally very advanced (Lewison 1980). In spite of a dismal five-year survival of less than 30% (Nyström 1922), local recurrences were common. A locally "radical" treatment, that is, the classical radical mastectomy of Halsted, often supplemented by radiotherapy was necessary to keep as many patients as possible free of recurrence during their short survival. Since that time, an increasing number of women present themselves with smaller, "earlier" tumors, in which local control is more easily achieved even with less mutilating procedures. In spite of this, breast cancer mortality did not decrease. This and other factors have led to a general acceptance that breast cancer in most instances is disseminated at the time of clinical detection, and that this dissemination rather than the given local treatment is the determinant of failure. This has also directed present interest to systemic treatment.

The increasing concern about the psychologic and social trauma inflicted on women by the mastectomy in addition to the cancer itself (Keynes 1937; Morris 1979) has led to increased use of breast-conserving treatment. This can be accomplished either by radiotherapy or by a local excision of the tumor. Usually a local excision of the tumor is combined with local radiotherapy in order to minimize the risk that a recurrence in the breast will necessitate the mastectomy that was meant to be avoided by this therapeutic approach.

Even if breast cancer undoubtedly is a generalized disease more often than not at the time of diagnosis, present adjuvant cytotoxic chemotherapy still has to prove its effect on survival and cure in the majority of the patients [e. g., in postmenopausal women and in patients with a massively involved axilla (Bonadonna et al. 1983)]. Until an effective systemic treatment is available, women should at least be given the best opportunity for a local control of the disease (Baum 1982). Therefore, various combinations of surgery and radiotherapy still have to be used in order to achieve as good a cosmetic and functional result as possible with a low risk for local and regional recurrences, which tend to appear early and thus shorten the disease-free interval.

Some Basic Concepts of Radiotherapy and Radiobiology

The basis for the use of ionizing irradiation is the ability to destroy neoplastic cells while leaving the normal tissues more or less intact. Such a difference in radiosensitivity could be caused by a higher sensitivity to the irradiation per se. The malignant cells of some types of lymphosarcoma and of seminoma of the testis, for instance, are often very sensitive and can be eradicated with low doses of radiation that leave the surrounding tissues unharmed. More often, however, the sensitivity of the neoplastic cells to ionizing radiation is very similar to that of the surrounding normal tissues. In such cases, obvious differences in radiosensitivity between the malignant and normal tissues may be explained by differences in the ability of different tissues to rebuild the cell population that had been reduced by the irradiation.

A fatally injured cell may remain virtually intact and may even divide one or a few times before it undergoes lysis. Low, single doses of radiation cause few injuries, which can be repaired and are thus not lethal. When the dose is increased, injuries are accumulated and when they exceed the repair ability of the cells, they do not survive. Above this threshold value, the fraction of cells killed by a single dose of radiation is *proportional* to the dose. If the logarithm of the proportion of surviving cells after a single dose is plotted graphically against the dose of radiation, the curve obtained is characterized by an initial plateau corresponding to the threshold dose (Fig. 20.**1**). At higher doses, there is a linear relation between the dose and the log-survival of cells. The broader the plateau and the less steep the slope of this survival curve, the more resistant are the cells.

The slope and the configuration of the curve varies with the oxygen tension of the cells. Anoxic or hypoxic cells have a less steep slope than well-oxygenated cells and hence are relatively more restistant to radiation. Cells in

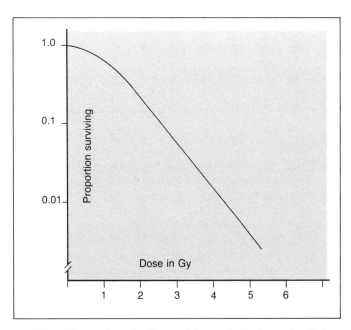

Fig. 20.**1** Proportion of cells surviving a single dose of radiation.

and late complications of normal tissues tend to increase with increasing doses of the individual fractions, especially if given over a short period of time (Kim et al. 1975). If the recovery is less complete for the neoplastic cells, their number will decrease with each fraction until, hopefully, no cell survives. This recovery is caused by the repair of radiation injuries in the cells and by the replacement of killed cells through repopulation.

Further, during the fractionated treatment, the tumor will shrink; hence, through the diffusion from the existing blood vessels, oxygen will reach even previously hypoxic areas. Through reoxygenation, previously radioresistant cells in hypoxic areas may become sensitive to the irradiation.

The optimal doses, the number of the fractions, and the intervals between them have yet to be elucidated for individual types of tumor and different tissues. Based on clinical and some experimental experience, most radiotherapists fractionate the doses from one to several times a week with total treatment times ranging from a few to several weeks. Mathematical models have been introduced to correlate the effects of radiation in normal tissues with dose, time of treatment and pattern of fractionation, and such models have at least in part been successful to compare effects on normal tissues of treatments with different fractionation scedules (Ellis 1969; Cohen and Creditor 1983). Still much empirical work remains before we know the optimal treatment of different tumors in different tissues.

hypoxic areas of a tumor may, therefore, survive the treatment and constitute the origin of a regrowth of the tumor. Hypoxic cells become increasingly more common when the size of the tumor increases, but may be present in tumors as small as a few millimeters in diameter because the cells grow out of their blood supply.

Fractionation of the Treatment

Usually, in external beam therapy, the treatment dose is not delivered in one session, but the treatment is divided in several sessions over a long period of time. There are several reasons why fractionated treatment generally is to be preferred to single-dose treatment. One reason is that normal tissues usually have a higher ability to recover than neoplastic cells. Even if the single lethal dose is similar for normal and for neoplastic cells, fractionated doses may allow the normal tissue to recover to a greater extent between the fractions. It has been shown that early

The relation between the total dose of irradiation and the effect on both normal and neoplastic tissues is best described by a sigmoid curve (Fig. 20.**2**). Therefore, two different doses of radiation have not a linear relation to the effect even if the individual doses and pattern of fractionation is similar. A small increase in dose will cause a considerable difference in response on the steep slope of the sigmoid curve. Efficient radiotherapy is based on the concept that the sigmoid curves of the dose response for normal tissues and for the tumor are separated. The gap between these curves constitutes the therapeutic width. The wider the gap, the greater the possibil-

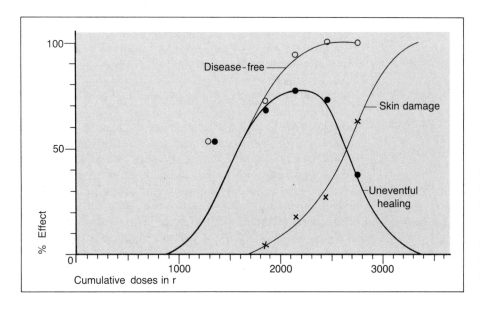

Fig. 20.**2** Relation between dose of irradiation and tissue effects. Open circles denote effect on tumor, x denote effects on normal tissues. The resultant curce (solid black circles) indicate cancer cure without tissue lesions. Courtesy of M. Strandqvist: Studien über die kumulative Wirkung der Röntgenstrahlen bei Fraktionierung. Acta Radiol suppl. 55, 1944

ity to eliminate the tumor while preserving the normal tissues and, conversely, if the gap is small, the tumor cannot be eliminated without a high risk of damage to normal tissues.

Size of Tumor and Dose

The larger the tumor, the higher is the dose required to eliminate the last cancer cell. One of the reasons for this is the exponential relationship between dose of radiation and proportion of cells surviving each dose. As has already been referred to, large tumors are more prone to have hypoxic areas where malignant cells may survive and later repopulate the area than small tumors. The relation between dose and size of tumor has been studied in breast cancer (Calle et al. 1973; Fletcher 1973; Timothy et al. 1979). Although a dose of 50 Gy (5000 rad) given over five weeks will eliminate more than 90% of remaining subclinical foci after surgery for an adenocarcinoma of the breast, a dose of 89 to 90 Gy in eight weeks will only control 56% of primary tumors larger than 5 cm (Calle et al. 1973).

The tolerance of normal tissues decreases with increasing volume of the irradiated area. Large tumors generally require higher doses to larger volumes than smaller tumors. The size of dose and the size of the target volume required to treat large tumors tends to diminish or eliminate the gap between the necessary dose to destroy the tumor and the possible dose with respect to the tolerance of normal tissues.

Systemic Effects of Radiotherapy

A radiation sickness syndrome and a depression of hematopoietic cells, including the granulocytes, the various types of lymphocytes, and the platelets are the most frequently encountered systemic effects of radiotherapy.

Radiation sickness is more likely to appear if large volumes, including the abdomen, are treated than if small, peripherally located regions are included in the treatment volume. Besides volume of treatment and anatomical site, the size of individual fractions are also related to the incidence of the sickness. The patients psychologic condition is also of importance both for sickness and the fatigue that are common complaints of patients undergoing radiotherapy.

True radiation sickness decreases rapidly when radiotherapy is interrupted. If such symptoms continue for more than a couple of days thereafter, other causes should be searched for. Radiation sickness can often be relieved by a reduction of the individual doses or by mild antiemetic drugs.

In primary breast cancer, the areas of interest for irradiation include the breast, or, after a mastectomy, the chest wall and the regional lymph node regions, that is, the axillary, supraclavicular, and internal mammary regions. Generally, irradiation of these areas gives little discomfort to the patient. Some fatigue and some nausea may be experienced. Rarely, the treatment has to be interrupted

or the doses reduced due to such general symptoms. The postoperative depression has been reported to be markedly increased in some patients who undergo postoperative radiotherapy (Morris 1979). Whether this is due to any somatic effects of the radiation itself or to the fact that postoperative radiotherapy means a prolongation of the treatment period, or both, is not known. Radiotherapy also induces a fall in blood pressure, which is most pronounced in elderly patients and in those with an initially high pressure (Larsson et al. 1976). A fall in blood pressure could be responsible for some of the general effects of radiotherapy.

Effects on Hematologic and Immunologic Cells

Radiotherapy may reduce the number of circulating granulocytes and various types of lymphocytes and thrombocytes. This is caused both by the direct irradiation in bone marrow and by irradiation of circulating blood within the irradiated volume. The effects on granulocytes and thrombocytes are usually mild and a rapid recovery is seen after the termination of radiotherapy. The effect on lymphocytic populations, on the other hand, is very long-lasting (Blomgren et al. 1981).

This has led to the assumption that radiotherapy might increase the risk for distant metastases and of death by a reduction of the immunocompetency (Stjernswärd et al. 1972). Support for an increased rate of pulmonary metastases after radiotherapy might be found in non randomized studies in which the reason some of the patients received radiotherapy and others did not is not entirely accounted for (Dao and Kovaric 1962). There is also experimental evidence for an enhanced rate of metastases in some tumor systems after local radiotherapy (e. g., de Ruiter et al. 1982; Baker et al. 1981). Stjernswärd (1974) also compiled some results from selected trials that seemed to give evidence for a decreased survival in patients who in addition to surgery had been treated with radiotherapy. This was used as an argument in the debate on the value and dangers of radiotherapy in breast cancer. The routine use of any treatment modality should be challenged continously. Undoubtedly, postoperative radiotherapy, sometimes with suboptimal techniques, had been used indiscriminately, just as the surgical radical mastectomy. This debate, especially in the United States, was used in the effort to establish the new medical speciality, medical oncology (Ansfield 1976; Lipsett 1981).

Stjernswärd's conclusions have, however, been criticized for several reasons. The depression of the number of circulating lymphocytes and of their reactivity after radiotherapy have been shown to lack prognostic significance (Baral et al. 1979; Petrini et al. 1980). The applicability of the statistical methods used by Stjernswärd to compile data from several studies in which not only radiotherapy but also the type of surgery varied between the treatment arms has been questioned (Levitt et al. 1977). The treatment techniques used in some of these studies also gave suboptimal doses in the internal mammary region, which is believed to be of importance (Fletcher 1976; Fletcher and Montague 1978). There were also other defects in these trials and in the use of data from them (Levitt and McHugh 1977; Wallgren 1977). Several well-controlled, randomized studies with a prolonged follow up have, however, shown that the rate of metastases is not increased in irradiated patients (Høst and Brennhovd 1977; Wallgren et al. 1978; Cancer Research Campaign 1976).

Local Complications

Any therapeutic procedure includes a calculated risk for some complications that may have to be accepted if adequate treatment is to be given. In this respect, radiotherapy does not differ from surgery. Therefore, the indications for radiotherapy, as well as for surgery, should be very strict and have to be questioned from time to time.

The region of interest in the treatment of carcinoma of the breast is highly irregular, and a very meticulous technique of radiotherapy has to be applied in order to avoid overdosage or underdosage that may increase the risk for complications or endanger the result of the treatment. Various complications may occur in tissues that are included in the irradiated volume. Such side effects may appear during or closely after the irradiation, or their appearence may be delayed for several years.

The complications may be very late in onset and, therefore, only detected after long periods of follow up. In locally advanced breast cancer, large volumes used to be irradiated to high doses. Long-term follow up has revealed that late sequelae such as severe fibrosis of the breast and necrosis of the skin continue to appear even after ten years (Spanos et al. 1980).

Often the skin over the breast or the chestwall has to be included in the target volume, for example, in inoperable or recurrent breast cancer. The acute reactions in the skin consist in an erythema that may increase to a moist desquamation. As late sequelae, dryness and thinning of the skin and telangiectasias may occur. This is unavoidable if the "biologic" dose is sufficiently high, but considerations concerning the dose-time relationship may reduce their appearance (Withers et al. 1978). To avoid a very high skin dose in patients treated with a tumorectomy only, the dose in the tumor bed is often "boosted" using implantation of radioactive sources, for example, ^{192}Ir (Weber and Hellman 1975).

A mild tracheitis and esophagitis are common complaints during the radiation of supraclavicular and internal mammary node regions. The proximity between the lymph nodes and these organs make such discomforts unavoidable, but these symptoms subside rapidly after the treatment and leave no sequelae.

Fibrosis is a late sequela after irradiation. Fibrosis of the breast may occur if single doses are high, especially in large, pendulous breasts (Harris et al. 1979). Fibrosis of the axilla may cause stiffness of the shoulder and an increased tendency to arm edema. The surgical axillary dissection without radiotherapy caused a higher frequency of arm edema (12%) than radiotherapy alone to the axilla without surgery (4%) in a randomized study (Kaae and Johansen 1977). On the other hand, the addition of radiotherapy to an axillary dissection increases the frequency of arm edema. We found that at a mean time of four years after treatment, the volume of the arm increased with at least 10% in 10% of only surgically treated patients compared with in 16% to 18% of irradiated patients (Swedborg and Wallgren 1981).

The lung is radiosensitive and as an effect of irradiation of the lung, radiation pneumonitis and fibrosis may occur. Acute symptoms may occur if large volumes are irradiated. The symptoms consist of a nonspecific cough and dyspnea. Such symptoms are rarely seen after regular postoperative radiotherapy in breast cancer. Vascular lesions and late fibrosis may cause shrinkage of the lung with a reduced vital capacity and a reduced perfusion of the irradiated parts of the lung (Notter et al. 1979; Racovec et al. 1974). Some degree of fibrosis is often seen in chest x-rays, but the chest is frequently symptom free. It is important to recognize radiation fibrosis so that such changes are not mistaken for metastases.

Osteitis and osteonecrosis may also occur as a late effect in ribs and in the bone of the shoulder girdle. High absorbed doses are required to cause severe osteitis (Langlands et al. 1977). The ratio between the dose absorbed in bone to that in soft tissues is very high in low-voltage irradiation from traditional x-ray tubes compared with that in high-voltage irradiation from ^{90}Co sources or from modern electron accelerators. Therefore, osteitis following radiotherapy is more common in conventional x-ray therapy than after treatment with high-voltage equipment.

Other rare side effects include lesions of the cervical plexus, which can be avoided after careful treatment planning in which the relation between dose, number of fractions, and overall treatment time is considered (Cohen and Svensson 1978).

Radiation Equipment and Treatment Planning
Different Types of Radiations

All types of radiation used in radiotherapy transfer their energy to the tissues through ionization of molecules, mainly water molecules. Through the ionization, highly reactive ions are eventually created that are responsible for most of the effects in tissues.

There are two kinds of ionizing radiation, namely, the electromagnetic or photons (x-rays and gamma rays) and the particulate (such as electrons or beta particles, alpha particles, neutrons, and protons). One basic difference between the particulate and the electromagnetic radiations is that the particulate radiations have a limited range of penetration into the tissues which is proportional to the initial energy and also depends on the type of particles. Electromagnetic radiation, on the other hand, decreases exponentially. The treatment can be delivered as *external* beam treatment or from *implanted* radiation sources.

In the x-ray tube, electrons are accelerated through an electrical field. The electrons strike a target, usually made of tungsten. When they are absorbed their energy is emitted as electromagnetic radiation with a maximal energy corresponding to the energy of the electrons. The energy of x-rays are, therefore, often measured in electron volts (eV). The voltage can also be used to qualify the radiation obtained. Most of the energy of the electrons is emitted as heat. Cooling of the target is essential. Filters made of, for instance, aluminium and copper, remove the "softest" radiations that increase the mean energy of the x-rays and make them more penetrating. At the same time, the output from the x-ray tube decreases.

In ordinary x-ray tubes, the maximum energy can only with difficulty be increased beyond a few hundred thousand electron volts (keV) because of electrical isolation problems. In the past x-ray tubes were the main treatment sources. The low-energy radiation obtained from these have several disadvantages that can be overcome in modern electronic accelerators. Radiotherapy delivered from standard x-ray tubes can, therefore, hardly be compared with modern treatment.

In the low-energy range, the maximum absorption of the energy is in the most superficial tissues, that is, in the skin. Deep-sited tumors only receive the dose that the skin tolerance permits. Cross-firing from several directions increases to some extent the ratio between tumor and skin dose. Originally, the dose of radiation was given as "skin erythema dose." In the low-energy range, the absorption of energy is very heterogenous in different tissues. The absorption in bone may be several times greater than that in soft tissues. This fact, being a prerequisite of diagnostic x-rays, is a disadvantage in therapeutic radiology. This increases the risk of radiation osteitis and tumors surrounded by bony structures receive a lower dose than calculated. Another disadvantage is that low-energy radiation spreads in all directions when interacting with tissues. At the borders of the "fields", the absorbed dose, therefore, diminishes diffusely and the fields become ill-defined.

The energy of electromagnetic radiation is absorbed in tissues, as already has been mentioned, through ionization of molecules. In the first step, electrons absorb the energy and these cause further ionizations. When the energy of the electromagnetic radiation is high, these electrons continue forward in the direction of the original electromagnetic beam into the tissues. Only at some depth under the surface is there a "saturation" of electrons. This is the reason why the maximal absorption of energy from high energy photon beams is not in the skin, but at some depth, the so-called build-up depth. This depth ranges from approximately 0.5 cm when the mean energy is about 1 MeV (e. g., radiation from a ^{60}Co source) to several centimeters, for example, radiation from 20 MV machines have a build-up depth of about 3 cm. This means that the dose can no longer be prescribed according to the visible skin reaction. The fields are better delineated because of the forwardly directed secondary electrons. At these energies, the absorption is also approximately equal in different tissues per weight unit.

Before modern electron accelerators for radiotherapy were constructed, high-energy radiation could be obtained from radium. Radium was, however, very expensive and the small amounts that were available could mainly be used for contact or close distance treatment. Radium emits both beta-radiation (electrons) and gamma-radiation. Gamma-radiation is equivalent to x-rays but consists of a few, distinct energies instead of a continous spectrum of energies.

In nuclear reactors, large amounts of radioactive isotopes can be produced. This has made it possible to build equipment where the radiation is not produced as a result of electron capture in a target, but originates in unstable isotopes. Radioactive cesium (^{137}Cs) and cobalt (^{60}Co) are the most commonly used artificially produced isotopes. The half-life of ^{60}Co is 5.3 years and the mean energy of the electromagnetic radiation (gamma-radiation) corresponds to about 1 MeV. Because of the limited half-life, the source has to be exchanged after some years when the treatment times have become uneconomically long. The cobalt unit consists of a small mass of ^{60}Co (approximately 2×2 cm) in a receptacle made of protective material. Through a "diaphragm" that can be operated from a radiation-protected room, the radiation leaves the unit. The radiation field can be shaped by means of shielding lead blocks.

The cobalt unit is a reliable tool since no complicated electronics are required. The radiating area of the source is, however, fairly large, which gives poorly delineated fields.

Electron accelerators, such as the betatron and the linear accelerators, also produce radiation with high energy. In practical use are machines with maximum energies ranging from 3 MeV to more than 40 MeV. In these machines, electrons are accelerated to a high energy and, as in the x-ray tube, are caught in a heavy metal target from which a continous spectrum of x-rays of different energies are emitted. The radiation of the lowest energies is filtered away. The mean energy of the x-rays is lower than the maximum energy of the electrons. A 3 MeV machine produces photons with similar penetration as the cobalt unit. Since the focus can be made very small, the fields are well delineated.

Besides x-rays, these machines can also deliver electrons suitable for therapeutic use. High-energy electrons reach a limited depth in the tissue that is determined by their energy. The energy absorption is fairly equal from the surface to this defined depth with little of the energy deposited beyond. Electron beams are, therefore, suitable for the treatment of superficially located tumors when there is need to protect underlying tissues. Electron beams with an energy of 6 to 9 MeV have suitable physical characteristics for the treatment of the chest wall postoperatively.

Interstitial Implants

Implants of natural radioactive sources, mainly radium, have been used in the treatment of breast cancer for more than 60 years (Keynes 1929). As the dose of any electromagnetic radiation diminishes with the square of the distance from the source, implants give a very high dose in the immediate vicinity of the source with a rapid fall-off of the dose. Radium may be used in the shape of needles that have to be removed after a few days. The handling of the needles and the care of the patients with the needles in situ implies a certain exposure to the staff. Besides, damage of the coverage of the needles might allow radon to leak from the needles, which increases the radiation hazards.

Artificially produced radioactive isotopes are now being used. For instance, iridium (^{192}Ir) may be obtained as "seeds" in thin plastic tubes. Under local or general anesthetic, a series of parallel rigid steel guide tubes can be inserted through the tumor at a distance of approximately 1 cm from each other in one or several planes. Their position can be checked in a radiograph. When their positions are correct, they are replaced by flexible plastic tubes. The tubes containing the seeds of ^{192}Ir are then inserted and fixed in these tubes (Pierquin et al. 1976; Levene 1977; Weber and Hellman 1975). In this way, controlled and adequate dosage is possible with a minimum contact with the radioactive sources by the staff.

Dose of Radiation

The dose of radiation is measured as the amount of energy absorbed per unit weight of tissue. The unit, gray (Gy), is the absorption of 1 J/kg. In many countries, the older unit of rad (Radiation Absorbed Dose) is still in use (1 rad = 0.01 Gy). The biologic effects of the same dose varies with the characteristics of the radiation. Within the mentioned energies, the biologic effects are similar. X-rays, especially from ordinary x-ray tubes, used to be measured in the roentgen (R) unit. This is a measure of exposure rather than absorbed dose, since it is defined as the number of ionizations per volume of air. One R equals to 2.58×10^{-4} coulomb per kilogram of air. Exposure dose should be replaced by absorbed dose.

Treatment Planning

Modern radiotherapy requires meticulous treatment planning in order to deliver high doses to the tissues considered to be involved in the malignant disease ("target" volume) while sparing the surrounding tissues as much as possible.

The planning is a multistep procedure. The regions of interest have to be defined. In the individual patient, these regions have to be located accurately. The planning of the absorbed doses in the tissues is performed by dosimetrists under the supervision of physicists who may suggest the optimal combination of treatment fields, energies, and types of radiation. The radiation therapist is responsible for the treatment in the patient. Finally, the set up of treatment fields in the individual patient requires the co-operation of the radiation therapist, the physicist, and technical assistants. Often the fields are marked on the skin of the patient using a special x-ray machine that "simulates" the treatment machine. Special fixation tools are often used to make it possible to repeat the treatments with an acceptable accuracy. The dose of radiation given during each treatment session may be monitored and the location of the treatment fields should be checked regularly during the treatment period by means of x-ray films that are sensitive for the used energy of radiation.

A staff of physicists and engineers is essential for a continous supervision of the modern high-voltage machines. Computers are often used for the treatment planning. Computer assisted planning is a rapid way of performing the calculations necessary to add the doses from several fields, to make corrections for example, for oblique angles of the beams to the skin and make it possible to test several combinations of energies and beams in the same time as it takes to make a manual planning. Information from CAT scans can be transferred directly into the planning computer, which increases the accuracy. Further, in many departments, computerized, so-called "check and confirm" systems have been installed. These are used to check that all subsequent treatments to a patient are given in the same way as was initially planned.

The Target Volumes in Primary Breast Cancer

The target volumes compose the breast (and postoperatively, the chest wall), the lymph node regions of the axilla, the supraclavicular fossa, and the internal mammary region.

The region of the breast and the chest wall are delineated interiorly by the lung and the pleura. These regions can be treated in different ways (Mansfield et al. 1978). Two tangential, opposing fields of photon radiation (gamma-radiation from a ^{60}Co source or 4 to 6 MV x-rays from an accelerator are suitable) can encompass the breast and the chest wall. Often the internal mammary nodes are included within these fields. The anterior part of the lung has to be included in the treated volume, but this usually causes little discomfort for the patient. By means of a special applicator, the divergence of the rays from a cobalt unit into the lungs can be eliminated (Fletcher et al. 1973). Tilting of the opposing fields outwards may achieve the same goal (Svensson et al. 1980).

Postoperatively, the chest wall may be irradiated using high energy electrons. The width of the chest wall should be measured in several points. If the width of the chest wall is underestimated, the dose to the lung can be considerable and cause radiation pneumonitis (Persson et al. 1972). Significant lung damage can be prevented if the point where the absorbed dose is 50% of the maximally absorbed dose is no closer to the pleura than 5 mm (Notter et al. 1979). By means of "tissue-equivalent" material, differences in the width of the chest wall can be compensated for.

The axillary lymph nodes are located in the anterior half of the axilla. The nodes of the apex of the axilla are found just under the middle of the clavicle (Fletcher and

Montague 1978). They are in continuity with the nodes of the supraclavicular fossa, which are found in the medial half of the fossa at a depth of 0.5 to 1 cm under the skin. The deep cervical nodes are located close to the midline. The axilla and the supraclavicular fossa can be treated using an anterior direct field that should go well over the midline in order to encompass the deep cervical nodes. The apex of the lung has to be included in this field as well as a rim of lung tissue laterally towards the axilla if the axillary nodes are to be treated. The dose in the deep portions of the axillary lymph nodes can be increased by means of an opposing posterior field.

The internal mammary nodes are generally located at the sternal edge at a depth of 3 to 4 cm. The nodes of the first three interspaces are the most frequently involved. Many of the commonly used treatment techniques give an uncertain dose in the region of these nodes, and this may be the cause for discrepancies between the results of reported series (Fletcher and Montague 1978). The position of the lymph nodes may be visualized by injecting radiopaque dye into the sternum, which opacifies the internal mammary veins (Fletcher and Montague 1978) or by internal mammary lymphoscintigraphy (Ege 1976). Such investigations have shown that these nodes may be located further laterally and deeper than previously anticipated. The use of a direct, anterior radiation field with sufficient energy of radiation and a sufficient width is a safe way to treat these nodes (Fletcher and Montague 1978). Planning of the treatment by means of lymphoscintigraphy (Rose et al. 1979) or ultrasound or CAT scan (Munzenrider et al. 1979) may also be used in order to avoid underdosage of involved internal mammary nodes if other treatment techniques are used than the direct field.

The combination of direct anterior and posterior fields to treat the lymph node regions and tangential opposing fields or electron beams to treat the chest wall or the breast causes problems along the junctions of the fields, with risks for over or underdosage along these. Different techniques have been proposed to solve this problem (Fletcher et al. 1973; Svensson et al. 1980; Lichter et al. 1983).

Effects of Radiation on the Normal Breast

The normal glandular tissue of the breast is radiosensitive. A single dose of radiation exceeding 3 Gy is sufficient to prevent the development of a breast if given to a young girl, an effect previously seen when radiation was used in the treatment of pectoral hemangiomas (Kolar 1967). A dose of 15 Gy in three fractions will prevent the tender swelling caused by the administration of estrogens to men with prostatic carcinoma (Moss and Brand 1969).

Ionizing radiation to breast tissues is carcinogenic and this has been established in several series of women accidentally exposed to radiation or in whom benign breast disorders were treated with irradiation (Baral et al. 1977; Boice et al. 1977; McGregor et al. 1977; Shore et al. 1977). There is still some doubt if the breasts of young women are more sensitive to radiation than those of elderly women. In one of the reported series consisting of women who had been treated for postpartum mastitis, it was suggested that the rate of radiation-induced cancers decreased if the dose of radiation increased over 4 Gy (Shore et al. 1977). This is consistent with a decrease of the carcinogenic effect due to the masking of cell death at high doses. This important finding seems to be supported by the fact that there are few reported late new cancers in breasts that have been irradiated to high doses for carcinoma (Rissanen 1968; Amalric et al. 1982; Clark et al. 1982). When tangential-beam radiotherapy is used to treat breast cancer, the medial half of the contralateral breast receives a significant dose of radiation. However, the frequency of second breast cancers in patients treated with radiotherapy, which might be radiation induced, does not seem to exceed the frequency of second cancers in only surgically treated patients (Levitt and Mandel 1983). Since the latency period for radiation-induced tumors is long, long-term follow-up studies over several decades should be undertaken in women treated with breast-conserving therapy, including radiotherapy.

Treatment of Primary Breast Cancer – Techniques and Results

Long-term follow up of breast cancer patients reveals that the disease is very heterogenous. Rapidly fatal cases are not uncommon but late recurrences even after several decades occur. There has been no long-term follow-up report that has convincingly shown that breast cancer patients even after several decades have no excess mortality compared with an age-matched population. Extrapolations and mathematical modeling, however, indicate that approximately 30% to 40% of an unselected breast cancer group may be considered cured in the sense that they are subject to normal mortality only (Rutqvist and Wallgren 1983). Even in node-negative cases, at most 50% to 60% may belong to the cured group (Rutqvist et al. 1983).

All therapeutic actions in breast cancer should be judged against this long perspective. Reports of treatment results after a few years are, therefore, of limited value. It is also important to recognize that even if a woman is not cured by the initial treatment, she may live for a long time before any recurrence appears and with possible treatment-induced sequelae. Differences in local treatment are not expected to change survival drastically (Mansfield 1976). This is in most patients already determined by the presence or absence of occult metastases and possibly to factors pertaining to the host-tumor relationship. So far, systemic treatment as the logical modality for a systemic disease has only proved to be beneficial for a minority of patients (Levitt and Potish 1981). While ongoing studies on adjuvant systemic treatment in breast cancer mature, it is still important to use the local treatment that gives the best local result, cosmetically and functionally, and that gives the patient the best opportunity to escape a local recurrence (Baum 1982). Whether more extensive local treatment may also increase the survival for some patients will be discussed below.

Radiotherapy in Locally Advanced Breast Cancer

The first patients with breast cancer who were treated with radiotherapy had locally advanced or recurrent disease. Since these early days, patients with "inoperable" breast cancer have been referred for radiotherapy. In advanced cases, it is possible to observe that breast cancer often is a radiosensitive disease. In this group of patients, whatever the definition of "inoperability" we use, the prognosis is poor and the majority of patients will die from the disease. Still, after radical radiotherapy only, a substantial proportion of patients remain free of local recurrence. Keynes (1937) showed that interstitial radium implantation could also be used in the palliative treatment of inoperable breast cancer, but that in his group of patients only 24% survived for more than five years.

At the Foundation Curie, Baclesse introduced the so-called "protracted" treatment. External x-ray treatment was given in high doses over a sufficiently long time to prevent severe acute skin reactions. His data indicated that only 15% of his patients were "clinically healed" after 10 to 20 years (Baclesse 1959). Very high doses have to be used to control such large tumors locally. In the experience of the Foundation Curie, a dose of 80 to 90 Gy given over 10 to 14 weeks achieved a 56% local control rate if the tumor exceeded 5 cm in diameter (Calle et al. 1973). However, severe late complications consisting of a progressive fibrosis of the breast with necrosis of the skin occur frequently after such high doses (Spanos et al. 1980). A combination of external beam therapy to the breast and the lymph node regions and interstitial iridium implants to increase the dose in the tumor when the local reaction after external radiotherapy has subsided appears to give a fair chance for a local control with a possibly lower rate of late complications (Alderman 1976). Some patients with initially inoperable tumors become technically operable after radiotherapy. At surgery, residual tumor can be identified after a preoperative dose of 60 to 70 Gy in approximately 75% of the cases (Zucali et al. 1976). The identification of tumor after irradiation is no proof that it is viable. Most relapses occurred in distant areas. In this group of patients, the prognosis of survival was determined by the extent of the disease. Patients with involved supraclavicular lymph nodes fared the worst and those without any clinical suspicion of lymph node metastases fared the best. The inflammatory type of carcinoma gave a survival that was as poor as for those with supraclavicular extension of the disease. When the tumor could be operated on, the survival was also better than when it was only treated with radiotherapy (Zucali et al. 1976).

The poor prognosis in this group of patients has prompted many attempts to combine systemic treatment with a locally efficient treatment (radiotherapy and/or surgery). In several series, it has been shown that radiotherapy may be combined with cytotoxic chemotherapy without unacceptable toxicity (Bedwinek et al. 1983; Buzdar et al. 1981; De Lena et al. 1981; Rubens et al. 1980). Compared with an historical control series of patients who had been treated with radiotherapy only, Bedwinek et al. (1983) and Rubens et al. (1980) found that adriamycin before, concomittent with, or after radiotherapy delayed the onset of disease progression, but with insignificant influence on survival. Similarly, Harris et al. (1983) found that the addition of systemic therapy to radiotherapy decreased both local and distant failure rates. In inflammatory carcinoma, a twice-daily fractionated irradiation increased the locoregional control (Barker et al. 1980). The addition of FAC (fluorouracil, adriamycin, cyclophosphamide) chemotherapy did not improve the local control further, but the patients treated with FAC had a slightly longer survival than those of a historical control group (Buzdar et al. 1981).

A randomized comparison between surgery and radiotherapy after adriamycin-vincristine chemotherapy showed no difference in overall relapse rate or survival. The locoregional relapse rate was, however, high in both groups (De Lena et al. 1981).

Thus, the results are poor after any treatment combination in this group of patients both concerning locoregional and distant control of the cancer. A small percentage of patients who present themselves with inoperable disease will, however, have a long disease-free period after local treatment only. The addition of chemotherapy has not clearly prolonged survival but may reduce the local and distant failure rates. Ongoing trials evaluate endocrine, cytotoxic, and radiotherapeutic treatment in locally advanced breast cancer. Until the results from such trials indicate otherwise, it seems reasonable to recommend a combination of both systemic treatment and a vigorous local treatment consisting of radiotherapy and surgery whenever possible, in an effort to improve at least the locoregional control of the disease (Montague and Fletcher 1983).

Preoperative radiotherapy decreases the possibility to evaluate the differentiation of tumor cells and to measure the contents of estradiol receptors in the tumor (Bressot et al. 1982), which might be of clinical importance for the stratification of patients for endocrine and other treatments. Fine needle aspirates of the tumor yield material that is suitable not only for diagnosing breast cancer (Franzén and Zajicek 1968), but which may also be used for the determination of estradiol receptors (Silfverswärd et al. 1980) and for the determination of the distribution of DNA in individual cells that may also serve as a prognostic guide (Auer et al. 1980).

Radiotherapy in Operable Breast Cancer

Numerous nonrandomized and randomized studies on the treatment results of various local treatment combinations in "early" breast cancer have been published. A thorough review of the literature up to 1975 has been given by Mansfield (1976).

Radiotherapists were among the first to use randomized trials in order to study various combinations of treatment in breast cancer. Many of the earlier studies have been rightfully criticized because of various errors of both statistical and technical nature (Fisher 1973; Fletcher 1976; Levitt and McHugh 1977; Wallgren 1977; Raventos 1977). Conclusions concerning differences as well as lack of differences have to be cautiously interpreted, but it seems to be possible to derive some facts from these studies.

Radiotherapy Replacing Surgery

Even if the radical mastectomy has remained the treatment of choice in most countries until the very last years, already in the 1920s systemic replacement of surgery by interstitial irradiation was introduced by Keynes in London (1929, 1937). A few years later, Baclesse in Paris (1959) and Mustakallio (1945) in Helsinki showed that external beam irradiation with or without surgery might give survival rates comparable to radical surgery. McWhirter in Edinburgh (1955) introduced systematic irradiation instead of a surgical dissection of the axilla.

George Keynes, a surgeon at the St. Bartholomew's Hospital in London, systematically treated patients with breast cancer using radium needles in the breast and the lymph node regions (Keynes 1929, 1937). He observed that residual tumor remained in approximately 50% of the cases who were later operated on because of a palpable tumor after irradiation. This he, probably correctly, believed to be due to the great tumor mass. He therefore suggested that the bulk of the tumor should be removed as conservatively as possible before radiation. The advantage of the conserving treatment is that the mutilation was slight compared with radical surgery. Keynes believed that the fear of mutilating surgery might partly be responsible for the fact that many women did not come for treatment soon enough.

Baclesse initiated the breast-conserving treatment at the Foundation Curie in Paris. At this institution, his works have been continued by Calle and co-workers (Calle et al. 1978), and have subsequently been introduced at several other French centers (Pierquin et al. 1975; Verhaeghe et al. 1980; Amalric et al. 1982). Mustakallio, a radiotherapist of Helsinki, started in the 1940s to employ conservative therapy when he successfully treated some patients who refused a radical operation (Mustakallio 1945, 1972). Breast-conserving treatment was later introduced on the American continent; first in Canada (Peters 1967; Clark et al. 1982; Poisson et al. 1976), but later also in the United States (e. g., Crile et al. 1980; Cope et al. 1977; Hellman et al. 1980; Bedwinek et al. 1980; Montague et al. 1979). The extent of the surgical excision as well as the doses and fields of irradiation vary from one center to the other. At least for small stage I tumors, reported survival results seem comparable to those after radical surgery. In a nonrandomized comparison of women treated with a radical mastectomy, Rissanen and Holsti (1974) found that the survival was poorer after breast-conserving treatment if the tumor was > 2 cm in diameter.

The results of randomized trials from the Guy's Hospital in London (Atkins et al. 1972; Hayward 1981) and from the National Cancer Institute of Milan (Veronesi 1981) have been reported. The Guy's Hospital trials included patients who were older than 50 years of age with T1 (up to 2 cm) or T2 (2 to 5 cm) tumors and without (N0) or with (N1) palpable axillary lymph nodes. The patients were either treated with a radical mastectomy or a wide excision of the tumor including a 3 cm margin but without an axillary dissection. The patients of both groups were treated with radiotherapy from a 300 kV x-ray unit with fields covering the axilla and the supraclavicular fossa and the dose was 25 to 27 Gy in the apex of the axilla in 12 to 18 days. After excision of the tumor, "tylectomy", the breast and the internal mammary nodes were treated to a dose of 35 to 38 Gy in three weeks using a 6 MeV linear accelerator. In addition, all patients were given a short, postoperative course of thiotepa. The results of this trial showed that there were more local and regional recurrences in the patients treated with a tylectomy plus radiation than after the radical mastectomy. Most of these recurrences occurred in the axilla of patients with N1 tumors. Thus, the low dose of irradiation used was clearly insufficient to control the disease in the axilla of these patients. The patients with N1 tumors also had more distant metastases and a poorer survival after tylectomy than after radical surgery (Atkins et al. 1972). The entry of patients with stage II disease into the trial was stopped, but a new series consisting of patients without clinically involved axillae was started using the same surgical and radiologic treatment principles as in the first series, but probably no thiotepa was given.

In the second series, there were significantly more local recurrences, distant metastases and a worse survival after tylectomy plus radiation than after radical mastectomy plus radiation (Hayward 1981). A comparison between the patients of the first and the second series who had been treated with a radical mastectomy and who clinically had no lymph node metastases revealed a lower local control rate in the second series. The main local problem was in the axilla. The cosmetic result was sometimes bad when big lumps were removed from small breasts with the wide excision. Edema was more frequent after the radical mastectomy than after the wide excision. These trials are interesting since they seem to challenge the concept that local control of the disease does not matter in breast cancer. The results of the Guy's Hospital trials do not easily fit into the generally accepted model that implies that the fate of breast cancer patients is not influenced by the radicality of the local treatment.

The results from the Milan study are easier to interpret than those from the Guy's Hospital trials. In this trial, only patients with T1 (up to 2 cm) and N0 tumors were included. The patients were treated either with a radical mastectomy or a quadrantectomy plus an axillary dissection. After quadrantectomy, the breast was irradiated with high-energy photons to a dose of 50 Gy with a "boost" of 10 Gy to the scar. The patients who were found to have lymph node involvement at surgery were similarly treated in both groups, either with radiotherapy, with adjuvant chemotherapy, or no further treatment. So far, the recurrence-free survival and the survival for all patients and for those with and without histopathologically involved lymph nodes are very similar in the two treatment groups.

A third randomized trial on mastectomy versus breast-conserving treatment including radiotherapy to the breast has been performed at the Institut Gustave Roussy at Villejuif and some preliminary results have been reported (Sarrazin et al. 1982). This study included patients with tumors not exceeding 25 mm. In case axillary node metastases were found at biopsy, a full axillary dissection was done. The breast was treated with 45 Gy in 4.5 weeks with a boost of 15 Gy to the scar. At five years, there are similar survival and recurrence-free survival rates in both groups. Approximately 5% of the patients in both groups have experienced a local recurrence.

The related trials and several nonrandomized studies show that the frequency of local recurrence depends on the size of the tumor, the extent of the surgical excision, and the dose of irradiation. In Toronto, 154 patients with breast cancer were treated by an excision only without radiation (Clark et al. 1982). At five years, 24% of these patients had relapsed in the breast, and at ten years the figure had increased to 26.5%. In patients who had been treated with radiotherapy to the breast after the excision of the tumor (generally to a dose of 40 Gy in three weeks), the relapse rate in the breast was lower, 7.6% at five and 16.3% at ten years. These groups were not equivalent since there were more patients with less advanced tumors (i. e., smaller tumors and noninvasive cancers) among those who had not received any radiotherapy. Similar results can also be derived from a smaller study from Montreal (Poisson et al. 1982).

The studies from Finland indicate that 24% of the patients with T1 tumors and 28% of those with T2 tumors had a relapse in the breast at five to ten years after the treatment. After excision of the tumor, the breast had been treated with 180 to 250 kV x-rays to an estimated dose of 25 to 35 Gy in two weeks (Rissanen and Holsti 1974), which thus seems to be too low a dose to control remaining cancer of the breast.

In an analysis of patients treated with breast-conserving techniques in several American centres, Bedwinek et al. (1980) showed that the frequency of recurrence in the breast was higher if less than an excision (i. e., incision or a needle biopsy) had been done. In these patients, increasing the dose of radiation over 50 Gy in five weeks by means of iridium implants reduced the frequency of breast recurrence to the same level as in patients who had been treated with an excision of the tumor followed by 50 Gy in five weeks to the breast.

The only reason to perform an excision of the tumor instead of a radical mastectomy is the better cosmetic result. A surgical excision alone seems to be effective to control local disease in approximately 70% to 75% of patients with "small" breast cancers according to the Canadian experience (Clark et al. 1982; Poisson et al. 1982). A limited excision of the tumor with adequate radiotherapy seems, however, to offer the best chances for a local control and a good cosmetic result in most patients with localized breast cancer (Bedwinek et al. 1980). Clearly, more studies are required to delineate the groups of patients for whom breast-conserving treatment

is suitable, both considering the tumor and patient characteristics. Several such studies are presently underway. To detect recurrence after breast-conserving treatment, serial mammograms are of value (Bloomer et al. 1976; Libshitz et al. 1977).

McWhirter introduced the treatment of breast cancer by means of a simple mastectomy supplemented by postoperative radiotherapy to the axilla in 1940 in Edinburgh because of a shortage of experienced surgeons during the war (Mansfield 1976). The simple mastectomy plus radiotherapy subsequently became one of the most common forms of treatment of operable breast cancer in the United Kingdom (Baum et al. 1972).

Several trials have been conducted aiming at a comparison between the McWhirter technique and the radical mastectomy without radiotherapy. In Copenhagen, Kaae and Johansen (1962, 1974, 1977) compared an extended radical mastectomy with a simple mastectomy plus radiotherapy in 1951 to 1957. The postoperative radiotherapy was given to the supraclavicular fossa, the axilla, and the skin flaps and the dose in the axilla was approximately 40 Gy in three weeks. Six hundred sixty-six patients were allocated to the two treatment groups by their date of birth. Some patients were found to be inoperable or were not treated according to the protocol for various other reasons leaving 425 patients for subsequent analyses. These show no differences in survival or in recurrence-free survival. The frequency of local and regional recurrence was not higher in the simple mastectomy group than in the extended radical mastectomy group (Kaae and Johansen 1974). In the group of patients who had been treated with the extended radical mastectomy without radiotherapy and who had confirmed lymph node metastases, the frequency of axillary node recurrence was as high as 13% at five years and that of supraclavicular recurrence was 15%. As an advantage of the McWhirter technique, there were fewer patients with arm edema in the simple mastectomy group than in the extended radical mastectomy group.

In the region of the southeast of Scotland around Edinburgh, a trial comparing a classical radical mastectomy with a simple mastectomy plus "radical" radiotherapy was conducted in 1964 to 1971 (Bruce 1971; Langlands et al. 1980). After the simple mastectomy, radiotherapy was given to the axilla, the supraclavicular fossa, and to the chest wall by high-voltage x-ray beams. The dose in the axilla was 42.5 Gy in ten fractions over four weeks. All patients under 60 years underwent a surgical or radiological castration as well. One thousand ninety-nine patients were randomly allocated to the two treatment groups before surgery, but 512 had to be withdrawn because the breast tumor was found to be benign. A further 89 cases were withdrawn, for example, patients refusing castration. With a follow-up time of up to 12 years, 30 patients belonging to the simple mastectomy group had experienced an axillary recurrence, 19 of whom had initially been classified as node negative. In the radical mastectomy group, seven women had an axillary recurrence, and only two of them had stage I disease at presentation. The total number of patients with locoregional recurrences was, however, not greater in the simple mastectomy group since there were fewer cases with supraclavicular recurrence after radiotherapy. The given radiotherapy was thus not as efficient as the radical mastectomy to eradicate axillary metastases. Interestingly, there was a significantly better survival in the radical mastectomy group compared with the simple mastectomy group, and this survival benefit seems to be confined to patients with stage I tumors. As in the Danish trial, a surgical dissection of the axilla gave a higher frequency of arm edema than the simple mastectomy plus radiotherapy (Bruce 1971). On the other hand, those treated with radiotherapy more often failed to abduct the arm beyond a right angle (4% vs 14%). This was thought to be due to fibrosis possibly caused by the high dose of radiation given per fraction. Apart from giving more late complications, the high frequency of axillary recurrence after radiation in this study may cast some doubt on the effectiveness of treating breast cancer with fewer high doses instead of using daily doses of about 2 Gy each.

In Manchester, patients with stage II breast cancer (T1–2, N1) were randomly allocated to a radical mastectomy or to a simple mastectomy with postoperative radiotherapy in 1970 to 1975 (Lythgoe et al. 1978). In addition to the local treatment, premenopausal and perimenopausal patients were castrated. The postoperative radiotherapy was given with two different techniques, which both gave a dose in the axilla that was probably less than 37 Gy in three weeks. There was no difference in survival or in the frequency of locoregional recurrence or distant metastases between the groups. The frequency of axillary recurrence has not been presented making it impossible at the present time to compare the efficiency of the two treatment modalities in controlling the disease in the axilla.

The NSABP (protocol No. B-04) also compared a radical mastectomy with a simple (total) mastectomy plus radiotherapy in patients without or with clinically involved axillary lymph nodes in 1971 to 1974. A third treatment arm, a simple mastectomy without radiotherapy, was included in the study of patients without clinically involved nodes (Fisher et al. 1977, 1980, 1981). The radiotherapy was to be given to a dose of 45 Gy in 25 fractions over five weeks to the internal mammary and supraclavicular regions at a depth of 3 cm. The chest wall was irradiated with tangential portals to 50 Gy. Patients with a clinically negative axilla were to be treated to that region to a dose of 50 Gy in the midaxilla. In patients with a clinically positive axilla, a boost of an additional 10 to 20 Gy should be given.

After a follow-up time of 26 to 62 months, there was no difference in recurrence-free survival or overall survival between the treatment groups. In patients with clinically negative nodes, 6 of 354 patients treated with a radical mastectomy had failed in the axilla and there was a similar frequency (5 of 282) of axillary relapses among those treated with a mastectomy with radiotherapy. During the same period of follow up, axillary tumor growth had resulted in an axillary dissection in 49 of 344 patients who had been treated with a total mastectomy without radiotherapy. When there were clinically positive nodes, axil-

lary recurrence occurred less often (3 of 227) after a radical mastectomy than in patients who had been treated with radiotherapy to the axilla (15 of 244). In clinically node-negative and node-positive patients, radiotherapy reduced the frequency of chest wall and supraclavicular recurrence.

The actual doses of radiotherapy varied in this trial. Seventeen per cent of the node negative patients and 61% of the node-positive patients were considered at an evaluation of the doses to have been given a too low dose in the axilla (Fisher et al. 1980). No correlation was found in this retrospective study between dose given and the frequency of recurrence. Mainly from statistical reasons, Potish et al. (1981) have warned against drawing the conclusion from this trial that the dose of irradiation does not matter. There are always reasons to believe that noncompliance in clinical trials do not occur at random, but from reasons that cannot be considered to be independent of the outcome (Coronary Drug Research Group 1980; Wallgren et al. 1979).

Radiotherapy in Addition to Surgery

There are several studies that have compared the result of the same surgical procedure in breast cancer with or without radiotherapy.

A simple mastectomy with or without postoperative radiotherapy was studied in patients without clinically involved nodes in the already mentioned Manchester study (Lythgoe et al. 1978) and as a part of the NSABP study (Fisher et al. 1977, 1980, 1981) as well as in a multicenter study sponsored by the Cancer Research Campaign in Britain. The latter study recruited 2243 evaluable patients in 1970 to 1975; 24% of whom had clinically involved nodes (Cancer Research Campaign 1976, 1980). The radiation techniques and the doses were allowed to vary in this study, but the aim was to irradiate the internal mammary, the supraclavicular, and the axillary regions as well as the chest wall. Also in this trial, an analysis of the given doses failed to reveal any relation between dose and freedom from locoregional recurrence (Cancer Research Campaign 1980).

All these three studies show that postoperative radiotherapy reduced the frequency of locoregional recurrence. In the NSABP study, as mentioned before, 49 of 344 patients with clinically negative nodes and who had been treated with a mastectomy alone developed histologically proved metastases in the axilla after an average of 36 months. The cumulative percentage of axillary disease at four years was approaching 20% (Fisher et al. 1977); that is, not too far from what might be the expected frequency of histologic involvement in clinically node negative patients. It should be noted that in one third of the patients who were treated with a total mastectomy, at least a partial axillary dissection may have been performed. Lymph nodes were retrieved in this proportion of cases and in 10% were more than five nodes found (Fisher et al. 1977). Unfortunately, the numbers of cases with involved lymph nodes in the different treatment groups have not been given. This information might be helpful in the evaluation of the efficacy of radiotherapy. Radiotherapy in these patients reduced the incidence of axillary recurrence to the same extent as the surgical dissection. Similarly, the Cancer Research Campaign (1976) study demonstrated that radiotherapy reduced the frequency of recurrence in the axilla, the supraclavicular region, and in the chest wall.

In the 1976 report from the Cancer Research Campaign trial, the number of patients who had confirmed axillary recurrence in the "wait and see" group was 110, whereas 19 of the patients who had been treated with radiotherapy had failed in the axilla after the same period of follow up. The reduction of axillary recurrence after radiotherapy in this population consisting mainly of patients without a clinical suspicion of nodal involvement at treatment seems to be of the same order of magnitude as in the NSABP study.

The Cancer Research Campaign study, the NSABP study, and the Manchester study do not give any indication that it should be deleterious to leave the axilla untreated until cancer growth becomes clinically obvious.

There are several studies in which all patients have been treated with a radical mastectomy or a modified radical mastectomy and in which some patients in addition have been treated with radiotherapy. From the results of the already mentioned studies, the addition of radiotherapy should be expected to decrease the frequency of recurrence in the irradiated regions. The extent of this reduction should be expected to vary according to the dose of radiotherapy, the extent of disease, and possibly with the radicality of the surgical procedure. There is one randomized study comparing the efficacy of radical and modified radical mastectomy, which did not show any difference in recurrence-free survival for stage I and II breast cancer patients (Turner et al. 1981). One study, however, indicated that more local recurrences occurred after a modified than a classical radical mastectomy in stage III patients (Baker 1981). Even after a meticulous radical mastectomy in a carefully selected series of patients, 3% of the patients without axillary lymph node metastases and 22% with nodal involvement had local-regional recurrence within ten years (Haagensen 1971).

The classical trial in which the value of the addition of radiotherapy to radical mastectomy was studied was performed in Manchester in 1949 to 1955 and comprised 1461 patients (Paterson and Russel 1959; Easson 1968). Unfortunately, this was not a strictly randomized trial, since the patients were allocated to the treatment groups according to whether their date of birth was odd or even, and the treatment option was thus known before the patient was entered into the study. It is stated that "Many post-operative cases were dealt with outside the experiment as a matter of free choice by one or other method, or in other ways as seemed indicated" (Patterson and Russel 1959). The study was divided into two subsets according to the type of radiotherapy (the "quadrate" and the "peripheral" series). Possibly as a result of the method of allocation to the treatment groups, there were more patients allocated to the "watch" group (393) than to the radiotherapy group (327, P = 0.05) in the "quad-rate" series. The number of patients with axillary node involvement was higher in the radiotherapy groups (66%) than in the watch groups (62%), although this difference was not statistically significant (P = 0.18).

The "quadrate" technique that was used during the first years of the study aimed to irradiate only the anterior chest wall and the axilla. The "peripheral" technique that was used thereafter included the supraclavicular fossa, the internal mammary nodes, and the axilla in the region of interest. The radiotherapy was given by means of 250 kV x-rays and the dose aimed at was 32 to 40 Gy in three weeks.

In the Manchester study there were fewer local-regional recurrences among the patients who were treated with radiotherapy (19% within 10 years) compared with the patients of the watch groups (32%). Of the patients of the watch groups, 37% subsequently had radiotherapy for recurrent disease. The local recurrences were controlled by treatment to such an extent when they appeared, so that at death 16% of the patients of both groups had locally growing cancer. It should be remembered that a local-regional recurrence was defined in this study as tumor regrowth in the skin flaps of the chest wall, in the supraclavicular fossa, and in the axilla, although not all of these regions were treated in every patient. Unfortunately, the distribution of recurrence in these three regions in the patients who had been treated with the two different radiation techniques has not been published. This information might be of interest in order to evaluate the efficacy of the given radiotherapy.

There was no significant difference in the frequency of distant metastases between the irradiated and the "watched" patients of the Manchester study. Since the frequency of locally growing cancer was the same irrespective of the initial treatment at death, the recommendation from this trial was that the patients could be spared an immediate postoperative radiotherapy that could as safely be given when and if a local-regional recurrence appeared.

The National Surgical Adjuvant Breast Project (NSABP) in the United States performed in 1961 to 1968 was a multicenter study that aimed to evaluate the merits of postoperative radiotherapy and perioperative chemotherapy (thiotepa) in addition to a radical mastectomy (Fisher et al. 1970). The protocol was changed during the period of investigation, eliminating the treatment arm of premenopausal women to be treated with only a radical mastectomy, since another study had indicated that the addition of thiotepa to surgery in this group might be beneficial. In order to increase the number of premenopausal controls, 142 premenopausal patients were added to the study at analysis. These had been treated either with thiotepa (87 women) or only surgically (55 women) in another clinical trial that aimed to evaluate oophorectomy in early breast cancer.

Since this was a multicenter study, the radiotherapy techniques varied, but the aim was to administer a "therapeutic dose of radiation" to the internal mammary chain, the apex of the axilla, and the supraclavicular region. The chest wall was not irradiated.

One thousand eighthundred eighty-two patients were entered into this study. Of these patients, 569 (30%) were excluded because they were considered inelegible, and 210 (11%) because data were incomplete, leaving 1103 patients or 59% for analysis. In the radiotherapy group only 470 of 915 patients or 51% were retained. Although the exclusion of patients according to some of the reasons listed in the report from this study (benign lesions, inelegible according to protocol) possibly would not bias the results, it is more difficult to accept that the exclusion of patients due to reasons related to the treatments (e. g., refused by patient, physician chose not to give adjuvant therapy, complications of surgery preventing initiation of adjuvant therapy according to protocol) would be unrelated to the fate of the patients as has been proposed (Fisher 1973). If it were possible to withdraw such a great proportion of patients from a randomized trial retrospectively and claim that this would not bias the results, then prospective, randomized studies would be unnecessary at all.

Due to the change of the protocol, it is difficult to calculate to what extent the exclusion of patients might have affected prognostic subgroups differently. However, according to the number of patients presented for the calculation of three-year survival rates, it can be seen that 36% of the radiotherapy patients had no axillary node metastases and 36% of them had more than three axillary node metastases. The corresponding figures for the combined control groups are 45% without metastases and 29% with more than three metastases. The difference in distribution is statistically significant (P = 0.05) and may be an indication that the exclusion of patients may have caused systemic errors.

In the radiotherapy group of the NSABP study, there were fewer regional recurrences than in the control groups. After a follow-up period ranging from 18 months to 5 years, there were 23 supraclavicular recurrences in 548 control patients compared with 2 of 406 irradiated women. The chest wall was the first location for recurrent disease in 28 of the radiotherapy patients (6.9%) compared with 50 of the control patients (9.1%). The reduction of recurrence in the nonirradiated chest wall may be of some importance, since it indicates that some of these recurrences really are retrograde outgrowth from foci in the lymphatics (Auchincloss 1958).

The reported results of the Manchester and the NSABP study did not show any statistically significant difference in survival between the irradiated patients and their controls, but there was a numerical survival advantage to the controls of both series, and especially in the premenopausal groups. These two studies constitute the fragile basis for the proof that Stjernswärd (1974) presented to indicate a worse survival after radiotherapy.

One German and two Scandinavian trials have also been designed to study the merits and dangers of the addition of radiotherapy to a radical or a modified radical mastectomy.

The German trial was conducted in Heidelberg in 1969 to 1972 and 142 patients were included in the study. Eighty-four of the patients received postoperative radiotherapy and 58 did not. So far, there is no difference in survival rates between the two treatment arms (Schumacher 1982).

In Oslo, two sequential trials were conducted in 1964 to 1972 including together 1088 patients (Høst and Brennhovd 1975, 1977; Høst 1981). A Halsted type of radical mastectomy was performed in all patients. By random numbers, 547 of the patients were allocated to be treated with postoperative radiotherapy as well. In 1964 through 1967, the radiotherapy was given by means of an x-ray unit with tangential fields to cover the internal mammary nodes and the chest wall and with appositional beams to cover the supraclavicular fossa and the axilla. The dose in the supraclavicular region was approximately 36 Gy (skin dose). The tangential fields were irradiated by 26 Gy each, which gave a dose of 25 to 31 Gy in the skin of the chest wall. The dose in the internal mammary nodes was probably negligable. The treatment was given in four weeks. This irradiation decreased the frequency of recurrence in the supraclavicular fossa from 6.8% in nonirradiated patients to 1.4%. In patients with lymph node involvement, the reduction of supraclavicular recurrence was 14.1% to 2.8%. Axillary recurrences were few in both treatment arms. In spite of the low dose to the chest wall, radiotherapy decreased the frequency of chest wall recurrence in patients with axillary node metastases from 15.2% to 8.2%. There were no differences in survival rates between the two treatment groups, neither for the total group nor for patients with or without axillary node metastases.

In 1968 through 1972, postoperative radiotherapy in the Oslo trial was given with a cobalt unit. The internal mammary region was treated with a direct appositional beam that also included the supraclavicular fossa and the apex of the axilla. The given dose was 57 Gy in 20 fractions over four weeks, which gives a dose of 50 Gy at a depth of 3 cm. Although the internal mammary region was treated to a very insignificant dose during the first four years of this study, the direct field gave a dose in this region that should have been sufficient to control more than 90% of microscopic disease (Fletcher and Montague 1978).

The high-voltage radiotherapy reduced the frequency of regional metastases in stage II patients from 16.3% at five years to 4.2% (P < 0.01; Høst 1981). Interestingly, the cumulative incidence of distant metastasis was lower in the group treated with radiotherapy than in the control group (Høst 1981). The survival seemed to be enhanced in patients with nodal metastases and especially when the tumor was centrally or medially located. However, the numbers of patients were small in these subgroups and the differences were not statistically significant. Still, this has been considered as a support for the hypothesis that metastases in lymph nodes might constitute a focus for further spread of cancer in some cases (Fletcher and Montague 1978). In the opinion of others, such an interpretation of data is merely a manifestation of the "classical conceptual rationalism", the representatives of which only look for corroborative evidence to support their belief (Baum 1982).

The second Scandinavian trial that aimed to study the value of radiotherapy in addition to surgery is our own, which was performed in Stockholm in 1971 to 1976. All patients of this study were operated on by a modified radical mastectomy and the surgery was performed in five surgical departments in Stockholm. The preoperative evaluation, all radiotherapy, and the follow up was done in collaboration with the surgeons in one department. This study was originally designed to study whether preoperative radiotherapy was advantageous to postoperative radiotherapy, but included also a nonirradiated control group. Patients with operable breast cancer were included in the study if the diagnosis was confirmed by a preoperative fine needle aspiration biopsy (Wallgren et al. 1978; Strender et al. 1981).

The radiotherapy was individually planned to give a dose of 45 Gy in five weeks to the internal mammary, the supraclavicular and the axillary regions, and also to the breast and postoperatively to the chest wall. Preoperatively, usually tangential ^{60}Co fields were used to irradiate the breast and the internal mammary region. Postoperatively, the chest wall and the internal mammary nodes were irradiated in most cases with a high-energy electron beam. During the first two years of the study, the aim was to irradiate both sides of the internal mammary node chains, but subsequently, only the ipsilateral chain was to be included. Due to unforeseen technical reasons, this change of policy resulted in an underdosage even in the ipsilateral internal mammary nodes in many patients who were treated during the later period and especially in those who were treated with the electron beam. The distribution of the doses were thus not equivalent in the preoperatively irradiated and in the postoperatively irradiated patients (Strender et al. 1981).

The analyses of the Stockholm trial after a follow-up time of six to ten years revealed that preoperative and postoperative radiotherapy to the same extent significantly increased the recurrence-free survival (Strender 1982). This difference in recurrence-free survival increases up to the tenth year of follow up. The reduction of recurrence is most pronounced in local-regional areas. Local-regional recurrences have been detected in 83 patients who were treated with surgery only at the first sign of a relapse. In 24 of these, distant metastases were concurrently detected. In the preoperatively irradiated patients, the corresponding figures were 25 and 12, respectively, and in postoperatively irradiated 23 and 13.

There is at the present time no significant difference in survival rates between the treatment groups. However, as in the Oslo trial, patients who had medial tumors and especially those who were treated early during the trial, when the internal mammary nodes should have been "adequately" irradiated, showed an improved survival after radiotherapy.

It is not an easy task to sum up the results of the reported trials. All trials have defects in treatment techniques, or in the randomization process and the number of patients is too low to permit conclusive analyses of subgroups of interest.

Local Disease and Radiotherapy

All reported trials seem to indicate that radiotherapy reduces the frequency of recurrence in irradiated areas. After a radical mastectomy, recurrence in the axilla seems to be a minor problem. Even low doses, as for instance the dose used in the first Oslo trial to treat the chest wall, seems to give some reduction of recurrence. It is possible that irradiation of the lymph node regions alone will also reduce the frequency of chest wall recurrence. "Adequate" doses, that is, of the magnitude of 40 to 50 Gy, are necessary to reduce significantly the frequency of recurrence from microscopic disease. Macroscopic disease, which is present in most of the cases with palpable axillary lymph nodes, is less well controlled by radiotherapy of such a dose level than by an axillary dissection. Local radiotherapy may supplement less radical surgical procedures to reduce the frequency of recurrent disease. The combination of less radical surgery and radiotherapy may give a better cosmetic and functional result than the radical mastectomy. In most cases, a local or regional recurrence is only an indication of the severity of the disease, or it may sometimes be controlled when it appears, but for the woman a local recurrence is a catastrophy that should be avoided.

Decreased Survival After Radiotherapy?

If only the trials are considered in which the randomization protocol seems to have been followed strictly and in which few patients have been excluded from analysis, there is no evidence that radiotherapy decreases survival. In the trials from Guy's Hospital and from Edinburgh a decreased survival may be explained by the poorer local control of the disease in the group treated by less radical surgery plus radiotherapy.

Are There Any Indications That Radiotherapy Improves Survival?

The overwhelming impression from all the quoted trials is that at least in the majority of patients the extent and radicality of the local treatment do not influence survival. However, there is some evidence that there is a subset of breast cancer patients where the disease remains local and regional for very prolonged periods of time and where a local undertreatment, whether by surgery or radiotherapy or both, might be deleterious to survival.

The Guy's Hospital trials (Atkins et al. 1972; Hayward 1981) showed lower survival rates in patients treated with a wide excision plus radiotherapy, which was unable to control the regional disease in a substantial proportion of the patients. These results seem to be corroborated by similar findings in the Edinburgh trial (Langlands et al. 1980). In this trial, axillary node recurrences occurred in patients considered as clinically node negative in spite of a dose of 42 Gy. In the NSABP study, a dose of 50 Gy in a similar clinical group of patients reduced the frequency of axillary recurrence to the same extent as a surgical dissection (Fisher et al. 1977). Differences in patient selection and/or in treatment techniques may explain the difference.

The second Oslo trial and our own trial from Stockholm seemed to indicate that there may exist a small subset of patients with metastases in the internal mammary nodes in whom "adequate" irradiation might influence the course of the disease (Høst and Brennhovd 1977; Strender et al. 1981).

A multicenter study on extended radical mastectomy versus a radical mastectomy showed no overall survival benefit after the superradical type of surgery (Lacour et al. 1976; Lacour et al. 1983). However, in the subgroup of patients with medially located tumors and axillary node involvement, there seemed to be a survival benefit for the patients who were treated with an internal mammary dissection (Lacour et al. 1976). In a recent update of this trial, no analysis of the survival of this subset was presented referring to the paper by Peto et al. (1977), in which a warning is given against subgroup analyses when there is no overall difference. It is certainly true that repeated subgroup analyses are likely to find some spuriously significant results. On the other hand, if the analysis of the same subgroups in several trials indicate that there are similar differences, this finding should at least be considered of significant interest. In the published studies, the statistical power, that is, the ability to find even great differences in subgroups and even more to negate these differences, is low due to the design and the small number of patients.

The Villejuif subset of patients included in this trial have been separately reported (Sarrazin 1982). This showed that patients with inner quadrant tumors and axillary node involvement had a worse survival if they were treated with a radical mastectomy only compared with if they were treated with an internal mammary dissection or with radiotherapy. In contrast to this, a separate analysis of the Milan group of patients included in this multicenter trial showed no benefit of the internal mammary dissection in any subset according to site or size of tumor, or axillary node involvement (Veronesi and Valagussa 1981).

The analysis of patients with medial tumors in the Cancer Research Campaign study (1980) also showed no difference between the two treatment arms (simple mastectomy or simple mastectomy plus radiotherapy). It thus does not support the hypothesis that radiotherapy to the internal mammary nodes would influence survival. Likewise, in the NSABP study on radical mastectomy versus simple (total) mastectomy with or without radiotherapy (protocol B-04), the patients with central or inner quadrant tumors and clinically negative nodes had the same survival if they were treated with a simple mastectomy with or without radiotherapy. When there were clinically positive nodes and the tumor was medially located, there was an almost significantly increased mortality in patients who had been treated with a mastectomy plus radiotherapy in comparison with those who were treated with a radical mastectomy. If the tumor was located in the lateral half of the breast, the survival was similar in both treatment groups. In this trial the situation is a little more complex, since in some patients radiotherapy did not eradicate metastases as well as the surgical axillary dissection.

It would be necessary to design a sufficiently large randomized study comprising patients with involved axillary nodes and medially located tumors only in order to finally reject or corroborate the hypothesis that irradiation of involved internal mammary lymph nodes might increase survival in some patients. This selection of patients is essential to avoid a dilution of the study population with cases that are less likely to have metastases in the internal mammary nodes.

Radiotherapy and Adjuvant Chemotherapy

Patients who have a fairly advanced local breast cancer have a high likelihood of local-regional recurrence and for distant metastases as well. Since postoperative radiotherapy decreases the frequency of recurrence within the irradiated areas and local and regional recurrence tend to appear before distant metastasis, radiotherapy will increase the recurrence-free survival (e. g., Strender et al. 1981; Tapley et al. 1982). Adjuvant cytostatic chemotherapy seems to be less efficient to prolong the recurrence-free interval if the tumor stage is advanced (Bonadonna and Valagussa 1983). In a retrospective comparison, Chu and Kiel (1982) found that postoperative radiotherapy was as efficient as adjuvant chemotherapy in patients with more than three axillary lymph node metastases, both in terms of recurrence-free and overall survival. In some series of patients who have been treated with adjuvant chemotherapy, this treatment seems to be less efficient in postmenopausal than in premenopausal women. This may or may not be related to difficulties for the majority of postmenopausal women to tolerate necessary doses (Bonadonna and Valagussa 1981). In our own ongoing trial, patients with axillary node metastases are treated either with radiotherapy postoperatively or with adjuvant chemotherapy of the same type as in the Milan study (Wallgren et al. 1981). There are 287 evaluable postmenopausal women in this study with a mean follow-up time of 48 months. At 48 months, 41% of the women in the chemotherapy group have experienced relapse compared with 34% in the radiotherapy group. This difference is due to the lower local control rate in the chemotherapy group. In this group, 36 patients of 147 have had a local-regional recurrence compared with only 13 of 140 women in the radiotherapy group.

The combination of postoperative radiotherapy and adjuvant chemotherapy has been attempted to increase both local and distant control of the disease. In a retrospective study, Holland et al. (1980) found that 27 patients who were treated with both radiotherapy and adjuvant chemotherapy had a worse recurrence-free survival than patients who were treated with the same type of chemotherapy alone. Using a similar chemotherapy regimen, Carey et al. (1979) found little effect of radiotherapy on the recurrence-free survival. Allen et al.

(1981), using another type of chemotherapy, believed that there might be a survival benefit for subsets of patients who were treated with both chemotherapy and radiotherapy. In a randomized trial comparing L-PAM and CMF chemotherapy, the patients were also randomized to receive radiotherapy or not (Cooper et al. 1981). The results have been reported after a short follow up. Radiotherapy in addition to L-PAM possibly increased and radiotherapy in addition to CMF possibly decreased the recurrence-free survival. After radiotherapy, the patients received less amounts of the drugs, at least during the first few courses. A longer follow up of this trial is essential to evaluate the effect of radiotherapy in addition to cytostatic chemotherapy.

There is obviously much room for improvement of the adjuvant treatment. The routine use of postoperative radiotherapy has been criticized among other things because it may not improve survival (for the majority of patients) and because local recurrences might be treated equally well when they appear. The same critique must of course be applied to adjuvant chemotherapy, not because the ideas of generalized disease may be wrong, but because the treatment that we can offer is not efficient enough and has only marginal effects on survival. The toxicity of a prolonged treatment with chemotherapy is generally much more severe than that of radiotherapy. The value of the combination of local radiotherapy with systemic treatment still has to be evaluated. There are problems of sequencing the various treatment modalities in an optimal way which have to find their solutions.

Radiotherapy in the Treatment of Recurrent and Metastatic Disease

Castration

A radiological castration is an alternative to a surgical oophorectomy. The estrogen levels decrease after a radiation-induced castration over several weeks and cannot be further reduced after a subsequent surgical oophorectomy (Diczfalusy et al. 1959). There is no indication that castration by means of either procedure is preferable in terms of responses.

Local and Regional Recurrence

Local and regional recurrence of the malignant disease is a common event even after radical surgery and correlates to the extent of the disease (Haagensen 1971). Even if the majority of these patients eventually will die from their disease, local freedom from cancer is essential in order to improve the quality of survival. Radiotherapy given in sufficiently high doses may control local disease (Chu et al. 1976). In general, though, local recurrence can be controlled in approximately only 50% of the cases (Toonkel et al. 1983), which is a lower figure than what can be controlled by prophylactic radiation. The addition of chemotherapy to an efficient local treatment (surgery and/or radiotherapy) prolonged the time to the next

historical control series, in which the patients had been only locally treated (Buzdar et al. 1979).

Distant Metastases

Although 30% to 70% of patients with distant metastases respond to various endocrine and cytotoxic manipulations, the overall survival is poor once distant metastases have appeared. The median survival after treatment with the most efficient of presently available cytostatic chemotherapy regimens is less than two years (Bonadonna and Valagussa 1983). The overall survival from the detection of metastases has probably not increased after the introduction of combination chemotherapy (Paterson et al. 1981; Powles et al. 1980). Any treatment, therefore, should be considered as palliative. Radiotherapy is an excellent tool for the palliative treatment of metastatic symptoms.

Painful bone metastases that do not respond to medical treatment can often be treated with a palliative effect using a short period of radiotherapy. A single dose of radiation of approximately 8 to 12 Gy may give as good palliation as protracted treatment. A single treatment spares the patient the trouble of getting to a hospital more than once (Delclos and Montague 1973; Penn 1976).

Choroidal metastases are not infrequent in breast cancer. They may be detected when they are small, due to the decrease in visual acuity. Such cases may be "early" metastatic cases with an expected survival sometimes of several years. Radiation therapy will improve the visual acuity in almost all cases and is, therefore, of a definite palliative value (Mewis and Young 1982).

Cerebral and meningeal metastases also have a grave prognosis. They often do not respond well to medical treatment. Radiotherapy, possibly given in combination with intrathecal methotrexate (Yap et al. 1982), may relieve the depressing symptoms.

Present Principles for Treatment of Breast Cancer in Stockholm, Sweden

The Stockholm Health Care region has a population of 1.5 million inhabitants. Every year about 900 new cases of breast cancer are detected. Active screening for breast cancer using single-view mammography is performed in one area. Abundant mammographic resources are available and the general concern about breast cancer is high. As a result, many small cancers are discovered and only 35% of the cases have axillary node involvement.

According to a regional management program for breast cancer, most of the patients are seen preoperatively by a multidisciplinary team consisting of surgeons, plastic surgeons, oncologists (radiation and medical), radiologists, and cytologists/pathologists. The diagnosis is generally obtained by fine needle aspiration biopsy cytology and a staging mammography is available.

When the tumor is small (≤ 2 cm) and the woman wants to have her breast preserved, a wide excision with at least 1 to 2 cm free margins is done, which gives a cosmetically acceptable result. An axillary level I dissection is done in these cases. Postoperative radiotherapy is given by means of tangential high-voltage beams to a dose of 50 Gy in five weeks.

The majority of patients are surgically treated by a modified radical mastectomy. When the tumor is smaller than 30 mm and there are no lymph node metastases, no further routine treatment is given. When there are lymph node metastases, or when the tumor is larger than 30 mm, postoperative radiotherapy has long been the standard treatment, since the risk for local-regional recurrence is high in these patients. The early results of adjuvant chemotherapy challenged the role of radiotherapy. A randomized trial comparing 12 monthly cycles of adjuvant chemotherapy (CMF) with postoperative radiotherapy is going on at the present time. Preliminary results from this trial indicate that adjuvant chemotherapy reduces the frequency of relapses more than radiotherapy in premenopausal patients. In postmenopausal patients, radiotherapy gives a similar recurrence-free survival as chemotherapy, but with fewer side effects. In the postmenopausal women, addition of tamoxifen for two years seems to further prolong the recurrence-free time both in patients given chemotherapy and radiotherapy (Wallgren et al. 1981).

When the breast cancer is considered inoperable because of local disease (including supraclavicular metastases), premenopausal and young postmenopausal patients are treated initially with chemotherapy (adriamycin, cyclophosphamide, fluorouracil). If the tumor becomes operable after a few courses, surgery is performed. Otherwise, radiotherapy is given with the aim of making surgery possible. Adjuvant chemotherapy is continued for at least one year. Postoperative radiotherapy is usually given when the tumor is operated on after chemotherapy. With this combined approach, we hope to be able to reduce both local and disseminated recurrences.

In elderly postmenopausal patients with advanced disease, the treatment is individualized. Determination of the receptor contents is performed by means of fine needle aspiration from the tumor. Usually, the initial treatment consists of tamoxifen sometimes combined with radiotherapy.

References

Alderman, S. J.: Combination teletherapy and iridium implantation in the treatment of locally advanced breast cancer. Cancer 38: 1936–1938, 1976

Allen, H., R. Brooks, S. E. Jones, E. Chase, R. S. Heusinkveld, G. F. Giordano, S. J. Ketchel, R. A. Jackson, S. Davis, T. E. Moon, S. E. Salmon: Adjuvant treatment for stage II (node positive) breast cancer with adriamycin-cyclophosphamide (AC) ± radiotherapy (XRT). In S. E. Salmon, S. E. Jones: Adjuvant Therapy of Cancer III. Grune & Stratton, New York 1981

Amalric, R., F. Santamaria, F. Robert, J. Seigle, C. Altschuler, J. M. Kurtz, J. M. Spitalier, H. Brandone, Y. Ayme, J. F. Pollet, R. Burmeister, R. Abed: Radiation therapy with or without primary limited surgery for operable breast cancer. A 20-year experience at the Marseilles Cancer Institute. Cancer 49: 30–34, 1982

Ansfield, F. J.: Adjuvant radiotherapy for breast cancer. J. Am. Med. Assoc. 235: 67–68, 1976

Atkins, H., J. L. Hayward, D. J. Klugman, A. B. Wayte: Treatment of early breast cancer: A report after ten years of a clinical trial. Br. Med. J. 1: 423–429, 1972

Auchincloss, H., Jr.: The nature of local recurrence following radical mastectomy. Cancer 11: 611–619, 1958

Auer, G., T. Caspersson, A. Wallgren: DNA content and survival in mammary carcinoma. Anal. Quant. Cytol. 2: 161–165, 1980

Baclesse, F.: Roentgen therapy alone in cancer of the breast. Acta Un. Int. Cancer 15: 1023–1026, 1959

Baker, D., D. Elkon, M.-L. Lim, W. Constable, H. Wanebo: Does local x-irradiation of a tumor increase the incidence of metastases? Cancer 48: 2394–2398, 1981

Baker, R. R.: A comparison of modified radical mastectomy to radical mastectomy in the treatment of operable breast cancer. In E. F. Lewison, A. C. W. Montague: Diagnosis and Treatment of Breast Cancer. International Clinical Forum. Williams & Wilkins, Baltimore 1981

Baral, E., H. Blomgren, K. Ideström, A. Wallgren, S. Ogenstad, B. Petrini, C. Silfverswärd, J. Wasserman: Prognostic relevance of radiation induced immune suppression in breast carcinoma. Acta Radiol. Oncol. 18: 313–320, 1979

Baral, E., L. E. Larsson, B. Mattsson: Breast cancer following irradiation of the breast. Cancer 40: 2905–2910, 1977

Barker, J. L., E. D. Montague, L. J. Peters: Clinical experience with irradiation of inflammatory carcinoma of the breast with and without elective chemotherapy. Cancer 45: 625–629, 1980

Baum, M.: Scientific empiricism and clinical medicine. In M. Baum, R. Kay, H. Scheurlen: Clinical Trials in Early Breast Cancer. 2nd Heidelberg symposium. Heidelberg, December 14–17, 1981. Birkhäuser Verlag, Basel 1982

Baum, M., M. H. Edwards, C. J. Margarey: Organization of clinical trial on national scale: Management of early cancer of the breast. Br. Med. J. 4: 476–479, 1972

Bedwinek, J. M., C. A. Perez, S. Kramer, L. Brady, R. Goodman, G. Grundy: Irradiation as the primary management of Stage I and II adenocarcinoma of the breast. Analysis of the RTOG breast registry. Cancer Clin. Trials 3: 11–18, 1980

Bedwinek, J. M., G. A. Ratkin, G. W. Philpott, M. Wallack, C. A. Perez: Concurrent chemotherapy and radiotherapy for nonmetastatic Stage IV breast cancer. A pilot study by the Southeastern Cancer Study Group. Am. J. Clin. Oncol. (CCT) 6: 159–165, 1983

Blomgren, H., E. Baral, C. Jarstrand, B. Petrini, L.-E. Strender, A. Wallgren, J. Wasserman: Effect of external radiation therapy on the peripheral lymphocyte population. In J. B. Dubois etc: Immunopharmacologic Effects of Radiation Therapy. Raven Press, New York 1981

Bloomer, W. D., A. L. Berenberg, B. N. Weissman: Mammography of the definitely irradiated breast. Am. J. Radiol. 118: 425–428, 1976

Boice, J. D. Jr., R. R. Monson: Breast cancer in women after repeated fluoroscopic examinations of the chest. J. Natl. Cancer Inst. 59: 823–832, 1977

Bonadonna, G., A. Rossi, G. Tancini, P. Valagussa: Adjuvant chemotherapy in breast cancer (Letter to the editor). Lancet 1: 1157, 1983

Bonadonna, G., P. Valagussa: Dose-response effect of adjuvant chemotherapy in breast cancer. N. Engl. J. Med. 304: 10–15, 1981

Bonadonna, G., P. Valagussa: Chemotherapy of breast cancer: Current views and results. Int. J. Radiat. Oncol. Biol. Phys. 9: 279–297, 1983

Bressot, N., F. Veith, J. Saussol, H. Pujol, M. Lavie, M. Granier, J. Gary-Bobo, H. Rochefort: Presurgical radiotherapy decreases the concentrations of estrogen and progesterone receptors in human breast cancer: A 200-patient study. Breast Cancer Res. Treat. 2: 117–183, 1982

Bruce, J.: Operable cancer of the breast. A controlled clinical trial. Cancer 28: 1443–1452, 1971

Buzdar, A. U., G. R. Blumenschein, T. L. Smith, C. K. Tashima, G. N. Hortobagyi, H. Y. Yap, J. U. Gutterman, E. M. Hersh, E. A. Gehan: Adjuvant chemoimmunotherapy following regional therapy for isolated recurrences of breast cancer (Stage IV NED). J. Surg. Oncol. 12: 27–40, 1979

Buzdar, A. U., E. D. Montague, J. L. Barker, G. N. Hortobagyi, G. R. Blumenschein: Management of inflammatory carcinoma of the breast with combined modality approach – An update. Cancer 47: 2537–2542, 1981

Calle, R., G. H. Fletcher, B. Pierquin: Les bases de la radiotherapie curative des epitheliomas mammaires. J. Radiol. Electrol. 54: 929–938, 1973

Calle, R., J. P. Pilleron, P. Schlienger, J. R. Vilcoq: Conservative management of operable breast cancer. Ten years experience at the Foundation Curie. Cancer 42: 2045–2053, 1978

Cancer Research Campaign: Management of early cancer of the breast. Report on an international multicentric trial supported by the Cancer Research Campaign. Br. Med. J. 1: 1035–1038, 1976

Cancer Research Campaign: Cancer Research Campaign (King's/Cambridge) trial for early breast cancer. A detailed update at the tenth year. Lancet 2: 55–60, 1980

Carey, R. W., D. Sohier, S. Kaufman, S. A. Weitzman, R. M. Kelley, R. A. Lew, E. Halpern: 5-drug adjuvant chemotherapy for breast cancer. Cancer 44: 35–41, 1979

Chu, A. M., K. Kiel: Comparison of adjuvant postoperative radiotherapy and multiple-drug chemotherapy (CMF-VP) in operable breast cancer patients with more than four positive axillary lymph nodes. Cancer 50: 212–218, 1982

Chu, F. C. H., F.-J. Lin, J. H. Kim, S. H. Huh, C. J. Garmatis: Locally recurrent carcinoma of the breast. Results of radiation therapy. Cancer 37: 2677–2681, 1976

Clark, R. M., R. H. Wilkinson, L. J. Mahoney, J. G. Reid, W. D. MacDonald: Breast cancer: A 21 year experience with conservative surgery and radiation. Int. J. Radiat. Oncol. Biol. Phys. 8: 967–975, 1982

Cohen, L., M. Creditor: Iso-effect tables for tolerance of irradiated normal human tissues. Int. J. Radiat. Oncol. Biol. Phys. 9: 233–241, 1983

Cohen, L., H. Svensson: Cell population kinetics and dose-time relationship for post-irradiation injury of the brachial plexus in man. Acta Radiol. Oncol. 17: 161–166, 1978

Cooper, M. R., A. L. Rhyne, H. B. Muss, C. Ferree, F. Richards, II, D. R. White, J. J. Stuart, D. V. Jackson, V. Howard, A. Shore, C. L. Spurr: A randomized comparative trial of chemotherapy and irradiation therapy for stage II breast cancer. Cancer 47: 2833–2839, 1981

Cope, O., C. A. Wang, A. Chu, C. C. Wang, M. Schultz, B. Castleman, J. Long, W. D. Sohier: Limited surgical excision as the basis of a comprehensive therapy for cancer of the breast. Am. J. Surg. 131: 400–407, 1976

Coronary Drug Project Research Group: Influence of adherence to treatment and response of cholesterol on mortality in the Coronary Durg Project. N. Engl. J. Med. 303: 1038–1041, 1980

Crile, G. Jr., A. Cooperman, C. B. Esselstyn, R. E. Hermann: Results of partial mastectomy in 173 patients followed for from five to ten years. Surg. Gynecol. Obstet. 150: 563–566, 1980

Dao, T. L., J. Kovaric: Incidence of pulmonary and skin metastases in women with breast cancer who received postoperative radiation. Surgery 52: 203–212, 1962

Delclos, L., E. D. Montague: Metastasis for breast cancer. In: G. H. Fletcher: Textbook of Radiotherapy. 2nd edition. Lea & Febiger, Philadelphia 1973

Diczfalusy, E., G. Notter, F. Edsmyr, A. Westman: Estrogen excretion in breast cancer patients before and after ovarian irradiation and oophorectomy. J. Clin. Endocrinol. Metab. 19: 1230–1244, 1959

Easson, E. C.: Post-operative radiotherapy in breast cancer. In A. P. M. Forrest, P. B. Kunkler: Prognostic Factors in Breast Cancer. Livingstone, Edinburgh 1968

Ege, G. N.: Internal mammary lymphoscintigraphy. Radiology 118: 101–107, 1976

Ellis, F.: Dose, time and fractionation: A clinical hypothesis. Clin. Radiol. 20: 1–7, 1969

Fisher, B.: Cooperative clinical trials in primary breast cancer: A critical appraisal. Cancer 31: 1271–1286, 1973

Fisher, B., E. Montague, C. Redmond, B. Barton, D. Borland, E. R. Fisher, M. Deutsch, G. Schwartz, R. Margolese, W. Donegan, H. Volk, C. Konvolinka, B. Gardener, I. Cohn, G. Lesnik, A. B. Cruz, W. Lawrence, T. Nealon, H. Butcher, R. Lawton: Comparison of radical mastectomy with alternative treatments for primary breast cancer. A first report of results from a prospective randomized clinical trial. Cancer 39: 2827–2839, 1977

Fisher, B., E. Montague, C. Redmond, M. Deutsch, G. R. Brown, A. Zauber, W. F. Hanson, A. Wang: Findings from NSABP protocol No. B-04 – Comparison of radical mastectomy with alternative treatments for primary breast cancer. I. Radiation compliance and its relation to treatment outcome. Cancer 46: 1–13, 1980

Fisher, B., N. H. Slack, P. J. Cavanaugh, B. Gardner, R. G. Ravdin: Postoperative radiotherapy in the treatment of breast cancer. Results of the NSABP clinical trial. Ann. Surg. 172: 711–732, 1970

Fisher, B., N. Wolmark, C. Redmond, M. Deutsch, E. R. Fisher: Findings from NSABP protocol No B-04: Comparison of radical mastectomy with alternative treatments. II. The clinical and biologic significance of medial-central breast cancers. Cancer 48: 1863–1872, 1981

Fletcher, G. H.: Clinical dose-response curves of human malignant epithelial tumors. Br. J. Radiol. 46: 1–12, 1973

Fletcher, G. H.: Reflections on breast cancer. Int. J. Radiat. Oncol. Biol. Phys. 1: 769–779, 1976

Fletcher, G. H., E. D. Montague: Does adequate irradiation of the internal mammary chain and supraclavicular nodes improve survival rates? Int. J. Radiat. Oncol. Biol. Phys. 4: 481–492, 1978

Fletcher, G. H., N. du V. Tapley, E. D. Montague, G. R. Brown: Management of localiszed breast cancer. In G. H. Fletcher. Textbook of Radiotherapy. 2nd edition. Lea & Febiger, Philadelphia 1973

Franzén, S., J. Zajicek: Aspiration biopsy in diagnosis of palpable lesions of the breast. Acta Radiol. 7: 241–262, 1968

Haagensen, C. D.: Diseases of the Breast. 2nd ed. WB Saunders Company, Philadelphia 1971

Harris, J. R., M. B. Levene, G. Svensson, S. Hellman: Analysis of cosmetic results following primary radiation therapy for stage I and II carcinoma of the breast. Int. J. Radiat. Oncol. Biol. Phys. 5: 257–261, 1979

Harris, J. R., J. Sawicka, R. Gelman, S. Hellman: Management of locally advanced carcinoma of the breast by primary radiation therapy. Int. J. Radiat. Oncol. Biol. Phys. 9: 145–149, 1983

Hayward, J.: The surgeon's role in primary breast cancer. Breast Cancer Res. Treat. 1: 27–32, 1981

Hellman, S., J. R. Harris, M. B. Levene: Radiation therapy of early carcinoma of the breast without mastectomy. Cancer 46: 988–994, 1980

Holland, J., O. Glidewell, R. G. Cooper: Adverse effect of radiotherapy on adjuvant chemotherapy for carcinoma of the breast. Surg. Gynecol. Obstet. 150: 817–821, 1980

Høst, H.: Adjuvant radiation therapy. In E. F. Lewison, A. C. W. Montague: Diagnosis and Treatment of Breast Cancer. International clinical forum. Williams & Wilkins, Baltimore 1981

Høst, H., I. O. Brennhovd: Combined surgery and radiation therapy versus surgery alone in primary mammary carcinoma. I. The effect of orthovoltage radiation. Acta Radiol. (Ther.) 14: 25–32, 1975

Høst, H., I. O. Brennhovd: The effect of post-operative radiotherapy in breast cancer. Int. J. Radiat. Oncol. Biol. 2: 1061–1067, 1977

Kaae, S., H. Johansen: Breast cancer: Five year results: Two random series of simple mastectomy with postoperative irradiation versus extended radical mastectomy. Am. J. Roentgenol. 87: 82–88, 1962

Kaae, S., H. Johansen: Ablatio mammae und postoperative Strahlentherapie des Mammakarzinoms. Strahlentherapie 147: 375–380, 1974

Kaae, S., H. Johansen: Does simple mastectomy followed by irradiation offer survival comparable to radical procedures? Int. J. Radiat. Oncol. Biol. Phys. 2: 1163–1166, 1977

Keynes, G.: The treatment of primary carcinoma of the breast with radium. Acta Radiol. 10: 393–401, 1929

Keynes, G.: Conservative treatment of cancer of the breast. Br. J. Radiol 2: 643–647, 1937

Kim, J. H., F. C. H., Chu, B. Hilaris: The influence of dose fractionation on acute and late reactions in patients with postoperative radiotherapy for carcinoma of the breast. Cancer 35: 1583–1586, 1975

Kolar, J.: Hypoplasia of the growing breast after contact x-ray therapy for cutaneous angiomas. Arch. Dermatol. 96: 427–430, 1967

Lacour, J., P. Bucalossi, E. Caceres, G. Jacobelli, T. Koszarowski, M. Le, C. Rumeau-Rouquette, U. Veronesi: Radical mastectomy versus radical mastectomy plus internal mammary dissection. Cancer 37: 206–214, 1975

Lacour, J., M. Le, E. Caceres, T. Koszarowski, U. Veronesi, C. Hill: Radical mastectomy versus radical mastectomy plus internal mammary dissection. Ten year results of an international cooperative trial in breast cancer. Cancer 51: 1941–1943, 1983

Langlands, A. O., W. A. Souter, E. Samuel: Radiation osteitis following irradiation for breast cancer. Clin. Radiol. 28: 93–96, 1977

Langlands, A. O., R. J. Prescott, T. Hamilton: A clinical trial in the management of operable cancer of the breast. Br. J. Surg. 67: 170–174, 1980

Larsson, L. E., J. Lindahl, B. Unsgaard: Fall in blood pressure during radiation therapy. Acta Radiol. Ther. Phys. Biol. 15: 241–251, 1976

De Lena, M., M. Varini, R. Zucali, D. Rovini, G. Viganotti, P. Valagussa, U. Veronesi, G. Bonadonna: Multimodal treatment for locally advanced breast cancer. Results of chemotherapy–Radiotherapy versus chemotherapy–surgery. Cancer Clin. Trials 4: 229–236, 1981

Levene, M. B.: Interstitial therapy of breast cancer. Int. J. Radiat. Oncol. Biol. Phys. 2: 1157–1161, 1977

Levitt, S. H., J. Mandel: Breast irradiation and future risk of carcinogenesis. Front. Radiat. Ther. Oncol. 17: 131–142, 1983

Levitt, S. H., R. B. McHugh: Radiotherapy in the postoperative treatment of operable cancer of the breast. Part I. Critique of the clinical and biometric aspects of the trials. Cancer 39: 924–932, 1977

Levitt, S. H., R. B. McHugh, C. W. Song: Radiotherapy in the postoperative treatment of operable cancer of the breast. Part II. A re-examination of Stjernswärd's application of the Mantel-Haenzel statistical method. Evaluation of the effect of the radiation on immune response and suggestions for postoperative radiotherapy. Cancer 39: 933–940, 1977

Levitt, S. H., R. A. Potish: The case for adjuvant CMF chemotherapy in breast cancer. Has it been made? Cancer Clin. Trials 4: 363–369, 1981

Lewison, E. F.: Changing concepts in breast cancer. Cancer 46: 859–864, 1980

Libshitz, H. I., E. D. Montague, D. D. Paulus: Calcifications and the therapeutically irradiated breast. Am. J. Roentgenol. 128: 1021–1025, 1977

Lichter, A. S., A. F. Benedick, J. van de Geijn, T. N. Padikal: A technique for field matching in primary breast irradiation. Int. J. Radiat. Oncol. Biol. Phys. 9: 263–270, 1983

Lipsett, M. B.: Postoperative radiation for women with cancer of the breast and positive axillary lymph nodes: Should it continue? N. Engl. J. Med. 304: 112–114, 1981

Lythgoe, J. P., I. Leck, R. Swindell: Manchester regional breast study. Preliminary results. Lancet 1: 744–747, 1978

Mansfield, C. M.: Early breast cancer. Its history and results of treatment. In A. Wolsky: Experimental Biology and Medicine. Monographs on Interdisciplinary Topics. Vol. 5. Karger, Basel 1976

Mansfield, C. M., K. Ayyangar, N. Sunthralingam: Comparison of various radiation techniques in treatment of the breast and chest wall. Acta Radiol. Oncol. 18: 17–24, 1978

McGregor, D. H., C. E. Land, K. Choi, S. Tokuoka, P. I. Liu, T. Wakabayashi, G. W. Beebe: Breast cancer incidence among atomic bomb survivors, Hiroshima and Nagasaki, 1950–1969. J. Natl. Cancer Inst. 59: 799–811, 1977

McWhirter, R.: Simple mastectomy and radiotherapy in the treatment of breast cancer. Br. J. Radiol. 28: 128–139, 1955

Mewis, L., S. E. Young: Breast carcinoma metastatic to the choroid. Ophthalmology 89: 147–151, 1983

Montague, E. D., G. H. Fletcher: The need for every modality treatment to prevent catastrophic local and regional failures in advanced breast cancer. Int. J. Radiat. Oncol. Biol. Phys. 9: 419–420, 1983

Montague, E. D., A. E. Gutierrez, J. L. Barker, N. du V. Tapley, G. H. Fletcher: Conservative surgery and irradiation for the treatment of favorable breast cancer. Cancer 43: 1058–1061, 1979

Morris, T.: Psychological adjustment to mastectomy. Cancer Treat. Rev. 6: 41–61, 1979

Moss, W. T., W. N. Brand: Therapeutic radiology. Rationale, technique, results. 3rd edition. C. V. Mosby, S. Louis 1969

Munzenrider, J. E., I. Tchakarova, M. Castro, B. Carter: Computerized body tomography in breast cancer. I. Internal mammary nodes and radiation treatment planning. Cancer 43: 137–150, 1979

Mustakallio, S.: Über die Möglichkeiten der Röntgentherapie bei der Behandlung des Brustkrebses. Acta Radiol. 26: 503–511, 1945

Mustakallio, S.: Conservative treatment of breast carcinoma. Review of 25 years of follow-up. Clin. Radiol. 23: 110–116, 1972

Nevin, J. E., J. T. Baggerly, T. K. Laird: Radiotherapy as an adjuvant in the treatment of carcinoma of the breast. Cancer 49: 1194–1200, 1982

Notter, G., D. Lindell, K. J. Wikterlöf: Strahlenreaktion in Lungen und Pleura bei Mammakarzinompatienten. Fortschr. Geb. Röntgenstr. Nuklearmed. 112: 571–584, 1979

Nyström, G.: Kräftsjukdomarne i Sverige. Statistiska undersökningar utförda på uppdrag av Svenska Cancerföreningen. Svenska Tryckeribolaget, Stockholm 1922

Paterson, A. H. G., O. Szafran, F. Cornish, A. W. Lees, J. Hanson: Effect of chemotherapy on survival in metastatic breast cancer. Breast Cancer Res. Treat. 1: 357–363, 1981

Paterson, R., M. H. Russel: Clinical trials in malignant disease. Part III Breast cancer: Evaluation of postoperative radiotherapy. J. Fac. Radiol. 10: 175–180, 1959

Penn, C. R. H.: Single dose and fractionated palliative irradiation for osseous metastases. Clin. Radiol. 27: 405–408, 1976

Persson, J.-E., K. J. Wikterlöf: Physical aspects on dose planning in treatment of mammary carcinoma. Acta Radiol. (suppl) 313: 122–126, 1972

Peters, M. V.: Wedge resection and irradiation. An effective treatment in early breast cancer. J. Am. Med. Assoc. 200: 144–145, 1967

Peto, R., M. C. Pike, P. Armitage, N. E. Breslow, D. R. Cox, S. V. Howard, N. Mantel, K. McPherson, J. Peto, P. G. Smith: Design and analysis of randomised clinical trials requiring prolonged observation of each patient. II. Analysis and examples. Br. J. Cancer 35: 1–39, 1977

Petrini, B., J. Wasserman, E. Baral, H. Blomgren, A. Wallgren: Radiotherapy, immunoreactivity and recurrence of breast cancer. Lancet 1: 606–607, 1980

Pierquin, B., F. Baillet, J. F. Wilson: Radiation therapy in the management of primary breast cancer. Am. J. Roentgenol. 127: 645–648, 1976

Poisson, R., C. Larose, S. Charlebois, A. Pagacz, J. P. Mercier, R. N. Lawson: Preliminary report on the individualized non-mutilating treatment of operable breast cancer. Clin. Oncol. 2: 55–71, 1976

Poisson, R., S. Legault, J. Mercier: Pilot study on the individualized non-mutilating treatment of breast cancer. Symposium on Fundamental problems in breast cancer. Jasper, Alberta, Canada 1982

Potish, R. A., J. Boen, S. H. Levitt: Statistical interference in the analysis of radiation compliance and its relation to treatment outcome. Cancer Clin. Trials 4: 475–481, 1981

Powles, T. J., R. C. Coombes, I. E. Smith, J. M. Jones, H. T. Ford, J.-C. Gazet: Failure of chemotherapy to prolong survival in a group of patients with metastatic breast cancer. Lancet 1: 580–582, 1980

Racovec, P., S. Plesnicar, A. Janezic: Veränderung der Lungenfunktion nach Strahlentherapie des Brustkrebses. Strahlentherapie 148: 339–346, 1974

Raventos, A.: Clinical trials of adjuvant radiation therapy for breast cancer. Cancer 39: 941–944, 1977

Rissanen, P. M.: A comparison of conservative and radical surgery combined with radiotherapy in the treatment of stage I carcinoma of the breast. Br. J. Radiol. 42: 423–426, 1968

Rissanen, P. M., P. Holsti: Vergleich zwischen konservativer und radikaler Chirurgie, kombiniert mit Strahlentherapie bei der Behandlung des Brustkrebses im Stadium I. Eine Untersuchung an 866 Patienten im Zeitraum von 10 Jahren. Strahlentherapie 147: 370–374, 1975

Rose, C. M., W. D. Kaplan, A. Marck, W. D. Bloomer, S. Hellman: Parasternal lymphoscintigraphy: Implications for the treatment planning of internal mammary nodes in breast cancer. Int. J. Radiat. Oncol. Biol. Phys. 5: 1849–1853, 1979

Rubens, R. D., S. Sexton, D. Tong, P. J. Winter, R. K. Knight, J. L. Hayward: Combined chemotherapy and radiotherapy for locally advanced breast cancer. Eur. J. Cancer 16: 351–356, 1980

de Ruiter, J., S. J. Cramer, P. Lelieveld, L. M. van Putten: Comparison of metastatic disease after local tumor treatment with radiotherapy or surgery in various tumor models. Eur. J. Cancer Clin. Oncol. 18: 281–289, 1982

Rutqvist, L.-E., A. Wallgren: Long term survival of 458 young breast cancer patients. Cancer (in press) 1985

Rutqvist, L.-E., A. Wallgren, N. Nilsson: Is breast cancer a curable disease? A study of 14 731 women with breast cancer from the Cancer Registry of Norway. Cancer 53: 1793–1800, 1984

Sarrazin, D., M. Le, H. Mouriesse, G. Contesso, F. Fontaine, R. Arriagada, M. Tubiana: Radiotherapeutic studies on breast cancer at Villejuif. Cancer Bull. 34: 242–249, 1982

Schumacher, M.: Assessing treatment effects over time. In M. Baum, R. Kay, H. Scheurlen: Clinical Trials in Early Breast Cancer. 2nd Heidelberg symposium. Heidelberg December 14–17, 1981. Birkhäuser Verlag, Basel 1982

Shore, R. E., L. H. Hempelmann, E. Kowaluk, P. S. Mansur, B. S. Pasternack, R. E. Albert, G. E. Haughie: Breast neoplasms in women treated with x-rays for acute postpartum mastitis. J. Natl. Cancer Inst. 59: 813–822, 1977

Silfverswärd, C., J. Å Gustafsson, S. A. Gustafsson, B. Nordenskjöld, A. Wallgren, Ö. Wrange: Estrogen receptor analysis on fine needle aspirates and on histologic biopsies from human breast cancer. Eur. J. Cancer 16: 1351–1357, 1980

Spanos, W. J., Jr., E. D. Montague, G. H. Fletcher: Late complications of radiation only for advanced breast cancer. Int. J. Radiat. Oncol. Biol. Phys. 6: 1473–1476, 1980

Stjernswärd, J.: Decreased survival related to irradiation postoperatively in early operable breast cancer. Lancet 2: 1285–1286, 1974

Stjernswärd, J., M. Jondal, F. Vanky, H. Wigzell, R. Sealy: Lymphopenia and change in distribution of human B and T lymphocytes in peripheral blood induced by irradiation for mammary carcinoma. Lancet 1: 1352–1356, 1972

Strender, L. E.: Clinical and immunological aspects on adjuvant therapy in primary breast cancer. Thesis. Stockholm 1982

Strender, L. E., A. Wallgren, J. Arndt, O. Arner, J. Bergström, B. Blomstedt, P. O. Granberg, B. Nilsson, L. Räf, C. Silfverswärd: Adjuvant radiotherapy in operable breast cancer. Correlation between dose in internal mammary nodes and prognosis. Int. J. Radiat. Oncol. Biol. Phys. 7: 1319–1325, 1981

Svensson, G. K., B. E. Bjärngard, R. D. Larsen, M. B. Levene: A modified three-field technique for breast treatment. Int. J. Radiat. Oncol. Biol. Phys. 6: 689–694, 1980

Swedborg, I., A. Wallgren: The effect of pre- and postmastectomy radiotherapy on the degree of edema, shoulder joint mobility, and gripping force. Cancer 47: 877–881, 1981

Tapley, N. duV., W. J. Spanos, Jr., G. H. Fletcher, E. D. Montague, S. Schell, M. J. Oswald: Results in patients with breast cancer treated by radical mastectomy and postoperative irradiation with no adjuvant chemotherapy. Cancer 49: 1316–1319, 1982

Timothy, A. R., J. Overgaard, M. Overgaard, C. C. Wang: Treatment of early carcinoma of the breast. Lancet 2: 25–26, 1979

Toonkel, L. M., I. Fix, L. H. Jacobson, C. B. Wallach: The significance of local recurrence of carcinoma of the breast. Int. J. Radiat. Oncol. Biol. Phys. 9: 33–39, 1983

Turner, L., R. Swindell, W. G. T. Bell, R. C. Hartley, J. H. Tasker, W. W. Wilson, M. R. Alderson, I. M. Leck: Radical versus modified radical mastectomy for breast cancer. Ann. R. Coll. Surg. 63: 239–243, 1981

Verhageghe, M., J. C. Laurent, G. Depadt, A. Delabelle, M. Madelain: Justification de l'association systematique de mastectomie partielle avec curage axillaire suivie d'irradiation pour le traitement des petits cancers du sein. Chirurgie 106: 118–126, 1980

Veronesi, U., R. Saccozzi, M. Del Vecchio, A. Banfi, C. Clemente, M. De Lena, G. Gallus, M. Greco, A. Luini, E. Marubini, G. Muscalino, F. Rilke, B. Salvadori, A. Zecchini, R. Zucali: Comparing radical mastectomy with quadrantectomy, axillary dissection and radiotherapy in patients with small cancers of the breast. N. Engl. J. Med. 305: 6–11, 1981

Veronesi, U., P. Valagussa: Inneficacy of internal mammary nodes dissection in breast cancer surgery. Cancer 47: 170–175, 1981

Wallgren, A.: Breast cancer. Int. J. Rad. Oncol. Biol. Phys. 2: 385–387, 1977

Wallgren, A., O. Arner, J. Bergström, B. Blomstedt, P.-O. Granberg, L. Karnström, L. Räf, C. Silfverswärd: Preoperative radiotherapy in operable breast cancer. Cancer 42: 82–87, 1978

Wallgren, A., B. Baral, U. Glas, M. Kaigas, L. Karnström, B. Nordenskjöld, N.-O. Theve, N. Wilking, C. Silfverswärd: Adjuvant breast cancer treatment with tamoxifen and combination chemotherapy in postmenopausal women. In S. E. Salmon, S. E. Jones: Adjuvant Therapy of Cancer III. Grune & Stratton, New York 1981

Wallgren, A., B. Mattsson, L. Karnström: Treatment departure and survival analysis in a randomized trial on the value of pre- and postoperative radiotherapy. In H. R. Scheurlen, G. Weckesser, I. Arnbruster: Clinical Trials in "Early" Breast Cancer. Springer Verlag, Berlin 1977

Weber, E., S. Hellman: Radiation as primary treatment for local control of breast carcinoma. J. Am. Med. Assoc. 234: 608–611, 1975

Withers, H. R., H. D. Thames, B. L. Flow, K. A. Mason, D. H. Hussey: The relationship of acute to late skin injury in 2 and 5 fraction/week gamma-ray therapy. Int. J. Radiat. Oncol. Biol. Phys. 4: 595–601, 1978

Zucali, R., C. Uslenghi, R. Kenda, G. Bonadonna: Natural history and survival of inoperable breast cancer treated with radiotherapy and radiotherapy followed by radical mastectomy. Cancer 37: 1422–1431, 1976

Chapter 21

Hormonal Treatment of Breast Cancer

N. O. Theve, K. Carlström, H. Sköldefors and N. Wilking

Introduction

Hormonal therapy of breast cancer has been used for many decades. By changing the hormonal milieu of the tumor, some breast cancer patients may achieve beneficial therapeutic effects. However, in spite of extensive research, the underlying mechanism of action of hormonal therapy is poorly understood. Hormonal manipulation has generally been the first line treatment in disseminated breast cancer, often with high remission rates of long duration. The side effects of hormone therapy are less prominent compared with chemotherapy.

The hormonal environment can be changed by ablation of endocrine glands or by addition of certain exogenous hormones or hormonally active drugs.

In recent years, new drugs have been introduced that interfere with the production and mode of action of steroids. The antiestrogens are compounds that compete with estradiol in the tumor cell, thereby blocking the action of estradiol. Another agent, aminoglutethimide, inhibits the synthesis of all adrenal steroids. This agent has been used as a replacement for surgical adrenalectomy.

Guidelines for selecting patients who are likely to respond to hormonal therapy have become more reliable with the discovery of estrogen and progesterone receptor proteins in the tumor tissue

Historical Background

More than 100 years ago it was observed that mammary carcinoma in some cases was hormone dependent. Sir Astley Cooper in 1829 recorded a woman with advanced breast cancer who had a slight regress of the tumor at the beginning of each menstrual period (Cooper 1835). Schinzinger in 1889 suggested that oophorectomy could improve the prognosis in premenopausal women since the outcome of breast cancer was better in postmenopausal women compared to premenopausal patients.

The first report on the practical use of this hypothesis was published in 1896 by Beatson, who the year before had performed castration in two young women with advanced disease. In both cases excellent regression was observed. This report started the era of ablative hormonal treatment in breast cancer.

In 1905 Lett published nearly 100 cases of inoperable breast cancer treated by oophorectomy. The overall rate of improvement was 36.4%. However, women over 50 years of age rarely responded. The mortality rate was high, a little over 6%.

A way to avoid this high operative mortality was to perform castration by irradiation, and this technique became the method of choice until the 1940s (Ahlbom 1930).

The next step in ablative surgery, adrenalectomy, was based on two observations. First, Schimkin and Wyman (1945) reported that adrenalectomy could decrease the incidence of mammary tumors in experimental animals. At the same time, Huggins and Scott (1945) performed bilateral total adrenalectomy in men with prostatic carcinoma. However, since hormonal maintenance therapy was not available at this time, the postoperative mortality rate was high. In 1951 when cortisone was available for replacement therapy, Huggins and Bergenstal reported the beneficial effect of bilateral adrenalectomy in women with advanced breast cancer. Two out of six patients with disseminated disease responded to this treatment. This report was followed by similar publications demonstrating the beneficial effect of adrenalectomy in advanced disease.

An alternative to castration and adrenalectomy was hypophysectomy which was first performed by Luft and Olivecrona (1953). They reported regression in one of nine patients treated in this way. The benefits of hypophysectomy were confirmed in subsequent reports (Luft and Olivecrona 1958; Pearson and Ray 1959; Hamberger et al. 1961).

Additive hormonal treatment of advanced breast cancer was introduced in 1939 by Loeser, who reported a favorable effect of androgen treatment in 1944. Haddow and co-workers demonstrated similar effects in patients treated with estrogens. Progesterone was introduced by Taylor and Morris in 1951. Corticoids as single therapy or in combination with ablative surgery were introduced during the same decade.

A major problem with hormonal therapy has been to predict which patient will benefit from the treatment. To some degree it has been possible to select patients by clinical criteria, such as "disease-free" interval, age, site of metastases, and response to previous hormonal therapy.

In 1961, Folca in England reported that breast cancer tumors that accumulated estrogens were more likely to respond to endocrine manipulation.

In 1966, Jensen et al. demonstrated the existence of an estrogen binding protein, the estrogen receptor, in breast cancer tissue. A few years later the same group was able to show that there was a correlation between the presence of this protein in the tumor and the response to endocrine manipulation.

A new class of compounds, the antiestrogens, was introduced during the 1960s. Today, tamoxifen is the antiestrogenic drug of choice in clinical use owing to its efficacy and lack of side effects. Another new drug undergoing clinical trials is aminoglutethimide used as "medical adrenalectomy."

Endocrine Control of the Breast

The hormonal control of normal and neoplastic breast tissue depends primarily on steroid hormones, notably estrogens, and a protein hormone, prolactin. The *steroid hormones* are structurally related to cholesterol from which they are formed by stepwise oxidative degradation. Cholesterol with its 27 carbon atoms is thus transformed into 21-carbon steroids including *gestagens* and *corticosteroids*, into 19-carbon steroids, *androgens* and, finally, into 18-carbon steroids, the *estrogens*.

The transformation in the different steroidogenic organs are stimulated by the appropriate pituitary hormone; by luteinizing hormone (LH) (interstitial cell-stimulating hormone, ICSH) in the gonads and by adrenocorticotropic hormone (ACTH) and probably also other pituitary factors in the adrenal cortex. The regulation of the fetoplacental steroidogenesis is still rather obscure.

One fraction of the biologically active steroids in the circulation is strongly bound to specific steroid-binding globulins originating from the liver. *Sex hormone-binding globulin (SHBG)* binds testosterone, other 17β-hydroxy androgens and estradiol-17β; *corticosteroid binding globulin (CBG, transcortin)* binds corticosteroids and progesterone. Another fraction is loosely bound to albumin. Only a minor fraction (1% to 3%) is free in the circulation and only this fraction is considered biologically active. Altering the steroid-binding globulin capacity by, for example, liver affection, will change the free steroid levels and hence also the biological activity (Dunn et al. 1981; Laurell and Rannevik 1979; Moll et al. 1981).

The steroids undergo metabolic transformation in the target organs as well as peripherally, notably in the liver, kidney, intestines, and skin. Metabolic transformations preceding excretion involve various reductions and conjugations mainly with glucuronic and sulfuric acids. Most of these transformations take place in the liver. Although the glucuronic acid conjugates are considered merely as excretory products, the steroid sulfates are also important intermediates in steroid biosynthesis. They are not only formed by peripheral metabolism, but are also directly secreted from the adrenal cortex and to a certain degree also from the gonads. Urinary excretion of steroid conjugates is the main excretory pathway in the human, and the fecal route is of minor importance in normal conditions (Adlercreutz and Martin 1980; Baulieu et al.

1965; Diczfalusy and Levitz 1970; Givens 1978; Roberts and Lieberman 1970; Roy 1970; Taylor 1971; Vihko and Roukonen 1975).

The levels of a biologically active steroid are thus affected by several factors: the hypothalamic-pituitary function including trophic hormones; the steroidogenic tissue and its interaction with pituitary hormone stimulation; steroid-binding globulin activity; peripheral metabolism; enterohepatic circulation; and renal function. It should be pointed out that in half of these points (steroid-binding globulin activity, peripheral metabolism, and enterohepatic circulation), one single organ, namely the liver, is of vital importance.

Steroid Hormones in Healthy Individuals

The endocrine situation is different in fertile, nonpregnant women, pregnant women, postmenopausal women, and men. Since breast cancer is most frequent among perimenopausal and postmenopausal women, their endocrinology will be discussed more in detail with special reference to the adrenocortical sex hormone biosynthesis. The other categories will be dealt with more briefly.

Fertile Nonpregnant Women

The ovary and the adrenal cortex are the main sources of steroid hormones in normally menstruating women. Direct ovarian secretion is responsible for the main part of estrogens and progesterone in the circulation, and peripheral estrogen formation is of limited importance. Many good reviews have been written on the menstrual cycle (e. g., Naftolin and Tolis 1978; Erickson 1978).

Estradiol-17β is considered as the terminal biologically active estrogen having the strongest affinity to the estrogen receptors. The two other "classical" estrogens, estrone and estriol, also bind to the estrogen receptors, but with a weaker affinity (Lippman et al. 1977). The biologic potency of estrone is approximately 0.10 and of estriol 0.01 of that of estradiol-17β (Emmens 1969). Although estradiol-17β is of 100% ovarian origin in young women, the corresponding figure for estrone is 60%, the remaining part being formed by peripheral aromatization of androgens. Estriol is not secreted by the ovary, but is a secondary metabolite formed from the other estrogens in the liver (Chang and Judd 1981; Crilly et al. 1981). Levels of estrogens and progesterone during the menstrual cycle are given in Table 21.**1**. The direct ovarian secretion of estradiol-17β is obviously sufficient to maintain necessary estrogenic effects in women of fertile age.

The androgens in the fertile woman originate from the ovaries and the adrenal cortex, the latter being the main source. Direct ovarian secretion is responsible for 20% of the peripheral testosterone, the remaining part being formed by peripheral conversion of 4-androstene-3, 17-dione and dehydroepiandrosterone. 4-Androstene-3, 17-dione has a mixed ovarian and adrenal origin (about 30%

Table 21.**1**   Serum levels of estrogens, progesterone and androgens in menstruating and postemenopausal woman. Values from the reviewers' laboratory

	Menstruating women			Postemopausal women
	Follicular	Midcycle	Luteal	
Estradiol-17β (pmol/L)	90–480	500–1300	380–800	20–100
Estrone, unconjugated (pmol/L)	90–300	400–1000	300–600	80–300
Estrone, total (mainly estrone sulfate) (nmol/L)	1–6	9–20	5–10	0.5–3
Progesterone (nmol/L)	0.3–8.2	0.3–8.2	15–120	0.3–4.5
Testosterone (nmol/L)	0.4–2.8	0.4–2.8	0.4–2.8	0.3–2.6
4-androstene-3,17-dione (nmol/L)	3–11	3–11	3–11	1–6
Dehydroepiandrosterone (nmol/L)	10–40	10–40	10–40	< 60 years: 7–26 > 60 years: 5–16
Dehydroepiandrosterone sulfate (nmol/L)	1900–8000	1900–8000	1900–8000	< 60 years: 600–5500 > 60 years: 250–3500

and 70%, respectively), whereas dehydroepiandrosterone and its sulfate are of entirely adrenal origin. The ovarian androgen synthesis is not as dependent on gonadotrophins as is the formation of estrogens and progesterone. The regulation of the adrenal androgen biosynthesis will be dealt with below (Chang and Judd 1981; Crilly et al. 1981; Givens 1978).

In most target tissues, testosterone exerts its strong androgenic potency via its reduced derivative, 5α-dihydrotestosterone. 4-Androstene-3, 17-dione and dehydroepiandrosterone and its sulfate are weak androgens, but may be of importance as testosterone precursors due to their high peripheral levels (Table 21.**1**) (Crilly et al. 1981; Dorfman 1969; Givens 1978).

Pregnant Women

The endocrine situation in the pregnant woman is characterized by the enormously increased levels of estrogens and progesterone, synthesized in the fetoplacental unit. At midgestation and in late pregnancy, progesterone is synthesized in the placenta and estrogens are formed in the placenta from fetal and maternal precursors. Several good reviews have been written on this subject to which the reader is referred for further information (e. g., Diczfalusy 1975).

Perimenopausal and Postmenopausal Women

The perimenopause comprises the period in a woman's life in which her cyclic ovarian activity gradually ceases, leading into the menopause. This unstable endocrine situation is further complicated in most cases by the concomitant decline in the adrenocortical androgen synthesis, sometimes called the "adrenopause" (Crilly et al. 1981). The perimenopause is characterized by shortened cycle length, shortened length of the luteal phase, and marked menstrual irregularity. The levels of ovarian steroids and gonadotrophins are highly variable, sometimes even from one day to another (Chang and Judd 1981; Korenman et al. 1978).

The transition of the perimenopausal stage into the menopause means the definite cessation of cyclic ovarian activity and cyclic ovarian-hypothalamic-pituitary interaction. The postmenopausal ovary no longer secretes significant amounts of estrogens and progesterone, and due to this, follicle-stimulating hormone (FSH) and LH levels are elevated. The ovarian stroma is, however, still active and is responsible for a considerable amount (40%; 20% by direct secretion) of the peripheral testosterone. The ovarian production of other androgens is rather limited in the menopause, and thus the role of the adrenal cortex as the main androgen source is further increased. The adrenal contribution to the peripheral 4-androstene-3, 17-dione is increased to 80% in the postmenopausal woman, whereas dehydroepiandrosterone and its sulfate are of 100% adrenal origin (Chang and Judd 1981; Crilly et al. 1981; Korenman et al. 1978). Furthermore, the estrogens in the postmenopausal woman arise almost entirely by peripheral conversion of adrenal androgens (Siiteri and Seron-Ferré 1978; Vermeulen 1976). *The activity of the adrenal cortex is therefore responsible for almost all of the sex steroids in the postmenopausal woman,* except for a certain part of the testosterone. This strongly motivates a more detailed discussion on adrenal androgen biosynthesis.

Although the regulation of adrenal glucocorticoid synthesis is reasonably well understood, the regulation of adrenal androgens is an enigma. Adrenocorticotropic hormone raises adrenal androgen and glucocorticoid levels, and intact ACTH secretion is a prerequisite for adrenal androgen secretion. However, there are important differences in the regulation of adrenal androgens and glucocorticoids. First, they are produced in two different zones in the adrenal cortex: androgens in the *zona reticularis* and glucocorticoids in the *zona fasciculata.* Second, adrenal androgen levels, in contrast to glucocorticoids, are strongly age dependent, being low in childhood, increasing to maximal levels at 25 to 35 years, and decreasing dramatically to low levels at 50 to 60 years. Third, administration of certain drugs selectively increases adrenal androgen levels without any concomitant increase in glucocorticoids (Carlström and Fredricsson 1980). There is further evidence for the existence of a specific, hitherto unidentified, adrenal androgen stimulating hormone (AASH), and the subject has been extensively reviewed by Grumbach et al. (1978) and by Parker and Odell (1981).

Some workers have suggested the age-related specific decrease in adrenal androgens to be secondary to the fall in estrogens due to the menopause (Abraham and Maroulis 1975; Korenman et al. 1978). However, oophorectomy has no effect on dehydroepiandrosterone and its sulfate, and no differences in these steroids are found between postmenopausal and age-matched menstruating women (Crilly et al. 1981). Finally, an identical fall in adrenal androgens also takes place in males, a fact that has been frequently overlooked. Thus, a hypothesis indicating a direct association between ovarian estrogen and adrenal androgen production is not valid.

The decline in adrenal androgens seems to be an entirely age-related phenomenon, involving usually only the adrenal cortex and perhaps also the pituitary. It has been discussed whether this "adrenopause" is a result of an isolated decline in adrenal androgen synthesis or the result of declining ACTH levels that are still able to maintain normal cortisol values due to the age-related decrease in metabolic clearance rate (Crilly et al. 1981; West et al. 1961). An age-related decrease in the *zona reticularis* (Parker and Odell 1978) as well as the above-mentioned differencies in regulation of adrenal androgens and glucocorticoids may indicate the former as the most likely explanation.

The estrogen levels in postmenopausal women depend on two main factors: The supply of substrate, that is, adrenal androgens, and the rate of conversion, that is, peripheral aromatization. It is now well established that high estrogen levels in postmenopausal women are associated with high levels of androgens (Botella-Lluisa et al. 1979; Calanog et al. 1977; Carlström et al. 1979; Vermeulen and Verdonck 1979). The exact regulation of the peripheral aromatization is unknown; it is independent of any known hypothalamic or pituitary factor. Increased peripheral estrogen synthesis has been associated with obesity, hepatic disease, hyperthyroidism, and aging (Siiteri and Seron-Ferré 1978). Fat tissue has been considered as the main site of peripheral estrogen synthesis, but recent findings suggest that the liver may play a major role. The increased peripheral estrogen synthesis observed in obese women would thus reflect change in liver function caused by the obesity rather than increased amounts of fat tissue. The subject has been excellently reviewed by Siiteri and Seron-Ferré (1978).

Aromatization of 4-androstene-3, 17-dione to estrone is the main pathway for postmenopausal estrogen biosynthesis. Estradiol-17β is formed almost entirely by reduction of estrone (Chang and Judd 1981), and its serum levels are lower than those of estrone in postmenopausal women (see Table 21.1). Estrone sulfate is by far the most abundant estrogen in the circulation (Crilly et al. 1981; Sköldefors et al. 1978). Estrogen target tissues, including breast carcinomas, easily transform estrone sulfate into estradiol-17β (Vignon et al. 1980; Wilking et al. 1980; and references cited therein). Estrone sulfate may therefore play an important role as a prehormone for the terminal biologically active estrogen, at least in postmenopausal women and other subjects with low peripheral estradiol-17β levels.

Males

The testis is the main androgen source in the male. Peripheral testosterone levels show a certain age-dependent decline that is in no way as dramatic as the menopause drop ef estrogens (Crilly et al. 1981; Sköldefors et al. 1978). There are no important differences in the adrenocortical steroids in males and females. The estrogens in the male arise in part from direct testicular secretion of estradiol-17β by the Sertoli cells and from peripheral conversion of testicular and adrenal 4-androstene-3, 17-dione. The peripheral estrogen levels are higher in older males than in postmenopausal women due to the gonadal contribution in the male. The estrogen levels decrease somewhat between 50 to 60 years, probably due to the concomitant decrease in adrenal androgens (Sköldefors et al. 1976, 1978).

Steroid Hormones in Breast Cancer Patients

Although extensive work has been devoted to this subject for many years, no valid evidence has emerged for an association between certain hormonal changes and breast cancer, with one single exception. Conflicting results are rather common and many of the studies have included poor age matching, sampling for too short a time after surgery when stress effects still persist, and unspecific analytic methods. The latter is the case in the studies that have resulted in the so-called "estriol hypothesis" on a "protective" effect of estriol. The subject has recently been reviewed by Nisker and Siiteri (1981).

Recently Siiteri and co-workers (Nisker and Siiteri 1981) described lower sex hormone-binding globulin (SHBG) activity and a larger fraction of free, non-protein-bound estradiol-17β in breast cancer patients compared with strictly matched controls. Breast cancer may thus be associated with higher levels of the biologically active estradiol-17β fraction, despite there being no difference in total unconjugated estradiol. This very interesting observation draws further attention to the role of the liver in the etiology of breast cancer, since SHBG is synthesized in the liver and its level can be affected by sex hormones and obesity (Nisker and Siiteri 1981). Changes in SHBG capacity may perhaps be one of the links between nutritional status and breast cancer.

How to Select Patients for Hormonal Therapy

The overall response to hormonal manipulation in advanced breast cancer seldom exceeds 30% even with the most efficient therapeutic modalities. There has been a constant search for factors and tests to find those patients who are likely to respond to hormonal treatment. Presently one of the best ways of predicting response to hormonal therapy is by observing the course of the disease. Factors such as age and menopausal status play an important role. Premenopausal women under 35 years of age are less likely to benefit from hormonal manipulations than women between 35 years of age and the menopause. The perimenopausal group of patients is also known to have a lower response rate than patients more than five years after the menopause.

Another important factor is the disease-free interval. Patients with a short or nonexistent disease-free interval seldom respond to hormonal manipulations.

Site of metastases is another important factor. Soft tissue metastases are known to have a better response than osseous metastases. Visceral metastases are least likely to respond.

If the patient has had a prior response to hormonal therapy, the likelihood for a new response is much better than if the patient has failed on prior hormonal therapy.

Beside these clinical observations, a great deal of work has been dedicated to a search for biochemical or morphologic indicators of hormonal dependency. The discovery of the estrogen receptor, a protein that binds estradiol-17β and thereby induces the hormone-dependent events in the cell, has been of a major importance. This scientific breakthrough started with the observation by Folca (1961) that tumors accumulating synthetic estrogens also responded to adrenalectomy. This observation together with the work of Jensen et al. (1962, 1966) and Toft and Gorski (1966) initiated intensive investigation in the field of response prediction. Within a few years it was possible to correlate the presence of estrogen receptor and the response to hormonal ablation (Jensen et al. 1971). The presence of estrogen receptor has not only been correlated to better response, but also to better prognosis, at least concerning disease-free survival (McGuire 1978). If the tumor is estrogen-receptor rich, the likelihood of response is around 50% to 60%. If the tumor is estrogen-receptor poor, the response, however, is around 5% to 10%. The analysis of another steroid receptor in the cell cytoplasm, the progesterone receptor, has added more information. If both estrogen and progesterone receptors are present in sufficient amounts in the cell cytoplasm, the prediction of response is around 80%. In Fig. 21.**1,** a model for the receptor mechanism is given.

In conclusion, the discovery of the estrogen and progesterone receptors has added more information to the basic understanding of steroid hormone action within the cell. It has also provided valuable information about prognosis and prediction of response. The steroid receptor analysis in combination with the earlier mentioned clinical criteria gives us a fair chance to select patients for hormonal therapy.

Hormone Therapy

Ablative Treatment

Hormonal ablative therapy has been used for many decades in advanced breast cancer. It involves the ablation of the ovaries, adrenals, or pituitary. The purpose is to deprive the patient of hormones that might promote the growth of the cancer cells. Both surgical and radiation castration are known to reduce the serum levels of estrogens, especially in premenopausal women. Adrenalectomy in the same way reduces the source of steroid hormones, especially in postmenopausal women. Pituitary ablation reduces both the levels of steroid releasing hormones and prolactin, the latter being a controversial hormone in the pathogenesis of breast cancer.

Different Ablative Procedures

Castration

This, the oldest method of endocrine treatment, is an effective method of palliation in advanced disease in premenopausal women. Since Beatson's (1896) pioneer work, a great number of investigations have been reported. Both therapeutic and prophylactic castration have been used.

Castration can be accomplished either by surgery or by radiation. Both procedures are comparable concerning the clinical response and the reduction in steroid levels (Diczfalusy 1959; Stein 1969; Lee 1971). Initially there

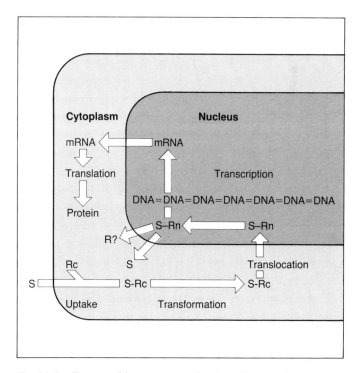

Fig. 21.**1**   The steroid receptor mechanism. The steroid (S) binds to the steroid cytoplasmatic receptor (Rc), thus forming a steroid-receptor complex (S-Rc). This receptor complex is transformed and translocated into the nucleus (S-Rn). The receptor complex is then bound to the genome. This induces transcriptive processes in the nucleus. The mRNA is then translated in the protein synthesis process.

was a high mortality risk with surgical castration in patients with advanced breast cancer. In 1905, Lett reported nearly 100 cases of oophorectomy with an operative mortality of 6%, and Lee and Hory reported in 1971 a mortality rate of 4%. The same figure has been reported by Taylor (1962) and Fracchia et al. (1969). The high operative mortality increased the interest in castration by irradiation. In 1922, de Courmelle introduced this procedure. This method became the procedure of choice until the mid 1940s, when safer surgical and anesthetic techniques were introduced. The effect of surgery is immediate, and reduction of the estrogen production is considerably faster than with irradiation. Surgical castration also allows exploration of the abdomen for metastases. The ovaries contain metastatic cancer in up to 25% of the cases (Fracchia et al. 1969; Lee and Hory 1971). Castration by irradiation is an effective alternative when time is not critical or when the surgical procedure is dangerous for the patient. After castration in premenopausal women symptoms of menopause occur. Hot flashes, weight gain, and mental disturbance are as common after castration as after the natural menopause. These symptoms should not be reduced by replacement therapy with hormones. Instead, tranquilizers or clonidine may be used and they may give some relief.

Therapeutic Castration

Oophorectomy has generally been the initial procedure in the palliation of advanced disease in premenopausal women. In postmenopausal patients, beneficial effects are rarely seen (Lett 1905; Taylor 1962; Fracchia 1969). In Taylor's series from 1962, only one postmenopausal woman responded.

Barlow et al. (1969) could find in a review of the literature only 16 postmenopausal women who had responded to castration. Today it is generally accepted that postmenopausal women are not candidates for this procedure. In several large series, objective tumor regression has been reported in about 30% of the cases. In a series of 481 patients from the Memorial Hospital, 34.5% of premeno-

pausal women had objective regression. In the one-year postmenopausal group, there were no responders (Fracchia 1969). In 1975, Veronesi reported an overall response rate of 29.5% after oophorectomy in 639 patients with advanced breast cancer. The average remission time was 16 months. Nineteen percent of the responders lived five years or more. The remission time can sometimes be very long, in some cases up to 25 years. Age is also of importance. Thirty-three percent of premenopausal women above 35 years of age responded, but only 17.9% of women under 35 years of age showed any response (Veronesi 1975). However, other reports have failed to confirm these observations (Mosley 1974; Puga 1976). The highest remission rates, about 40%, are found in cases with soft tissue and bone metastases (Taylor 1962; Veronesi et al. 1975). In patients with lung and visceral metastases, the response rate is lower, 26% and 9% (Taylor 1962; Fracchia 1969; Veronesi 1975). Some of the major studies are summarized in Table 21.**2**.

Prophylactic Castration

This procedure was suggested by Taylor in 1935. The poor results of mastectomy in young women with breast cancer and the benefits of oophorectomy in some premenopausal women with advanced disease was the rational background to this procedure. In 1939, Taylor presented a study where he compared mastectomy alone and mastectomy in combination with prophylactic castration. Castration was performed by irradiation. He concluded that "Artificial menopause cannot be demonstrated as an advantage when employed as prophylactic procedure in patients, who are submitted to radical operation." Since then, several prospective clinical trials have been carried out to test the value of prophylactic castration.

In England, the Manchester trial was reported by Cole in 1964. Patients with breast cancer who were premenopausal, at the menopause, or within two years of their last menstrual period, were included. The patients were allocated in two groups and one group was castrated by ovarian irradiation. The other group served as a control group. Ovarian irradiation did not significantly increase the ten-year survival, even if there was a trend in favor of the irradiated group.

In the Oslo trial (Nissen-Meyer 1964), there was only a small difference between the group receiving ovarian irradiation plus small doses of corticosteroids and the noncastrated group. In postmenopausal patients, the effect of ovarian irradiation was surprising. After four years, there was a statistical difference between the irradiated and non irradiated groups concerning both survival and recurrence rate. Nissen-Meyer recommended prophylactic ovarian radiation for patients up to the age of 70.

In 1969, Fracchia et al. presented another study in which 201 patients were analyzed with 100 patients in the prophylactic castration group and 101 in the therapeutic castration group. All the patients had stage I or II carcinoma at the time of radical operation. There was no statistical difference in length of survival between the two groups. Prophylactic castration resulted in a slightly

Table 21.**2** Objective remission after surgical oophorectomy in 6 reported studies

Author	No. of cases	No. of remission	% remission
Pearson et al. (1955)	75 pre-menopausal	33	44
	21 post-menopausal	2	10
Taylor (1962)	381	113	30
Hall (1963)	282	69	24.5
Fracchia (1969)	442 pre-menopausal	140	32
	85 post-menopausal	3	3.5
Veronesi (1975)	550	162	29.5
Puga (1967)	381	113	30

longer recurrence-free interval. He concluded that patients who might be cured by radical mastectomy could be spared an unnecessary procedure.

The National Surgical Adjuvant Breast Project reported in 1970 a prospective study of prophylactic castration (Ravdin et al. 1970). Premenopausal patients with operable breast cancer were treated by radical mastectomy and about 50% underwent oophorectomy. Three hundred fifty-seven patients entered the trial. There were 154 patients in the oophorectomy group and 203 in the control group (some of the latter received chemotherapy). After three years, there was no significant difference either in survival or recurrence rate between the two groups.

In 1979, Meakin and co-workers presented a trial in which following mastectomy, patients with operable breast cancer underwent postoperative irradiation of the chest wall and axillary region. They were then randomized to castration by irradiation or castration by irradiation and prednisone. Seven hundred five patients were included and were followed up to ten years. Only in premenopausal women 45 years or older did castration by irradiation and prednisone significantly delay the recurrence and improve the survival. No benefit was observed in postmenopausal women.

Because of this conflicting and meager evidence, prophylactic castration cannot be recommended today. In premenopausal women, it seems wise to delay this procedure until the time of recurrence. Perhaps further studies may change the concepts about prophylactic castration if the patients are selected according to the content of steroid receptors in the tumor.

Adjuvant Therapy to Castrated Patients

As a supplementary therapy to castration, Beatson (1896) prescribed thyroid substance for his patients. Loeser (1954) did not find any support for this treatment. In another study under the aegis of the Cooperative Breast Cancer Group, 218 premenopausal women with metastatic carcinoma were studied. The effect of surgical castration was not enhanced by the addition of thyroid substance (O'Bryan et al. 1974).

Additional androgen or corticosteroid therapy starting immediately after castration have also been used (see Additive Hormonal Treatment).

Oophorectomy has also been combined with chemotherapy. In 1977, Ahmann et al. reported a randomized study in 75 patients who received either early chemotherapy following oophorectomy or delayed chemotherapy after the appearance of metastatic disease after oophorectomy. Those treated with early chemotherapy had a better response rate, both in terms of survival and disease-free interval.

In a similar study with 42 premenopausal women with advanced breast cancer, Brunner (1977) showed that chemotherapy plus oophorectomy gave a response rate of 75%, whereas chemotherapy alone gave a response rate of 43%. The difference, however, was not statistically significant.

In another study from South Africa, Falkson et al. (1979) found that in a group of premenopausal women, the response rate for patients treated by oophorectomy and chemotherapy as a first treatment following the appearance of metastases was significantly higher and longer than the response rate achieved by oophorectomy alone.

Adrenalectomy

There is no evidence that the adrenal cortex secretes estrogen, but it is well established that androstenedione is secreted by the cortex and converted to estrogens in peripheral tissue. In the postmenopausal woman, this pathway is responsible for almost 100% of the circulating estrogens; therefore castration has very little – if any – influence on the estrogen levels in postmenopausal women. However, adrenalectomy will strongly reduce the estrogen levels.

Adrenalectomy was first tried by Atkins as early as 1948 in six patients with advanced breast cancer. Cortisone was not available at that time and total adrenalectomy would have been followed by the death of the patient in addisonian crisis. Therefore, he performed subtotal adrenalectomy by removing one adrenal completely and three fourths of the other. Two patients showed some improvement, but the margin of safety of the adrenal function was too narrow and the benefits in terms of regression were too small, and he abandoned the operation. In 1952, a year later, cortisone had become available for clinical use, and Huggins and Bergenstal reported the results of total adrenalectomy in patients with advanced disease. In six cases with advanced breast cancer, two patients improved, one patient had moderate benefit, and in three cases there was no demonstrable evidence of regression. Since then several clinical series have been reported (Huggins and Dao 1954; Fracchia et al. 1959; Hellström and Frankson 1958; Dao and Nemoto 1965; Moore et al. 1974; DeWitt et al. 1979; Moseley et al. 1980). Both premenopausal and postmenopausal women have responded to this treatment. The largest series has been reported from the Memorial Hospital in New York by Fracchia et al. (1967). In 500 cases, 40% had subjective benefit and 41% had objective reduction of the tumor for six months or more. In Table 21.**3**, some larger reported studies are summarized.

Surgical Procedure

Both the transabdominal and posterior route have been used. Nash and Robbins (1973) compared the two routes and found very little difference in mortality. The posterior approach seems to give a higher blood loss and a higher rate of pulmonary complications. The abdominal approach permits exploration of the abdomen, and also oophorectomy can be performed through the same incision (Barlow and Meggitt 1968).

Initially, the postoperative mortality was high, between 9% and 29% (Taylor 1962; Fracchia 1967; Dao 1978). With improved surgical and anesthetic technique, the surgical mortality has declined. Presently, the operative

Hormonal Treatment of Breast Cancer

Table 21.**3** Objective remission after surgical adrenalectomy in 8 reported studies

Author	No. of cases	No. of remission	% remission
Dao and Higgins (1955)	100	39	39
Hellström and Frankson (1959)	233	100	42
MacDonald (1962)	690	196	28.4
Fracchia (1967)	500	178	36
Dao et al. (1967)	207	83	40
Barlow and Meggitt (1968)	280	112	40
Brown et al. (1975)	95	44	46
de Witt and Hardwick (1979)	100	65	65

mortality is around 5% (Fracchia 1967; Galbut et al. 1976).

Castration is indicated in premenopausal women and can be performed simultaneously with the adrenalectomy. In postmenopausal women, there is no indication for oophorectomy.

Substitution therapy with cortisone or one of its analogues is absolutely necessary and should start on the day of operation. The maintenance dose corresponds to 25 mg cortisone acetate or equivalent twice a day. Mineral corticoids are rarely necessary unless the patient develops postural hypotension. The best indication that the patient is adequately substituted is her sense of well-being. If the patient develops anorexia, nausea, or loss of energy, these are signs of adrenal insufficiency. This can be corrected by a small increase in the dosage. Severe stress, as in intercurrent cholecystitis or appendicitis, may cause adrenal crisis that has to be treated vigorously. Patients who are to undergo major surgical operations must be prepared as if they were to have an adrenalectomy. Even for minor surgical operations, the cortisone dosage should be increased prior to the operation. A patient in adrenal crisis should be treated with cortisone acetate or cortisol and some vasopressor agent. In addition to this, the shock should be controlled with intravenous colloid solutions.

Selection of Patients

Selection of patients for adrenalectomy has been based on clinical criteria, such as disease-free period, age, extent of metastases, and response to previous hormonal therapy. Most of these criteria are unreliable (Dao 1978). One criterion that can be of some use for predicting subsequent response to adrenalectomy seems to be prior response to surgical castration. About 40% of those patients who responded to castration responded to subsequent adrenalectomy (MacDonald 1962; Fracchia 1969). This has not been confirmed in other reports (Brown 1975; DeWitt 1979). Also, age has been said to influence response rate; patients under 45 years of age have a lower

response to adrenalectomy (Brown 1975; Moseley et al. 1980). Today, the determination of estrogen receptor (ER) protein is the most effective predictor for response. About 50% to 60% of the ER-positive tumor patients have a probability of response. After the introduction of estrogen receptor assays, most adrenalectomies are performed in patients with ER-positive tumors (see How to Select Patients for Hormonal Therapy). Adrenalectomy has also been used as adjuvant therapy to mastectomy (Dao 1975), but this procedure has not been generally accepted.

Adrenalectomy has been combined with chemotherapy. In 1971, Wilson et al. showed that adrenalectomy combined with systemic fluorouracil markedly improved the response rate in women with a short, free interval and with visceral metastases. A similar study was presented by Moore et al. in 1974 showing that the objective response rate for adrenalectomy without chemotherapy was 40% and with chemotherapy 58%. In 1979, Oberfield et al. reported a study in 31 patients with advanced disease. These patients were treated by adrenalectomy-oophorectomy and randomized either for combined therapy or no chemotherapy. He did not find any significant difference in response or survival.

Hypophysectomy

An alternative to castration and adrenalectomy for advanced breast cancer is hypophysectomy. The aim of this procedure is to influence the growth of the tumor cells by changing the hormonal environment. In 1953, Luft and Olivecrona reported the first results of hypophysectomy in nine patients with advanced breast cancer. In one case there was a marked regression. Subsequent reports confirmed the palliative effect of hypophysectomy in disseminated breast cancer (Pearson and Ray 1959; Luft and Olivecrona 1958). Removal of the pituitary gland causes a suppression of the ovaries, thyroid, and adrenals. Within four to six weeks after hypophysectomy, there are clinical manifestations of hypothyroidism (Lee et al. 1965). Menstruation ceases and clinical manifestations of menopause ensue in premenopausal women. The ovaries become greatly reduced in size.

It is still an open question whether the response to hypophysectomy is always associated with a decrease in steroid hormones or releasing hormones. Bates et al. (1976) were unable to correlate the clinical response to the postoperative hormone levels.

Prolactin has been discussed as a growth-promoting hormone in breast cancer. One of the aims with hypophysectomy has been to reduce this hormone. However, McMillin et al. (1977) did not find any correlation between prolactin levels and tumor response. On the contrary, clinical remission may be seen after pituitary stalk sections, an operative maneuver that increases the prolactin level (Newsome et al. 1977).

Surgical Procedure

Different methods have been developed.

Transfrontal Hypophysectomy

This was originally used. By open craniotomy and retraction of the cortex, the pituitary was exposed. The hypophyseal stalk was divided and the pituitary removed by suction or curettage. Mortality rate varies between 1.2% to 17% (Dunbar 1967; Edelstyn et al. 1968; Newsome et al. 1971).

Transsphenoidal Hypophysectomy

This has a lower mortality rate and is less disturbing for the patient. The procedure dates from the beginning of the century, but it was not accepted until reported by Hamberger et al. (1961) and Riskaer et al. (1961). The mortality rate varies from 1% to 7% (Hamberger 1961; Escher 1967; Richards 1974) and the procedure is equally effective as by the transfrontal approach (Collins 1974; Bates 1976).

Implantation of Radioactive Isotopes

This technique for hypophyseal destruction is an alternative method. Both ^{198}Au and ^{90}Y have been used. The procedure is simple and well tolerated. Mortality rate is low (Collins 1974; Piotrowski 1979).

Other methods for hypophysectomy have been described, such as cryohypophysectomy, pituitary stalk section, and ultrasonic heat destruction. The different types of hypophysectomy have been described by Robin and Dalton (1977).

The complications associated with hypophysectomy include cerebral spinal fluid fistula, meningitis, visual loss, and insomnia. One of the most disturbing complications is the development of *diabetes insipidus*. About 10% of the patients need permanent use of pitressin.

After hypophysectomy, the patient requires substitution with cortisone and thyroid hormones and sometimes antidiuretic hormones. Disturbances in carbohydrate metabolism have been minimal after hypophysectomy. If the cortisone maintenance dose is adequate, the glucose

Table 21.**4** Objective remission after hypophysectomy in nine reported studies

Author	No.	Response rate %	Surgical procedure
Luft et al. (1958)	54	50	Transfrontal
McDonald (1962)	340	33	Transfrontal
Pearson and Ray (1960)	333	43	Transfrontal
Bateman (1962)	35	33	Transsphenoidal
Fracchia (1971)	100	323	Transsphenoidal
Robin (1975)	108	24	Transsphenoidal
Notter (1959)	48	33	^{90}Y implantation
Scheer (1967)	467	19	^{90}Y implantation
Henningsen and Piotrowski (1976)	558	17	^{198}Au implantation

tolerance tests are normal. Insulin requirements for diabetes mellitus do not change (Dao 1972).

Objective regression has been reported in 50% to 70% of the cases. Duration of remission following hypophysectomy is similar to that after adrenalectomy. Metastatic lesions of all sites have been shown to regress after hypophysectomy in about 40% of the patients. In a retrospective study, the Joint Committee on Endocrine Ablative Procedures of the American College of Physicians and the American College of Surgeons emphasized that the results of hypophyseal and adrenal ablation was similar (MacDonald 1962). In Table 21.**4** some major series are summarized.

Selection and prediction of patients for hypophysectomy are the same as for adrenalectomy (see Table 21.**4**).

Additive Hormonal Treatment

The concept that breast cancer is hormone dependent and the observation that sex hormones could suppress experimental mammary tumors led to clinical trials in humans with androgens and estrogens. In 1939, two reports were published about the effect of androgen in advanced breast cancer (Loeser; Ulrich). In 1943, Biden reported regression of advanced breast cancer after administration of stilbesterol. The following year, Haddow and co-workers (1944) presented a number of cases with advanced breast cancer treated with synthetic estrogens.

Estrogens

Estrogen therapy of breast cancer has been used mostly in postmenopausal women even though premenopausal women may respond to very high dose of estrogens. In women more than five years after the menopause, the administration of estrogens in high doses has been the primary endocrine therapy for metastatic breast cancer. Objective remission has been reported in 31% to 37% of the cases (Council on Drugs 1960; Cooperative Breast Cancer Group 1964; Stoll 1964; Kennedy 1965; Beex 1981). In ER-positive tumors, the response rate increases to about 60%. Objective remission differs according to site of involvement. The response in descending order is as follows: skin and soft tissue, 34% to 45%; pulmonary, 30% to 40%; osseous, 20% to 30% (Council on Drugs 1960; Kennedy and Nathanson 1953; Kennedy 1974). The median duration of response to high-dose estrogen therapy is approximately 18 months.

Mode of Action

It has been difficult to give a satisfactory explanation as to how estrogens, considered to be growth-promoting hormones in breast cancer tumors, could cause regression in advanced breast cancer in postmenopausal women. In premenopausal women, estrogens are rarely effective, even at very high doses (Kennedy 1953), and the same holds for women less than five years after the menopause (Stoll 1973). Some hypotheses have been postulated about the mode of action.

1. Estrogen may interact with insulin leading to inhibition of glucose transport into the tumor cell (Lacho 1975)
2. Excessive estrogen administration may completely translocate the cytoplasmic estrogen receptor into the nucleus, thereby causing the tumor to mature, differentiate and stop proliferating (Hilf 1979)
3. Local cytotoxic effect (Hilf 1979).

Drugs

The most commonly used estrogen is diethylstilbestrol (DES), 5 mg orally three times a day. Another estrogen preparation that has been used is ethinylestradiol, 1 mg orally three times a day. A positive correlation between response and dose has been reported for DES (Carter 1977).

Withdrawal response, or rebound regression, has been seen in hormonal therapy. When estrogen therapy is discontinued because of relapse after primary response, about 30% of the patients will develop second tumor regression (Baker et al. 1972; Kauffmann and Escher 1961; Nesto 1976).

Side effects are considerable when estrogens are given in high doses and 10% to 15% of the patients have to discontinue the treatment (Kennedy and Nathanson 1953). Nausea and vomiting are the most common early side effects. Increased nipple, areolar, and axillary pigmentation are frequent. This can be alleviated by increasing the dose stepwise.

Fluid retention is seen in one third of the patients and is more common with advanced age. This complication is especially dangerous in patients with known cardiac disease. The treatment consists of low salt diet and, when necessary, administration of diuretics.

Breakthrough or withdrawal bleeding in postmenopausal women occurs in about 40%. Bleeding during therapy could often be controlled by sharply increasing the dose of estrogens. Urinary incontinence is another effect of large doses of estrogens. These symptoms occur primarily in older women who have borne children.

The most serious complication of estrogen therapy is an exacerbation or "flare" of the disease. This can also be seen with other hormones, especially androgens. In one third of patients with flare, hypercalcemia is seen (Kennedy 1953; Muggia and Heineman 1970). (See under Hypercalcemia in Breast Cancer).

Androgens

Based on animal experiments (Murlin et al. 1939; Lacassagne and Reynaud 1939), androgens were tried as palliative treatment of advanced breast cancer. In 1939, two reports were published about the effects of androgens in advanced breast cancer (Loeser; Ulrich). Further reports established the palliative value of androgens both in premenopausal and postmenopausal women. Various side effects were noted including hypercalcemia in patients with osseous metastases (Farrow and Woodward 1942; Adair and Herman 1946; Council on Drugs 1960; Cooperative Breast Cancer Group 1962).

The Council on Drugs reported a remission rate of 20% in 160 premenopausal and 21.9% in 420 postmenopausal women. In 1962, the Cooperative Breast Cancer Group (CBCG) presented the results of androgen therapy in 564 postmenopausal women. In this trial the response rate was equivalent, 21.5%. Almost identical remission rates have been published in other series (Kennedy 1965; Stoll 1969). Androgens have been used especially in women with bone metastases. In premenopausal women, the pain of bone metastases is reduced in over 80% of the cases (Stoll 1969). Also in postmenopausal women, androgens are effective in patients with skeletal metastases (Ward 1976; Stoll 1969; Westerberg 1980). The response rate of soft tissue metastases is reported to be 16% to 25% (CBCG 1962; Stoll 1969). As with all kinds of endocrine manipulation, visceral metastases have a lower rate of remission, 11% to 18% (Kennedy 1965; Stoll 1969; Westerberg 1980). Patients may experience a general sense of well being, relief of pain, increased appetite, and weight gain. The androgenic hormones also stimulate erythropoiesis.

Side Effects

These are associated with the physiologic effect of male hormones. The most distressing symptom is virilization including acne, hirsutism, and sometimes increased libido, and clitoral hypertrophy. The masculinizing symptoms depend on which androgenic drug is used. With previously used agents, such as testosterone propionate or methyltestosterone, they occur in about 50% (Kennedy and Nathanson 1953). Hypercalcemia occurs more frequently with androgens than with estrogens (Kennedy and Nathanson 1953).

The mode of action of androgens still remains unclear. Androgens cause involution of normal breast tissue, probably by inhibiting the gonadotropins FSH and LH. It is also assumed that androgens exert their effect on the tumor cells. These conclusions are based on experiments with cancer cells in culture and the demonstration of androgen receptors (Lippman and Huff 1976; Maass et al. 1975). It is also possible that androgens may be converted to estrogens in some tumors, but whether this has any clinical implication is uncertain (Nisker and Siiteri 1981). Toxic effects are the same as with high doses of estrogens.

Drugs and Dosage

Testosterone propionate was the first androgen in use. The drug was given intramuscularly, 100 mg in oil three times weekly. As mentioned above, the side effects were severe. Several new drugs have been introduced in recent years including dimethyltestosterone and testololactone, but none has been less virilizing and more effective than fluoxomesterone (Halotestin®) (Talley et al. 1973; Falkson et al. 1974). Fluoxomesterone is given at a dosage of 20 to 30 mg daily by mouth. Regression rates are similar to the other compounds, and virilization is very unusual when used for a trial period of three months (Stoll 1958; Cooperative Breast Cancer Group 1961).

Progestins

Since the beginning of the 1950s, progestins have been used in the treatment of metastatic mammary cancer (Kardinal and Donegan 1979). Progestins have been used both as single-drug therapy and in combination with other hormonal additive treatments, such as estrogens and antiestrogens. Many of the early reports of the results of progestin treatment were unable to show any definite benefit of progestin therapy when compared with estrogen and androgen therapy. During the last decade, some interesting reports have been published where the therapeutic results of high-dose progesterone treatment have shown higher response rates (Pannuti 1979) than low-dose therapy. High-dose progestin treatment has also been used in combination with different cytotoxic therapies.

Mode of Action

Different modes of action of the progestins have been suggested. Progestins might interfere with the nuclear binding of the estrogen receptor complex thereby modifying the estrogen-induced response in the cell (Clark 1977). It is also known from in vitro studies on human endometrium that the progestins may reduce the content of estrogen receptor within the cell (Tseng 1977).

Another possible way of interacting with the hormonal-dependent tumor cell may be through binding to the progesterone receptor. Whether this mode of action plays any major role in the therapeutic response of progestins is still unknown.

Clinical Results with Progestin Therapy

The progesterone agents most commonly used during the past few years have been megestrol acetate (Megase®), medroxyprogesterone acetate (Depo Provera®, Farlutal Depo®) and hydroxyprogesterone caproate (Delalutin®). Some of the reports on the effects of these compounds are summarized in Table 21.**5**.

During the past few years, special interest has been focused on the use of high-dose medroxyprogesterone acetate and some of the clinical result of this mode of therapy are given in Table 21.**6**.

As seen from the tables, it seems that high-dose progesterone therapy is to be preferred in comparison with low-dose progesterone therapy. Progesterone therapy shows a similar response pattern as other additive therapies in that soft tissue lesions are most likely to respond and visceral lesions are least likely to respond. When evaluating response rate and menopausal status, it seems that the response rate in premenopausal women is lower than with ablative therapy and antiestrogen therapy. In the perimenopausal and the postmenopausal period, progesterone seems to follow the same pattern of response as other additive therapies (De Lena 1979). Progestins have also been used in combination with other hormonal therapies, such as estrogen (Crowley 1965) and antiestrogens (Mouridsen 1979).

However, it has been hard to prove that combining progesterone therapy with other hormonal additive treatments has been superior to the use of single-drug therapy with either substance. High-dose medroxy progesterone acetate has also been used in combination with different cytotoxic agents. These observations are still too preliminary to justify any definite conclusions.

Table 21.**5** Low-dose progesterone treatment of advanced breast cancer

Author	Dose (mg/day)	No. of patients	Response rate (%)
Stoll (1967)	200–400 PO	12	16
Segaloff et al. (1967)	100 PO	23	0
Goldenberg (1969)	100 PO	108	9
Klaasen et al. (1976)	200–300 PO 1,600/week IV	40	5

Table 21.**6** High-dose progesterone treatment of advanced breast cancer

Author	Dose (mg/day IM)	No. of patients	Response rate %
Mattson (1978)	1,000	25	28
De Lena et al. (1979)	1000–1500	81	28
Pannuti et al. (1979)	500	46	43
Pannuti et al. (1979)	1,500	46	45

Dosage

Several different dose levels have been used in progesterone treatment of metastatic breast cancer. The most commonly used dose of megestrol acetate (Megasel®) has been 40 mg orally four times a day. Medroxyprogesterone acetate (Depo Provera®, Farlutal Depo®) has in low-dose treatment been used in doses of 100 to 400 mg intramuscularly three times weekly or orally, 100 to 300 mg daily. In high-dose medroxyprogesterone treatment, the doses have varied from 500 mg to 1,500 mg intramuscularly daily during a period of 30 days and after that 500 mg to 1,500 mg a week. Hydroxyprogesterone caproate (Delalutin®) has been used in 1,000 mg intramuscular doses weekly or 500 mg intramuscularly two or three times weekly.

Side Effects

The side effects of progesterone treatment have been relatively few. Fluid retention, nausea, and vomiting have been observed in low-dose progesterone treatment. More severe side effects have been observed in high-dose medroxyprogesterone therapy such as Cushing-like syndrome, tremor, sweating, and gluteal abscesses due to the intramuscular injection.

Conclusions

Progesterone therapy has been used in advanced breast cancer for almost 30 years. With the use of high-dose progesterone therapy in the form of medroxyprogesterone acetate, more promising results have been achieved comparable with high-dose estrogen therapy or antiestrogen therapy. The high-dose progesterone therapy might prove to be of value as a second-line therapy in patients that have failed on antiestrogen therapy.

Corticosteroids

Corticosteroids have been used in the therapy of breast cancer for three decades. They have been given alone or in combination with other hormonal or cytotoxic agents. The corticosteroids also have a definite place in replacement therapy after adrenalectomy and hypophysectomy. When used alone, corticosteroids have been known to cause objective remission of metastatic mammary carcinoma in soft tissue, bone, and viscera. Complete remissions have been rare, and objective regressions have only been temporary. The response rate when using corticosteroids as a single drug has been less than 20% in most published material (Donegan 1979). More interesting results have been achieved with corticosteroids when used in combination with cytotoxic agents or in the treatment of special metastatic sites such as brain metastases and lung metastases. Another therapeutic use for corticosteroids has been in hypercalcemia occurring both spontaneously and in association with hormonal treatments (see Hypercalcemia in Breast Cancer).

Mode of Action

Some of the therapeutic responses seen with corticosteroid treatment such as improvement in cerebral symptoms due to brain metastases as well as improvement in pulmonary symptoms due to metastatic lesions has been ascribed to reduction in inflammation and edema. Responses in these metastatic lesions are associated with the use of glucocorticoids with potent anti-inflammatory activity, whereas the glucocorticoids that have more sodium-retaining potential are less effective. More specific modes of action have been discussed, and corticosteroids produce a reduction of circulating estrogens secondary to a suppression of adrenocortical androgen synthesis. It is well known that ACTH is suppressed, thereby reducing estrogen precursors in the serum. Receptors for glucocorticoids have also been found in breast cancer. Other modes of action have been discussed, and the role and mechanism of corticosteroid therapy in breast cancer is excellently reviewed by Geimer and Donegan (1980).

Clinical results

The clinical results of corticosteroids as a single agent in breast cancer therapy are less impressive than with antiestrogens, high-dose estrogens, androgens, and ablative maneuvers. The response rates range from only a few percent up to 30% to 35%. Most authors seem to agree that objective response is less than 20% and short lasting (Geimer 1980). However, corticosteroids play a major role in the treatment of certain metastatic lesions and in the treatment of hypercalcemia. In patients with brain metastases associated with increased intracranial pressure and neurologic symptoms, corticosteroids may rapidly decrease symptoms. Improvement is often seen within 24 hours. The regression of the cerebral symptoms does not seem to correlate with any generalized regression of the tumor burden.

Similar results have been described with pulmonary metastases when the patient presents with dyspnea and respiratory distress. As with brain metastases, it seems that edema produced around the tumor plays the major role in the appearance of the acute symptoms.

The treatment of hypercalcemia is another major indication for corticosteroids and is covered later in the chapter.

Corticosteroids have been used in combination with chemotherapy in advanced breast cancer, and in some reports the addition of corticosteroids has been associated with higher response rates. There is still disagreement about the definite advantage of adding corticosteroids to different chemotherapeutic regimens. Some authors have claimed that corticosteroids may be very useful in combination with chemotherapy in patients with bone marrow involvement where the use of chemotherapy alone may induce severe bone marrow depression (for references, see Geimer 1980).

Glucocorticoids As Adjuvant Agents

Glucocorticoids, especially prednisone, have been used in combination with irradiation (Meakin 1979; Nissen-Meyer 1964). No statistically significant advantage of the addition of corticosteroids has been reported.

Corticosteroids have also been used in combination with adjuvant chemotherapy. From the limited material, it is hard to draw any definite conclusion as to the advantage of adding corticosteroids to adjuvant chemotherapy.

Glucocorticoids As Replacement Therapy

Corticosteroids are a necessary replacement for steroid hormones after adrenalectomy and hypophysectomy as well as during treatment with aminoglutethimide. For further information, see the pertinent parts of this chapter.

Dosage

Of the corticoids, prednisolone is the most commonly used agent in a dose varying from 10 mg and upwards. The low dose has been used in adjuvant situations and has been combined with oophorectomy or cytotoxic therapy. Higher doses of prednisolone might be used in pulmonary metastases or in the initial treatment of hypercalcemia.

Dexamethasone has been used especially in patients with symptoms due to cerebral metastases. A dose of 8 to 12 mg dexamethasone has been administered intravenously followed by 4 mg intramuscularly four times daily until maximum response has been obtained. One can often reduce the dexamethasone dose within a few days.

Side Effects

The side effects of corticosteroids are well known and are closely related to the dose used. With low doses, such as prednisolone 10 mg a day, the side effects are usually mild. However, after a few months most patients develop cushingoid appearance. When higher doses are used, complications including sleeplessness, psychotic symptoms, gastric or duodenal ulcers, and infections may appear. These potential complications must be weighed in relation to the therapeutic situation. The situation is different when adjuvant therapy is required, and corticosteroids may be used for periods over several years.

Hormone Suppressors

Aminoglutethimide (AG)

This drug was first introduced in 1958 as an anticonvulsant. The drug was withdrawn in 1966 after reports that it caused adrenal insufficiency (Camacho et al. 1966). Cash et al. (1967) proposed to use this effect of AG to perform medical adrenalectomy in patients with advanced breast cancer. This group reported in 1967 a single patient with advanced disease who had dramatic relief of bone pain after administration of the drug for four years. In 1973 Griffiths et al. presented a study with nine postmenopausal patients with metastatic breast cancer treated with AG and dexamethasone. Three patients responded with objective remission and two had stabilization of their disease. Since then, several studies have been carried out and many clinical trials are in progress.

Mode of Action

Aminoglutethimide inhibits the biosynthesis of estrogens in two ways. In the adrenal gland, AG blocks the enzymatic conversion of cholesterol to pregnenolone (and reduces the production of all steroids in the gland and even the major estrogen precursor, androstenedione.) In peripheral tissues, AG inhibits the aromatization of androstendione to estrogens. By this dual action, estradiol is decreased to levels similar to those seen after surgical adrenalectomy in postmenopausal women (Santen et al. 1978). Initially cortisone secretion is decreased by AG. This inhibition is compensated by a reflex rise in ACTH. Glucocorticoids are used concurrently to suppress endogenous ACTH by negative feedback activation. The usual replacement dose of 1 mg of dexamethasone cannot prevent the increase in ACTH level. It has been shown in pharmacokinetic studies that AG accelerates the metabolism of dexamethasone as opposed to hydrocortisone (HC) (Santen et al. 1977). This can be compensated by increasing the dose of dexamethasone two or three times or by using HC to prevent the reflex rise in ACTH. In contrast to surgical adrenalectomy, AG preserves androgen secretion.

After withdrawal of AG-HC treatment, adrenal recovery is rapid. Eighteen hours after stopping AG-HC treatment, the cortisol plasma levels were normal (Worgul and Santen 1982).

In summary; AG in combination with glucocorticoid replacement uniformly blocks adrenal steroidogenesis and estrogen production but preserves androgen secretion.

Clinical Results

In unselected postmenopausal patients with advanced breast cancer, a response rate of 30% to 40% has been reported. In patients with ER-rich tumors, the response rate is about 50%.

Bone and soft tissue metastases responded most frequently. Patients who had had regression from additive hormonal treatment responded more frequently to AG-HC. Some clinical results are summarized in Table 21.7.

Table 21.7 Objective tumor regression in postmenopausal women with advanced breast cancer treated with AG + glucocorticoid

Reference	No.	Response (%)
Patients with unknown estrogen receptor status		
Griffiths et al. (1973)	9	3 (33)
Wells et al. (1978)	50	19 (38)
Gale et al. (1976)	65	21 (33)
Misbin (1977)	134	33 (24)
Smith (1978)	52	17 (33)
Mason et al. (1980)	112	22 (20)
Savaraj and Trone (1980)	26	13 (50)
Patients with estrogen receptor rich tumors		
Lawrence et al. (1980)	45	22 (48)
Holdaway et al. (1980)	11	7 (63)

Aminoglutethimide plus hydrocortisone have been compared with major endocrine ablative procedures. Harvey et al. (1979) compared hypophysectomy and AG plus HC in postmenopausal women with advanced breast cancer. They found that the results were comparable, and in some patients the medical treatment was safer and produced more profound endocrine suppression than hypophysectomy.

In another study comparing medical and surgical adrenalectomy in postmenopausal women with ER-rich metastatic breast cancer, AG-HC therapy produced regression as frequently and for a similar duration as that induced by surgical adrenalectomy.

Aminoglutethimide does not block estrogen production in premenopausal women (Santen et al. 1980) and no objective regression was seen in 18 premenopausal women (Harris 1982).

Aminoglutethimide-hydrocortisone has also been compared with tamoxifen in a small number of patients (Santen 1982). Preliminary data indicate that AG-HC may produce bone healing more frequently than does tamoxifen.

New trials are in progress to study the effect of AG combined with other treatment modalities. A randomized trial is being performed in England to study the use of AG-HC as adjuvant therapy.

Indications for Therapy

Prime candidates for AG-HC therapy are postmenopausal women with inoperable, recurrent, or metastatic carcinoma of the breast. Contraindications include patients with ER-poor tumors, the presence of central nervous system metastasis, metastatic involvement of more than 30% of the liver, and rapidly progressive lymphangitic metastases to the lungs. Premenopausal status is at present a contraindication for therapy with AG.

Dosage

Santen et al., with a great experience in the use of AG, recommended the following drug regimen: 250 mg of AG twice daily for the first two weeks and then 250 mg four times a day. Large doses of hydrocortisone, 100 mg daily, are administered for the first two weeks with 60 mg given at night followed by 20 mg at 8 am and 5 pm. After two weeks, hydrocortisone is reduced to 40 mg daily, 20 mg in the evening, 10 mg in the morning, and 10 mg at 5 pm.

If there are signs and symptoms of orthostatic hypotension or hyponatremia, 9-α-fluorohydrocortisone, 0.05 to 0.10 mg daily, is administered.

The most practical marker of the endocrine function is the measurement of dehydroepiandrosterone sulfate (DHEA-S) plasma levels. This steroid, which represents the major 17-ketosteroid, is highly protein bound and has a blunted diurnal variation compared with cortisol. Over a three-month period, the level should fall to 20% of the basal value. Treatment should be continued for at least 8 weeks in order to assess response.

Side Effects

These are usually mild and transient and are mostly seen during the first weeks of treatment. The drug is well tolerated during prolonged administration. Approximately 40% of the patients develop lethargy and 10% develop ataxia, dizziness, and sometimes nystagmus. In about 5% of the patients, side effects of AG necessitated cessation of the drug (Harris 1982; Santen et al. 1980). Facial fullness develops in a few patients. Rarely, patients develop weight gain, leg cramps, or blood dyscrasias.

When AG treatment is terminated, there has been no evidence of remaining adrenal insufficiency.

Aminoglutethimide also has an inhibitory effect on thyroxine secretion. Initially there is a reduction in thyroxine level resulting in a reflex rise in TSH. This rise in TSH is sufficient to compensate for the decrease in thyroxine production. Goiter does not develop in patients treated with AG (Santen 1980).

The medical adrenalectomy regimen of AG-HC is a suitable alternative to surgical adrenalectomy. It is simple and free from the risk of surgical mortality.

The adrenal blockage is reversible, and even after prolonged treatment with AG-HC, no maintenance steroid therapy is required. This is important if the patient is subsequently to receive chemotherapy, which is poorly tolerated in adrenalectomized patients.

Antiprolactins

The role of prolactin in the growth of breast cancer in humans is unclear. In breast cancer of experimental animals, this hormone seems to be of importance. Prolactin inhibitors, such as levodopa and bromocriptine, have been tried in advanced disease in humans without any significant response being reported (Engelman et al. 1975; European Breast Cancer Group 1972; Settatree 1980). At present, it seems that antiprolactin drugs play no role in the treatment of human breast cancer.

Antigonadotropins

Danazol, an antigonadotropin, has been used in benign breast disease (Greenblatt 1980) and in animal experimental tumors (Trope et al. 1979). There is an increasing interest in the use of danazol in advanced breast cancer. At present, several clinical trials are in progress. Perhaps this drug will be useful in the treatment of hormone-sensitive mammary cancer.

Antiestrogens

Reduction of the estrogen-induced growth promotion of the hormone-dependent breast cancer is essential. Ablative maneuvers and additive treatments in the form of, for example, oophorectomy, adrenalectomy, or aminoglutethimide, produce an estrogen reduction at the target cell. Another possible way of interfering with the estrogen-induced response is by addition of drugs that block the estrogen action at the tumor cell level. In this form of treatment, the so-called antiestrogens play a major role. In this part of the chapter the antiestrogens are described as agents that reduce the response to estrogen in the target tissue. The substances that will be further described are more or less antagonistically active when used in the treatment of breast cancer. Three nonsteroidal antiestrogen compounds have been used in clinical trials during the last 15 to 20 years Herbst (1964) was the first to report on the effects of clomiphene citrate in the treatment of breast cancer. Due to the high percentage of side effects of this antiestrogen, only a few clinical reports have been presented. Nafoxidine, another nonsteroidal antiestrogen, has been studied in several clinical reports (Legha 1976; EORTC Breast Cancer Group 1972). Side effects have also been troublesome with this drug. The most extensively used antiestrogen has been tamoxifen, a drug very closely related to clomiphene. With tamoxifen, the side effects have been much less disturbing than with the other antiestrogens.

Mode of Action of Nonsteroidal Antiestrogens

Antiestrogens have been described both to alter the hormonal environment of the treated woman (Czygan 1972; Willis 1977) and to interfere with estradiol-17β on the tumor cellular level (Koseki 1977). The interference with estradiol-17β in the tumor cell has been most extensively studied. The antiestrogens appear to compete with estradiol-17β for the ER binding site. After binding to the ER, the antiestrogen-receptor complex, as with the estradiol-17β receptor complex, is transported into the nucleus of the tumor cell. The receptor complex then binds to special nuclear acceptor sites of the chromatin. Whether there are separate binding sites in the tumor cell nucleus for the antiestrogen receptor complex and the estradiol-17β receptor complex is still not clear. After binding to the chromatin, the estradiol receptor complex induces certain changes within the cell that include synthesis of RNA and thus induction of protein synthesis. The antiestrogen receptor complex is able to induce the same kind of response. However, the response as measured by protein synthesis is much lower than for the natural estrogen estradiol-17β (Koseki 1977). In animal tumor systems using 7-12-dimethylbenzantrazene-(DMBA)-induced breast cancer, antiestrogens have been shown both to cause regression of established tumors as well as protecting the animal from developing tumors when exposed to DMBA (Nicholson 1975; Jordan 1976). In human inoperable breast cancers, it has been possible to show by the use of fine needle biopsy that the antiestrogen causes a significant reduction in ^{3}H-labeled thymidine incorporation in breast cancer tumors that respond to antiestrogen therapy (Nordenskjöld 1975).

The effects of antiestrogens on the hormonal environment in the treated patients have also been studied. Serum levels of estrogens, androgens, adrenal androgens, gonadotropins, and prolactin have been investigated during treatment with tamoxifen (Willis 1977; Szamel 1979; Wilking 1982; Groom 1976). These studies, although inconclusive, seem to indicate that tamoxifen does not cause any remarkable change in the hormonal environment. It has been shown that tamoxifen is capable of inhibiting prostaglandin synthesis in vitro in malignant breast cancer tissue (Ritchie 1977). Prostaglandins have been discussed as possible mediators of bone resorption in the metastatic lesions, and this might indicate an additive effect of tamoxifen in bone metastases.

Estrogen-like effects, such as vaginal cornification (Bochardo 1981), and estrogen-like induction of serum proteins (Sakai 1978; Levin 1981) have been observed during tamoxifen treatment. This weak estrogen effect may well be explained by the effects of the tamoxifen-estrogen receptor complex (Koseki 1977). It is uncertain if these observations have any clinical significance.

Clinical Results

Clomiphene Citrate

There are few reports on the use of clomiphene citrate in the treatment of advanced breast cancer (Herbst 1964; Hecker 1974). The overall response rate in unselected patients has been 30% to 40%, which is comparable to ablative maneuvers. Clomiphene does not seem to differ from the other antiestrogens with regard to its effects on different sites of metastases as well as its effect correlated to age.

Dosage

Daily doses of clomiphene citrate varying from 200 to 300 mg have been used in the clinical trials reported.

Side Effects

The most common side effect with clomiphene has been visual disturbance. Nausea, tinnitus, and loss of equilibrium have been described (Legha 1976; Hecker 1974). Although clomiphene has produced remission rates comparable to those obtained with other antiestrogens and additive treatments, it is no longer available for clinical use.

Nafoxidine Hydrochloride

The initial interest in nafoxidine was focused on its contraceptive properties, but the drug did not show sufficient efficacy as an antifertility agent. In 1965, the clinical trials on the drug in the treatment of disseminated breast cancer started (Legha 1976). In two major clinical trials (EORTC 1972; Legha 1976), the clinical results measured by objective remissions were around 35%. This means that nafoxidine produces clinical response in advanced breast cancer in about the same proportion of patients as clomiphene and tamoxifen.

Dosage

The most common dose has been 60 mg three times daily orally.

Side Effects

Dermatologic toxicity has been the major problem when using nafoxidine. Most patients treated for more than one or two months have developed ichthyosis (Legha 1976). Many of the patients have also suffered from cutaneous photosensitivity even after indirect sunlight. Some of these side effects can be reduced by a dose reduction to 90 to 120 mg/day. Apart from the cutaneous side effects, other side effects such as gastric disorders have been described. A few cases of liver toxicity and hypercalcemia have also been reported. Due to the side effects, the present use of nafoxidine is limited.

Tamoxifen Citrate

The most widely used antiestrogen in the treatment of breast cancer is tamoxifen. Its antiestrogenic properties have been studied for more than 15 years. The first clinical trial with tamoxifen in advanced breast cancer was presented by Cole in 1971. This study has been followed by a number of clinical trials. The result of the major clinical trials have been reviewed by Mouridsen et al. in 1978. The majority of the clinical trials with tamoxifen have been in advanced breast cancer in postmenopausal women. There is also a fairly large clinical experience with the use of tamoxifen in advanced breast cancer in premenopausal women, as well as the use of tamoxifen as an adjuvant treatment after radical surgery. In Table 21.**8**, the overall response rate in terms of objective remission is given.

Table 21.**8**

No. of patients	Complete remission	Partial remission	No. change	Progressive disease
3089	216	812	509	1492

Response rate (complete remission + partial remission) = 33%

(Adapted from Patterson 1981.)

As seen from this table, the response rate of tamoxifen in terms of complete and partial remission is similar to the other antiestrogens and comparable to high-dose estrogen therapy and ablative surgery. If the patient has had a prior response to endocrine therapy, the likelihood of responding to tamoxifen increases to nearly 70%. Even if the patient has failed on prior endocrine therapy, around 15% respond to tamoxifen treatment (Mouridsen 1978). The response rate of tamoxifen with regard to metastatic site is similar to other hormonal treatments. Soft tissue metastases are most likely to respond, whereas bone and visceral metastases show a lower response rate. Similarly, tamoxifen induces a higher rate of response in postmenopausal patients compared with perimenopausal patients. In patients over 70 years of age, the response rate is almost 50% (Mouridsen 1978).

The response of tamoxifen has also been correlated to the existence of ER protein within the tumor cell and the response rate in the receptor-rich patients has been around 50%. Between 10% and 15% of the ER-poor patients have responded to tamoxifen therapy (Furr 1979). This means that tamoxifen has shown a surprisingly high response rate in patients who have a low ER content of their tumor.

Tamoxifen has been used as an adjuvant agent after radical surgery. Experience is not extensive, although there are many on-going trials. (Palshof et al. 1980; Hubay 1980; Fisher et al. 1981; Wallgren et al. 1981; Baum 1983).

Tamoxifen has also been used in combination with cytotoxic therapy as well as with other hormonal agents. Combinations with other agents such as progestins and androgens have not shown any clear advantage over the respective single drugs. In combination with cytotoxic agents, some new reports (Fisher et al. 1981) have shown a statistically significant advantage of the addition of tamoxifen to the cytotoxic regimen, at least for women over 50 years of age. Other reports (Heuson 1976; Cavalli 1978) support this opinion.

Experience with tamoxifen in premenopausal women is not extensive. Some reports have shown response rates around 30% (Meakin 1978; Yoshida 1978).

If tamoxifen treatment is compared with endocrine ablation and endocrine addition, the result in advanced breast cancer shows that tamoxifen has a high response rate, a long duration of response, and is effective both in premenopausal and postmenopausal women (Pearson 1980).

Dosage

The doses used in the majority of the clinical trials with tamoxifen have varied from 10 mg twice daily to 40 mg twice daily. The most commonly used dose has been 10 mg three times daily or 20 mg twice daily.

Side Effects

The main advantage of tamoxifen treatment in comparison with high-dose estrogen therapy, androgen therapy, and other antiestrogens has been the relatively few and mild side effects. In the review article by Mouridsen et al. (1978), only 2.6% of the patients were unable to tolerate the therapy. The most common side effects have been nausea and vomiting as well as hot flushes. These side effects have been observed in around 10% of the treated patients. A mild thrombocytopenia has also occurred. In most patients, this phenomenon has been transient.

"Tumor flares" have been discussed as a side effect of tamoxifen treatment. It is still very controversial whether or not this flare is an indication of tumor stimulation. Hypercalcemia is another phenomenon that is observed in many patients during hormonal treatment. In most patients, neither tumor flare nor hypercalcemia seem to be associated with tumor progression. If hypercalcemia occurs, it should be treated in a proper manner (see Hypercalcemia in Breast Cancer). When the patient is normocalcemic, the tamoxifen treatment may be started again.

Conclusions

Of the nonsteroidal antiestrogens that have been used, namely, clomiphene, nafoxidine, and tamoxifen, the latter substance has by far gained the most clinical interest as a therapeutic tool in the treatment of breast cancer. The response rate of the nonsteroidal antiestrogens is comparable to the bestknown additive hormonal treatments as well as to ablative surgical maneuvers. When considering the limited number of side effects, tamoxifen has taken the place of first line hormonal treatment of advanced breast cancer in the postmenopausal women.

Hypercalcemia in Breast Cancer

Hypercalcemia is a complication of advanced breast cancer. There is no obvious correlation between the extent of clinically detected bone metastases and the degree of elevation of serum calcium levels. If unrecognized, hypercalcemia may result in death. Therefore, it is vital to be aware of this syndrome.

The principal symptoms of hypercalcemia are anorexia, nausea, vomiting, weakness, obstipation, polyuria, renal failure, somnolence progressing to coma and finally vascular collapse and death.

Hypercalcemia has been reported to occur in up to 40% of patients with advanced disease (Kennedy 1953; Graham et al. 1963). In most cases hypercalcemia is spontaneous and unassociated with prior hormonal therapy, although in 5% the condition is induced by hormonal manipulation (Kennedy et al. 1953; Muggia and Heineman 1970).

Hormonally induced hypercalcemia generally starts within two weeks after the beginning of hormonal treatment (Swaroop and Kvant 1973). When hypercalcemia occurs shortly after the start of additive hormonal treatment, it has often been interpreted as evidence of exacerbation or "flare" of the disease. Hypercalcemia has been observed after all forms of hormonal treatment, but the highest incidence has been reported after androgenic drugs (Kennedy and Nathanson 1953).

The management of the situation is to stop the hormone administration, correct the hypercalcemia, and change the treatment plan. The management of the hypercalcemia ultimately depends on the ability to control the disease but can be immediately treated in different ways. Immobilization can aggravate the hypercalcemia and activity of the patients should be increased. Sodium excretion promotes calcium excretion and infusion of normal saline may be sufficient in mild cases to correct serum calcium levels. The effect can be enhanced by diuretics (furosemide). Corticosteroids can reverse the condition. After an initial daily dose of 100 to 200 mg hydrocortisone or equivalent, the maintenance dose is 20 to 50 mg prednisone daily. If these measures fail, EDTA, sodium sulfate, or sodium phosphate may produce a response.

Mithramycin, an antitumor antibiotic, is effective in a variety of hypercalcemic states in malignant diseases. Mithramycin seems to interfere temporarily with the osteoclastic function resulting in a rapid reduction in serum calcium. A single injection of 25 µg/kg body weight of mithramycin can correct the hypercalcemia (Perlia et al. 1970).

Calcitonin is a peptide hormone that has also been used in the management of hypercalcemia of malignancy. No major side effects have been reported (Vaughan and Vaitkevicius 1974).

The management of hypercalcemia in breast cancer has been excellently reviewed by Davis (1973).

Hypercalcemia is a serious and lethal complication in breast cancer if not recognized and treated without delay. Long-term control of this condition can only be achieved by treating the underlying malignancy.

Future Approach to Endocrine Therapy

Steady progress is occurring in the hormonal therapy of breast cancer. During the last decades, our knowledge of the mechanism of action and metabolism of steroid hormones has increased considerably. Estrogen and other steroid receptor proteins have been demonstrated in breast cancer tissue. The presence or absence of these proteins has made it possible to predict hormonal dependency of the tumor. Although the assay of estrogen receptor proteins has increased the possibilities to predict hormone sensitivity, only about 60% of patients with ER-rich tumors will respond to hormonal manipulations. Analysis of other hormone receptor proteins, such as progesterone and androgen receptors, might be one way to improve the selection of patients for hormonal therapy.

Recently it has been demonstrated that the nuclear content of DNA of the tumor cell correlates well to the prognosis and the content of ER proteins. The estimation of the DNA pattern might be an additional refinement in the prediction for identifying patients suitable for hormonal therapy (Auer et al. 1980; Theve et al. 1982).

New hormonal agents with improved therapeutic effect have been developed. Antiestrogens, of which tamoxifen has been the most studied and used, have been demonstrated to be as effective as estrogens in postmenopausal women with ER-rich tumors. In addition, a remarkably high portion of women with ER-poor tumors respond to this drug (15%). Recently it has been reported that there is also a fairly high response rate in premenopausal women with advanced disease, although present data are less extensive. Therefore, the role of tamoxifen in premenopausal women has to be fully elucidated, especially whether or not this drug could replace oophorectomy.

Aminoglutethimide (AG) is another new hormonal compound under clinical evaluation. In several reports its value has been demonstrated in advanced disease. Aminoglutethimide causes a reversible inhibition of the biosynthesis of the adrenal steroids and thereby produces a medical adrenalectomy. That this inhibition is reversible is of great value if the patient is subsequently to receive chemotherapy that is poorly tolerated in adrenalectomized women. According to current data, the response rate and duration of remission appear quite similar to major surgical endocrine ablation by adrenalectomy or by hypophysectomy.

Following the introduction of these new drugs, the major ablative maneuvers have been less frequently used, and further current trials will show if surgical hormonal ablation will be obsolete in the future.

Hormonal treatment in breast cancer may also be used prophylactically. In recent studies, adjuvant postoperative tamoxifen treatment with or without chemotherapy seems to increase the recurrence-free survival significantly in patients with ER-rich tumors. In patients with ER-poor tumors, the recurrence-free survival is slightly, but not significantly, increased.

Various combinations of new hormonal agents have been tried, but the results are still inconclusive. Clinical trials are also in progress to evaluate the combination of endocrine therapy and chemotherapy. Other new drugs, such as antiprolactins and antigonadotropins, have shown antitumor activity in experimentally induced animal tumors. So far, no significant therapeutic effect has been demonstrated in human mammary cancer.

To improve the treatment of breast cancer, further clinical, randomized studies are necessary to evaluate the new modalities of hormonal therapy and its use in combination with other therapeutic tools.

References

Abraham, G., G. B. Maroulis: Obstet. Gynecol. 5: 271, 1975

Adair, F. E., J. B. Herrman: Ann. Surg. 123: 1023, 1946

Adlercreutz, H., F. Martin: J. Steroid Biochem. 13: 231, 1980

Ahlbom, H.: Act. Radiol. 11: 614, 1930

Ahman, D. L.: N. Eng. J. Med. 297: 356, 1977

Atkins, H. J. B.: Ann. R. Coll. Surg. 38: 133, 1966

Auer, G.: Eur. J. Cancer 16: 1, 1980

Baker, L. H.: Cancer 29: 1268, 1972

Barlow, D., B. F. Meggitt: Br. J. Surg. 55: 59, 1968

Barlow, J. J.: N. Eng. J. Med. 280 12: 633, 1969

Bateman, G. H.: J. Laryng. & Otolaryng. 75: 442, 1962

Bates, T.: Europ. J. Cancer 12: 775, 1976

Baulieu, E. E.: Rec. Progr. Hormone Res. 21: 411, 1965

Baum, M.: The Lancet. Saturday 5. February: 157, 1983

Beatson, G. T.: Lancet 2: 104, 1896

Beex, L.: Cancer Treat. Rep. 65: 179, 1981

Biden, W. M.: Brit. Med. J. July: 57, 1943

Boccardo, F.: Oncology 38: 281, 1981

Botella-Lluisa, J.: Maturitas 2: 7, 1979

Brown, P. W.: Arch. Surg. 110: 77, 1975

Bruhner, K. W.: Cancer 39: 2923, 1977

Camacho, A. M.: J. Pediat. 6: 852, 1966

Calanog, A.: Am. J. Obstet. Gynecol. 129: 553, 1977

Carlström, K.: Acta Obstet. Gynecol. Scand. 58: 179, 1979

Carlström, K & B. Fredricsson: Int. J. Androl. 3: 417, 1980

Carter, B.: Jama 237: 2079, 1977

Cash, R.: J. Clin. Endocrinol. Metab. 27: 1239, 1967

Cavalli, F.: Medical oncology 5, Abstract 17, 1978

Chang, R. J. & H. J. Judd: Clin. Obstet. Gynecol. 24: 181, 1981

Clark, J. H.: In Biochemical action of progesterone and progestines. Ed. by E. Guipide, NY Acad. Sci. 286: 161, 1977

Cole, M. P.: Brit. J. Surg. 51: 216, 1964

Cole, M. P.: Brit. J. Cancer 25: 270, 1971

Collins, W. F.: Clin. Neurosurg. 21: 68, 1974

Cooper, A.: Lectures on the principles and practice of surgery. London. H. Renshaw 356, Strand p 346, 1835

Cooperative Breast Cancer Group: JAMA 188: 1069, 1964

Council on Drugs: JAMA 172: 1271, 1960

Crilly, R.: Clin. Endocrinol. Metab. 10: 115, 1981

Crowley, L. G. & J. MacDonald: Cancer 18: 436, 1965

Czygan, P.-J. & K. D. Schulz: Gynecol. Invest. 3: 126, 1972

Dao, T. L. & T. Nemoto: Surg. Gynecol. Obstet. 121: 1257, 1965

Dao, T. L. & C. Huggins: Jama 165: 1793, 1957

Dao, T. L.: Annual review of Med. 23: 1, 1972

Dao, T. L.: Int. J. Radiation Oncology Biol. Phys. 4: 473, 1978

Dao, T. L.: Surg. Clin. N. Amer. 58: 801, 1978

Dao, T. L.: Prognostic factors in Breast Cancer. Edinburgh, E. & S. Livingstone Ltd: 177, 1967

Dao, T. L.: Cancer 35: 478, 1975

Davis, H. L.: Oncology 28: 126, 1973

De Lena, M.: Cancer Chemother. Pharmacol. 2: 175, 1979

Dewitt, J. E. & J. M. Hardwich: Am. J. Surg. 137: 629, 1979

Diczfalusy, E.: In Vokaer, R. and G. de Bock (Edits): Reproductive Endrocrinology. Pergamon Press, Oxford 1975

Diczfalusy, E.: J. Clin. Endocrin. 19: 1230, 1959

Diczfalusy, E. & M. Levitz: In Bernstein, S. and S. Solomon (Edits): Chemical and Biological Aspects of Steroid Conjugation. Springer Verlag, Berlin–Heidelberg–New York p 291, 1970

Dorfman, R. I.: In R. I. Dorfman (Edit): Methods in Hormone Research Vol. II A. Bioassay Academic Press, New York p 151, 1969

Dunbar, H. S.: Major Endocrine Surgery for treatment of carcinoma of the breast in advanced stages. Ed. M. Dargent and C. Romieu, Lyon p 33, 1977

Dunn, Y. F.: J. Clin. Endocrinol. Metab. 53: 58, 1981

Edelstyn, G.: Clin. Radiology 19: 426, 1968

Emmens, C. W.: In R. I. Dorfman (Edit): Methods of Hormone Research. Vol II A. Bioassay. Academic Press, New York p 4, 1969

Engelsman, E.: Brit. Med. J. 2: 714, 1975

EORTC Breast Cancer Group: Europ. J. Cancer 8: 387, 1972

Erickson, G. F.: Clin. Obstet. Gynecol. 21 (1): 31, 1978

Escher, G. C.: Major Endocrine Surgery in the treatment of the carcinoma of the breast in advanced stages. Ed. Darget & C. Romeu, Lyon, p 109, 1967

Europ. Breast Cancer Group: Europ. J. Cancer 8: 155, 1972

Falkson, G.: Cancer Chemother. Rep. 58: 939, 1974

Falkson, G.: Cancer 43: 2215, 1975

Farrow, J. H. & F. E. Adair: Science 95: 654, 1942

Fisher, B.: N. Eng. J. Med. 305: 1, 1981

Folca, P. J.: Lancet 2: 796, 1961

Fraccia, A. A.: Cancer 12: 58, 1959

Fraccia, A. A.: Surg. Gynecol. Obstet. 125: 747, 1967

Fraccia, A. A.: Surg. Gynecol. Obstet. 128: 1226, 1969

Fraccia, A. A.: Surg. Gynecol. Obstet. 124: 270, 1969

Fraccia, A. A.: Surg. Gynecol. Obstet. 133: 241, 1971

Furr, B. J.: Pharmacological and Biochemical Properties of Drug Substances, p. 355, 1979

Galbut, D. L. & M. K. Wallach: Am. J. Surg. 131: 267, 1976

Gale, K. E.: Clin. Res. 24: 376, 1975

Geimer, N. F. O., W. L. Donegan: Rev. End. Cancer, Aug, 6: 5, 1980

Givens, J. R.: Clin. Obstet. Gynecol. 21 (1): 115, 1978

Grumbach, M. M.: In James, VHT, M. Serio, G. Giusti and L. Martini (Edit): The Endocrine Function of the Human Adrenal Cortex. Academic Press, New York, Vol 18, p. 583, 1978

Goldenberg, I. S.: Cancer 23: 109, 1969

Graham, W. P.: Surg. Gynecol. Obstet. 117: 709, 1963

Greenblatt, R. B.: Fertility Sterility 34, 3: 242, 1980

Griffiths, C. T.: Cancer 32: 31, 1973

Groom, G. V. & K. Griffiths: J. Endocrin. 70: 421, 1976

Haddow, A.: Brit. Med. J. II: 393, 1944

Hamberger, C. A.: Archives of otolaryng. 74: 2, 1961

Hall, T. C.: Cancer Chemother. Rep. 31: 47, 1963

Harris, A.: Aminoglutethimide (Orimetene®). Proc. Internat. Symp., Basel. Ed. F. J. A. Paesi, Ciba-Geigy, p. 156, 1982

Harvey, H. A.: Cancer 43: 2207, 1979

Hecher, E.: Europ. J. Cancer 10: 747, 1974

Hellström, J. & C. Frankson: Endocrine aspects of breast cancer. Edinburgh & Livingstone, 1958

Henningsen, B. & W. Piotrowski: Prophylaxe und Therapie von Behandlungsfolgen bei Karzinomen der Frau. Ed. D. Schmähl, Thieme Verlag, Stuttgart, p. 85, 1979

Heuson, J. C.: Cancer Treatment Reports 60: 1463, 1976

Herbst, A. L.: Cancer Chemotherapy Reports 43, 1964

Hilf, R.: Rev. End. Rel. Cancer, p. 11, Febr. –79

Holdaway, I. M.: Brit. J. Cancer 41: 136, 1980

Hubay, C. A.: Surgery 87: 494, 1980

Huggins, C. & W. W. Scott: Ann. Surg. 122: 1041, 1945

Huggins, C. & D. M. Bergenstal: Cancer Res. 12: 134, 1952

Huggins, C. & T. L. Dao: Ann. Surg. 140: 497, 1954

Jensen, E. V.: Steroid Dynamics, Acad. Press New York, p. 133, 1966

Jensen, E. V.: Therapy Nat. Cancer Inst. Monogr. 34: 55, 1971

Jordan, V. C.: Eur. J. Cancer 12: 419, 1976

Kardinal, C. G., W. L. Donegan: Cancer in the Breast. Major problems in clinical surgery, p. 361, 1979

Kauffman, R. J. & G. C. Escher: Surg. Gynecol. Obstet. 113: 635, 1961

Kennedy, B. J.: Surg. Gynecol. Obstet. 120: 1246, 1965

Kennedy, B. J.: Semin Oncol. 1: 119, 1974

Kennedy, B. J. & I. T. Nathanson: JAMA 152: 1135, 1953

Kennedy, B. J.: Cancer Res. 13: 445, 1953

Klassen, D. J.: Cancer Treat. Rep. 60: 251, 1976

Korenman, S.: Clin. Endocrinol. Metab. 7: 625, 1978

Koseki, Y.: Endocrinology 101: 1104, 1977

Lacassagne, A. & A. Raymond: Compt. Rend. Soc. de Biol. 131: 586, 1939

Lacho, L.: J. Cellular Physiol. 86: 673, 1975

Laurell, C.-B. & G. Rannevik: J. Clin. Endocrinol. Metab. 49: 719, 1979

Lawrence, B. V.: Cancer 45: 786, 1980

Lee, M. C.: J. Clin. Endocrinology 15: 1228, 1965

Lee, Y. T. & J. M. Hori: Cancer 27(6): 1374, 1971

Lee, Y. T.: Surg. Gynecol. Obstet. 132: 871, 1971

Lehga, S. S.: Cancer 38: 1535, 1976

Lett, H.: Lancet 1: 227, 1905

Loeser, A.: Acta Un. Int. Cancer 4: 375, 1939
Loeser, A.: Brit. Med. J. 21: 1380, 1944
Lippman, M.: Cancer Res. 36: 4595, 1976
Lippman, M.: Cancer Res. 37: 1901, 1977
Luft, R. & H. Olivecrona: J. Neurosurg. 10: 301, 1953
Luft, R. & H. Olivecrona: Endocrine Aspects of Breast Cancer. Edinburgh & Livingstone, p. 27, 1958
Mason, R. C.: Trans. Biochem. Soc. 8: 301, 1980
Mattson, W.: Acta Radiol. Oncol. 17: 387, 1978
McDonald, J.: Surg. Gynecol. Obstet. 115: 215, 1962
McGuire, W. L.: Cancer Res. 38: 4289, 1978
McMillan, J. M.: Cancer 39: 2254, 1977
Meakin, J. W.: Can. Med. Assoc. J. 120: 1221, 1979
Misbin, R. J.: Ann. Int. Med. 86: 828, 1977
Moll, G. W.: J. Clin. Endocrinol. Metab. 52: 68, 1981
Moore, F. F.: Surg. 76: 376, 1974
Moseley, H. S.: Am. J. Surg. 128: 143, 1974
Moseley, H. S.: Am. J. Surg. 140: 164, 1980
Mouridsen, H.: Cancer Treatment Rev. 5: 131, 1979
Muggia, F. M. & H. O. Heineman: Ann. Intern. Med. 73: 281, 1970
Murlin, J. R.: Arch. Path. 28: 777, 1939
Naftolin, F. & G. Tolis: Clin. Obstet. Gynecol. 21(1): 17, 1978
Nash, A. C. & G. F. Robbins: Surg. Gynecol. Obstet. 137: 670, 1978
Nesto, R. W.: Cancer 38: 1834, 1976
Newsome, J. F.: Am. Surg. 174(5): 769, 1971
Nicholson, R. I. & M. Golder: Europ. J. Cancer 11: 571, 1975
Nisker, J. A. & P. K. Siiteri: Clin. Obstet. Gynecol. 24(1): 301, 1981
Nissen-Meyer, R.: Clin. Radiol. 15: 152, 1964
Nissen-Meyer, R.: Acta radiol. Suppl. 249, 1965
Nordenskjöld, B.: Proc. Symp. on Hormonal Control of Breast Cancer. Alderley Part, 24th Sept. p. 43, 1975
Notter, G.: Acta Radiol. Suppl. 184: 1, 1959
O'Bryan, R. M.: Cancer 33: 1082, 1974
Oberfield, R. A.: Surg. Gynecol. Obstet. 148: 881, 1979
Palshof, T.: Rev. on Endocrine Rel. Cancer Suppl. Oct., p. 57, 1978
Palshof, T.: Recent Results Cancer Res. 71: 185, 1980
Panutti, F.: Europ. J. Cancer 15: 593, 1979
Parker, L. N. & W. D. Odell: J. Clin. Endocrinol. Metab. 47: 600, 1978
Patterson, J. S.: Gan no Rinsho (Japanese J. of Cancer Clinics) Suppl. (Nov.): 157, 1981
Pearson, O.: Arch. Intern. Med. 95: 357, 1955
Pearson, O. & S. Ray: Cancer 12: 85, 1959
Perlia, C. P.: Cancer 25: 389, 1970
Pietrowski, W.: In Recent results in cancer res. Endocrine treatment of breast cancer. Ed. B. Henningsen, F. Linder, C. Steichele, Springer Verlag, 1980
Pritchard, K. J.: Ann. Int. Med. 89: 721, 1978
Puga, F. J.: Arch. Surg. 111: 877, 1976
Ravdin, A. G.: Surg. Gynecol. Obstet. 131: 1055, 1970
Richards, S. H.: Proc. of Roy Soc. Med. 67: 889, 1974
Riskaer, N.: Arch. Otolaryng. 74: 983, 1961
Ritchie, G.: Symp. the Antioestrogen and Breast Cancer, King's College Cambridge, p. 40, 1977
Roberts, K. D. & S. Lieberman: In S. Bernstein, and S. Solomon (Edits): Chemical and Biological Aspects of Steroid Conjugation. Springer Verlag, Berlin–Heidelberg–New York, p. 219, 1970
Robin, P. E.: Brit. J. Surg. 62: 85, 1975
Robin, P. E. & G. A. Dalton: Breast cancer management. Early and late. Ed. B. Stoll, W. Heinemann, Medical Books Ltd., London, 1977

Roy, A. B.: In: S. Bernstein and S. Solomon (Edits): Chemical and biological Aspects of steroid conjugation. Springer-Verlag, Berlin–Heidelberg–New York, p. 74, 1970
Santen, R. J.: J. Clin. Endocrin. Metab. 45: 469, 1977
Santen, R. J. & S. A. Wells: Cancer 46: 1066, 1980
Santen, R. J.: J. Clin. Endocrin. Metab. 51: 473, 1980
Savaraj, N. & B. Troner: Med. Pediatr. Oncology 8: 251, 1980
Scheer, K.: Major Endocrine Surgery in the Treatment of Carcinoma of the Breast in advanced Stages. Ed.: M. Darget, C. Romeiu, Lyon, Simep Editions, p. 94, 1967
Schimkin, M. B. & R. S. Wyman: J. Nat. Cancer Inst. 6: 187, 1945
Schinzinger, A.: Verh. Deutsch. Ges. Chir. 18: 28, 1889
Segaloff, A.: Cancer 20: 1673, 1967
Settatree, R. S.: Rev. End. Rel. Cancer Suppl. 5, 63, 1980
Siiteri, P. K. & M. Serón-Ferré: In: James V. H. T., M. Serio, G. Giusti and L. Martini (Edits): The endocrine function of the human adrenal cortex. Vol. 18, Academic Press, New York, p. 251, 1978
Sköldefors, H.: Acta Obstet. Gynecol. Scand. 55: 119, 1976
Sköldefors, H.: Int. J. Androl. 1: 308, 1978
Smith, I. E.: Lancet 2: 646, 1978
Smith, I. E.: Aminoglutethimide (Ormitene®). Proc. Int. Symp., Basel. Ed. F. J. A. Paesi, CIBA-GEIGY, p. 139, 1982
Stein, J. J.: Cancer 21: 1350, 1969
Stoll, B. A.: Med. J. Aust. 1: 70, 1958
Stoll, B. A.: Med. J. Aust. 1: 980, 1964
Stoll, B. A.: Brit. Med. J. 3: 338, 1967
Stoll, B. A.: Brit. Med. J. 3L446, 1973
Swaroop, S. & M. Kvant: JAMA 223: 913, 1973
Szamel, I.: Cancer Treatment. Rep. 63: 1202, 1979
Sakai, F.: J. Endocr. 76: 219, 1978
Talley, R. W.: Cancer 32: 315, 1973
Taylor, G. W.: Surg. Gynecol. Obstet. 68: 452, 1939
Taylor, S.: Surg. Gynecol. Obstet. 115: 443, 1962
Taylor, S. G. & R. S. Morris: Med. Clin. North. Am. 35: 351, 1951
Taylor, W.: Vitam. Horm. 29: 201, 1971
Theve, N. O.: Acta Chir. Scand. 148: 239, 1982
Toft, D. & J. Gorski: Proc. Nat. Acad. Sci. 55: 1581, 1966
Tseng, L.: Ann. N. Y. Acad. Sci. 286: 190, 1977
Trope, C.: Cancer Treat. Rep. 63: 1221, 1979
Ulrich, P.: Acta Un. Int. Cancer 4: 377, 1939
Vaughan, C. B. & V. K. Vaitkevicius: Cancer 34: 1268, 1974
Vermeulen, A.: J. Clin. Endocrinol. Metab. 42: 247, 1976
Vermeulen, A. & L. Verdonck: Steroid Biochem. 11: 897, 1979
Vignon, F.: Endocrinology 106, 1079, 1980
Vikho, R. & A. Roukonen: J. Steroid. Biochem. 6: 353, 1975
Veronesi, U.: Surg. Gynecol. Obstet. 141: 569, 1975
Wallgren, A.: Adjuvant Therapy of Cancer III. Ed. S. E. Salmon, S. E. Jones. Grune and Stratton, p. 345, 1981
Ward, H.: In: Proc. Symp. Hormonal Control of Breast Cancer, Mocclesfield, 1976
Westerberg, H.: Cancer Treat. Rep. 64: 117, 1980
Wells, S. A.: Ann. Surg. 187: 475, 1978
West, G. D.: J. Clin. Endocrinol. Metab. 21: 1197, 1961
Wilking, N.: Europ. J. Cancer 16: 1338, 1980
Wilking, N.: Acta Chir. Scand. 148: 345, 1982
Willis, K. J.: Brit. Med. J. 1: 425, 1977
Wilson, R. F.: Progress Reprot. Cancer 28: 962, 1971
Wilson, R. F.: Cancer 24: 1322, 1696
Worgul, J. T. & R. J. Santen: Aminoglutethimide. Proc. Int. Symp. Base. Dec. 1980. Ed. F. J. A. Paesi, CIBA-GEIGY, p. 91, 1982.
Yoshida, M.: Cancer & Chemotherapy 5: 1, 1978

Chapter 22

Chemotherapy and Management of Disseminated Disease

R. Cantor

Introduction

Although controversy may persist regarding the primary management of potentially curable breast cancer, there can be little argument that the majority of patients will ultimately die of metastatic involvement. The biologic unpredictability of cancer is never better underscored than when one considers the seemingly endless risk that these patients face. However, the palliative management of disseminated breast cancer has long been one of the most satisfying areas of oncology and developments in both cytotoxic and hormonal management during the past decade have been among the brightest and most potentially rewarding in all of medicine. Today, the majority of patients with hematogenous metastases can look forward to objective remittence of their disease with improved quality and quantity of life. The rationale for a palliative approach to these patients is rooted in a legacy of empiric data starting with Beatson's report in 1896 of remission following oophorectomy in premenopausal women with advanced disease. The explosion of knowledge that followed during the first half of the 20th century led to a wealth of largely uncontrolled information. The process of digesting and resynthesizing this information, subjecting it to controlled studies, and objectively measuring responses while prospectively identifying and controlling variables has been one of medicine's more significant clinical advances. Thus, today's cancer therapist can call on an amalgam of the tradition of the past fused to the more concrete knowledge of the present when deciding how to attempt palliation. In the process he must recognize the heterogeneity of this disease and consider both the rate and pattern of spread, the predominant sites of involvement, and the biologic predictability of responsiveness.

Chemotherapy

The past decade has seen significant advances in the management of metastatic adult solid tumors. Many of the most dramatic advances have been in the less frequent malignancies such as lymphoma, ovarian cancer, and testicular cancer. Of the more common malignant diseases, metastatic breast cancer has become a keystone disease offering significant responses to a variety of cytotoxic agents used as either single agents or in combination. Although many difficult issues have been addressed by carefully designed randomized prospective studies, many points remain unclear. When evaluating a patient for systemic intervention, one must once again consider the biologic heterogeneity of disease, the disease-free interval and rate of progression, sites of involvement, patient's general condition, and prior therapies and responses. These must be considered in light of the patient's goals and expectations as well as her abilities to understand and tolerate anticipated drug toxicities. Such an approach broadened by appropriate insights regarding the specifics of chemotherapy should allow for an intelligent and optimistic attempt at therapeutic remission.

Documented responses to single agent chemotherapy go back several decades. Much of the data, however, are quite deficient as they generally measured response rates only, with little concern for either quality or duration of life. Table 22.1 offers respresentative data.

Table 22.1 Single agent therapy

Drug	Response rate (%)	Median duration (months)	Reference
Melphelan	23	3.5–5.8	Carter (1976)
Cyclophosphamide	34	3.5–5.8	Carter (1976)
5-Fluorouracil	26	3.5–5.8	Carter (1976)
Methotrexate	34	3.5–5.8	Carter (1976)
Vincristine	21	3.5–5.8	Carter (1976)
Vinblastine	40	3.5–5.8	Yap et al. (1983)
Adriamycin	40–50	7–8	Gottlieb (1974) Hoogstraten (1976) Tormey et al. (1977)

Much of these data were collected in a nonrandom fashion and response criteria were often too broad and subjective. As a generalization, the alkylating agents cyclophosphamide, melphelan, thiotepa, and chlorambucil are regarded as interchangeable. Cyclophosphamide has enjoyed the most frequent use because of its oral availability and relatively predictable and short-lived bone marrow suppression. The other first-line cytotoxic agents are the antimetabolites 5-fluorouracil and methotrexate, the vinca alkaloids, and the anthracycline antibiotic adriamycin.

Adriamycin was the last of these first-line agents to be introduced into clinical practice, and is the most active single agent yet available. Unfortunately, it is also the most toxic of breast cancer antineoplastics frequently causing profound nausea and vomiting, alopecia, and cytopenias. Various schedules have been attempted to try to decrease toxicity and increase patient acceptance. Dose-response studies suggest that high-dose therapy can probably be tailored to an every three-to-five-week schedule (Knight et al. 1979), but lower doses given more frequently are unfortunately associated with a significant loss of efficacy (Creech et al. 1980), despite a lesser incidence of cardiomyopathy. Thus, a variety of effective single-agent drugs with varying toxicities and different mechanisms of actions are currently available. Several second-line agents such as asparaginase (Yap et al. 1979) and mitomycin (Godfrey 1979) also show significant single-agent responses. However, responses to single agents are generally short-lived and incomplete, and only rarely associated with meaningful prolongation of life. Table 22.2 summarizes the mode of action of the commonly used chemotherapy agents.

The parallels to Hodgkin's disease are too similar to ignore. Here, too, exists a disease that has evidenced responsiveness to a variety of different agents manifesting as short-term incomplete responses. As experience with the Mustargen-Oncovin-procarbazine-prednisone (MOPP) regimen accumulated, a similar well-controlled prospective study emerged from the National Cancer Institute. This study (Canellos et al. 1976) carefully compared single agent treatment with L-phenylalanine mustard to a cyclical combination of cyclophosphamide, methotrexate, and 5-fluorouracil (CMF) and documented a superior response rate (53% VS. 21%) with survival advantage. Data with other relatively similar combinations began to emerge from other centers (Mouridsen et al. 1977; Greenspan 1969) clearly documenting higher response rates, improved survival, and for the first time, consistent complete response in about 25% of responding patients. This data generally showed a doubling of survival in patients who manifested a measurable partial response compared with nonresponders. Complete responders manifested a threefold increase of median survival.

Adriamycin-based combinations were studied most actively by the various cooperative groups and at M. D. Anderson Hospital in Houston. When adriamycin was substituted for methotrexate and compared with CMF (Smalley et al. 1977), it evidenced a higher response rate

Table 22.**2** Mechanism of action

Agent	Mechanism
Melphelan Cyclophosphamide	Alkylate DNA by forming covalent bonds with nucleic acid, usually at the N^7 position of guanine. This may lead to inaccurate base pairing, single-strand breakage, and cross linking. Act on cells both in and out of cell cycle, but more active against rapidly dividing cells.
5-Fluorouracil	Antimetabolite that binds thymidylate synthetase and inhibits DNA synthesis. Also interferes with RNA function.
Methotrexate	Antifolate antimetabolite that inhibits dihydrofolate reductase, thus diminishing the synthesis of purine nucleotides and thymidylate. This inhibition can be reversed by administration of a reduced folate such as leucovorin.
Vincristine Vinblastine	Plant alkaloids that cause metaphase arrest by binding to tubulin, thus affecting the microtubule spindles which chromosomes migrate along during mitosis.
Adriamycin	Fungal produced antibiotic which acts by intercalation of DNA, producing oxidation-reduction reactions, chelating divalent cations, and reacting directly with cell membranes.

with little difference in median survival. This combination did, however, offer more efficacy in the two particularly poor strata of disease: hepatic and lymphangitic pulmonary involvement. Unfortunately, attempts at adding adriamycin to CMF did not particularly improve responses or survival (Tranum et al. 1978). Further efforts at increasing responses, particularly complete responses, by alternating cycles of non-cross-resistant agents have also yielded little to date (Brambilla et al. 1978). At this time, it would appear that either of these three drug regimens offer the patient the maximal potential benefit.

However, this is not to say that all patients to be treated with chemotherapy require multiagent treatment. Combination therapy should be used for patients who present with explosive disease, marrow infiltration, hepatic involvement, poor general condition, and short disease-free interval. Patients who show less ominous prognostic factors should first be considered for hormonal intervention and are also reasonable candidates for sequential single-agent chemotherapy.

One may also consider the possibility of a combined approach using both hormonal intervention and chemotherapy. There seems to exist a reasonable amount of data to justify this approach in the premenopausal patient. The Mayo group (Ahmann et al. 1977) compared oophorectomy alone with oopherectomy plus cyclophosphamide, fluorouracil, and prednisone. The group treated with a combination of drugs yielded higher response rates and improved survival with median disease control of 53 weeks vs 17 weeks. The median survival of 131 weeks was also significantly better than 88 weeks in the oophorectomy-alone group. The Swiss Cooperative Group used CMF plus vincristine and prednisone (CMFVP) chemotherapy as their control and oophorectomy as a variable and found little significant difference in responses or survival.

A similar study using cytoxan, adriamycin, and fluorouracil (CAF) also failed to reveal any differences (Arraztoa and Ramirez 1981). Unfurtonately, none of these studies were justified by receptor data and it is quite likely that significant benefit in receptor-positive patients may be seen in future protocol investigation. To date, there are no impressive data suggesting benefit using both modalities concurrently in the postmenopausal patient, but once again adequate receptor statistics are lacking.

Hormonal Intervention

Soon after Beatson's report of the beneficial effects of oophorectomy, several others followed (Boyd 1900). These documented in larger numbers that about one third of premenopausal patients could benefit from oophorectomy. What is most remarkable about this work is how little was known about endocrine or ovarian function at that time. Estrogen was not identified until 1929 (Doisey 1929), and it wasn't until 1938 that diethylstilbesterol was produced (Dodds et al. 1938). The potential role for additive hormonal therapy in postmenopausal patients was not conclusively documented until Maddow's work was published (Maddow et al. 1944). This, coupled with Ulrich's two reported cases documenting responses to androgens (Ulrich 1939), opened the door for additive hormonal therapy and provided widespread acceptance for this modality. As endocrinology and pharmacology developed, the numbers of various agents and procedures proliferated, and despite relative disparities certain criteria and patterns of responsiveness became clear when looking for probable hormonal dependence.

Most studies suggest that a disease-free interval of less than two years predicts against hormonal response. Biologically explosive disease also is unlikely to benefit by hormonal manipulation. Stratification by sites of metastases also clearly predicts for unresponsiveness in patients with central nervous system involvement or with all but indolent hepatic spread. Thus, the sites most likely to respond are the soft tissues, lymph nodes, lungs, and skeleton. Although most responses are less than complete, they generally persist for six to twelve months and provide a clear survival advantage. Close to 50% of hormonal responders will then respond again to further hormonal manipulation (Kennedy et al. 1964), adding further to their survival advantage.

However, as we shall soon see, with the advent and maturation of cytotoxic therapy, it became increasingly clear that a more precise method was needed to predict for hormonal responses. Attempts to discriminate responsiveness on the basis of hormonal profiles was the first scientific thrust into this area. These investigations were based on unproved postulates about hormone metabolite excretion and prospective analysis of even the most sophisticated discriminate profiles failed to confirm predictability.

Hormone Receptors

As newer cytotoxic agents became available and the efficacy of combination chemotherapy progressively developed, enthusiasm for hormonal intervention began to lessen. The inability to predict for responsiveness and the need to wait for two to three months to determine hormonal response seemed unacceptable to many clinicians. What was clearly needed was some mechanism that could predict that a response to hormonal manipulation was likely. By the late 1950s, a great deal of work was occurring in the areas of hormone uptake by target tissues. The initial report of labeled estrogen uptake by human breast cancer soon followed (Folca et al. 1961). In their patients they documented higher uptake in metastases at the time of adrenalectomy in responsive patients compared with nonresponders. The pieces began to fall more clearly into place by 1967 when Jensen demonstrated that the primary tumors of patients which could accumulate in vitro radioactive-labeled estrogen predicted for in vivo hormonal responsiveness and that the absence of uptake was associated with refractiveness to hormonal intervention. Jensen documented that there existed in the cytoplasm of these responsive tumors a specific receptor protein. He was later able to document that there existed in hormonal target tissue a two-step mechanism whereby the receptor was transferred to the cell's nucleus (Jensen et al. 1968).

Although there still exists considerable uncertainty regarding the exact interactions that follow, the currently held concensus is that bound estrogen in the plasma passes through the cell membrane by diffusion and is actively retained in the cytoplasm where it binds to its specific receptor to form an activated complex. This transformed molecule is then translocated to the nucleus where there exists nuclear acceptor sites on the chromatin (Puca et al. 1974). Transcription is effected at the level of DNA and messenger RNA is coded to alter protein synthesis. It is this new message which initiates tumor cell regression.

A wide variety of other hormonal receptors have been identified in human breast cancer. These include progesterone, androgen, prolactin, thyroid hormone, insulin, glucocorticoid, and calcitonin. Receptors for retinoids and vitamin D have also been elucidated. The roles, interactions, and implications of most of these remain speculative. The best studied has been the progesterone receptor. In mammalian species this receptor would appear to be estrogen dependent and regulated. It has been speculated that the presence of this receptor might then increase the predictability of hormonal responsiveness as its quantification should indicate the presence of malignant cells sophisticated enough to express an estrogen-triggered stimulus via a nuclear-mediated event.

As a generalization, about 50% of all primary tumors contain estrogen receptor. If metastases are analyzed, this figure falls a little (Allegra et al. 1980). Postmenopausal patients are more likely to have estrogen-receptor-positive tumors and quantification confirms higher values than in premenopausal women (Maguire et al. 1975; Lippman and Allegra 1978). This disparity was first thought to be due to the inability to recognize and measure bound receptors in endogenously estrogen-rich premenopausal patients. However, as more sophisticated methods were developed to unbind and measure presaturated receptor, this disparity persisted. This may reflect other hormonal interactions or just be further evidence for the heterogeneity of this disease.

There seems to be no relationship between tumor size, location, or nodal status and the presence of receptors. Those factors associated with low receptor status are obesity, poor cellular differentiation, and the presence of lymphocytic infiltration (Siebert and Lippman 1982). The lowest rates for receptor positivity are seen in perimenopausal patients (Kiang and Kennedy 1977). It is interesting to note that ER-negative tumors tend to have higher rates of tritiated thymidine incorporation than ER-positives (Silvestrini et al. 1979), and that receptor-negative patients show recurrence of tumor growth both sooner and more often than otherwise comparable ER-positive patients (Hahnel et al. 1979).

Clinical response to endocrine therapy is correlated to the presence and amount of estrogen receptor protein. About 60% of Er-positive tumors will respond compared with less than 10% of ER-negative tumors. Subsequent loss of response in initially responsive ER-positive patients is usually due to the development of receptor-negative clones, and analyses of receptor from emerging new sites of disease have documented this (Allegra et al. 1980). The 40% incidence of hormonal failure of initial therapy in ER-positive patients is not totally clear, but in about half of these cases it can be documented that only the cytoplasmic receptor is present with minimal to undetectable amounts of nuclear receptor (MacFarlane et al. 1980). In this circumstance, one would expect the progesterone receptor to likewise be absent. Close to 50% of ER-positive patients will be found to be PR-positive. These patients have a response rate in the range of 70% to 80% (Bloom et al. 1980; McGuire 1980). Response rates for ER-positive PR-negative and the converse generally run in the 30% range.

Response rates generally are higher for postmenopausal women, and within the groupings by menopausal status younger premenopausal and younger postmenopausal patients manifest lesser response rates than their older counterparts (Dao 1972). Response rates are generally similar whether one uses ablative, additive, or antiestrogenic intervention if one stratifies patients according to menopausal status, receptor characteristics, and predominate sites of involvement. Soft tissue disease is the most responsive with response rates usually in the 70% range. This falls to about 40% for ER-positive patients with bone disease. Responses with visceral disease vary, but generally are in excess of 50% for parenchymal lung and pleural metastases. Indolent liver involvement may be quite responsive (Lippman 1980), but aggressive hepatic, pulmonary lymphangitic, and central nervous system metastases are usually unresponsive.

Attempts to predict subsequent responses to chemotherapy on the basis of receptor data are controversial. Several studies have suggested a strong correlation (Kiang et al. 1978; Samal et al. 1980; Young et al. 1980), but at present there is not yet enough data to clarify this issue. It is possible that this information will be understandable when analyzed by sites of involvement or in relation to which cytotoxic agents were used.

The presence of receptors predicts for responsiveness but does not direct the choice of therapy. The role of ablative surgery other than oophorectomy is debatable and diminishing, particularly in view of recent advances with antihormone therapy. The choice of agents for conventional additive hormonal therapy is usually a matter of physician preference and patient tolerance. Current choices in terms of antihormonal intervention include the antiestrogen, tamoxifen, or medical adrenalectomy with aminoglutethimide.

Surgical adrenalectomy was first used by Huggins in 1952. Responses in ER-positive tumors occur about 50% of the time. The procedure carries with it significant morbidity and a life-long need for exogenous steroid replacement. This operation can now be mimicked medically with aminoglutethimide and controlled prospective results are similar to either adrenalectomy or hypophysectomy (Harvey et al. 1979; Santen et al. 1982). The mechanism of action of this agent mimics surgery by first suppressing de novo steroid synthesis via the inhibition of the conversion of cholesterol to pregnenolone. This inhibition is relatively complete yet reversible once the drug is stopped in terms of cortisol production, but less so for adrenal androgens. The adrenal gland produces no estrogens, but the adrenal androgen, androstanedione, is converted by peripheral aromatization to estrone and estradiol. Aminoglutethimide also acts to block this aromatase-mediated reaction, thus effectively eliminating endogenous estrogen production.

The role for the use of antiestrogens logically followed the elucidation of the estrogen receptor. These agents are amino-ether polycyclic phenols and are structurally similar to synthetic estrogens. Early studies were done with clomiphene, nafoxidine, and tamoxifen; but the first two have been rejected because of excessive toxicity. Initially, it was believed that this agent functioned by competitively binding to cytoplasmic estrogen receptor. However, it is now clear that this complex does translocate to the nucleus and current studies are looking at the probable existence of a specific antiestrogen receptor site. Further evidence for the likelihood of a direct effect is the lack of elevation of follicle-stimulating levels in premenopausal patients treated with this agent (Pritchard et al. 1981).

Radiation Therapy

It must be remembered that radiotherapy has a continuing role in patients with disseminated disease. Localized and short-term treatment to patients with bone metastases can particularly offer pain relief. Cutaneous recurrence can be treated with either conventional x-ray or electron beam therapy. Excellent palliation may be provided for those with cerebral metastases. The ovaries can also be radiated when ablative hormonal therapy is indicated; however, a worsening of marrow suppression and possibly immunosuppression may occur when x-ray and chemotherapy are used concomitantly or even sequentially. The reader is referred to Chapter 20 on radiation treatment for a substantive review of the overall role of radiation therapy.

Adjuvant Therapy

If one perceives breast cancer as a systemic disease at presentation, then the role of surgery becomes less imperative. Surgery can be viewed as an attempt to achieve local control, assist in staging, and diminish tumor burden. By diminishing tumor burden, one might allow for an improved immune response to possible microscopic residuals. Paradoxically, it is quite clear from animal studies that size reduction of a tumor often leads to a kinetic stimulus for residual malignant cells. It is these rapidly growing cells that are most vulnerable to cytotoxic therapy.

In order to design a study to look at an adjunctive therapy, certain requisites must be met. First, a staging system that adequately predicts for risk is needed. Next, one requires an interventive therapy- – whether it be cytotoxic or hormonal – that has demonstrated responsiveness in the management of systemic disease. One then must carefully account for variables and monitor potential adverse effects while trying to account for results in an unbiased, randomized and prospectively controlled fashion.

The first attempt at an adjuvant study structured in this manner was by the NSABP (Fisher et al. 1975). This was stimulated by necessity, prior controversial studies looking at the role of prophylactic castration, and encouraging results with adjunctive chemotherapy in children with Wilm's tumors. The NSABP study used perioperative thiotepa in a randomized double-blind fashion comparing the Halsted radical mastectomy plus thiotepa with the operation alone. The drug was given immediately postoperatively and for the next two days in relatively small doses. Initially, no obvious survival difference was noted. However, careful observation of the data revealed that in the subset of premenopausal patients with four or more involved axillary nodes, there existed a 20% survival advantage that persisted for ten years. A similar study using six days of cyclophosphamide postoperatively in Scandinavia (Nissen-Meyer et al. 1978) likewise documented benefit in both disease-free and actual survival for all patients regardless of menopausal status.

The past decade has brought many other adjuvant studies to our attention. Most successful among these have been the NSABP trial in the United States (Fisher et al. 1978) and the National Cancer Institute study in Milan (Bonadonna et al. 1976). The NSABP study looked at the role of oral L-phenylalanine mustard (L-PAM) used in five-day courses every six weeks for two years. To date it has

revealed a persistent and statistically significant disease-free survival for premenopausal patients. Hopefully, this will translate into a survival advantage. This study, however, has failed to show any advantage for postmenopausal patients.

The Milan study used the conventional CMF regimen monthly for one year. Premenopausal patients stratified as having either one to three involved nodes or four or more have shown statistically significant improvement in both disease-free and absolute survival. The data for postmenopausal patients have been less clear. This group initially appears to have a transient disease-free survival benefit, which disappears at three years. However, when Bonadonna retrospectively segregated patients on the basis of percentage of ideal dose of drug received, he found that those patients who received 85% or more of the recommended dose indeed have both disease-free and survival advantages that are statistically significant and similar to the premenopausal group (Bonadonna 1981). There exist other smaller studies that seem to confirm this advantage. More recently, the Milan group has looked at a six-cycle CMF regimen. Initially it was felt that the results were virtually the same, but at the recent American Society of Clinical Oncology meeting, Bonadonna reviewed his six-year experience with the six-cycle regimen. The overall results for this program now suggest improved disease-free survival for all subsets of patients treated with the six-cycle program compared with the previous twelve-cycle study regardless of menopausal or nodal status.

The role of adjuvant hormonal therapy is still uncertain. Variable reports exist in the older literature regarding oopherectomy. The first attempt at a controlled randomized study (Cole 1970) utilized ovarian irradiation and revealed a prolonged disease-free interval without survival benefit. The Toronto study (Meakin et al. 1977) suggested improved survival and disease-free interval for all premenopausal women similarly treated, but this was statistically significant only for patients who were premenopausal but over 45 years of age and taking daily corticosteroids. There exist two significant studies (Hubay et al. 1980; Fisher et al. 1981) that imply that tamoxifen used with cytotoxic adjuvant therapy will add to the disease-free interval for patients who are receptor positive. However, follow-up is as yet short and the design of each study is easily criticized. There are currently several well-designed studies that should better address this issue.

At this time even the most optimistic among us can only speak of a projected 10% to 20% survival advantage with adjuvant therapies. Whether this can be improved by earlier initiation of therapy, more intense therapy with multiple or alternating non-cross-resistant regimens, changes in timing or duration of treatment, synergism with hormonal intervention, or perhaps the development of efficacious biologic response modifiers remains to be seen.

References

Ahmann, D. L., M. J. O'Connell, R. G. Hahn, et al.: An evaluation of early or delayed adjuvant chemotherapy in premenopausal patients with advanced breast cancer undergoing oophorectomy. N. Engl. J. Med. 297: 356–360, 1977

Allegra, J. C., A. Barlock, K. K. Huff, et al.: Changes in multiple or sequential estrogen receptor determinations in breast cancer. Cancer 45: 792–794, 1980

Arraztoa, J., C. Ramirez: Chemotherapy with and without hormone manipulations in the treatment of advanced breast cancer. A collaborative study of the Wisconsin Clinical Cancer Center and the Chilean Cooperative Group. Proc. Am. Assoc. Cancer Res. 435 (abstr.): C–40, 1981

Bloom, N. D., E. H. Tobin, B. Schreibman, et al.: The role of progesterone receptors in the management of advanced breast cancer. Cancer 45: 2992–2997, 1980

Bonadonna, G., P. Valagussa: Dose-response effect of adjuvant chemotherapy in breast cancer. N. Engl. J. Med. 304: 10–15, 1981

Bonadonna, G., et al.: Multimodal therapy with CMF in resectable breast cancer with positive axillary nodes: The Milan Institute Experience. In S. E. Salmon, S. E. James: Adjuvant Therapy of Cancer III. Grune and Stratton, New York, 1981

Boyd, S.: On oophorectomy in cancer of the breast. Br. Med. J. 1161, 1900

Brambilla, C., P. Valagussa, G. Bonadonna: Sequential combination chemotherapy in advanced breast cancer. Cancer Chemother. Pharmacol. 1: 35–39, 1978

Brunner, K. W., R. W. Sonntag, P. Alberto, et al.: Combined chemotherapy and hormonal therapy in advanced breast cancer. Cancer 39: 2923–2933, 1977

Canellos, G. P., S. J. Pocock, S. G. Taylor, et al.: Combination chemotherapy for metastatic breast carcinoma. Prospective comparison of multiple drug therapy with L-phenylalanine mustard. Cancer 38: 1882–1886, 1976

Carter, S. K.: Integration of chemotherapy into combined modality treatment of solid tumors. Cancer Treat. Rev. 3: 141–174, 1976

Cole, M. P.: Prophylactic compared with therapeutic x-ray artificial menopause. Second Tenovus Workship on Breast Cancer pp 2–11, 1970

Creech, R. H., R. B. Catalano, M. K. Shah: An effective low-dose adriamycin regimen as secondary chemotherapy for metastatic breast cancer patients. Cancer 41: 2073–2077, 1978

Dao, T. L.: Ablation therapy for hormone-dependent tumors. Ann. Rev. Med. 21: 1–18, 1972

Doisey, E. A., C. D. Veler, S. Thayer: Folliculin from urine of pregnant women. Am. J. Physiol. 90: 329–330, 1929

Fisher, B., et al.: Treatment of primary breast cancer with chemotherapy and tamoxifen. N. Engl. J. Med. 305: 1–6, 1981

Fisher, B., et al.: Ten year follow-up results of patients with carcinoma of the breast in a cooperative clinical trial evaluating surgical adjuvant chemotherapy. Surg. Gynecol. Obstet. 140: 528–534, 1975

Fisher, B., et al.: L-phenylalanine mustard (L-PAM) in the management of premenopausal patients with primary breast cancer. Cancer 44: 847–857, 1979

Folca, P. J., R. F. Glascock, W. J. Irvine: Studies with tritium labelled hexoestrol in advanced breast cancer. Lancet 2: 796–798, 1961

Godfrey, T. E.: Mitomycin-C breast cancer. In: Mitomycin-C: Current Status and New Developments. Academic Press, New York 1979

Gottlieb, J. A., S. E. Rivkin, S. C. Spigel, et al.: Superiority of adriamycin over oral nitrosoureas in patients with advanced breast carcinoma. Cancer 33: 519–526, 1974

Greenspan, E. M.: Combination cytotoxic chemotherapy in hormone resistant breast cancer. Proc. Am. Assoc. Cancer Res. 10: 15, 1969

Haddow, A. L., J. M. Watkinson, E. Patterson, P. C. Koller: Influence of synthetic oestrogens upon advanced malignant disease. Br. Med. J. 2: 393, 1944

Hahnel, R., T. Woodings, A. B. Vivian: Prognostic value of estrogen receptors in primary breast cancer. Cancer 44: 671–675, 1979

Harvey, H. A., R. J. Santen, J. Osterman, et al.: A comparative trial of transsphenoidal hypophysectomy and estrogen suppression with aminoglutethimide in advanced breast cancer. Cancer 43: 2207–2214, 1979

Hoogstraten, O., S. L. George, B. Sammal, et al.: Combination chemotherapy and adriamycin in patients with advanced breast cancer. Cancer 38: 13–20, 1976

Hubay, C. A., et al.: In H. T. Mouridsen, T. Palshof: Breast Cancer – Experimental and Clinical Aspects. Pergamon Press, Oxford 1980

Huggins, C., D. M. Bergenstal: Inhibition of human mammary and prostatic cancer by adrenalectomy. Cancer Res. 12: 134–141, 1952

Jensen, E. V.: Hormone receptor studies in human malignancy. In J. E. Harris, S. G. Taylor: Reviews on Endocrine Related Cancer. Stuart Pharmaceutical, Wilmington 1980

Jensen, E.: Hormone dependency of breast cancer. Cancer 47: 2319–2326, 1981

Kennedy, B. J., I. E. Fortuny: Therapeutic castration in the treatment of advanced breast cancer. Cancer 17: 1197–1202, 1964

Kiang, D. T., D. H. Frenning, J. Gay, et al.: Estrogen receptor status and response to chemotherapy in advanced breast cancer. Cancer 46: 2814–2817, 1980

Kiang, D. T., B. J. Kennedy: Factors affecting estrogen receptors in breast cancer. Cancer 40: 1571–1576, 1977

Knight, E. W., J. Horton, T. Cunningham, et al.: Adriamycin: Comparison of a five week schedule with a three week schedule in the treatment of breast cancer. Cancer Treat. Rep. 63: 121–122, 1979

Lippman, M. E., J. C. Allegra, E. B. Thompson, et al.: The relation between estrogen receptors and response rate to cytotoxic chemotherapy in metastatic breast cancer. N. Engl. J. Med. 298: 1223–1228, 1978

Lippman, M. E., J. C. Allegra: Quantitative estrogen receptor analyses: The response to endocrine and cytotoxic chemotherapy in human breast cancer and disease free interval. Cancer 46: 2829–2834, 1980

Lippman, M. E., J. C. Allegra: Estrogen receptor and endocrine therapy of breast cancer. N. Engl. J. Med. 299: 930–934, 1978

MacFarlane, J. K., D. Fleiszer, A. G. Fazekas: Studies on estrogen receptors and regression in human breast cancer. Cancer 45: 2998–3003, 1980

McGuire, W. L.: Current status of estrogen receptors in human breast cancer. Cancer 36: 638–644, 1975

McGuire, W. L., K. B. Horwitz: A role for progesterone in breast cancer. Ann. N. Y. Acad. Sci. 286: 90–100, 1977

McGuire, W. L.: The usefulness of steroid hormone receptors in the management of primary and advanced breast cancer. In H. T. Mouridsen, T. Palshof: Breast Cancer Experimental and Clinical Aspects. Pergamon Press, New York 1980

Meakin, J. W., et al.: In S. E. Salmon, S. E. James: Adjuvant Therapy for Cancer. Elsevier/North Holland Press, Amsterdam 1977

Mouridsen, H. T., T. P. M. Brahm, I. Rahbek: Evaluation of single drug versus multipledrug chemotherapy in the treatment of advanced breast cancer. Cancer Treat. Rep. 61: 47–50, 1977

Nissen-Meyer, R., et al.: Surgical adjuvant chemotherapy: Results with one short course of cyclophosphamide after mastectomy for breast cancer. Cancer 41: 2088–2098, 1978

Pritchard, K. I., A. Malkin, D. Malhen, et al.: The influence of tamoxifen on menstruation and serum hormone levels in premenopausal patients with metastatic breast cancer. Proc. Am. Assoc. Cancer Res. 144 (abstr.): 574, 1981

Puca, G. A., V. Sica, E. Nola: Indentification of a high affinity nuclear acceptor site for estrogen receptor of a calf uterus. Proc. Nat. Acad. Sci. U.S.A. 71: 979–983, 1974

Samal, B. A., S. C. Brooks, G. Cummings, et al.: Estrogen receptors and responsiveness of advanced breast cancer to chemotherapy. Cancer 46: 2925–2927, 1980

Santen, R. J., A. M. H. Brodie: Suppression of oestrogen production as treatment of breast carcinoma: Pharmacological and clinical studies with aromatase inhibitors. In B. J. A. Furr: Hormone Therapy. Clinics in Oncology (1, 77–130). WB Saunders, London 1982

Silvestrini, R., Diadene, M. G., Di Fronzo, G.: Relationship between proliferative activity and estrogen receptors in breast cancer. Cancer 44: 665–670, 1979

Smalley, R. V., J. Carpenter, A. Bartolucci, et al.: A comparison of cyclophosphamide, adriamycin, 5-fluorouracil (CAF) and cyclophosphamide, methotrexate, 5-fluorouracil. inerivstine, prednisone (CMFVP) in patients with metastatic breast cancer. Cancer 40: 625–632, 1977

Tormey, D., et al.: Breast cancer survival in single and combination chemotherapy trials since 1968. Proc AACR and ASCO 18: 64, 1977

Tranum, B., B. Hoogstraten, A. Kennedy, et al.: Adriamycin in combination for the treatment of breast cancer. Cancer 41: 2078–2083, 1978

Ulrich, P.: Testosterone (hormone male) et son role possible dans la traitement de certain cancers du sein. Acta Univ. Int. Cancer 4: 377, 1939

Yap, H. Y., R. S. Benjamin, G. R. Blumenschein, et al.: Phase II Study with sequential L-asparaginase and methotrexate in advanced refractory breast cancer. Cancer Treat. Rep. 63: 77–83, 1979

Yap, H. Y., G. R. Blumenschein, M. J. Keating, et al.: Vinblastine given as continuous five day infusion in the treatment of refractory advanced breast cancer. Cancer Treat. Rep. 64: 279–283, 1980

Young, P. C., C. E. Ehrlich, L. H. Einhorn: Relationship between steroid receptors and response to endocrine therapy and cytotoxic chemotherapy in metastatic breast cancer. Cancer 46: 2961–2963, 1980

Chapter 23

Secondary Lymphedema of the Arm

L. Clodius and M. Földi

In the following text, secondary arm lymphedema due to tumor obstructing the axillary lymphatic and venous outflow is not considered.

What Is Secondary Arm Lymphedema

For the Patient

Swelling of the arm, especially of the dorsum of the hand, is the most unpleasant long-term complication for the patient (Fig. 23.**1**). She can hide her chest wall or have her breast reconstructed to her esthetic satisfaction, but her hand, which might look like a boxing glove, will signal the loss of her breast to everybody. Her arm will suffer from acute and chronic tension pains, fluctuating and diffuse hyperalgesias, and hyperesthesias where it is swollen. The quality of her active life (sports, necessity to wear special clothing) is reduced additionally by the swelling and weight of her arm.

For the Surgeon

The determination of the cause for the swollen arm is most important. By exact and repeated axillary and supraclavicular palpation, tumor involvement of the axilla should be looked for, keeping in mind the preoperative and intraoperative findings of the axilla and the histologic report. If there is fullness of the deltopectoral sulcus, if there is evidence of a cutaneous collateral venous circulation around the axilla, if lymphedema is quickly progressive and involves mostly the upper arm, and if the patient complains of pain and weakness of her arm, axillary tumor growth must be considered and this diagnosis secured or ruled out by biopsy. But even in the absence of lymphedema, when operating and dissecting the axilla for radiation-induced infraclavicular brachial plexus palsy (Clodius 1977; Uhlschmid and Clodius 1978), we have found tumor in the axilla, causing neither lymphatic obstruction nor neurological symptoms.

For the Pathophysiologist (How to Understand Surgery for Lymphedema)

Lymphedema, which is high protein edema, is the swelling of the skin and subcutaneous tissues down to the deep fascia, due to lymph stasis.

During axillary dissection, lymph channels belonging to the deep lymphatic system are resected (Fig. 23.**2**). Subsequent and different clinical evolutions ultimately affect the arm (Fig. 23.**3**). In some patients who suffer acute arm edema following operation, there may be initial complete regression, but it may return following a latent phase of months or even many years (Table 23.**1**). Others never experience any arm swelling. Why do not all patients after axillary dissection develop a swollen arm? If there is a sufficient number of axillary lymph channels remaining or if a sufficient lymphatic collateral circula-

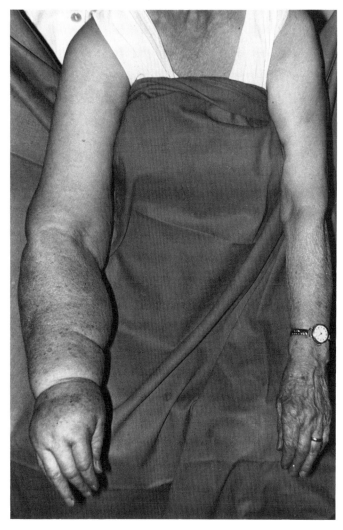

Fig. 23.**1** Typical clinical picture of a patient with secondary postmastectomy lymphedema. The swelling involves mainly the distal arm, where it has overstretched the skin to such a degree that above the wrist a second crease is visible.

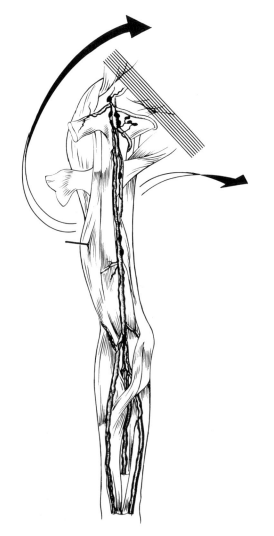

Fig. 23.**2** Schematic representation of the deep lymphatic system of the arm, which is blocked at the axilla. The two arrows represent the collateral lymphatic circulation around the axillary lymph block toward the anterior chest wall and toward the neck.

Table 23.**1** Lenght of latent phase in 1155 cases of arm lymphedema (Gregl et al. 1967)

Time of onset	Lymphedema present
4 month postoperative	40% of all cases
10 month postoperative	68% of all cases
3 years postoperative	89% of all cases

tion involving especially the cephalic lymph system (Kubik et al. 1981) is present, or if a sufficient number of lymphovenous anastomoses are open to handle the lymphatic load of the arm (Malek 1972), then there will be no swelling. Furthermore, the lymphatic transport capacity may be increased through the formation of lympholymphatic anastomoses at the operative site (Halsted 1921; Gray 1939/1940; Reichert 1926; Danese et al. 1962).

In addition to these compensatory lymph-vascular mechanisms, cells of the mononuclear phagocytic system will move into the affected area and along with those already present will rapidly divide (Spector and Ryan 1970). This invasion of cells is aimed at facilitating uptake and proteolytic breakdown of the extravascular accumulated proteins. This cellular mechanism, the "extralymphatic mastering of plasma-proteins" (Földi 1971), (a much underestimated system for the relief of lymphedema) is the basis for the pharmacologic therapy of lymphedema. Summarizing these pathophysiologic events, lymphedema is the combined failure of canalicular lymph drainage and of cellular extralymphatic handling of plasma proteins to cope with a normal lymphatic load.

Why does a patient develop arm lymphedema years following axillary dissection (Table 23.**1**)? Why does a single attack of erysipelas precipitate definitive swelling of an arm, hitherto unaffected by swelling? Experimen-

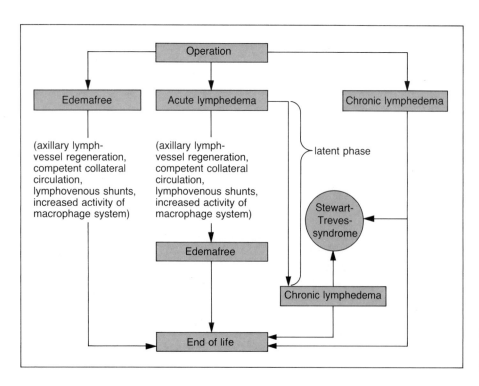

Fig. 23.**3** The possible clinical courses for the arm lymphedema following breast amputation, axillary dissection and/or radiation.

tally, if the deep lymphatics at the root of an extremity are blocked (Clodius and Wirth 1974; Clodius and Altorfer 1977) following an acute postoperative swelling, definitive lymphedema becomes evident after five to six months. However, during this clinically nonedematous latent period, lymphography will demonstrate the typical signs of obstructive lymph stasis; delayed filling of the lymphatics, localized dilatations of the superficial lymphatics, and reversed flow of the contrast medium from the deep towards the superficial lymphatic system (Fig. 23.**4**). In contrast to the lymphograms in definitive lymphedema, deep lymphatics are still visualized and there is no dermal back flow. The histologic pictures (Altorfer et al. 1977) show only a quantitative difference between the prelymphedematous and the manifest state: the lymph channels of both the epicutaneous and subcutaneous lymph systems are dilated, their walls swollen from intracellular and extracellular edema; multiple thrombi, consisting of fibrinoid materials are present in many smaller and larger lymph channels. The connective tissues are at first edematous and gradually sclerose. In one animal, areas of a typical proliferative tissue consisting of an abundance of blood and lymph capillaries and of fibroblasts were found. Histologically, the latent phase as well as manifest lymphedema can be regarded as a form of chronic inflammation (Gaffney and Casley-Smith 1981; Casley-Smith and Gaffney 1981). Why are these changes, summarized in Fig. 23.**5**, at times stable, at times quickly progressive (Fig. 23.**3**)? If the delicate equilibrium between lymphatic protein and water load and lymphatic transport capacity combined with the extralymphatic control of plasmaproteins is disturbed, by one or two remaining lymph channels decompensating under the increased lymphatic load, this ends the latent phase: high protein edema will become visible.

This most important concept of the latent phase has an important bearing on the evaluation of the results for lymphedema surgery. Did our surgical procedure really provide not only an improved but a permanently adequate lymphatic outflow? Was the obstruction completely relieved? Did we sufficiently reduce the relative lymphatic overload and establish definitively a stable balance between the amount of lymph produced and its outflow capacities or did we only return the swollen extremity to the state of latent lymphedema, during which the tissue damage progresses and from which swelling will recur sooner or later? Fig. 23.**6** demonstrates the problem and its mechanism in the experiment: to simulate the disturbances of lymph circulation in congenital annular growes, in the midthigh of the foreleg of a dog, all epifascial lymphatics are blocked by a ring of scar tissue. All of the lymph has to leave the extremity through one subfascial lymph channel. A few months following the lymphblock, the channel, and this is most important, in unobstructed healthy tissue dilates, as it is unable to carry all of the lymphatic load from the leg. This lymph channel, which is provided by nature, could be a well-functioning microsurgically transplanted lymph channel (Baumeister 1981) or a microsurgically constructed lymphovenous shunt (Yamada 1969; Sedlacek 1969; Degni 1974). Nevertheless, if the quantitative law of adequate

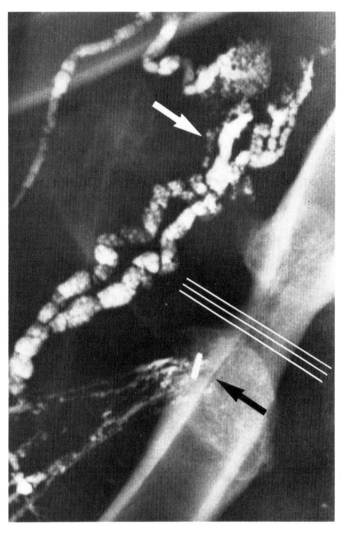

Fig. 23.**4** Experimental block of the deep lymphatic system where the periosteum was also scraped away (three white lines). The contrast medium flows through deep lymphatics toward the site of their interruption by a silver clip (black arrows). The white arrow points to the dilated lymphatics of the superficial system where the lymph flows in reverse direction.

lymph drainage is not fullfilled, if the quantity of the remaining or surgically constructed by-pass channels is inadequate, clinical swelling or lymphedema will be the result.

Arm Lymphedema and Venous Outflow

MacDonald (1948) and MacDonald and Osman (1955) published data on 55 patients who had resections of the axillary vein. This was performed to allow for a more radical excision that included the retrovenous lymph nodes. A statistical analysis of these patients showed no increase in arm swelling. In ten additional patients, cinevenograms were made; these showed that some patients who had lymphedema were free of axillary vein compression. To further substantiate this lack of correlation between venographic appearance and presence of lymphedema, Lobb and Harkins (1949) reported 70 instances of segmental axillary vein resection without lymphedema development. In case of an axillary venous

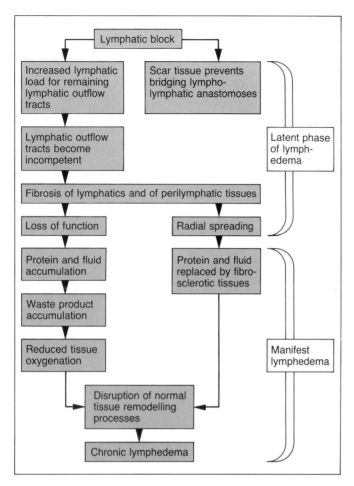

Fig. 23.**5** The pathologic events in the tissues following a lymph-block (from Clodius 1981)

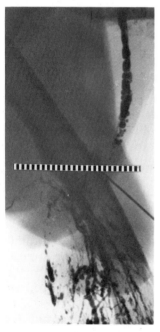

Fig. 23.**6** Lymphogram in experimental lymphedema. The horizontal line shows the site of the lymphatic block. In front of it, multiple dilated lymphatics. In normal tissues an unblocked lymph collector that has to carry all of the lymphatic load from the leg is visualized. But it dilates, since its lymphatic transport capacity is too small for its task.

obstruction, collateral venous circulation is always marked, unless inhibited by gross tumor growth. Elevation of venous pressure would lead to partial or complete blocking of peripheral lymphovenous shunts and to an increase of the lymphatic load, which can be handled by a normal lymphatic system, as it is able to increase its transport capacity by faster and stronger contractions of the lymph channels and by opening up of collateral lymphatics. The authors have never seen a patient whose arm lymphedema had benefited from an axillary venolysis.

Statistics

In the literature, the incidence of secondary arm lymphedema varies betwen 2.7% (Oppolzer 1962) and 72% (MacDonald 1948; MacDonald and Osman 1955). From Gregl's 1 155 patients, whose arms were all measured, one third (33.5%) were affected by arm lymphedema. Of these, 28% were mild (difference in circumference up to 2 cm), 48% moderate (difference in circumference 2 to 6 cm), and 24% were severe (more than 6 cm difference in circumference). It is interesting to note that the incidence of lymphedema in the group of patients with preoperative and postoperative radiation was 2.5 times higher than in patients with postoperative radiation only. In patients with severe lymphedema, postoperative axillary wound complication was present in 78%. Of the 1155 post-mastectomy patients of this series, eleven percent of the prospective lymphedema patients were found three years postoperatively to be still in the latent phase of their arm lymphedema.

After the age of 35, approximately 6% of the female population will develop breast cancer (Dunn 1969; Cutler et al. 1976; Strax 1969). If half of these patients are operated on and if one third of them is affected by lymphedema, 1% of the women after the age of 35 will have a swollen arm.

Conservative Therapy for Secondary Arm Lymphedema

The best therapy is prevention, since conservative therapy is a life-long task and operative therapy, as a rule, does not give good results.

For surgical prophylaxis we consider all of the following points important: Preoperatively, intraoperatively, and postoperatively there should be no intravenous injections or infusions into the arm on the operated side. Shaving of the axilla should be carried out immediately prior to surgery. The incision should not cross the axilla. If the pectoralis major has to be removed, the cephalic vein and the lymphbearing tissues around it must be carefully protected from direct and blunt trauma. Postoperatively, in order to prevent infection, adequate suction drainage is recommended. The drainage tubes should be left in place for about five days, not only to prevent hematoma formation but also to remove the lymph that leaves the cut lymphatic channels. Should a seroma or accumulation of lymph develop anyway, it is not evacuated by spreading the skin edges, but by needle aspiration under rigid asepsis. A moderate axillary compression dressing is applied to aid fast adherence of the mobilized skin; the shoulder is immobilized until healing is complete, since it is motion that produces increased scar formation (Blair 1924), preventing lympholymphatic anastomoses between cut lymphatics. Therefore, no early physiotherapy. We advocate the administration of preoperative antibiotics for three days. Haagensen (1974) stresses the importance of the postoperative care: "I dress my wounds myself. Even with wardpatients, for whom I act as first assistant while my residentsurgeon operates, I supervise the postoperative care of the wound."

If the surgeon knew which arms would develop secondary lymphedema, microsurgical prophylactic anastomoses between the cut lymph channels and veins in the distal axilla and distal to the anticipated field of postoperative irradiation are strongly advisable (Clodius 1977). By preoperative lymphography, with separate compression of the axillary lymphatics, the presence of cephalic lymph collectors could be determined. The authors have not been able to embark on such a program.

Should a swollen arm be treated at all – is it not just a cosmetic problem? Any high protein edema leads to tissue fibrosis and to the events outlined in Fig. 23.5 and to reduction of the function of the arm. In 10% of the patients affected with a lymphedema lasting longer than ten years, lymphangiosarcoma (Steward-Treves syndrome) (McConnel and Haslam 1959), with an average survival of 19 months (Woodward et al. 1972), is a threat. Without therapy, the arms increase in size and harden progressively (Clodius and Piller 1978).

The Patient's Own Care

The detailed education of the patient for the "do's" and "don'ts" (Table 23.2) is of utmost importance. Not only must the patient be motivated to care for her arm, but she must be proud to demonstrate at each visit to her physician at least a slightly thinner and/or softer arm. We refuse any therapy to patients who are not willing to cooperate in this way.

Drug Therapy

For high protein edemas, the benzopyrones frequently have been shown to be the stimulators of the macrophages (Földi and Zoltan 1965; Földi 1972; Bolton and Casley-Smith 1975; Casley-Smith 1976). Breakdown of the abnormally accumulated proteins is enhanced and tissue oxygenation is improved (Casley-Smith and Piller 1974; Clodius and Földi 1976; Piller 1976). The "protein poisoning of the tissues" as outlined in Fig. 23.5 can be halted. The protein fragments, unlike the protein that was dependent on the lymphatic system for its removal, can presumabely leave via the vascular system because of smaller size, a higher diffusion coefficient, and a concentration gradient from the tissues. It has been shown in experimental models of lymphedema that benzopyrones are still effective, even when the lymphatic system is

Table 23.**2** Rules for postmastectomy patients (in part adapted from Nelson, 1966)

Do not permit injections or blood specimens to be drawn from this arm or acupuncture.
Do not permit blood pressure to be taken on this arm.
Do not permit a lymphophlebogram or arteriogram without clear therapeutic indication.
Do not permit biopsies or removal of (remaining) lymphnodes without clear therapeutic indication.
Do not pick or cut cuticles or long nails.
Do not dig in the garden or work near thorny plants.
Do not reach into a hot oven.

Do wear loose-fitting rubber gloves when washing dishes.
Do wear a thimble when sewing.
Do apply a good lanolin-base hand cream several times daily.
Do wear a light breast prosthesis.

Do not permit heat or cold packs to be aplied to your arm.
Do not permit compressing the arm under anesthesia or when this is painful.
Do not permit rough, vigorous massage starting at the hand or forearm.
Do not permit surgery without conservative therapy for one year.
Do not permit long-term diuretics or glucocorticoids.

If any signs and symptoms of erysipelas develop, you must get an appropriate antibiotic immediatly.

completely occluded (Casley-Smith 1976; Casley-Smith and Gaffney 1981). The removal of the excess protein reduces the tendency for further fibrotic tissue formation. Removal of stagnant tissue fluid allows various cells to attain their normal functional capacity, since the conditions of metabolic acidosis associated with stagnating proteinaceous fluid are removed. The removal of excess protein, which is the stimulus for excess collagen formation, also allows for the restoration of the normal remodeling processes of the body to remove fibrosclerotic tissues: clinically this is diagnosed, using tissue tonometry, by softening of the arm (Clodius et al. 1976; Piller and Clodius 1976). The statistics of the clinical results of the use of benzopyrones have been reported (Clodius and Piller 1978, 1980; Piller and Clodius 1981). The calculated predictable time to 0 cm difference in circumference, using 100 mg Cumarin, one tablet each day, is 62 months for the upper arm, 133 months for the forearm, and 39 months for the wrist. This is not a staggering result. But without this ambulatory and cheap therapy, the difference in circumference of the arms increase by 1.3 cm per year (Clodius and Piller 1982). Tissue tonometry showed a gradual softening of the arms. After 17 months of therapy, the tissue tonometry was equal to the normal arm: both arms were of the same softness.

Long-term diuretics should be avoided: the problem of lymphedema is not a reduced renal excretion of water and sodium (Földi 1973). In order to reduce lymphedema, it is necessary to remove the excess of proteins that cause fluid retention. The diuretics shift Starling's equilibrium toward resorption, but resulting dehydration leads to compensatory mechanisms: secretion of aldosterone and antidiuretic hormone. This stimulates retention of water and sodium chloride.

Complex Physical Decongestive Treatment

There is never an absolute lymphatic block between the limb and its root in secondary arm lymphedema. Experimental studies (Clodius 1977) have proved that by creating a total lymph block, the extreme increase of tissue pressure causes skin to rupture and protein-rich edema fluid to leak out in such quantities as to be incompatible with life. Even if all lymphatic channels in the axilla are resected, reversed flow connections still remain between the lymphedematous territory and the bordering normal territory through the superficial dermal lymph plexuses and prelymphatic tissue channels situated in the dermis and in the adventitia of blood wessels (Kubik et al. 1981).

In the majority of cases lymphedema is not restricted to the arm, but involves the homolateral upper quadrant of the trunk; that is, the whole tributary zone of the axillary lymph nodes. This is a most important point to be considered in the technique of complex physical decongestive treatment.

Complex physical decongestive therapy originates from Winiwarter (1892). We apply the centrifugal, not centripetal, massage technique (on an inpatient basis, during which time the patient is fully educated how to optimally care for her arm) as described by Vodder (1957). It must always be started at those central regions of the trunk that border the lymphedematous territory in order to stimulate lymphangiomotoric activity to cope with the sudden increase of the lymphatic load to follow. The second step is the manual evacuation of the most central zone affected by lymphedema. Edema fluid has to be carefully offered to the normal lymphatics previously stimulated without overwhelming them; in this case they will be able to reabsorb and to transport it. As long as the trunk and the root of the extremity have not been freed from edema, no massage is applied to the limb itself. The third step is the evacuation of the proximal part of the upper arm, the fourth that of the distal part of the upper arm, the fifth that of the proximal part of the lower arm, and the sixth that of the distal part of the lower arm. The hand must be evacuated last. Massage is usually applied twice a day, its average duration is 45 minutes. This special massage technique is taught to masseurs, together with training in basic and clinical lymphology in four-week-courses.

The second constituent, quite equivalent to massage, of the treatment applied simultaneously with massage is the bandaging of the limb. During bandaging there is a special kind of remedial exercises and the limb is elevated during rest.

Pneumatic compressive devices are added to the treatment only after the necessary manual evacuation of the trunk and the root of the limb and then under very strict supervision: some patients do not tolerate these devices and react by reaccumulation of edema at the root of the limb. Patients with an additional brachial plexopathy should not be treated by pneumatic compression. Treatment is best controlled by at least weekly volume measurements and clinical examination. It ends with the prescription of elastic sleeves and gloves made to measure. The general principle is to prescribe the highest degree of compression the patient is able to tolerate. Elastic sleeves are never prescribed for patients beginning therapy. The goal of the sleeves is to compensate for the elastic insufficiency of the skin after the successful decongestion achieved by complex physical therapy.

It is a very important question whether the therapeutic effect that has been achieved can be maintained. Fig. 23.7 shows that it can. The figure demonstrates a further interesting fact: a second treatment, given after an interval of 15 months, leads to further decrease of the swelling.

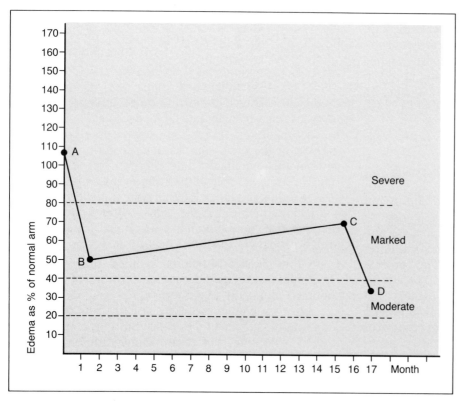

Fig. 23.**7** Amount of edema in percent of the normal arm. A: Before treatment. B: After a first course of treatment. C: 15 months after the first course of treatment but before the second treatment. D: After the second course of treatment.

Surgery for Secondary Arm Lymphedema

Selection of Patients

Only patients with differences in circumference of at least 8 cm for the upper and 6 cm for the lower arm are candidates for surgery, if they are tumor free. All patients are treated preoperatively for at least one year by conservative methods. In our patients there was no change of any conservative therapy before and after surgery. The results are hence uninfluenced by drugs (benzopyrones), elastic sleeves, or complex physiotherapy.

The Problems of Surgery for Lymphedema

In all our surgical attempts, as brilliant as they may be from a technical standpoint, we must distinguish between the biological problem of lymphedema (tissue poisoning by plasma proteins) and the many different surgical possibilities.

Operations to increase the lymphatic outflow from the arm, by-passing the axillary block through lympholymphatic anastomoses (Danese et al. 1962; Calderon et al. 1967; Danese et al. 1968), by microsurgical lymphovenous shunts (Crockett and Goodwin 1962; Yamada 1969; Sedlacek 1969; Degni 1974), or through transplants of lymph collectors (Baumeister 1981), besides providing for a sufficient quantity of outflow channels to master the entire load of the arm, must primarily receive a normal lymphatic inflow: tissue drainage through interstitial tissue channels, initial lymphatics, and lymph collectors must be intact, the functional tissue lymph system unit should not be damaged irreversibly (Clodius and Pepersack 1979; Clodius et al. 1981). In the case shown in Fig. 23.**8**, the lymphogram demonstrates multiple dilated and incompetent lymphatics, which technically can be anastomosed to small veins. The results, however, have been

such that O'Brien and Shafiroff (1979) advocate combining microsurgical lymphovenous shunts with excisions of lymphedematous tissues. Even if a localized lymph block is effectively by-passed through peripheral lymphovenous shunts, relieving completely subjective complaints and normalizing the Patent blue test, we have not observed an important reduction of swelling and fibrosis of the extremity (Clodius 1978; Clodius et al. 1981). But what the patient expects is a normal or only slightly swollen arm.

For more than a century, as outlined above, the traditional concept for the surgeon dealing with lymphedematous extremities consisted of the belief that only the epifascial lymph system was affected by lymphedema (Kondoléon 1912; Lanz 1911; Poirier et al. 1903; Sappey 1874; Thompson 1969). It was, therefore, considered that draining the epifascial lymphatics into the subfascial lymphatics across the barrier of the deep fascia represented a physiologic approach. By clinical lymphangiography and by experiment, it was demonstrated that this concept certainly for secondary lymphedema was wrong (Clodius 1977; Clodius and Wirth 1974; Crockett 1965; Gibson and Tough 1955; Watson 1963). In secondary lymphedema with which our patients are affected, the deep lymphatics are removed at the root of the extremity. The partially or totally interrupted deep outflow must be compensated by the epifascial lymphatics. However, under normal conditions, due to the unidirectional flow provided by the lymphatic valves, the epifascial lymph drains into the deep lymphatic system. Following a deep lymph block, the deep lymph collectors dilate massively and their wall becomes edematous. Between the cellular elements and the collagen fibers, protein-rich material leading to fibrosis is embedded and multiple thrombi occupy the lumen of the lymph channels (Altorfer et al. 1977). This is unfortunate because all or most of the lymph must be drained through the superficial lymphatics, which as the typical lymphogram reveals, become irregular, tortuous, and dilated (Fig. 23.**8**). There is dermal backflow of the contrast medium, which stag-

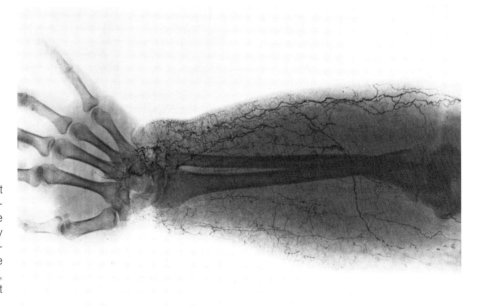

Fig. 23.**8** Typical lymphogram in manifest secondary arm lymphedema. The deep lymphatic system is no longer visualized. There is backflow of the contrast medium distally and into many small, dilated tortuous lymphatics of the subcutis and the skin. These are never outlined under normal conditions, since the reflux is prevented by competent valves.

nates. Unless lymphedema is operated in its latent period or prophylactically as stated above, microsurgical shunts must be performed with these diseased superficial lymphatics.

Results and Complications

The principles of the operation for secondary arm lymphedema are outlined on Figs. 23.**8** and 23.**9**, the details of our surgical technique having been described before (Clodius 1977). The important element is the resection of as much lymphedematous tissue as possible from the epifascial compartment of the arm (Winiwarter 1892; Sistrunk 1927), opening it along the longitudinal axis of the arm (Fig. 23.**9**). This resection carries an important functional element: the reduction of the lymphatic load. As a second step, the thickened deep fascia is removed (Kondoleon 1912, 1938). Following the excision of a large portion of subcutaneous lymphedematous tissue, the skin and the remaining small portion of the subcutis contain per tissue unit a much denser concentration of lymphatics

then the excised fibrosclerotic adipose tissue. The lymph plexus between subcutis and cutis now comes into close contact with the lymph-propelling forces of the muscle pump and of the arterial pulsations. Following additional removal of the thickened deep fascia, these lymphpropelling forces can act more directly.

As a third step of the operation (Fig. 23.**10**), the lateral longitudinal flap is de-epithelialized and buried between extensor and flexor muscles (Thompson 1967). By transposing superficial lymphatics within the flap toward the deep-blocked lymphatics, the rationale, in contrast to Thompson, is to drain lymph from the deep subfascial space toward the surface and laterally around the axillary block (Fig. 23.**9**, 23.**10**B). But this lymphatic by-pass will only function if a sufficient number of lympholymphatic anastomoses between the two systems develop.

Our experience consists of 171 patients with secondary postmastectomy lymphedema. Of these, 28 patients with severe lymphedema, treated conservatively without success for at least one year, were operated on. The amount of reduction of arm circumference is reported both for the

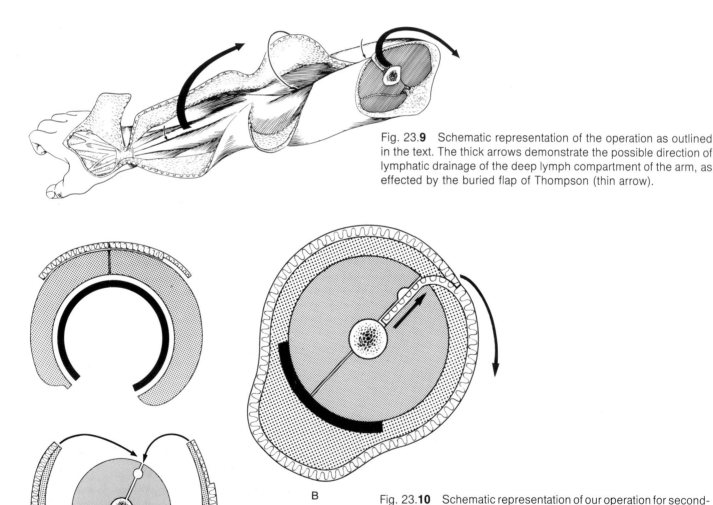

Fig. 23.**9** Schematic representation of the operation as outlined in the text. The thick arrows demonstrate the possible direction of lymphatic drainage of the deep lymph compartment of the arm, as effected by the buried flap of Thompson (thin arrow).

Fig. 23.**10** Schematic representation of our operation for secondary arm lymphedema on cross section. A: in the lower half of the picture the closure following removal of the skin, of fibrosclerotic subcutaneous tissues, and of deep fascia (as shown on the upper half) is seen. B: the lateral de-epithelialized flap of Thompson is inserted into the deep lymphatic compartment and the wound is closed. The arrows demonstrate the possible lymph drainage toward the skin if lympholymphatic anastomoses between the buried flap and the deep lymphatics are able to develop.

Table 23.**3** Long-term surgical results for patients with secondary arm lymphedema

Forearm circumference difference	Postoperative control in years (no. patients)			
	1–3	4–6	7–9	10–12
up to 3 cm	20	2	6	3
3 to 5 cm	6	6	3	3
5 to 6 cm	1	2	–	1
more than 6 cm	1*	–	–	–

* in this patient the arm was amputated elsewhere

upper and for the forearm in Table 23.**3**. Subjectively, there were 27 satisfied patients. They all resumed their normal preoperative occupation. In one patient, within less than two years, the swelling was even worse than preoperatively and her arm was amputated. This patient had been heavily irradiated around her shoulder and her neck, with irradiation changes of her lung and a fracture of the humerus, due to radiation, which healed uneventfully under conservative therapy. This patient might have benefited from the operation of Standard (1942) in which a flap from the inside of the upper arm is switched with a similar one from the chest wall. This procedure is only really suitable for patients who can no longer abduct the affected shoulder, but it certainly reduces the size of the limb and promotes lymph drainage (Hirshovitz and Goldan 1971).

Besides the mentioned amputation of the arm in one patient (error in surgical indication), there were immediate postoperative complications (error in surgical technique): in one patient there was a skin slough of a skinflap at the elbow that needed a split thickness skin graft and in a second patient there was delayed secondary wound healing. This complication rate compares favorably with the only other study on longterm results in such patients (Thompson and Wee 1981).

It is most important that the reader realizes that secondary arm lymphedema, as any extremity lymphedema, cannot be handled as a rule to the patient's satisfaction with one single therapeutic modality. The combination of therapeutic approaches is essentiel: the help and cooperation of the patients, a highly specialized and complex physiotherapy team and, the administration of benzopyrone drugs. Surgery, desirable as a prophylactic measure, is necessary only in the exceptional case.

Acknowledgment

The experimental basis for this work was made possible through generous grants of the Swiss National Fund.

References

Altorfer, J., Chr. Hedinger, L. Clodius: Light and electron microscopic investigation of extremities of dogs with experimental chronic lymphostasis. Folia Angiol. 25: 141, 1977

Baumeister, R. G. H.: Therapeutische Lymphgefäßtransplantation. Fortschr. Med. 99: 418, 1981

Blair, V. P.: The influence of mechanical pressure on wound healing. Illinois Med. 46: 249, 1924

Bolton, T., J. R. Casley-Smith: An in vitro demonstration of proteolysis by macrophages and its increase with coumarin. Experientia 3: 27, 1975

Calderon, G., B. Roberts, L. Johnson: Experimental approach to surgical creation of lymphatic venous communications. Surgery 61: 122, 1967

Casley-Smith, J. R., N. B. Piller: The pathogenesis of edemas and the therapeutic action of coumarin and related compounds. Folia Angiol 3 (suppl.): 33, 1974

Casley-Smith, J. R.: The functioning and interrelationships of blood capillaries and lymphatics. Experientia 32: 1, 1976

Casley-Smith, J. R.: The actions of the benzo-pyrones on the Blood-tissue-lymphsystem. Folia Angiol. 24: 7, 1976

Casley-Smith, J. R.: Functional fine structure of lymphatics. Experientia 32: 818, 1976

Casley-Smith, J. R., R. M. Gaffney: Excess plasma proteins as a cause of chronic inflammation and lymphedema: Quantitative electron microscopy. J. Pathol. 133: 243, 1981

Clodius, L., W. Wirth: A new experimental model for chronic lymphedema of the extremities. Chir. Plast. 2: 115, 1974

Clodius, L., L. Deak, N. B. Piller: A new instrument for evaluation of tissue tonicity in lymphedema. Lymphology 9: 1, 1976

Clodius, L., M. Földi: Eine neue Methode zur Herbeiführung eines numerisch erfaßbaren Gangräns am Kaninchenohr; die therapeutische Wirkung einer Behandlung mit Benzopyronen. Schweiz. Rundsch. Med. Prax. 65: 514, 1976

Clodius, L.: The experimental basis for the surgical treatment of lymphedema. In L. Clodius: Lymphedema. Thieme, Stuttgart 1977

Clodius, L., J. Altorfer: Die Erzeugung einer radikalen Lymphostase beim Hund. Erg. Angiol. 13: 47, 1977

Clodius, L.: Microlymphatic Surgery In R. K. Daniel, J. K. Terzis: Reconstructive Microsurgery. Little Brown, Boston 1978

Clodius, L., N. B. Piller: Conservative therapy for postmastectomy lymphedema. Chir. Plast. 4: 193, 1978

Clodius, L., W. Pepersack: Etude critique de la chirurgie du lymphoedème. Ann. Chir. Plast. 24: 217, 1979

Clodius, L., N. B. Piller: Das sekundäre Armlymphödem: Spontanverlauf, Resultate konservativer und operativer Therapie. Therapiewoche 30: 5182, 1980

Clodius, L., N. B. Piller, J. R. Casley-Smith: The problems of lymphatic microsurgery for lymphedema. Lymphology 14: 69, 1981

Clodius, L., N. B. Piller: The conservative treatment of post mastectomy lymphedema patients with Cumarin. In E. V. Bartos, D. Davidson: Progress in Lymphology. Avicenum Prague 1982

Crockett, A. T. K., W. E. Goodwin: Chyluria: Attempted surgical treatment by lymphatic-venous anastomosis. J. Urol. 88: 566, 1962

Crockett, D. J.: Lymphatic anatomy and lymphedema. Br. J. Plast. Surg. 18: 12, 1965

Cutler, S. J., S. S. Davesa, T. H. C. Barclay: The magnitude of the breast cancer problem. In G. St. Arneault, P. Band, L. Israel: Breast Cancer. Springer, Berlin/Heidelberg/New York 1976

Danese, C., J. M. Howard, R. Brower: Regeneration of lymphatic vessels. Ann. Surg. 156: 61, 1962

Danese, C., R. Brower: Experimental anastomoses of lymphatics. Arch. Surg. 84: 6–9, 1962

Danese, C., A. N. Papaioannou, L. E. Morales, S. Mitsuda: Surgical approaches to lymphatic blocks. Surgery 64: 821, 1968

Degni, M.: New technique of drainage of the subcutaneous tissue of the limbs with nylon net for the treatment of lymphedema. VASA 3: 329, 1974

Dunn, J. E.: Epidemiology and possible identification of high-risk groups that could develop cancer of the breast. Cancer, 23: 775, 1969

Földi, M., Oe. T. Zoltan: Über den Wirkungsmechanismus eines Melitolus-Präparates. Arzneim.-Forsch. 15: 899, 1965

Földi, M.: Erkrankungen des Lymphsystems. Witzstrock, Baden-Baden 1971

Földi, M.: Physiology and Pathophysiology of the Lymphsystem. Handbook of General Pathology. Springer, Berlin/Heidelberg/New York 1972

Földi, M.: Vitamin P and lymphatics. Angiologica 9: 375, 1972

Földi, M.: Sind Diuretika für die Behandlung eines Lymphödems geeignet? Herz Kreisl. 5: 429, 1973

Gaffney, R. M., J. R. Casley-Smith: Excess plasma proteins as a cause of chronic inflammation and lymphedema: biochemical estimations. J. Pathol. 133: 229, 1981

Gibson, T., S. Tough: A simplified one stage operation for the correction of lymphedema of the leg. Arch. Surg. 71: 809, 1955

Gray, H. J.: Studies of the regeneration of lymphatic vessels. J. Anat. 74: 309, 1939/1940

Haagensen, C. D.: Treatment for operable breast carcinoma. Surgery 76: 701, 1974

Halsted, W. S.: The swelling of the arm after operations for cancer of the breast, elephantiasis chirurgica, its cause and prevention. Bull. Johns Hopkins Hosp. 32: 309, 1921

Hirshowitz, B., S. Goldan: A bi-hinged chest-arm flap for lymphedema of the upper limb. Plast. Reconstr. Surg. 48: 52, 1971

Kondoleon, E.: Operative Behandlung der elephaniastischen Oedeme. Zentralbl. Chir. 39: 1022, 1912

Kondoleon, E.: Die Lymphableitung als Heilmittel bei chronischen Oedemen nach Quetschung. Münch. Med. Woschenschr. 59: 525, 1912

Kondoleon, E.: La pathogénie et le traitement de l'elephantiasis. Arch. Ital. Chir. 51: 464, 1938

Kubik, St., M. Manestar, G. Molz: Angioarchitecture of the lymphatic system. In M. Földi: Textbook of Lymphology. Schattauer, Stuttgart 1981

Lanz, O.: Eröffnung neuer Abfuhrwege bei Stauung im Bauch und unteren Extremitäten. Zentralbl. Chir. 38: 3, 1911

Lobb, A. W., H. N. Harkins: Postmastectomy swelling of arm with note on effect of segmental resection of axillary vein at time of radical mastectomy. West. J. Surg. 57: 550, 1949

MacDonald, I.: Resection of the axillary vein in radical mastectomy; its relation to the mechanism of lymphedema. Cancer 1: 618, 1948

MacDonald, I., K. Osman: Postmastectomy lymphedema. Am. J. Surg. 90: 281, 1955

Malek, R.: Lymphaticovenous Anastomoses. In: Handbuch der Allgemeinen Pathologie. Springer Verlag, Berlin/Heidelberg/New York 1972

McConnell, E. M., P. Haslam: Angiosarcoma in post-mastectomy lymphedema. Br. J. Surg. 46: 322, 1959

O'Brien, B., B. B. Shafiroff: Microlymphatic, venous and resectional surgery in obstructive lymphedema. World J. Surg. 3: 3, 1979

Oppolzer, R.: Zur Verhinderung des Armödems nach radikaler Mammaamputation. Wien Klin. Wochenschr. 74: 41, 1962

Piller, N. B.: Drug induced proteolysis. Br. J. Exp. Pathol. 57: 266, 1976

Piller, N. B., L. Clodius: The use of a tissue tonometer as a diagnostic aid in extremity lymphedema: A determination of its conservative treatment with benzo-pyrones. Lymphology 9: 127, 1976

Piller, N. B., L. Clodius: Benzopyrone (Venalot) as a conservative therapy for postmastectomy lymphedema. In H. Weissleder, V. Bartos, L. Clodius, P. Malek: Progress in Lymphology. Avicenum, Prague 1981

Poirier, P., B. Cueno, G. Delamere: The Lymphatics. Constable, London 1903

Reichert, F. L.: The regeneration of lymphatics. Arch. Surg. 13: 871, 1926

Sappey, P. C.: Anatomie, Physiologie, Pathologie des Vaisseaux Lymphatiques Considérés Chez l'Homme et les Vertebrés. Dela Laye, Paris 1874

Sedlacek, J.: Lymphovenous shunt as supplementary treatment of elephantiasis of lower limbs. Acta Chir. Plast. 11: 157, 1969

Sistrunk, W. E.: Contribution to plastic surgery. Ann. Surg. 85: 185, 1927

Spector, W. G., G. B. Ryan: The mononuclear phagocyte in inflammation. In R. von Furth: Mononuclear Phagocytes. University Press, Oxford 1970

Standard, S.: Lymphedema of the arm following radical mastectomy for carcinoma of the breast; new operation for its control. Ann. Surg. 116: 816, 1942

Strax, Ph.: Mass screening in control of breast cancer. In L. Venet: Breast Cancer. SP Medical and Scientific Books, New York/London 1979

Thompson, N.: The surgical treatment of chronic lymphedema of the extremities. Surg. Clin. North Am. 47: 445, 1967

Thompson, N.: The surgical treatment of advanced postmastectomy lymphedema of the upper limb. Scand. J. Plast. Surg. 3: 54, 1969

Thompson, N., J. T. K. Wee: Twenty years experience of the buried dermis flap operation in the treatment of chronic lymphedema of the extremities. Chr. Plast. 5: 58, 1981

Uhlschmid, G., L. Clodius: Eine neue Anwendung des frei transplantierten Omentums. Chirurgia 49: 12, 1978

Vodder, E.: Lymph-drainage. Kosm. Fachztg. Nr. 59, 1957

Watson, T. A., A. F. Bond, A. J. Phillips: Swelling and dysfunction of the upper limb following radical mastectomy. Surg. Gynecol. Obstet. 116: 99, 1963

Winiwarter, A.: Die elephantiasis. In: Deutsche Chirurgie. F. Enke, Stuttgart 1892

Woodward, A. H., J. C. Ivins, E. H. Soule: Lymphangiosarcoma arising in chronic lymphedematous extremitites. Cancer 30: 562, 1972

Yamada, Y.: Studies on lymphatic venous anastomosis in lymphedema. Nagoya J. Med. Sci. 32: 1, 1969

Chapter 24

Treatment of Local Recurrences and Postradiation Lesions

W. Mühlbauer and R. R. Olbrisch

Local Recurrences after Carcinoma of the Breast

Local recurrence after surgical treatment of mammary carcinoma may occur within the scar itself, sometimes only as small microscopic areas, within the operative field, in the chest wall, or in the axilla. These are early signs of a systemic dissemination. In more than 90% of local recurrences, a disseminated disease is present. They rarely originate from tumor cells left behind at the time of operation or surviving after radiation. From a biologic point of view they should be regarded as metastases and be treated accordingly (Bruce et al. 1970; Dao and Neomoto 1963; Marshall et al. 1974; Stjernswärd 1977). In most larger series the majority of local recurrences will be diagnosed within the first two years (75% according to Ungeheuer and Lüders 1978; 66% according to Heberer et al. 1981) In isolated cases, however, we have seen local recurrence and distant metastases thirty years or longer after primary treatment. To what degree postoperative radiation to the chest wall and the axilla could prevent local recurrence is questionable. (See Chapter 20, p. 189.) According to Turnball et al. (1978) and Weichselbaum et al. (1976), postoperative radiation significantly reduces the appearance of local recurrence from about 10%–15% to 5%. The survival rate, however, does not become better since this is dependent on disseminated disease that is uninfluenced by local radiation. To achieve the desired effect, high doses of at least 5,000 rads (50 Gy) must be given (Fletcher 1972). The recurrent tumor often shows a histologic picture of lower differentiation and wilder growth, thus being more malignant.

Local recurrence can often be easily diagnosed as nontender lumps with adjacent adherence within or under the skin. Excision biopsy and histology will rapidly confirm the diagnosis. In order to plan for therapy, the involvement of surrounding tissues such as muscles, ribs, and brachial plexus and possibly disseminated disease as well has to be checked.

Local Effect of Radiation

Any treatment with ionizing radiation necessarily causes damage to the skin and underlying structures even if this is not always seen macroscopically. The changes start in the small blood vessels as radiation-induced obliterative endarteritis. To this is added a general fibrosis of the tissue as well as direct damage to the cells with changes in their chromosomes, which prevent normal cell recovery and reproduction. Local lymphedema, increased hyalinization of elastic fibers and thrombosis of arterioles and venules with time causes disturbances of nutrition in local tissue. This gives rise to poorly healing ulcerations (Figs. 24.1, 24.2), which with time almost always become malignant (Robinson 1975). According to Schultz-Ehrenburg (1980), this happens after a latency period of 4 to 40 years. The appearance of these visible lesions is dependent on radiation dose, type of radiation, and modality of application. With modern high-voltage ther-

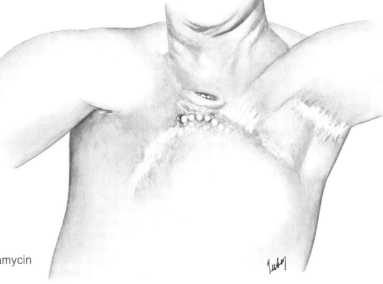

Fig. 24.**1** Radiation ulcers in the sternal region with gentamycin Palacos pearls after bilateral mastectomy.

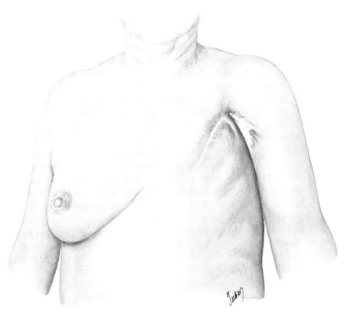

Fig. 24.**2** Radiation ulcer in the axilla after mastectomy with progressive paresis of plexus and pain.

apy, this type of lesion is seen less frequently. Depending on the quality of radiation, the maximum dose as an effective accumulation lies at a depth of 0.5 to 6 cm; this means that skin no longer receives the heaviest radiation. The risk of a carcinoma induced by radiation, however, increases with the accumulated dosage (Schultz-Ehrenburg 1980). Accordingly we speak of radiation sequelae when we have a so-called radiodermatitis; that is, an unelastic, hard, edematous, or already atrophic skin with telangiectasia and both depigmentration and hyperpigmentation or a true radiation ulcer with or without radiation-induced carcinoma. Other less frequent sequelae of radiation are radionecrosis of ribs or the clavicle as well as fibrosis of the pleural and pulmonary parenchyma. These will be difficult to distinguish from metastases and may also effect the heart. The not uncommon lesions of the brachial plexus also belong to this group. They produce progressive paralysis of motor or sensory function and severe night pains. Lymphedema of the arm with reduced mobility is another sequela of radiation. Skin metastases have a tendency to favor radiated skin areas. In premenopausal women, radiation is seen significantly to increase the rate of distant metastases and to decrease the survival time (Stjernswärd 1977). Other findings may also be related to radiation, such as long-standing lymphopenia, higher frequency of herpes zoster, and locally reduced hypersensitivity reactions in the irradiated skin area.

Indications for Treatment

In isolated local recurrences, surgical excision is the method of choice compared with radiation even when the patient has not had any previous radiation therapy. In cases in which there are also distant metastases, an excision of local recurrences reduces the tumor mass,

which itself allows a better effect of cytostatic treatment; but as the cancer in this state has already become systemic, the future might better be influenced through immunologic measures. The radiodermatitis, through its induration, may effect breathing or arm mobility and should be excised and replaced by smooth mobile skin which provides additional benefit as cancer prophylaxis. Painful, penetrating, sometimes itching radiation ulcers should in any case be surgically treated if only to relieve pain and to facilitate nursing care. Even if survival time were not improved, certainly it will dramatically improve the quality of life.

Indications for surgical revision or attention to a lesion of the brachial plexus after mastectomy and radiation should be very well defined and restricted to very special cases. The operation is technically difficult due to the altered anatomy resultant from radiation fibrosis, is time consuming and may be associated with extensive bleeding from the major vessels, and may even lead to loss of the entire arm. A relative indication for revision is provided by evidence of rapidly progressing paralysis, by severe pain that appears especially during the night, and by any suspicious metastases in the axilla. Absolute contraindications for surgical intervention are a poor prognosis from the underlying tumor, and poor general condition of the patient.

Surgical Treatment

Local recurrence or radiation sequelae should be treated as primary tumors, with adequate margins to the periphery and depth. The margins must be checked histologically using numerous frozen sections. If necessary, ribs, part of the sternum, or even the complete chest wall might have to be resected. Direct closure of the wound may not be possible. To cover the wound with a split-thickness skin graft is often possible, except where underlying chest wall is involved. Split-thickness grafts, in addition, allow early diagnosis of underlying future recurrences. Older textbooks often recommended covering the defect by the use of contralateral breast. This procedure is today abandoned because of the risk involved and the unnecessary mutilation. Most of the large defects have to be covered by well vascularized flaps. These might include:

1. *Free flaps with microvascular anastomosis.* These would be most useful. Most often, however, there would be problems finding good recipient vessels for anastomosis in the neighboring area. The use of larger free vessel grafts to elongate the vascular pedicle increases the risk of thrombosis. This is why, in our experience, this procedure is too insecure.

2. *Rotation flaps* from the surrounding area offer the safest method since their blood supply is locally intact (Olbrisch and Mühlbauer 1978). These flaps, sometimes bilobed (that is employing additional flaps to help cover the defect created by the original flap) from the neighboring area, are most useful in covering wound defects (Figs. 24.**1**, 24.**3**, 24.**4**). In doing this, we try to incorporate the

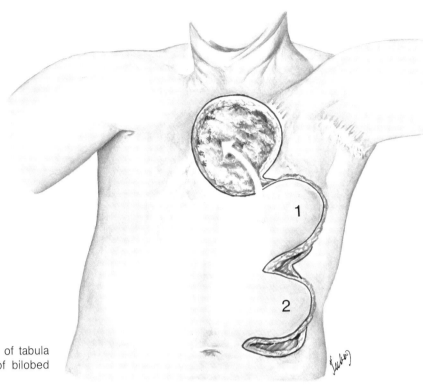

Fig. 24.**3** Excision of ulcer including resection of tabula externa of the sternum. Covered by means of bilobed rotation flaps.

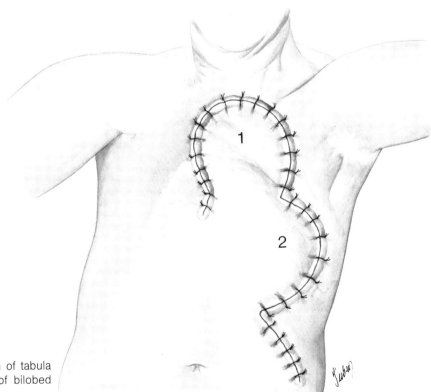

Fig. 24.**4** Excision of ulcer including resection of tabula externa of the sternum. Covered by means of bilobed rotation flaps.

axial vessels such as in the thoracoepigastric flap. Sometimes, however, necrosis in the margin of the flap may occur when occult radiation damage to the small intracutaneous and subcutaneous vessels have been overlooked during the operation. If the deep fascia is incorporated in the flap, a so-called fasciocutaneous flap, the circulation would be safer.

3. *Myocutaneous flaps* have an even better-established circulation and being thicker they are also more stable (Mühlbauer and Olbrisch 1977, Olivari 1976). Of special value in this regard is the latissimus dorsi myocutaneous flap (Figs. 24.**5**, 24.**6**). The donor area lies outside the radiated area. This flap shows a constant axial vessel and nerve supply through the thoracodorsal artery, vein, and

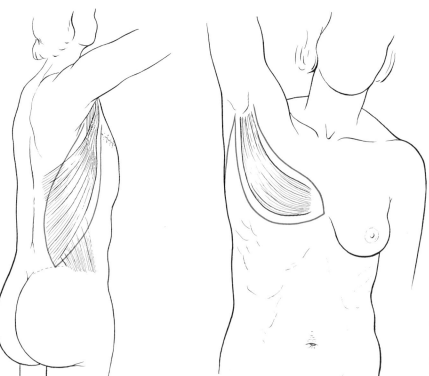

Fig. 24.**5** Schematic representation of a typical myocutaneous latissimus dorsi flap to cover defects at the anterior chest wall and axilla.

Fig. 24.**6** Schematic representation of a typical myocutaneous latissimus dorsi flap to cover defects at the anterior chest wall and axilla.

Fig. 24.**5**   Fig. 24.**6**

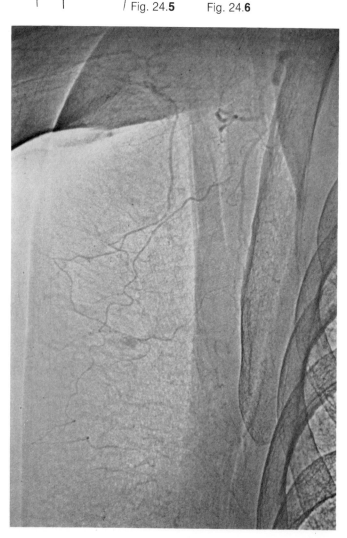

Fig. 24.**7** Preoperative visualization of the thoracodorsal vessels of the donor region of the latissimus dorsi myocutaneous flap by means of transvenous microangiography and xeroarteriography technique according to Kramann et al. (1980).

nerve (Fig. 24.**7**), making it possible to rely on a very narrow and long pedicle. It might even be used as an island flap. The turning point in the posterior part of the axilla makes it useful for covering defects in the shoulder area. Being so long and large, it could cover the complete anterior chest wall as far as the supraclavicular region. Because of the thickness and stability of the flap, it is possible to cover a defect of the chest wall up to a size 10 cm by 10 cm without any further stabilization. After larger resections of the chest wall, we first suture a free dermis graft or a dermis flap into the defect and then cover this with a large latissimus dorsi myocutaneous flap (Figs. 24.**8–11**). The latissimus dorsi, with its good circulation, also offers a very excellent cover for exposed vessels and the nerve plexus in the axilla. The thoracodorsal vessels might have been ligated in the course of a mastectomy or been damaged as a result of a penetrating radiation ulcer. For this reason we recommend always beginning the dissection to prepare the flap in the axilla in order to inspect the thoracodorsal vessels. If in doubt, an angiogram might be done. Particularly gentle and elegant is the transvenous microangiography and xeroarteriography technique according to Kramann et al. (1980). If the latissimus flap is not cut too broadly, it is possible to make a primary closure of the donor area particularly after undermining the wound edges on both sides. In other cases, part of the defect would have to be covered with split-thickness skin grafts. The missing latissimus dorsi muscle does not cause functional problems since its function is compensated by the other muscles of the shoulder and back.

4. *The greater omentum* might be used to cover larger defects of the chest wall and axilla either on a pedicle or as a free microvascular flap; the outer surface is then covered with split skin or a mesh graft. The omentum, however, is sometimes rather thin and may shrink con-

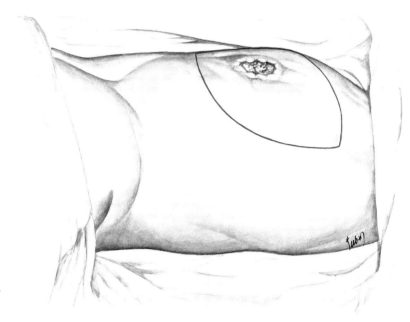

Fig. 24.**8** Ulcerated chest wall recurrence of carcinoma of the breast.

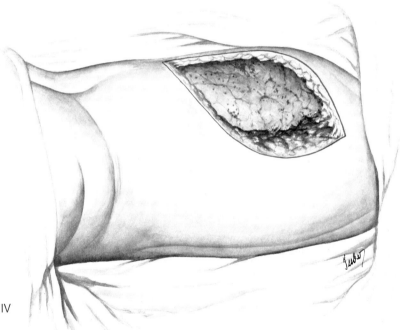

Fig. 24.**9** Resection of chest wall including ribs II to IV and pleura parietalis.

siderably so that its stability will not be sufficient in spite of massive fibrosis. Herniation of the abdominal wall where the pedicle goes through and symptoms of intestinal ileus as a sequela of transposition of the omentum have been reported. Because of these disadvantages and risks, the use of omentum is not a first choice for chest wall coverage.

5. *Distant flaps,* for instance tube flaps, have more historic interest in this age of myocutaneous, fasciocutaneous, and free flaps with microvascular anastomosis. They are also a very time-consuming procedure with many possibilities for complications. Despite extensive resection, at times radiated tissue may be left behind.

This will either be resolved by the adequate circulation of the cutaneous or myocutaneous flaps, through ingrowth of new vessels (biologic excision), or be sloughed by way of a longstanding fistulization without damaging the flap itself (Marino 1967).

6. *Surgical treatment of lesions in the brachial plexus.* The very restricted indications have already been discussed. The surgical revision of fibrotic scar tissue caused by radiation is difficult and connected with risk for extensive bleeding that might be difficult to control. This could even lead to loss of the arm (Figs. 24.**12**, 24.**13**). The operation is only to be considered where recurrences or fibrosed scar tissue caused by radiation have com-

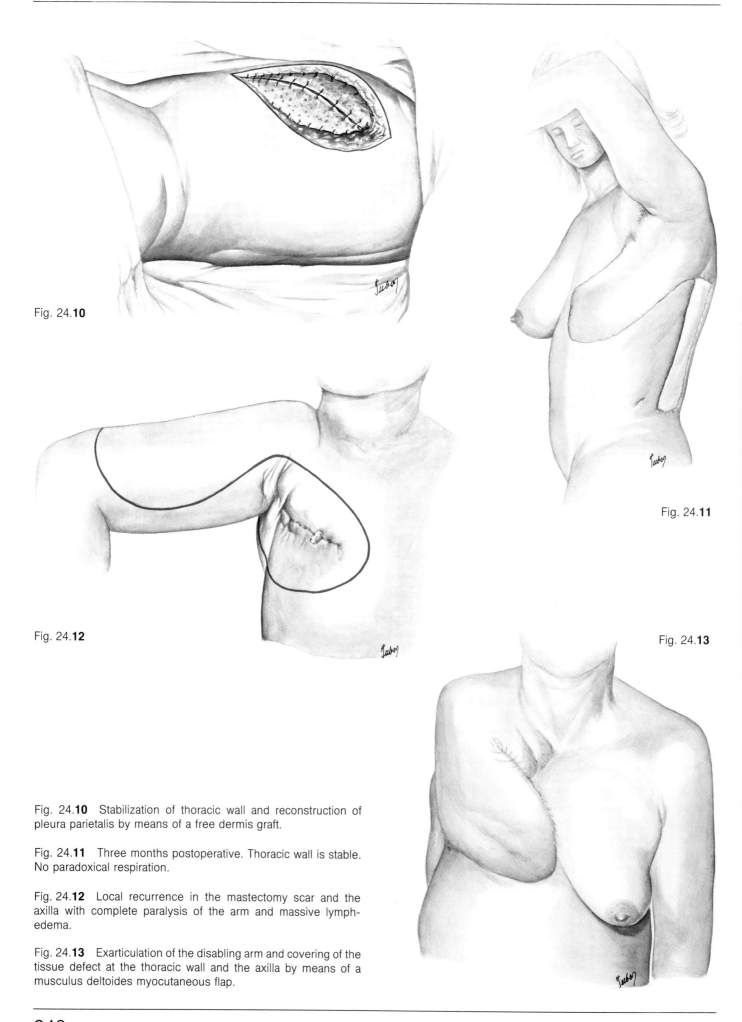

Fig. 24.**10**

Fig. 24.**11**

Fig. 24.**12**

Fig. 24.**13**

Fig. 24.**10** Stabilization of thoracic wall and reconstruction of pleura parietalis by means of a free dermis graft.

Fig. 24.**11** Three months postoperative. Thoracic wall is stable. No paradoxical respiration.

Fig. 24.**12** Local recurrence in the mastectomy scar and the axilla with complete paralysis of the arm and massive lymphedema.

Fig. 24.**13** Exarticulation of the disabling arm and covering of the tissue defect at the thoracic wall and the axilla by means of a musculus deltoides myocutaneous flap.

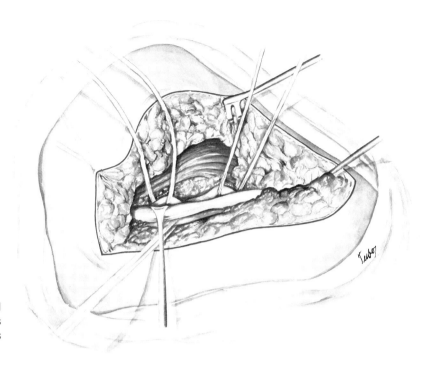

Fig. 24.**14** After excision of ulcer and of fibrosed scar tissue caused by radiation, surgical neurolysis of the brachial plexus is performed, which shows clear signs of compression on the nerve bundles.

pressed nerve bundles. This is, however, impossible to differentiate neurologically. The aim of the operation is to release the compression on the nerve bundles by performing a neurolysis. The "internal" of fascicular neurolysis is not to be recommended since it might lead to devascularization with damage to axial circulation causing secondary intrafascicular fibrosis. We restrict ourselves in this approach to longitudinal incision of the epineurium. From practice we have found the external scar contraction more common than direct radiation damage to the nerve with resultant atrophy. According to present experience, the result of surgical revisions will most often be a relief of pain that usually appears at night and sometimes a cessation or regression of the progressive paralysis, but very seldom reinervation (Figs. 24.**2**, 24.**14**, 24.**15**.)

Summary

Local recurrences are harbingers or signs of a systemic dissemination. Their frequency is reported to be 5% to 15%. When they occur, two thirds to three fourths of them will make their appearance in the first two years after primary treatment. Untoward effects of radiation include radiation dermatitis, ulceration, carcinoma induced by radiation, radionecrosis, and spontaneous fractures of the ribs or clavicles, pleural fibrosis, lesions of the brachial plexus, lymphedema of the arm, and reduction of arm movement. Surgical treatment consists of resection of local recurrences (partially to reduce the tumor mass when distant metastases are present) and resection of skin damaged by radiation, possibly with ulceration, to relieve pain, to faciliate care, to improve the quality of life, and to prevent malignant transformation.

The surgical treatment is basically the same as when dealing with a primary tumor; that is, histologically

confirmed resection into an area of healthy tissue. For wound closure, flaps are being used, for example, axial fasciocutaneous or combined myocutaneous from neighboring areas; free flaps utilizing microvascular technique or the abdominal greater omentum. Indications for surgical revision of damage to the brachial plexus are rapidly developing paralysis or cases with suspicious local recurrences in the axilla. The surgical revision of damage to the brachial plexus is restricted to external decompression. Even this carries a high risk and usually is not very successful.

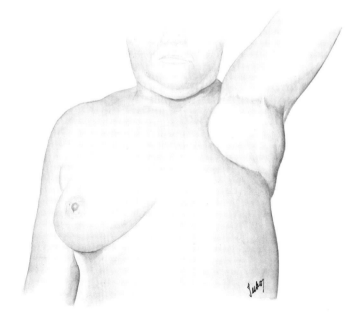

Fig. 24.**15** Six months after covering of the plexus fascicle and of the tissue defect by means of a latissimus dorsi myocutaneous flap. Almost free mobility of the shoulder joint.

References

Bruce, J., C. D. Carter, J. Fraser: Patterns of recurrent disease in breast cancer. Lancet 1: 433, 1970

Dao, T. C., T. Neomoto: The clinical significance of skin recurrence after radical mastectomy in woman with cancer of the breast. Surg. Gynecol. Obstet. 117: 447, 1963

Fletcher, G. H.: Local results of irradiation in the primary management of localized breast cancer. Cancer 29: 545, 1972

Heberer, G., W. Wilmanns, B. Günther, H. Sauer: Das Mammacarcinom – Operative und interdisziplinäre Aspekte. Chirurg 52: 212, 1981

Kramann, B., G. Ingianni, W. Mühlbauer, N. Christen: The value of transvenous xero-arteriography in plastic surgery. A preliminary report. Chir. Plast. 5: 93, 1980

Marino, H.: Biologic excision: Its value in the treatment of radionecrotic lesions. Plast. Reconstr. Surg. 40: 180, 1967

Marshall, K. A., A. Redefern, B. Cady: Local recurrence of carcinoma of the breast. Surg. Gynecol. Obstet. 139: 406, 1974

Mühlbauer, W., R. R. Olbrisch: The latissimus dorsi myocutaneous flap for breast reconstruction. Chir. Plast. 4: 27, 1977

Olbrisch, R. R., W. Mühlbauer: Mehrblättrige Lappen. Z. Plast. Chir. 2: 217, 1978

Olivari, N.: The latissimus flap. Br. J. Plast. Surg. 29: 126, 1976

Robinson, D. W.: Surgical problems in the excision and repair of radiated tissue. Plast. Reconstr. Surg. 22: 41, 1975

Schultz-Ehrenburg, U.: Der Strahlenschaden aus dermatologischer Sicht. Diagnostik 13: 298, 1980

Stjernswärd, J.: Adjuvant radiotherapy in breast cancer Cancer 39: 2846, 1977

Stjernswärd, J.: Evaluation of the role of routine use of postoperative radiotherapy in operable breast cancer. In U. Veronesi et al.: I Tumori della Mammella. Casa Editrice Ambrosiana, Mailand 1977

Turnball, A. R., A. D. B. Chant, R. B. Buchanan, D. T. L. Turner, J. M. Shepard, J. D. Fraser: Treatment of early cancer. Lancet 2: 7, 1978

Ungeheuer, E., K. Lüders: Chirurgische Behandlung des Mammakarzinoms. D. Ärzteblatt 4: 161, 1978

Weichselbaum, R. R., A. Marck, S. Hellmann: The role of postoperative irradiation in carcinoma of the breast. Cancer 37: 2882, 1976

Postmastectomy Reconstruction

H. Bohmert and J. O. Strömbeck

Principles and Techniques

Introduction

Over the last years, postmastectomy reconstruction of the female breast has become an accepted procedure in the therapy of breast carcinoma. Improved early diagnosis, especially in younger women, has given reconstruction an increasing importance in rehabilitation. Before reconstruction after cancer surgery could be recognized, however, some basic objections from an oncological viewpoint had to be refuted. The opinion that reconstruction could promote the risk of recurrence and impair healing was common. Furthermore, there was skepticism as to the esthetics of the reconstruction.

A pronounced change in both these objections has taken place (Urban 1982). An understanding of the limitations of radical surgery has given preference to the modified radical mastectomy as compared with standard radical mastectomy.

Extended knowledge of biology and behaviour of mammary cancer has given further impetus to breast-saving approaches in minor cancers, where lumpectomy and node dissection with radiation therapy is a viable alternative. Such therapy will give minimal deformity with possible comparable survival time. Quality of life and body image have to be taken into account when discussing therapy. This refers also to mastectomy with the possibility of later reconstruction. Today, there is a better understanding of the psychological burden brought on by radical mastectomy. The patient's wish for breast reconstruction is an important part of her rehabilitation. Leading oncologists have already stressed the importance of optimal physical and psychic rehabilitation.

The trend toward more limited surgery with preference for the modified radical mastectomy has also considerably facilitated the technical prerequisite of reconstruction. By preserving the pectoral muscles, the base for symmetry of the thorax is established. This makes it possible for a great number of women to have a breast contour established by rather simple techniques. Also in cases of severe deformities of the chestwall after radical surgery, procedures have been developed to balance the defect after mastectomy. Today, breast reconstruction is possible following any kind of cancer surgery.

Indications

Reconstruction after mastectomy is a relatively new procedure and there does not yet exist any strict rules for selection of patients and timing of the reconstruction.

Selection of Patients

Ideally, the surgical treatment of breast cancer should have the complete rehabilitation of the patient in view. All women who are to have an operation for a malignant breast lesion should be told of the possibility of reconstruction. Most women not only fear the grave disease but also the disfigurement braught about by the operation. The possibility of a reconstruction might be of considerable consolation.

So far, it is rather seldom that the surgeon suggests a later reconstruction. The negative attitude of earlier days based on doubts concerning cure rate and poor cosmetic results has fortunately over the last years switched to a more positive attitude.

As a principle, the patient with a breast tumor should have the same right to reconstruction as any other patient with a tumor where the operation causes a deformity. The patient herself, however, must decide on whether further surgery is worthwhile to restore her personal image. General experience points out that especially young, intelligent women with differentiated personality structure and pronounced body consciousness appreciate a reconstruction most and feel the loss of the breast as a considerable constriction to their personality.

Most patients in need of an operation are age 30 to 55, the age when breast cancer is most commonly seen. Reconstruction, however, is not restricted by age; general health, anesthetic risk, and particularly the patient's wish to have the operation are decisive. Information carefully given to the patient concerning what is to be expected and what is not possible to achieve is all important. This depends, in each individual case, on the anatomical situation after the mastectomy. The patient must be aware that in general it is not possible to reshape the original breast. She has to understand that the reconstructed breast never could become completely normal and that full symmetry rarely is to be obtained. The main aim of reconstruction is that she could count on regaining bodily integrity.

Timing of Reconstruction after Mastectomy

Before a reconstruction is considered, the patient's history and state of health has to be critically examined. Localization and size of the resected tumor as well as histology and state of the axillary nodes are important criteria when deciding on the time for reconstruction.

At best, there is a small tumor without nodal involvement; in the ideal case, only a microscopic cancer or even an in situ cancer. Depending on the findings, we choose the time for reconstruction one half to one year postmastectomy. When the nodes are involved, the patient usually will have chemotherapy or radiation. Reconstruction must wait at least until the adjuvant therapy is completed, most often even two years. Within this period of time, most local recurrences will appear. An early local recurrence after reconstruction would be a tremendous disappointment to the patient. The old concept that reconstruction has to wait until complete healing is obtained is not practical and not according to the demands of the patient. Urban (1973) and others believe that reconstruction can still be done after six months when the skin cover after the mastectomy has become soft and stretchable.

In case of distant metastasis, a reconstruction will as a rule not be considered. But there are exceptions when progress of the disease is not detectable or when the patient, in spite of the poor prognosis, urgently wishes the reconstruction. In such a case, the adequately informed patient should not be denied since a reconstruction might increase the quality of life, even if only for a relatively short period of time.

Primary reconstruction after mastectomy for cancer is a rare and special occurence. There are, however, patients who refuse to have the mastectomy unless a reconstruction is done simultaneously. The number of patients operated on in this way is too small to allow any conclusions as to the late results. This procedure is technically possible if the alternative is to be considered.

If this procedure is to be considered, the tumor should be small and there should be no suspicious nodes. The breast should be of normal size, offering a fair chance for symmetry. The patient should always be aware that the finding of a larger tumor than expected will postpone the reconstruction. Experience shows that patients having had an immediate reconstruction often are dissatisfied as they never had to live with the disfigurement caused by the mastectomy and are less apt to appreciate the reconstructed breast. In addition, two arguments against the primary reconstruction are: doubts concerning the circulation of the skin flaps with risk for impaired healing and secondly, absence of accurate staging. To avoid these difficulties many surgeons prefer a delayed primary reconstruction five days following mastectomy. The condition of the skin flaps in then easier to judge and staging is known. In most cases, however, the reconstruction will not be performed until the wounds have healed and the tissue has recovered. As a rule, it takes six to twelve months until the tissue becomes completely soft and stretchable.

Surgical Techniques

Concept of Breast Reconstruction

The plan for a reconstruction consists of substituting all tissues missing and bringing about breast symmetry in one or two operations. The following objects are to be accomplished:

1. Substitution of skin deficit
2. Rebuilding of the breast contour
3. Reconstruction of the anterior axillary fold with compensation of the excavation in the axilla
4. Compensation of the infraclavicular defect by substituting the pectoral muscles
5. Reconstruction of nipple and areola
6. Restoration of breast symmetry

Choice of Surgical Procedure

The choice among the different techniques is dependent on the prerequisites at hand after the amputation. The main problem usually is compensating for the skin loss caused by the mastectomy. Depending on the way the excision lines were placed at the mastectomy, there exists either a horizontal or vertical skin deficit. If the breast was excised in a horizontal ellipse, the skin deficit has a vertical orientation. This could easily be compensated for by advancing abdominal skin to the thoracic wall. If, however, the breast was excised in a vertical or oblique ellipse (the Halsted incision), the skin deficit will be horizontal, that is, in the direction of the thoracic circumference. As the circumference of the chest wall has hardly any excess skin, the insertion of a flap will usually be necessary to gain a sufficient amount of skin to make the desired projection possible.

Surgical Technique by Adequate Skin Cover

In each individual case it must be estimated if a flap is required. In favorable cases, there is a satisfactory skin cover to achieve a rebuilding of the contour without any tension. Even when using flap procedures, the technically more simple procedure as a principle should be given preference if this offers an esthetically satisfactory result. If the pectoral muscle still exists, the submuscular implantation of the prosthesis is favored.

Submuscular Implantation

In patients having had a modified radical mastectomy with preservation of the pectoral muscles, the submuscular implantation of the prosthesis is the method of choice.

The inferior border of the pectoral muscle does not reach to the inframammary crease, located between the sixth and seventh rib, but inserts on the fifth rib. This makes it necessary to utilize the adjacent muscles, that is, the oblique abdominal muscle, the serratus anterior, and the fascia of the rectus abdominis, to provide a cover for the prosthesis (Fig. 25.1). The incision is made at the level of the original submammary fold. It is often, however, easier to proceed from the lateral side starting in the area of the anterior axillary line perpendicular through to

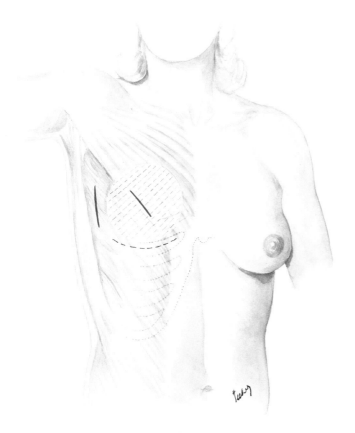

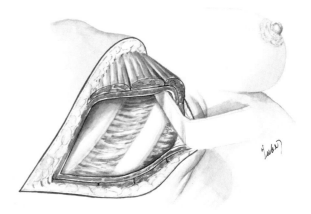

Fig. 25.**2** A transverse incision through the serratus anterior muscle in the anterior axillary line gives direct access to the submusculofascial pocket.

Fig. 25.**1** Submusculofascial implant position. Selection of incision location – pectoralis major approach or serratus anterior incision – must be individualized.

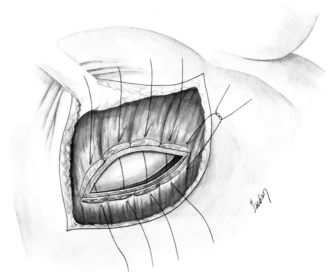

Fig. 25.**3** Preplaced sutures will protect the implant from damage by a needle before the insertion of the implant.

serratus muscle to reach the submuscular plane. Underneath the pectoral it is easy to dissect in a medial direction to the sternum and caudally to the insertion of the pectoralis at the fifth rib. In this area, a sharp dissection just over the periosteum makes it possible to carry on with the dissection in the right plane without damage to the muscular continuity (Fig. 25.**2**).

When the dissection is brought further caudally, the adjacent serratus and external oblique muscles as well as the anterior sheet of the rectus fascia will be elevated to form a pocket that reaches some 2 cm below the submammary fold. In this way, dislocation of the implant in a cranial direction is prevented (Fig. 25.**3**). In order to provide a satisfatory lateral cover, a mobilization of the latissimus dorsi is sometimes recommended.

Advancement of Abdominal Skin

If the mastectomy was done with a Stewart horizontal incision, it is possible to compensate for the skin defect by advancing the abdominal skin. For this purpose, the old scar is excised, and the abdominal skin undermined usually until the level of the umbilicus (Fig. 25.**4** and Fig. 25.**5**). The mobilized skin cover is advanced cranially and fixed at the periosteum of ribs in the level of the inframammary fold (Fig. 25.**6**). By additional undermining in the cranial direction, the pocket for the prosthesis is created (Fig. 25.**7**).

In selected cases, this procedure might also be used in patients with vertical or oblique scars if no tension in a horizontal direction is present. It might then be the method of choice, being an easy procedure leaving limited scars and giving a satisfactory esthetic result.

If the patient had radiation therapy, the skin circulation might be impaired and this procedure is usually not practical. The fixation sutures to the periosteum might cause circulatory disturbances affecting the skin area between the incision line in the mastectomy scar and the submammary crease. That is why the following modification is to be recommended. The incision is made 3 to 5 cm below the original submammary fold. Through the advancement maneuver, the wound edge and later the scarline will be located in the new submammary fold. The skin cover over the chest wall including the advanced abdominal skin will then be mobilized cranially to form a pocket for the prosthesis so that the mobilized abdominal

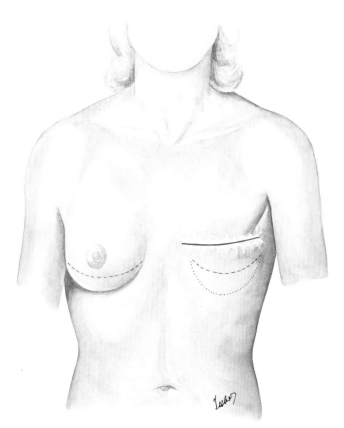

Fig. 25.**4** Reconstruction with the abdominal advancement flap. Markings of the chest wall include the transverse incision as well as the level of the submammary fold and the proposed extent of additional skin for reconstructing the breast.

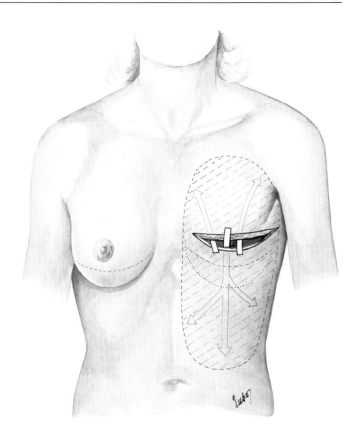

Fig. 25.**5** The abdominal skin is elevated off the fascia and the external oblique muscle and the rectus sheath down to the level of the lower abdomen.

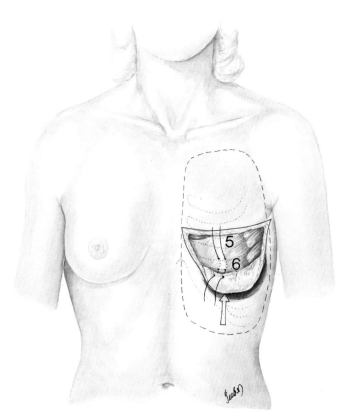

Fig. 25.**6** The flap is advanced upward and sutured to the periostium of the ribs and the fascia of the muscles to define the submammary fold.

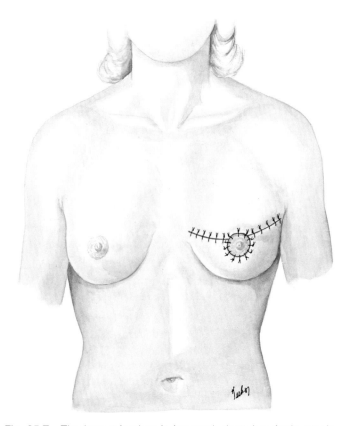

Fig. 25.**7** The breast implant is inserted; than the nipple-areola complex is reconstructed.

skin without tension could be sutured to the new created submammary fold. The wound edge is fixed to the advanced position with isolated stitches of resorbable suture material. The suture should grip the dermis and subcutaneous tissue that is tied to the periosteum of the rib. In this way, sinking of the submammary fold is prevented.

When using the abdominal advancement technique, the submuscular implantation of the prosthesis is recommended, especially in cases of radiation damaged skin. If the pectoral muscle is missing, the latissimus dorsi flap is to be preferred.

The Thoracoepigastric Flap

The thoracoepigastric flap can in certain reconstructive cases be the method of choice. This is especially true in cases with oblique and vertical postmastectomy scars, when the horizontal skin deficit is the main problem in creating a natural-looking breast. The skin flap substitutes for the skin area excised at the mastectomy and gives a sufficient skin cover to produce the wanted projection given by the prosthesis.

As the flap contains a reasonable amount of fat tissue, it offers an excellent protection for the prosthesis that even in most cases becomes surprisingly soft. The flap, however, could not substitute an inadequate skin cover in the cranial breast area. The infraclavicular contour defect in the medial-cranial area and the contour defect in the axilla with loss of the anterior axillary fold could not be corrected by this flap. In the axillary area, it might be possible to insert a distally de-epithelialized skin flap that in combination with a special prosthesis could eliminate the contour defect. The conclusive advantage in comparison with other flap techniques is that this procedure is technically simple and safe.

History of the Development of the Thoracoepigastric Flap

To restore an adequate skin and soft tissue cover of the defect after mastectomy is the most important prerequisite for successful breast reconstruction.

Because of the development of modern plastic surgical techniques, for example, the thoracoepigastric flap, this becomes feasible, and was the decisive breakthrough in breast reconstruction after mastectomy.

The results with the procedures used until then were unsatisfactory for two reasons: first because of insufficient resemblance to the natural breast and second because of extended and conspicous scars. That is why the techniques with use of tubed skin flaps or sharing of the remaining breast never were a success.

The impulse to the concept of breast reconstruction developed by the author was given by Pierer in 1967. He described, probably as the first in the world literature, a laterally based transposition flap derived from the epigastric area for breast reconstruction. The disadvantages were, however, obvious: insufficient size of the flap needed, poor circulation, and inconveniently placed conspicuous scars. To overcome these disadvantages, the author in 1972 developed a plan for a flap, which from many points of view seemed promising. A flap from the lateral abdominal wall, based medially in the epigastrium, has a safer circulation. The flap could, in this region, be made as broad as needed without any difficulty. The donor area could be primarily closed after extensive undermining.

The remaining scar is rather unconspicuously located. The advantage of this concept could soon be proved in practice, and the technique published by the author in 1974 as "lateral abdominal flap" was then recommended for breast reconstruction in cases with vertical and oblique postamputation scars.

This method was shortly after that reported and advocated in the United States by Höhler. Independently, Cronin et al. (1977) described a similar flap as "delayed flap" based on the work of Tai and Hasegawa (1974).

Anatomy of the Thoracoepigastric Flap

The author made studies of the vascular pattern of this in cadavers since they were not described in the literature. Selective angiographs were made in six patients before and after flap repair.

In dissection on cadavers, the flap was raised and the internal mammary artery dissected free where it leaves the subclavian artery. The vessels were visualized by injecting synthetic resin as well as by x-ray contrast. By means of the filling of the vessels with the synthetic material, a casting of the internal mammary artery and its branches could be prepared. The constant presence of a coarse branch from the superior epigastric artery running axial within the skin flap was demonstrated. Although the anatomical textbooks note a branch from the superior epigastric artery that perforates the rectus muscle and then directly branches into a fine vascular net, it now was demonstrated that this artery is a coarse vessel and runs in the subcutis laterally as far as the axillary line. It is most important for the use of this flap that it actually has an axial artery. The diameter of this artery corresponds to that of the musculophrenic artery, which also emanates from the internal mammary artery and runs laterally almost parallel to the lateral branch of the superior epigastric artery, as shown in the casts (Fig. 25.**8**). This axial vessel that feeds the flap and runs from the base to the apex could also be visualized with angiography in the anatomical preparations.

Preoperative and postoperative angiography in patients confirmed these findings. As result of this investigation, it could be shown that the flap has a vascular supply of its own and is a so called axial pattern flap. An axial pattern flap could without any danger have the length : width ratio of 2 : 1.

In addition to the lateral branch from the superior epigastric artery, the flap also receives three or four smaller branches perforating the rectus muscle coming from the internal mammary artery. These rami perforantes run through the medial part of the rectus muscle to subcutis and skin. The lateral branch of the superior epigastric artery bends off immediately after the entrance of the main branch of the superior epigastric artery and

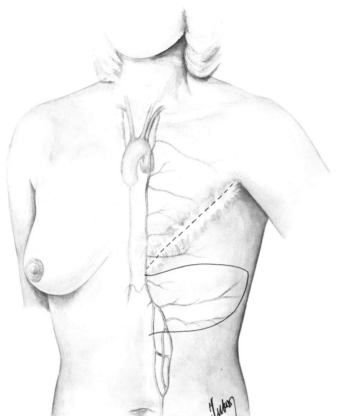

Fig. 25.**8** Anatomy and design of the thoracoepigastric flap. The flap is based on vessels from the superior epigastric artery, which perforate the rectus muscle and course laterally to the anterior axillary line.

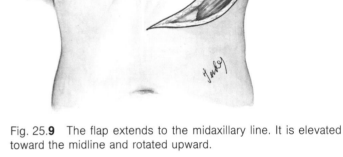

Fig. 25.**9** The flap extends to the midaxillary line. It is elevated toward the midline and rotated upward.

runs through the muscle perpendicularly and then horizontally through the skin. The entrance of the main branch of the superior epigastric artery lays some 3 cm distally and 2 cm from the midline between the costal angle and the xiphoid on the under surface of the rectus muscle. All vessels nourishing the flap should be carefully preserved. The preparation of the flap should not be carried further than to the middle of the rectus muscle.

Surgical Technique

The operation is done with the patient in a semisitting position. To decide the appropriate size of the flap, which as an average is 8 to 10 cm wide and 18 to 22 cm long, a pattern is used, first placed in the donor area for the flap. The size of the flap is dependent on the desired breast volume, the length and location of the scar, the defect of the axilla, if any, and also on the flexibility of the abdominal skin.

Once the desired size of the flap is determined, the pattern, cut to this size, is placed with its upper border in the original submammary area and with its medial end at the lateral border of the rectus muscle or rather on the midpoint of the rectus where the point of rotation of the flap will be. The lateral end of the pattern, which mostly reaches the midaxillary line, is rotated into the area of the postmastectomy scar (Fig. 25.**9**).

Now, if desired, some part of the apex of the flap could be de-epithelilized and buried under the skin. The pattern is

then returned to the horizontal position and its borders marked on the skin.

A delayed procedure is necessary only when the flap surpasses the midaxillary line. Another reason for a delay could be if the postmastectomy scar runs far below the submammary fold into the base of the flap. If this part of the scar it not more than 2 cm, it is of no significance. Longer scars in the base area could be a reason not to use this flap, or to do a delayed procedure.

After having marked the flap (size 18 to 23 × 8 to 12 cm) from the middle of the rectus muscle to the midaxillary line, the flap is mobilized starting at its apex. The flap is dissected off the muscles. The fascia of the serratus and the external oblique are included in the flap, which guarantees a better circulation, since the fascia has a vascular net on both sides.

When this dissection under the fasciae of the anterior serratus and external oblique abdominal muscles has reached the lateral border of the rectus sheath, it is decided if a further dissection medially is necessary. This could be done, without any danger to the circulation, to the middle of the rectus sheath. The perforating vessels to the flap penetrate more medially and should be preserved. In special cases, the rectus muscle could be completely divided in its caudal part to facilitate a good rotation of the flap. The postmastectomy scar is excised and the wound edges are widely undermined medially to

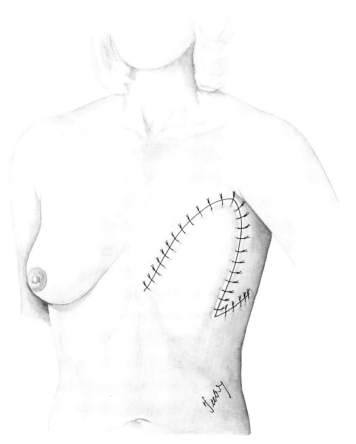

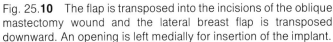

Fig. 25.**10** The flap is transposed into the incisions of the oblique mastectomy wound and the lateral breast flap is transposed downward. An opening is left medially for insertion of the implant.

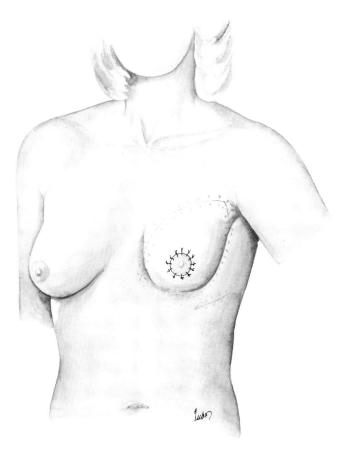

Fig. 25.**11** The submammary fold is defined in a second stage, when the nipple areola complex will be reconstructed.

the sternum, cranially to the clavicula, laterally to the midaxillary line, and caudally to the submammary fold.

The flap can now be transposed into position. The abdominal skin is undermined often to the level of the iliac bone to make primary closure of the donor area possible. If the pectoral muscle still exists, the prosthesis is placed under the muscle. After a radical mastectomy, however, the implant is placed directly under the skin flaps in the same operation. A protruding skin surplus is often seen medially over the sternum. This dog ear could not be excised until later, since otherwise the circulation in the base of the flap might be damaged. This correction could be done together with the nipple reconstruction. This flap will supply the extra skin and soft tissue that is needed to rebuild the breast contour with silicone implants (Fig. 25.**10** and 25.**11**).

Advantages of this Technique

The thoracoepigastric flap, being an axial pattern flap, has a safe circulation and can be rotated into an oblique or vertical position on the chest wall without delay. The flap can be cut to any desired size to cover a large area in the lower two thirds of the chest wall. The donor area can in all cases be closed primarily after undermining.

The scar in the donor area lays in a horizontal skin crease, is often hidden by the brassiere, and is not disturbing to the patient. The flap has thick skin and subcutaneous layers offering a good protection for an implant that

mostly stays surprisingly soft. The technique is simple and in comparison with the latissimus dorsi flap, a minor surgical procedure.

Disadvantages of the Technique

The flap is suitable for repairing the skin and soft tissue in the two lower thirds of the breast and cannot be used to substitute unstable skin in the upper medial part of the breast. When the skin is thin and the pectoral muscle is missing, the latissimus dorsi flap is the method of choice to eliminate the infraclavicular contour defect and rebuild the axillary fold. The thoracoepigastric flap cannot be used when the mastectomy incision is carried far below the submammary fold, sacrificing the axial vessels of the flap.

The thoracoepigastric flap is still a useful method in breast reconstruction even though the indications for its use have been reduced by the development of new techniques, such as the latissimus dorsi myocutaneous flap and the contralateral thoracoepigastric myocutaneous flap.

The Contralateral Thoracoepigastric Musculocutaneous Upper Rectus Flap

Based on the anatomical studies of the circular pattern of the thoracoepigastric flap showing an axial pattern, a new concept of breast reconstruction was developed.

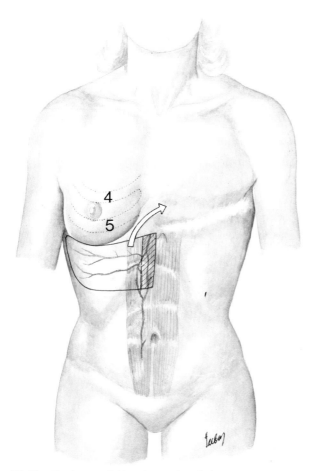

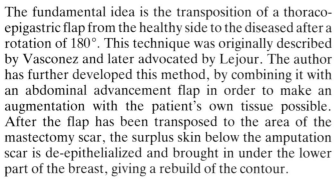

Fig. 25.**12** Design and blood supply of the transverse upper rectus flap. The flap is nourished by one or two perforators from the superior epigastric artery.

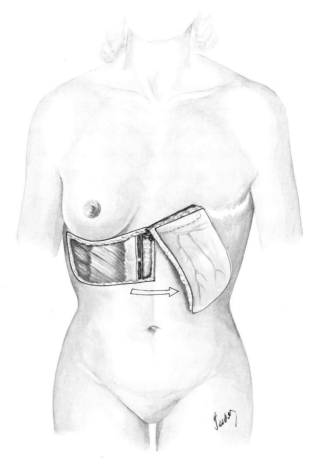

Fig. 25.**13** The flap is based on the medial portion of the rectus muscle including the superior epigastric vessels. It is rotated downward to the mastectomized side.

The fundamental idea is the transposition of a thoraco-epigastric flap from the healthy side to the diseased after a rotation of 180°. This technique was originally described by Vasconez and later advocated by Lejour. The author has further developed this method, by combining it with an abdominal advancement flap in order to make an augmentation with the patient's own tissue possible. After the flap has been transposed to the area of the mastectomy scar, the surplus skin below the amputation scar is de-epithelialized and brought in under the lower part of the breast, giving a rebuild of the contour.

In this way, a technique is developed that provides a satisfactory augmentation with autogenous tissue in a relatively simple way as compared with the lower rectus flap. In this procedure, a thoracoepigastric flap of 20 to 23 cm length and 10 to 12 cm width is outlined on the healthy side (Fig. 25.**12**).

In most cases, some 1 to 2 cm above the submammary fold is included in the flap. The mobilization of the flap starts as usual from the lateral end and is extended until the rectus sheath, which should be left intact in its lateral third. The middle and medial part of the rectus sheath and muscle are divided and the muscle elevated cranially. The rectus has to be divided in the midline until the posterior sheath of the rectus fascia and the rectus muscle with its sheath is divided caudally. When the myocutaneous flap is elevated, the nourishing vessels i. e., the

superior epigastric artery and vein could be seen on the posterior surface of the muscle (Fig. 25.**13**).

The vessels lay below the costal arch some 2 cm distal to the angle between the costal arch and the xiphoid and enters the rectus muscle one finger width further distally.

To make a total mobilization of the myocutaneous flap possible, its vascular stalk has to be completely visualized. Not until the muscle has been completely detached from the costal arch is it possible to bring the flap in position and after excision of the amputation scar to suture it to the cranial edge of the scar. The skin caudal to the amputation scar is de-epithelialized until the level of the donor defect, and after mobilization of the skin and subcutis in the lower chest wall and the upper abdomen, transposed underneath the flap. Its medial part is incised and doubled to exaggerate the contour in the central part of the breast (Fig. 25.**14**). Some periosteal stitches are placed in the level of the submammary fold to reinforce the contour and to prevent sinking of the flap. The donor area on the contralateral side is closed primarily, resulting in a scar within the submammary fold. The results are esthetically most pleasing (Fig. 25.**15** and 25.**16**).

The decisive advantage with this procedure is that all potential complications due to the silicone implant are avoided. In addition, the procedure has a positive psychological effect because the use of the patient's own tissue.

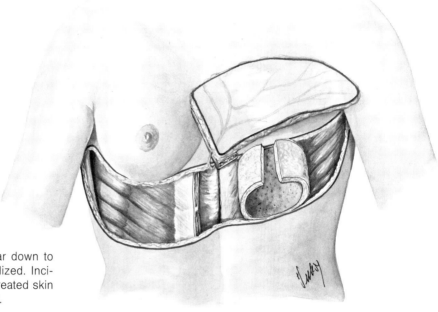

Fig. 25.**14** The skin from the mastectomy scar down to the level of the contralateral breast is deepithelized. Incisions are made medially and laterally and the created skin flaps are turned over to build the breast mound.

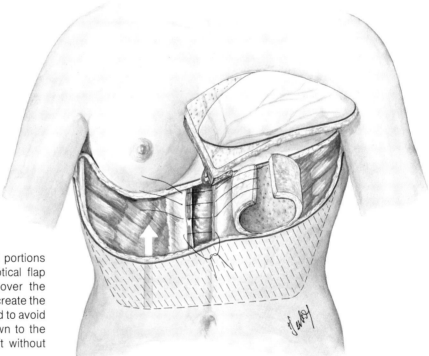

Fig. 25.**15** The medio-cranial and medio-caudal portions of the flap are deepithelized to achieve an elliptical flap design for optimal aesthetical reason. It will cover the deepithelized skin flaps from the abdomen which create the breast volume. The anterior rectus sheath is closed to avoid a hernie. The abdominal skin is undermined down to the level of the umbilicus to allow an abdominal lift without tension.

Nipple-Areolar Reconstruction

Without a nipple-areola complex a reconstructed breast does not look natural and therefore almost all patients want to have the nipple and areola reconstructed following reconstruction of the breast mound. The nipple reconstruction should not be performed until the breast has attained its final form, that is usually after three to six months. The position of the nipple-areola complex should be on the summit of reconstructed breast in the sitting position. In case of a "normal" breast the exact position can be measured from the sternal notch and xyphoid process to match the healthy side. Otherwise the position depends more on the visual effect than on direct measurements. For good symmetry it might be necessary to make adjustments in the size and configuration of the opposite side which could be performed at the same time as the nipple reconstruction. Selection of the technique for reconstruction of the nipple and areola must be carefully individualized.

Areolar Reconstruction

The donor area for the areola skin is selected to match the color of the contralateral areola. If the areola of the opposite breast is sufficiently large, part of it can be used

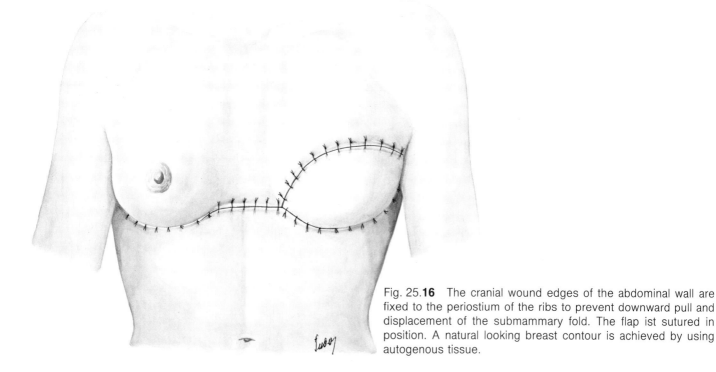

Fig. 25.**16** The cranial wound edges of the abdominal wall are fixed to the periostium of the ribs to prevent downward pull and displacement of the submammary fold. The flap ist sutured in position. A natural looking breast contour is achieved by using autogenous tissue.

for reconstruction, the concentric circle method. An outer circle of the large areola is removed as a thick split-thickness skin graft to give two areolas of equal size (Fig. 25.**17**).

The conjoined spiral method of sharing the areola is generally not used today because of the very conspicuous scars between the spirals. The usual donor site, however, is the upper inner thigh. A full thickness skin graft from

this area will give a light brown color once it matures. Grafts obtained from the labium minus will be the most pigmented. If an areola of a lighter pink tone is required, the postauricular area could be used (Fig. 25.**18**). Tattooing has been used for areola simulation, but there seems to be superior methods available.

Technique: Preoperatively the proper location and size of the areola is outlined. The skin in this area is denuded in the dermis and the free graft applied and sutured.

Nipple Reconstruction

If the opposite breast has a good sized nipple, nipple sharing is the method of choice. The top 3–4 mm of the donor nipple is amputated and used as a composite graft (Fig. 25.**19**).

If the nipple prominence is inadequate for sharing or the patient does not wish the normal nipple to be disturbed, labium minus grafts could give an adequate projection and pigmentation for reconstruction of the nipple. Other possibilities are using composite ear lobe grafts or grafts from the toe pulp (Fig. 25.**20**). To obtain nipple projection conchal cartilage grafts have been used successfully. Additionally, minute pieces of cartilage dispersed under the skin grafts in order to simulate Montgomery glands results in an even more natural appearing areola.

Also the local skin of the reconstructed breast might be used to fake a nipple prominence by a "mushrom procedure" or by multiple V–Y plasties (Fig. 25.**21**).

Banking the nipple-areola complex from the involved breast on a dermal bed in the groin for later transfer to the new nipple site is not used any longer because of the possibility of transferring tumor with the graft and because these grafts tend to lose pigmentation in the multiple transfers.

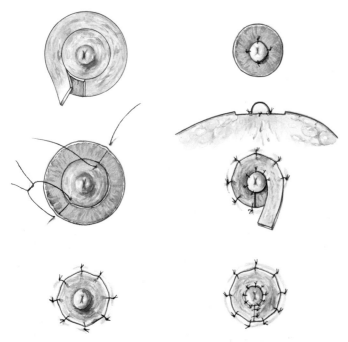

Fig. 25.**17** The areolagraft from the opposite areola is marked and the donor area closed by periareola reduction. Deepithelized area with reconstructed nipple in place is covered by the areola graft.

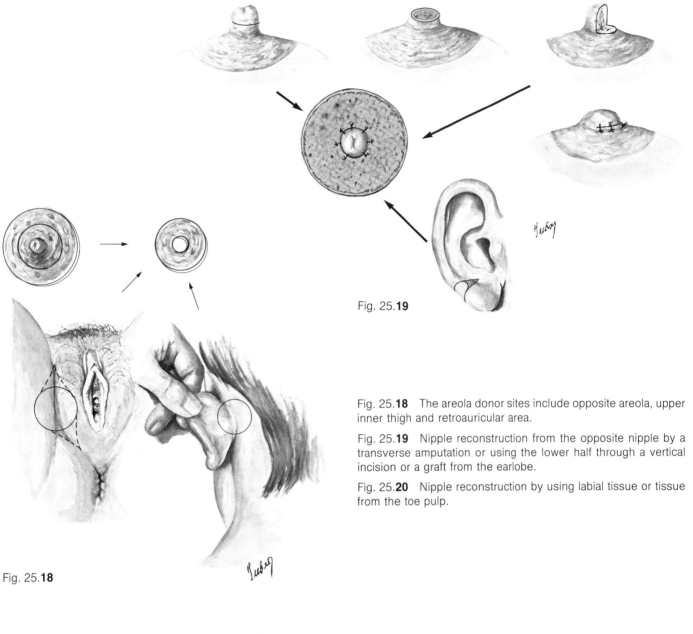

Fig. 25.**19**

Fig. 25.**18**

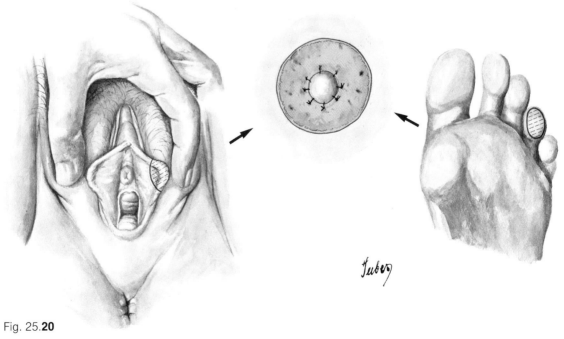

Fig. 25.**18**   The areola donor sites include opposite areola, upper inner thigh and retroauricular area.

Fig. 25.**19**   Nipple reconstruction from the opposite nipple by a transverse amputation or using the lower half through a vertical incision or a graft from the earlobe.

Fig. 25.**20**   Nipple reconstruction by using labial tissue or tissue from the toe pulp.

Fig. 25.**20**

253

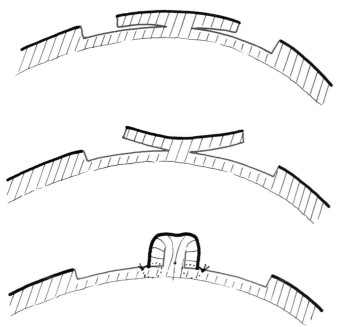

Fig. 25.**21** Nipple reconstruction with a local flap. Four V-shaped areas of skin a marked around a circle of 1 cm in diameter and elevated.

Special Techniques

One-Stage Complete Reconstruction after Modified Radical Mastectomy

A technique for a one-stage reconstruction has been described by Juri and Juri (1983) utilizing the principle of the abdominal advancement flap. In the ideal breast, the nipple should be at the same level as the inframammary fold. After a breast amputation, the skin area from the nipple to the submammary fold is missing and could be substituted by abdominal skin. The defect on the donor area could be closed by advancing the abdominal skin (Fig. 25.**22**).

Planning the operation:

1. The level of the submammary fold corresponding to the healthy side is outlined and on this line is marked the proper location for the nipple
2. The amount of skin needed to cover the lower pole of the breast is outlined below the level of the submammary fold with removal of a wedge with a side of 8 cm length and its apex pointing to the submammary fold. A small skin flap (1 × 4 cm) based upward from the apex of the wedge could be outlined to simulate a nipple when duplicated (Fig. 25.**23**).
3. If necessary, a breast reduction could be made at the same time on the healthy side using the same measurements to obtain a full symmetry

The operation consists of the following steps:

1. The epithelium of the areolar region is removed and the lower borderlines of the flaps are incised and then dissected free continuing in cranial direction underneath the pectoral muscle to give a good pocket for the implant (Fig. 25.**24**).
2. The abdominal skin with subcutaneous fat is undermined to the level of the umbilicus so that it could be advanced to cover the defect and is now anchored to the ribs in the level of the inframammary fold (Fig. 25.**25**).
3. The sides of the wedge excision are sutured together, an implant is introduced into the pocket, and the lower borders of the flaps are sutured to the submammary fold (Fig. 25.**26**).
4. The nipple and areola are reconstructed. The small local flap is rolled as a spiral to simulate the nipple and the de-epithelialized areola region is covered with a free full thickness skin graft. Juri and Juri (1983) use skin from the upper eyelids, but skin from the inner side of the upper thigh is most often used for this purpose (Fig. 25.**27**).

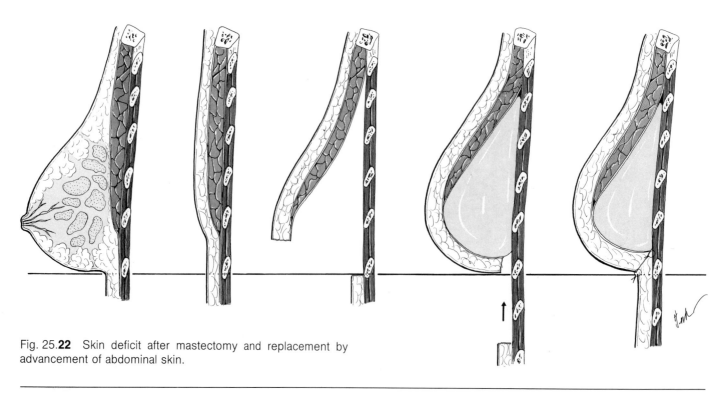

Fig. 25.**22** Skin deficit after mastectomy and replacement by advancement of abdominal skin.

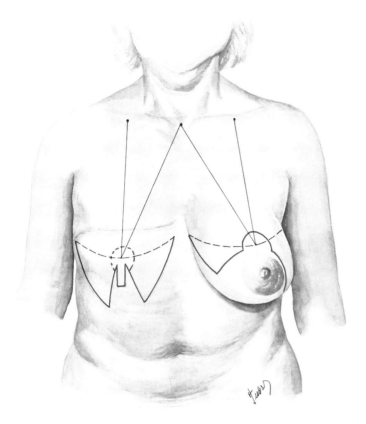

Fig. 25.**23** Preoperative planning according to Juri and Juri (see text).

Fig. 25.**24** Skin flaps incised and retromuscular pocket created.

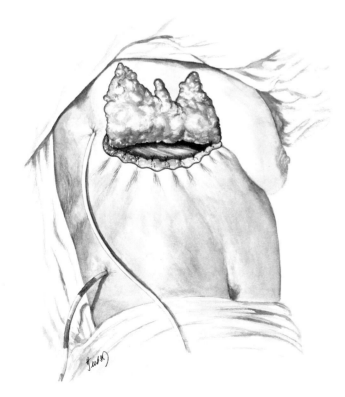

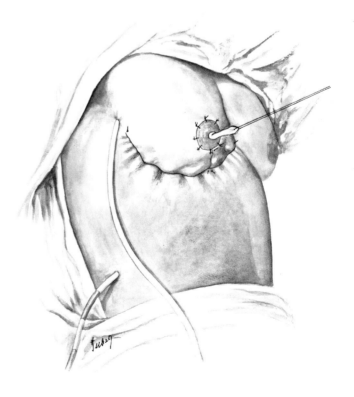

Fig. 25.**25** Abdominal skin advanced to the level of the inframammary fold where it is anchored.

Fig. 25.**26** Skin flaps sutured over the implant. Areolar reconstruction begun.

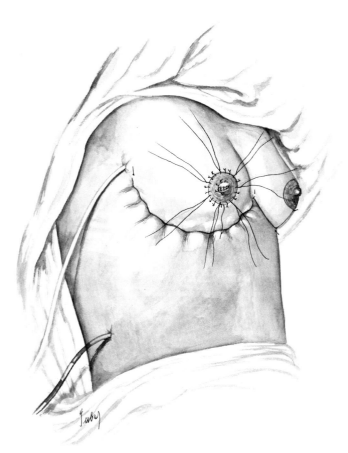

Fig. 25.**27** Reconstruction completed.

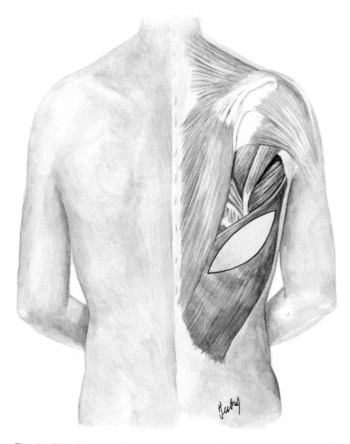

Fig. 25.**28** The position of the skin island to be transposed is calculated to fit into the post-mastectomy scar area.

If combined with a reduction mammoplasty on the other breast, this technique offers a complete reconstruction with full symmetry in one stage for patients having had a previous modified mastectomy through a transverse incision.

The Latissimus Dorsi Musculocutaneous Flap

In 1976, Olivari described the use of the latissimus dorsi muscle to provide coverage of defects of the anterior chest wall after radiation lesions. Although this technique actually was published by D'Este as early as 1912, Olivari has to be given credit for having opened up a new area of latissimus dorsi flap techniques. The use of latissimus dorsi to provide a better cover for the implant in breast reconstruction was popularized by Mühlbauer and Olbrisch in 1977 and especially by Bostwick et al. in 1979.

As the skin area over the muscle receives its circulation through perforating vessels, the overlying skin could be included in the flap. The latissimus dorsi myocutaneous flap thus provides tissue to substitute not only a missing pectoral major, but also breast skin, giving an excellent cover for a breast implant and a natural shape of the reconstructed breast.

Indications

The main indication for the latissimus dorsi myocutaneous flap is in patients having had a radical mastectomy, especially thin patients where the ribs stand out giving a deformity that is most obvious even with ordinary clothing. If the patient had additional radiation treatment, the flap adds to the safety of a reconstructive procedure. This flap may also be the method of choice if the other breast is somewhat large and the patient does not want to have the healthy side reduced.

Operative Technique

The first step has to be to make sure that the nerve and blood supply of the muscle have not been damaged at the mastectomy operation. Angiography is not necessary; it is enough just to check that the patient is able to contract the muscle.

The borders of the muscle are outlined prior to surgery with the patient in the sitting position. The size and position of the skin island is designed recognizing that the rotation point will be the posterior axillary fold. If the skin island is to be transferred to the area of an oblique mastectomy scar, the skin island will be an ellipse horizontally located below the scapula. Such a defect could be easily closed with a resulting scar being covered by the brassiere (Fig. 25.**28**).

The operation is made with the patient in the lateral position, which gives access to both donor and recipient areas simultaneously. The skin island is circumscribed and carried down to the muscle fascia preserving part of the surrounding subcutaneous tissue and the rest of the skin covering the muscle is dissected free. In the early

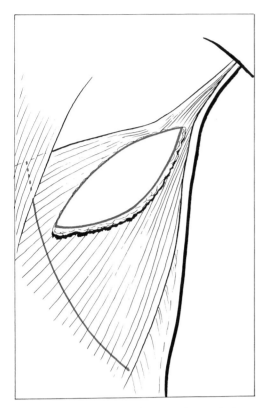

Fig. 25.**29** After the deep surface of the muscle has been dissected free the muscle is cut inferiorly.

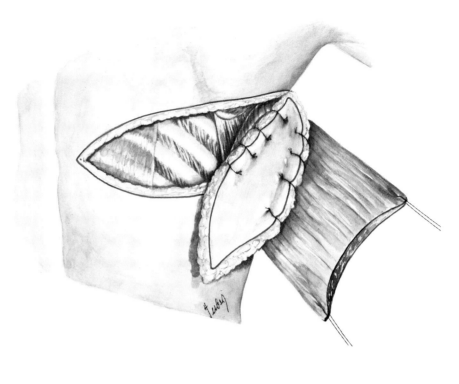

Fig. 25.**30** The musculocutaneous flap is raised.

part of the procedure, it might be helpful to anchor the borders of the skin island to the muscle with some interrupted stitches to prevent unnecessary tearing of the skin island during the preparation of the flap.

The anterolateral border of the muscle is identified and from here it is easy to free the deep surface of the muscle by blunt dissection, taking care to separate it from the serratus anterior muscle. The superior border of the latissimus dorsi is dissected free and detached from the lower angle of the scapula. The muscle is then cut inferiorly at a level to provide as much muscle as needed to cover the upper medial part of the chest wall (Fig. 25.**9**). After the medial aponeurotic attachments to the spine area have been cut, the flap is made free to rotate around its neurovascular stalk in the posterior axillary fold (Fig. 25.**30**).

The mastectomy scar is excised and a wide tunnel is made subcutaneously from the posterior axilla to the mastectomy area. The flap is brought through the tunnel to the postmastectomy wound (Fig. 25.**31**). The skin on the donor area is closed and the wound drained with a suction catheter.

At this point in the operation, it might be more convenient to reposition the patient to have her lying on her back, although this is not necessary if you wish to shorten the operation time.

The skin over the anterior chest wall is now undermined all the way to the clavicle, the sternum, and the submammary fold. The flap is now positioned and the cranial and medial edges are anchored to the subclavicular and sternal areas, respectively, under the skin flap (Fig. 25.**32**).

The inferior edge of the muscle flap is sutured to the region of the inframammary fold. The upper medial edge of the skin island is now sutured to the corresponding postmastectomy wound edge continuing with the lower edge from medial to lateral. Before the closure is completed, a prosthesis of appropriate size is introduced under the muscle flap from the lateral side, which is still open.

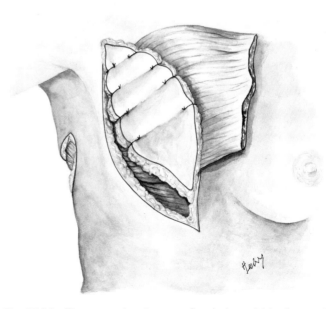

Fig. 25.**31** The musculocutaneous flap is brought to the post-mastectomy scar area through a subcutaneous tunnel.

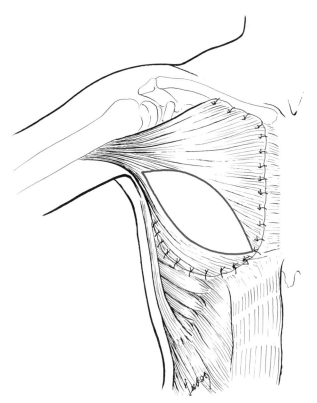

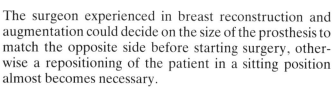

Fig. 25.**32** Anchoring of the edges of the latissimus flap under the skin flap.

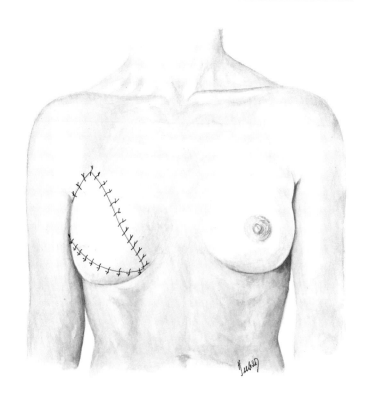

Fig. 25.**33** Suturing completed.

The surgeon experienced in breast reconstruction and augmentation could decide on the size of the prosthesis to match the opposite side before starting surgery, otherwise a repositioning of the patient in a sitting position almost becomes necessary.

It is important to secure the muscle flap to the chest wall lateral to the pocket to prevent dislocation of the prosthesis into the axilla. The anterior cavity is drained with suction catheter for 12 to 24 hours depending on outflow. A soft dressing is applied taking care not to apply any pressure on the pedicle of the flap (Fig. 25.**33**). Nipple-areola reconstruction is mostly delayed until a later stage.

Comments on the Latissimus Dorsi Musculocutaneous Flap

C. E. Horton and J. B. McCraw

The latissimus dorsi cannot adequately correct the total loss of the pectoralis major muscle. The quality of the anterior axillary fold reconstruction is not as good as one would like, because the fatty layer cannot easily by recreated by the limited bulk of the muscle.

It is a mistake to try to always position the skin island in the brassiere line, since this commits the skin position on the anterior chest, and it will only correct certain deformities because the skin overlaying the muscle is relatively immobile, due to the attachments of the perforating vessels. The skin, which is transposed anteriorly, will have a poor color match many times and will appear as a "patch". For some reason, the skin of the back tans more deeply than the breast skin and will frequently have numerous freckles or nevi unlike the normal breast skin.

Sensation is totally lacking in this flap and, although it does not cause problems, it is a deficiency of the reconstructive method. When the patient has had a thoracotomy which divides the muscle, the muscle is absolutely not usable distal to the scar.

Technical Considerations

Latissimus muscle should be carefully separated from the serratus anterior muscle and also completely separated from the teres major muscle, so that a "bulge" will be avoided in the axilla.

Adequate lateral closure is necessary to prevent implant dislodgement into the back.

Complications

Seroma formation is so common that it almost should not be called a complication. It occurs in at least 25% of the cases and can be a chronic problem which is difficult to eradicate.

Scar encapsulation around the implant is a concomitant in approximately 30% or more of the cases.

Only one infection occurred in a series of over 400 latissimus reconstructions.

The Transverse Rectus Abdominis Flap

This flap, first described by Hartrampf et al. (1982), contains the amount of skin and subcutaneous tissue usually resected in a lower abdominoplasty. It is carried on the contralateral or the ipsilateral rectus muscle nourished by the superior epigastric artery and transferred to the postmastectomy area to provide skin and tissue to build up a new breast without the use of an implant.

Indications

Patients with considerable tissue defects in the mastectomy area and a fair amount of surplus skin in the lower abdomen, almost in need of an abdominal plasty, are ideal candidates. An additional indication might be in patients refusing to have an implant or those in whom an earlier implant has caused considerable contracture with deformation and pain.

Operative Technique

The flap is designed as a horizontal ellipse giving sufficient tissue for the reconstruction, but also allowing an easy closure of the donor area. It is located in the lower abdomen with its upper border cranial to the umbilicus, which is circumscribed as a first step of the operation and left in place (Fig. 25.**34**). The lower border of the flap is incised down to the fascia of the abdominal wall and the dissection is carried cranially until the first major perforating vessels from the rectus are reached. They are usually midway between the symphysis and the umbilicus and have to be preserved.

The upper border of the flap is now incised down to the abdominal wall leaving some extra subcutaneous fat over the rectus sheath to save some more perforating vessels.

The lateral parts of the flap are dissected free extending medially until the borders of the rectus, which is to carry the flap. The dissection is then extended on the rectus sheath until the perforating vessels can be seen.

Now the upper abdominal skin is undermined over the deep fascia to a level above the costal margin.

Preparation of the stalk starts by incising the rectus sheath caudal to the perforating vessels and cutting the rectus muscle at this level (Fig. 25.**35**). The inferior epigastric artery running on the posterior surface of the muscle is ligated. The anterior rectus sheath is now incised on both sides of the perforating vessels leaving medially and laterally as much as possible of the rectus sheath to allow good closure. The central edge of the rectus sheath, which is attached to the rectus muscle, could be sutured to the muscle to prevent unnecessary tearing of the perforating vessels during the preparation of the flap. The rectus abdominis muscle with its anterior sheath is then dissected free up to the costal margin (Fig. 25.**36**). The viability of the flap has to be checked throughout the preparation. If, at an early stage, the circulation seems questionable, it could be considered to suture the flap back in place calling it a delayed procedure. If, however, the circulation becomes more than questionable at a later stage of the preparation, it might be considered to sacrifice the flap and convert the operation to an abdominoplasty.

With an adequate circulation, the flap is brought through a subcutaneous tunnel to the postmastectomy scar area that has been excised (Fig. 25.**37**). If necessary, for an adequate rotation, part of the upper rectus could be

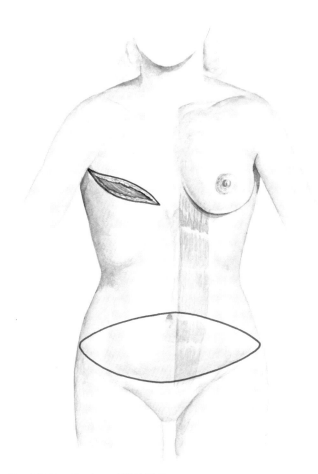

Fig. 25.**34**   Design of TRAM-flap.

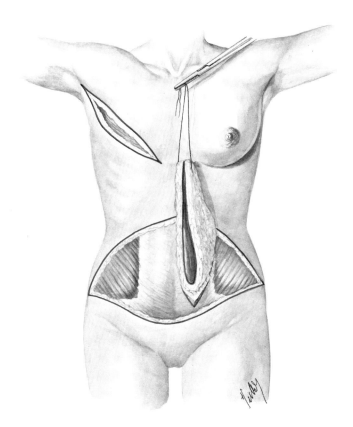

Fig. 25.**35**   Flap dissected to the rectus fascia. The caudal incision in the rectus muscle is seen.

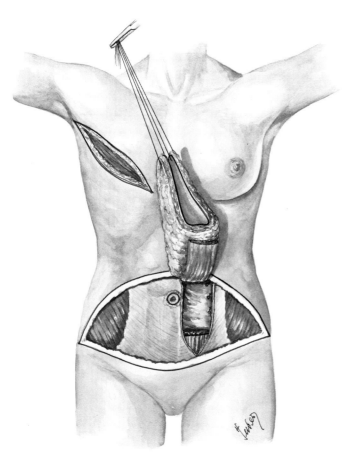

Fig. 25.**36**   Dissection of rectus muscle pedicle.

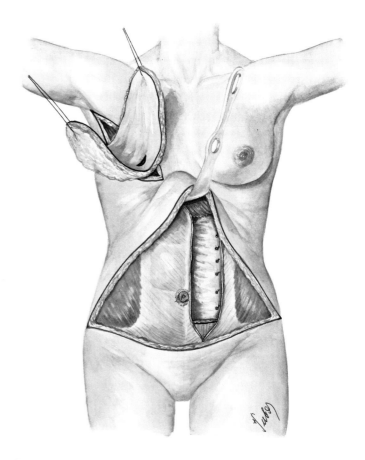

Fig. 25.**37**   The flap is brought to the area of the post-mastectomy scar through a tunnel.

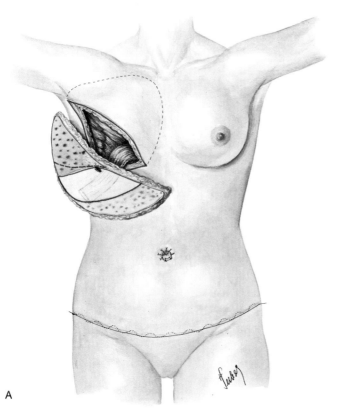

A

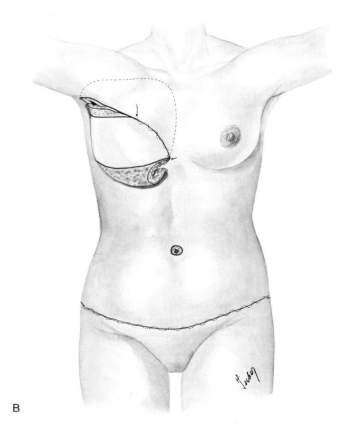

B

Fig. 25.**38** A, B   Part of the flap is de-epithelized and brought subcutaneously to build up the breast contour.

divided once the superior epigastric vessels have been identified (see p. 250). There is now a considerable amount of tissue at hand to build a breast. It has to be decided how much skin is needed and how much of the skin should be de-epithelialized and brought subcutaneously to build up the anterior axillary fold, the infraclavicular groove, and the inferior bulking of the breast (Fig. 25.**38**). This is a real challenge for a plastic surgeon to match the healthy breast (Fig. 25.**38**).

Closure of the donor area starts with direct closure of the fascial defect of the rectus sheath, which has to be very meticulous to prevent weakness of the abdominal wall and herniation (Fig. 25.**39**).

The abdominal wound is closed as in an abdominoplasty. The original umbilicus is usually so lateralized that it has to be resected and a false umbilicus simulated. Both operative areas have to be drained.

The advantage of this procedure is the large amount of tissue offered for reconstruction; the disadvantage is that it is a major procedure with complications and even complete loss of flaps reported.

Another point is that the large amount of transposed tissue makes it impossible to detect local recurrences at an early stage. Minor areas of fat necrosis are palpated as hard lumps and may cause further worry for the patient and the oncologist.

As an alternative, a vertical myocutaneous rectus abdominis flap (Robbins 1981) might be used either from the ipsilateral or contralateral side. The skin over the rectus is included in the flap. This will supply less tissue than the vertical rectus flap, but is a surgically simpler procedure when not too much tissue is needed. It could make it possible to rebuild a breast contour even without an implant. The main disadvantage is the rather conspicious vertical scar in the upper abdomen.

The surgical technique is basically similar to that of the transverse flap, the difference being that a skin island is left over the rectus sheath to be brought through a tunnel into the recipient area (Fig. 25.**40**).

Comments on the Transverse Rectus Abdominis Flap

C. E. Horton and J. B. McCraw

The lower transverse rectus abdominis flap, described by Hartrampf, Scheflan and Black, is a major advance in many respects and the very best reconstructive results with this technique are unsurpassed, when compared to other methods. It is an extremely demanding operation, from the technique standpoint, but is a salutary addition to our armamentarium. This technique is particularly helpful in the moderately obese patient, in which a large breast reconstruction is required.

It is unfortunate that the flap is denervated, both in the cutaneous and muscular portion, in the course of its elevation, because both the motor and sensory supply are derived from the intercostal system.

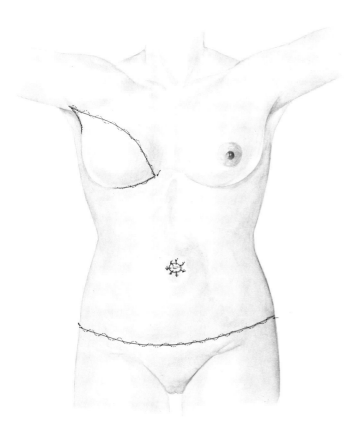

Fig. 25.**39** Closure completed.

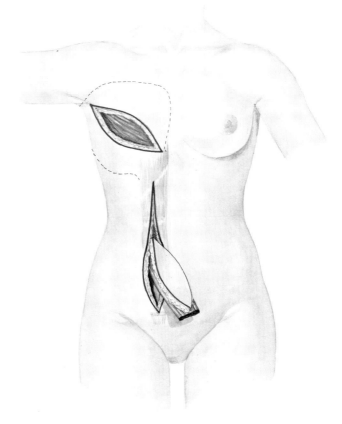

Fig. 25.**40** Design of vertical musculocutaneous rectus abdominis flap.

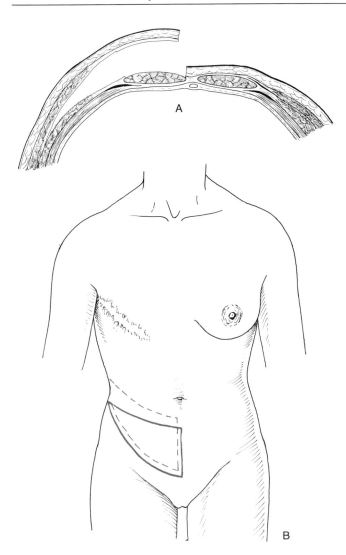

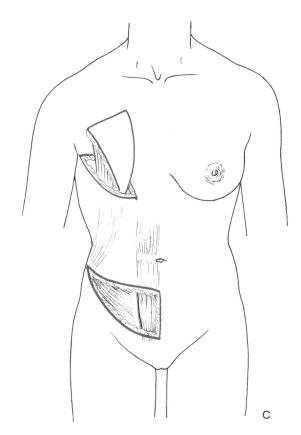

Fig. 25.**41** A, B, C Outline of external oblique musculocutaneous flap according to Marshal et al.

Technical Considerations

The lower midline scar is a common situation, and this absolutely prevents the use of the opposite side skin, since the fascial and subdermal plexus vessels will not traverse the lower midline scar.

Unless the new inframammary fold is placed at a sufficiently high level, it will be pulled too low by the abdominal closure.

Reshaping is a real problem. We cannot seem to get it right the first time, but that should not be a discouraging factor for this procedure in our early experience of 70 cases.

At the second operation, one reshapes the flap, treats the opposite breast and does the nipple reconstruction. It should be considered a two-staged operation, first, because it cannot all be done adequately in a single stage, and second, because only a few of our cases have required third stage.

Complications

This flap is obviously "cold sensitive", but our problems have almost always occurred in smokers. The stated incidence (Bostwick) of flap complications is 10% and this is probably a reasonable figure.

We certainly have had no total flap losses. We have had minor flap losses, when the flaps were placed into irradiated areas.

Hernias have occurred in our hands, only because of technical errors. We should have used a fascial or prosthetic replacement in tight closures and did not. In our initial cases, we had an 8% hernia rate which required a later repair. This was caused by a very tight closure in obese patients and is totally avoidable. If the closure is tight, particularly in an obese patient, prolene or marlex mesh should be used without hesitation.

Atelectasis has occurred in 12% of our patients by objective determinations.

Two patients sustained pulmonary emboli. Both resolved these problems without any difficulty with full heparinization. Although flap loss has not been a significant problem, flap stiffness and fat necrosis have been. We refer to "stiffness" as an entity, because it is a firm area related to fat. Fat necrosis is something more dramatic because it can form cysts and may cause sharply circumscribed dense scarring.

The External Oblique Abdominis Muscle Flap

In 1982, Marshall et al. reported the use of an external oblique abdominis myocutaneous flap in postmastectomy breast reconstruction. The flap is based laterally and nourished by the vessels entering the muscle from its lateral side. Perforating vessels to the skin makes it possible to use part of the overlying skin as an island. The flap is brought through a tunnel to the postmastectomy area and provides a considerable amount of tissue and might build up the contour even without the use of an implant (Fig. 25.**41**A–C).

Holle and Pierini (1983) have reported the use of the external oblique abdominis muscle to provide a better cover for an implant in reconstruction after a modified radical mastectomy. They use the part of this muscle caudal to the breast as an upwardly based muscle flap nourished by intercostal perforators (Fig. 25.**42**). When the muscle flap is turned over, the free muscle border can be sutured to the lower edge of the pectoral major muscle under which the pocket for the implant has been prepared. To provide additional skin to the lower part of the breast, Holle and Pierini recommend two large z-plasties, one medially and one laterally to reposition the skin from a horizontal to a vertical direction (Fig. 25.**43**A, B).

A simple and effective technique for breast reconstruction after modified radical mastectomy is the following:

1. A long horizontal incision is made in the level of the submammary fold down to the underlying muscle fascia.

2. The inferior border of the pectoralis major is incized horisontally and the plane between the pectoralis major and minor is dissected up to the level of the clavicle and medially to the sternum. The medial insertion of the pectoralis major on the sternum is cut so that the submuscular pocket opens widely downward all the way above the inframammary fold.

3. The abdominal skin is undermined from the submammary incision to the level just above the umbilicus to expose the externus oblique muscle and the rectus fascia.

4. A turn-over muscle flap consisting of the external oblique abdominis muscle and part of the adjacent rectus fascia is designed and prepared based cranially (Fig. 25.**42**). The length of the flap is first decided and a horizontal incision is made through the muscle and extended through the rectus fascia to the midline. The medial vertical incision line lies medially in the rectus fascia and the lateral one in the externus obliqus. The muscle flap is prepared including a superficial part of the rectus muscle and the dissection is advanced cranially until the sixth intercostal space (Fig. 25.**44**). The flap can now be turned over to cover the lower part of the breast (Fig. 25.**45**). This muscle flap constitutes an excellent submammary demarcation.

5. An implant is introduced under the pectoralis muscle and the edge of the turned-over external oblique muscle is sutured to the edge of the pectoral muscle over the implant (Fig. 25.**46**).

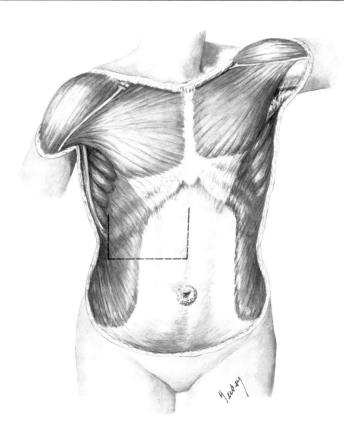

Fig. 25.**42**   Outline of external oblique turn-over muscular flap.

6. The skin incision is closed (Fig. 25.**47**).

7. If additional skin is needed in the lower part of the breast, this can be brought about by applying a full-thickness free skin graft to the surface of the turned-over muscle flap. In such a case, the inferior skin edge of the submammary incision is anchored to the chest wall. A suitable skin graft is removed from the other breast if a reduction mammaplasty is made at the same time. Otherwise the graft is removed from the lower abdomen and sutured in place (Fig. 25.**48**).

8. Nipple-areolar reconstruction is better made in a second stage when the shape of the breast has been established.

References

Baroudi, R., J. A. Pinotti, E. M. Keppke: A transverse thoracoabdominal skin flap for closure after radical mastectomy. Plast. Reconstr. Surg. 61: 547, 1978

Biggs, T. M., E. D. Cronin: Technical aspects of the latissimus dorsi myocutaneous flap in breast reconstruction. Ann. Plast. Surg. 6: 381, 1981

Birnbaum, L., J. A. Olsen: Breast reconstruction following radical mastectomy, using customized-designed implants. Plast. Reconstr. Surg. 61: 355, 1978

Bohmert, H.: Eine neue Methode zur Rekonstruktion der weiblichen Brust nach radikaler Mastektomie. Transactions 5. Tagung der Vereinigung der Deutschen Plastischen Chirurgen, München, Demeter Verlag 1974

Bohmert, H.: Plastic Surgery of the Head and Neck and the Female Breast. Thieme, Stuttgart 1975

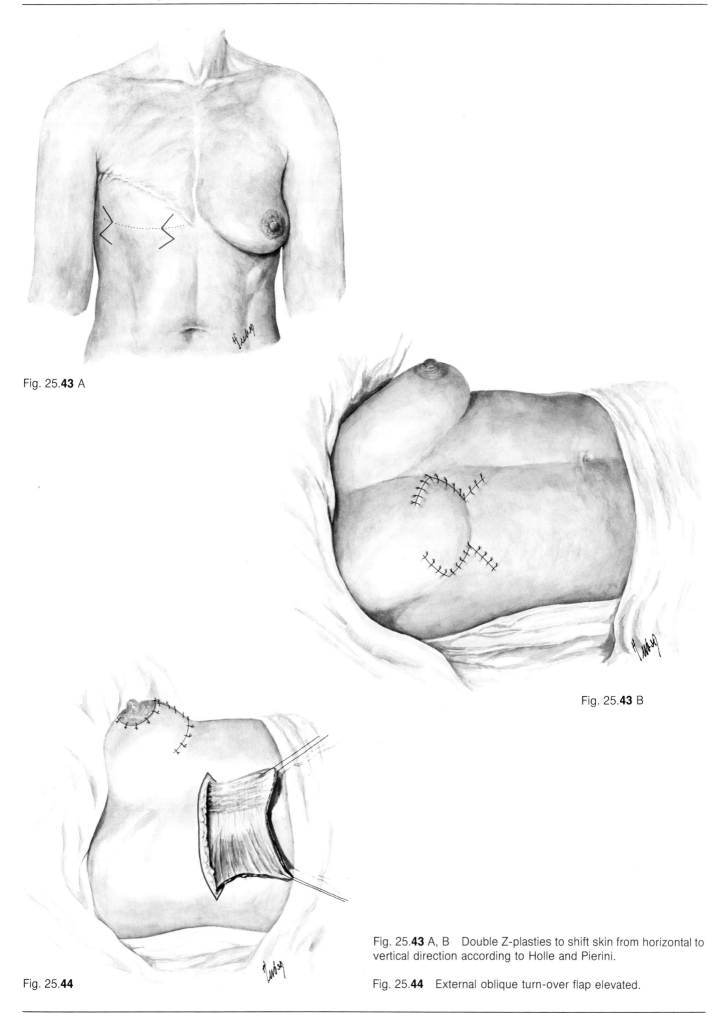

Fig. 25.**43** A

Fig. 25.**43** B

Fig. 25.**44**

Fig. 25.**43** A, B   Double Z-plasties to shift skin from horizontal to vertical direction according to Holle and Pierini.

Fig. 25.**44**   External oblique turn-over flap elevated.

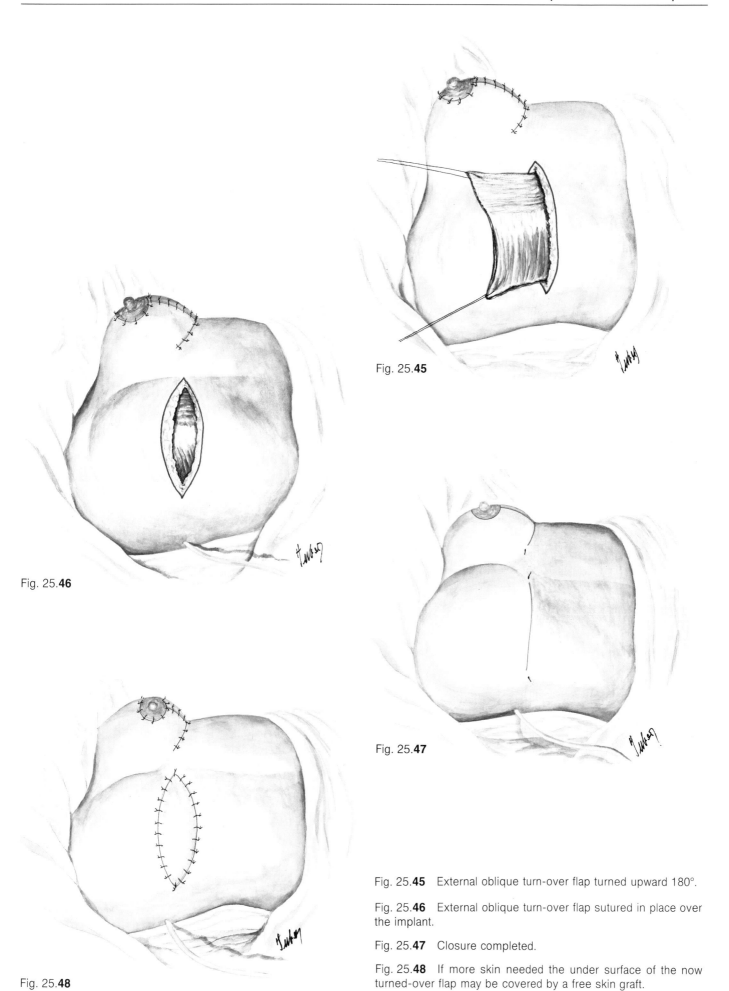

Fig. 25.**45**

Fig. 25.**46**

Fig. 25.**47**

Fig. 25.**48**

Fig. 25.**45**　External oblique turn-over flap turned upward 180°.

Fig. 25.**46**　External oblique turn-over flap sutured in place over the implant.

Fig. 25.**47**　Closure completed.

Fig. 25.**48**　If more skin needed the under surface of the now turned-over flap may be covered by a free skin graft.

Bohmert, H.: Personal method for reconstruction of the female breast following radical mastectomy. In: Transactions of the Sixth International Congress of Plastic and Reconstructive Surgery. Massom, Paris, New York 1976

Bohmert, H.: Refinements in Technique of Breast Reconstruction with thoracoepigastric and advancement flaps in 150 patients. In: Transactions Intern. Congr. Plast. Reconstr. Surg., Rio de Janeiro, 1979. Cartgraf, Sao Paulo 1980

Bohmert, H.: Experience in breast reconstruction with thoracoepigastric and advancement flaps. Acta Chir. Belg. 79: 105, 1980

Bohmert, H.: Breast Cancer and Breast Reconstruction. Thieme, Stuttgart, New York 1982

Bohmert, H.: Aufbauplastik nach Mastektomie. In H. Feiereis, H. E. Grewe: Brustkrebs der Frau. Hrsg. Marseille Verlag, München 1983

Bohmert, H.: Breast reconstruction with a contralateral thoracoepigastric myocutaneous flap. Transactions VIII. International Congress Plastic Surgery, Bibliotheque nationale de Quebec, Montreal 1983

Bostwick, J., L. O. Vasconez, M. J. Jurkiewicz: Breast reconstruction following radical mastectomy. Plast. Reconstr. Surg. 61: 682, 1978

Bostwick, J., H. L. Hill, F. Nahai: Repairs in the lower abdomen, groin, or perineum with myocutaneous or omental flaps. Plast. Reconstr. Surg. 63: 186, 1979a

Bostwick, J. III, F. Nahai, J. F. Wallace, L. O. Vasconez: Sixty latissimus dorsi flaps. Plast. Reconstr. Surg. 63: 31, 1979b

Bostwick, J.: Aesthetic and Reconstructive Breast Surgery. Saint Louis Mosby, 1983

Brown, R. G., L. O. Vasconez, M. J. Jurkiewicz: Transverse abdominal flaps and the deep epigastric arcade. Plast. Reconstr. Surg. 55: 416, 1975

Cronin, T. D., J. Upton, J. M. McDonough: Reconstruction of the breast after mastectomy. Plast. Reconstr. Surg. 59: 1, 1977

Davis, W. M., J. B. McCraw, J. H. Carraway: Use of a direct transverse thoracoabdominal flap to close difficult wounds of the thorax and upper extremity. Plast. Reconstr. Surg. 60: 526, 1977

De la Plaza, R.: Postmastectomy reconstruction by contralateral abdominomammary flap. Ann. Plast. Surg. 6: 97, 1981

Der Hagopian, R. P., P. C. Zaworski, E. V. Sugerbaker, A. S. Ketcham: Management of locally recurrent breast cancer adjacent to prosthetic implants. Am. J. Surg. 141: 590, 1981

D'Este, S.: La technique de l'amputation de la mamelle pour carcinome mammaire. Rev. Chir. (Paris) 45: 164, 1912

Dinner, M. I., H. P. Labandter, R. V. Dowden: The role of the rectus abdominis myocutaneous flap in breast reconstruction. Plast. Reconstr. Surg. 69: 209, 1982

Dowden, R. V., C. E. Horton, F. E. Rosato: Reconstruction of the breast after mastectomy. Surg. Gynecol. Obstet 149: 109, 1979

Georgiade, N. G.: Reconstructive Breast Surgery. Mosby, St. Louis 1976

Hartrampf, C. R., M. Scheflan, P. W. Black: Breast reconstruction with a transverse abdominal island flap. Plast. Reconstr. Surg. 69: 216, 1982

Hillelson, R. L., J. Glowacki, N. A. Healey, J. B. Mulliken: A microangiographic study of hematoma associated flap necrosis and salvage with isoxsurprine. Plast. Reconstr. Surg. 66: 528, 1980

Holle, J., A. Pierini: Breast reconstruction by a turn-over flap of the external oblique abdominis muscle and double Z-plasty of the abdominal skin. In: Transact. VIII Internat. Congress Plast. Reconstr. Surg., Montreal 1983

Juri, C., G. Juri: Mammary reconstruction in one surgical stage. In: Transactions of the VIII International Congress of Plastic Reconstructive Surgery, Montreal 1983

Lemperle, G.: Verschiedene Schwenk- und Verschiebeplastiken in der Brustchirurgie. In: Brustkrebs und Brustrekonstruktion. Thieme, Stuttgart, New York 1982

Leis, H. P., Jr.: Selective and reconstructive surgical procedures for carcinoma of the breast. Gynecol. Obstet. 148: 17, 1979

Lejour, M., H. Eder, A. De Mey, W. Mattheiem: Breast reconstruction at the Tumor Centre of the University of Brussels. A three year report. Acta Chir. Belg. 79: 135, 1980

Lejour, M.: Reconstruction of the breast with a contralateral epigastric rectus myocutaneous flap. Chir. Plast. 6: 181, 1982

Lewis, J. R., Jr.: Use of a sliding flap from the abdomen to provide cover in breast reconstruction. Plast. Reconstr. Surg. 64: 491, 1979

Marshall, D. R., E. J. Anspee, M. J. Stapleton: Soft tissue reconstruction of the breast using an external oblique myo-cutaneous abdominal flap. Br. J. Plast. Surg. 35: 443, 1982

Mathes, S. J., F. Nahai: Clinical atlas of muscle and musculocutaneous flaps. The C. V. Mosby Co., St. Louis 1979

Mathes, S. J., J. Bostwick: Rectus abdominis myocutaneous flap to reconstruct abdominal wall defects. Br. J. Plast. Surg. 30: 282, 1977

Mattheiem, W.: Modern trends in the treatment of breast cancer. Acta Chir. Belg. 79: 77, 1980

Maxwell, G. P., B. M. McGibbon, J. E. Hoopes: Vascular considerations in the use of a latissimus dorsi myocutaneous flap after a mastectomy with an axillary dissection. Plast. Reconstr. Surg. 64: 771, 1979

McCraw, J. B., D. G. Dibbell, J. H. Carraway: Clinical definition of independent myocutaneous vascular territories. Plast. Reconstr. Surg. 60: 341, 1977

McCraw, J. B., J. Bostwick, III, C. E. Horton: Methods of soft tissue coverage for the mastectomy defect. Clin. Plast. Surg. 6: 57, 1979

Millard, D. R., Jr.: Variations in the design of the latissimus dorsi flap in breast reconstruction. Ann. Plast. Surg. 7: 269, 1981

Millard, D. R., Jr.: Reconstruction mammaplasty using an economical flap from the opposite breast. Ann. Plast. Surg. 6: 374, 1981

Montandon, D.: Incidental discovery of recurrent breast carcinoma in patients seeking breast reconstruction. Br. J. Plast. Surg. 32: 318, 1979

Mühlbauer, W., R. Olbrisch: The latissimus dorsi myocutaneous flap for breast reconstruction. Chir. Plast. 4: 27, 1977

Olivari, N.: The latissimus flap. Br. J. Plast. Surg. 29: 126, 1976

Peters, C. R.: Recurrence of breast cancer in the reconstructed patient. Considerations and treatment. Proceedings 51st Annual Convention A. S. P. R. S., October 1982

Pierer, H.: Reconstruction of the breast after carcinoma operation. Transact. 4. Int. Congr. f. Plast. Reconstr. Surg. 1967

Piontec, R. W., K. R. Kase: Radiation transmission study of silicone elastomer for mammary prosthesis. Radiology 136: 505, 1980

Prpic, I., P. Martinac: Reconstruction of the breast as a primary and secondary procedure. In: H. Bohmert: Breast Cancer and Breast Reconstruction. Thieme, Stuttgart, New York 1982

Robbins, T. H.: Rectus abdominis myocutaneous flap for breast reconstruction. Aust. N. Z. J. Surg. 49: 527, 1979

Robbins, T. H.: Post-mastectomy breast reconstruction using a rectus abdominis musculocutanous island flap. Br. J. Plast. Surg. 34: 286, 1981

Rosato, F. E., E. E. Horton, G. P. Maxwell: Postmastectomy breast reconstruction. Curr. Probl. Surg. 17: 585, 1980

Schneider, W. J., H. L. Hill, R. G. Brown: Latissimus dorsi myocutaneous flap for breast reconstruction. Br. J. Plast. Surg. 30: 277, 1977

Snyderman, R. K., R. H. Guthrie: Reconstruction of the female breast following radical mastectomy. Plast. Reconstr. Surg. 47: 565, 1971

Tai, Y., H. Hasegawa: A transverse abdominal flap for reconstruction after radical operations for recurrent breast cancer. Plast. Reconstr. Surg. 53: 52, 1974

Urban, J. A.: Reconstruction after mastectomy. In R. K. Snyderman: Symposium on Neoplastic and Reconstructive Problems of the Female Breast. Mosby, Saint Louis 1973

Wolfe, L. E., T. M. Biggs: Aesthetic refinements in the use of the latissimus dorsi flap in breast reconstruction. Plast. Reconstr. Surg. 69: 788, 1982

Woods, J. E.: Breast reconstruction after mastectomy. Surg. Gynecol. Obstet. 150: 869, 1980

Chapter 26

Subcutaneous Mastectomy and Total Mastectomy with Reconstruction

C. E. Horton, J. B. McCraw and J. O. Strömbeck

Introduction and Indications

A safe, but efficient mastectomy without resulting deformity is needed for the patient who has a high risk of developing mammary cancer (Layton 1964). In the past if the general surgeon and the patient felt that breast disease potential was significant, a total mastectomy was recommended, accepted reluctantly, and the patient's breast was amputated leaving a linear scar and a flat chest. The lack of normal breast contour resulted in many defeminized patients with psychological disturbances. This was deemed too high a price for most patients and therefore a simple mastectomy was usually recommended as a last resort when the danger of developing malignancy appeared excessive. For years, conscientious physicians have attempted to find alternative methods that would remove breast disease potential and still allow retention of the normal breast form. Using modern reconstruction techniques, the realization of this objective seems near.

Although most general surgeons agree that there are cases that are best treated with prophylactic total breast extirpation, it is difficult to set firm guidelines for patient selection (Pennisi and Capozzi 1973). Most authorities would agree that women with a biopsy-proved proliferative histologic variant of fibrocystic disease represent a difficult clinical problem (Monson et al. 1976). Adequate observation by physical examination is unreliable in the patient with diffuse breast nodularity. Mammography and xeroradiography have limitations as well as drawbacks (Wolfe 1976). There is some concern that these techniques may influence the tumor development especially where metaplastic changes have already occurred. This inability to detect cancer of the breast in its incipient or preinvasive stage causes anxiety for patient and physician alike. It is in this clinical situation that some type of prophylactic mastectomy is acceptable.

The history of breast cancer in the contralateral breast or positive family history of breast malignancy adds substantially to the patient's cancer potential (Potter et al. 1968). Silicone injections, which produce breast lumps that are indistinguishable from cancer by physical examination, should be condemned and breasts that have been injected previously should probably be operated on to remove all breast tissue and injected silicone material (Bandeian et al. 1978). Cowden's syndrome is a familial hereditary condition in which all females are at high risk for breast cancer; therefore, prophylactic mastectomy is necessary for these patients.

Main indications for prophylactic mastectomy:

1. Family history of premenopausal breast cancer (mother, aunt, sister)
2. Patients who had one breast removed because of cancer and whose other breast shows cystic disease or intraductal hyperplasia or papillomas
3. Severe cystic disease with lobular neoplasia or intraductal hyperplasia
4. Cowden's syndrome

Subcutaneous Mastectomy

Since Rice and Strickler's original report (1951) on subcutaneous mastectomy using an inframammary approach, many papers have appeared recommending this technique. Many articles have been written advocating the operation of subcutaneous mastectomy and either immediate or delayed reconstruction of the breast. In the usual subcutaneous mastectomy, the breast tissue is dissected out through an inframammary approach leaving a rim of breast tissue under the nipple. A prosthesis is introduced in the pocket (Freeman 1962). Other techniques have been described for subtotal excision of breast tissue using an areolar incision. The efficacy of this operation depends on the zeal of the surgeon in attempting to eradicate all elements of breast tissue. Some surgeons may leave some of the breast tissue attached to the skin, whereas others attempt a more radical approach, leaving some breast tissue only under the areola. Since the blood supply to the nipple is impaired if breast tissue is removed from beneath the nipple, it is accepted that breast tissue must be left in this site or the nipple will undergo necrosis due to avascularity. Peripheral breast tissue and tissue near the axillary tail may also be difficult to remove through the inframammary approach. Goldman and Goldwyn (1973) reported that positive biopsies can be obtained after subcutaneous mastectomy performed on cadavers. Many surgeons have reported malignancies that have developed in the remnants of the breast tissue remaining after subcutaneous mastectomy. Pennisi et al. (1976), on the other hand, feel that a definite beneficial effect can be demonstrated for subcutaneous mastectomy. No statistics are available to show whether or not cancer potential is in any way a function of breast size. Women with small breasts have the same potential to develop breast cancer as do women with large breasts. Most authorities feel that breast cancer is not a localized disease, but that breast cancer potential exists throughout

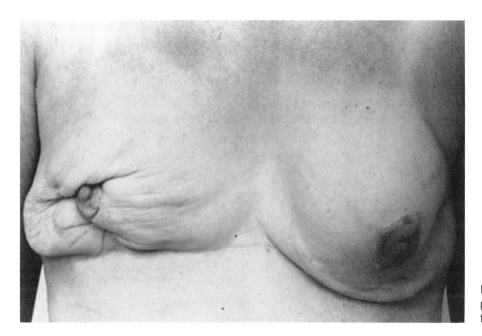

Fig. 26.**1** Wrinkling of skin after loss of prosthesis following subcutaneous mastectomy.

all elements of the breast tissue if the patient is susceptible to this type of malignancy. As long as breast tissue remains, the patient remains at risk to the formation of cancer. Subcutaneous mastectomy, with implantation of prosthesis in the subcutaneous pocket, carries a high morbidity and complication rate. Lynch et al. (1978) reported that at least 50% of all subcutaneous mastectomies have complications and must be reoperated. Schlenker et al. (1978) reported a high rate of early and late complications.

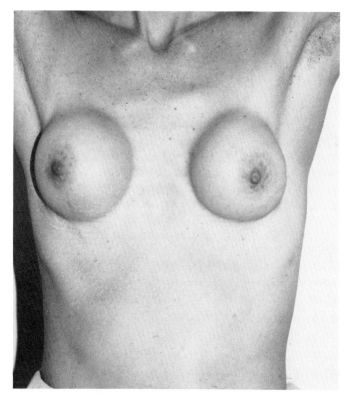

Fig. 26.**2** Mastodynia and capsular contracture after subcutaneous mastectomy.

Complications of the Subcutaneous Mastectomy

The complication rate of this operation varies with the enthusiasm of the surgeon. If all breast tissue is removed, the nipple and adjacent skin often becomes devascularized and necrotic. Skin flap necrosis causes exposure and loss of the prosthesis if it is placed on top of the pectoral muscle immediately beneath the skin flaps. Complications of the usual subcutaneous mastectomy can be classified according to the time of occurrence. Early complications include necrosis of the nipple and/or necrosis of the raised skin with resulting exposure of the prosthesis. Severe scarring and skin wrinkling are inevitably following these complications (Fig. 26.**1**). Even if the breast reconstruction is delayed after subcutaneous mastectomy, the remaining skin usually becomes so wrinkled and the nipple so malpositioned that the final cosmetic result is jeopardized. Late complications include implant displacement, wrinkling of excessive skin not tightened by a large enough implant, persistent mastodynia, severe capsular contracture with abnormal breast firmness (Fig. 26.**2**), and wrinkling of the implant with late pressure erosion through the skin. A general unsightly cosmetic appearance occurs all too frequently. Because of these complications, the subcutaneous mastectomy with simultaneous reconstruction with prosthesis has gotten a bad reputation.

To live up to the name of mastectomy, the skin has to be dissected off the gland leaving no glandular rests attached to the skin. The dissection is made in the same plane as when developing the skin flaps in an ordinary mastectomy. Since glandular offshoots sometimes may extend close to the skin, it is important that the surgeon has good access to the operative field to be able to inspect the under surface of the skin to be sure that no glandular rests are left behind. A submammary incision does not, in our opinion, give a satisfactory access. After a mastectomy, the skin is often very thin and does not, in most cases,

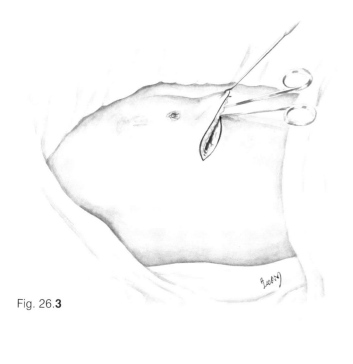

Fig. 26.**3**

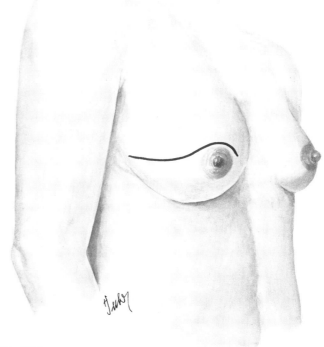

Fig. 26.**4**

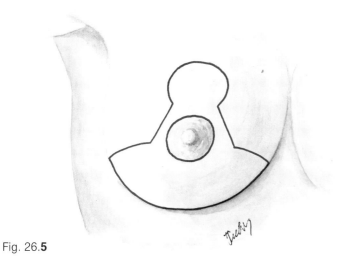

Fig. 26.**5**

Fig. 26.**3** Skin is dissected off the gland from an inframammary incision.

Fig. 26.**4** An hemiareolar incision extended laterally is recommended when no skin reduction has to be made.

Fig. 26.**5** If skin reduction is to be made the incisions are planned as in reduction mammaplasty.

offer a satisfactory cover for a prosthesis. If, however, the prosthesis is placed under the pectoralis muscle, the complication rate will drop and the results improve. The weak point of the operation will then be small glandular remnants underneath the nipple (Strömbeck 1982).

Operative Technique

From a long incision in the inframammary fold, it might be possible to dissect the skin off the gland (Fig. 26.**3**). In so doing, it is important not to sacrifice the small subcutaneous vessels around the areola and to leave some glandular tissue just beneath the nipple. The accurate dissection to remove the axillary tail may be difficult from that incision and the access to the operation field to secure hemostasis and to check that all glandular tissue really has been removed might be difficult. Even if, for

example, Pennisi has reported excellent results with this technique, we strongly feel that the submammary incision should not be recommended when doing a subcutaneous mastectomy.

A hemiareolar incision extended laterally (Fig. 26.**4**) gives an excellent access both for inspection and hemostasis. This incision for subcutaneous mastectomy is recommended for breasts of small and normal size (Strömbeck 1982). The gland could be dissected off the skin under direct vision in a plane leaving no glandular tissue behind. When dissecting the deep surface from the muscle, care should be taken not to damage the muscle tissue. If, however, the breasts are large and pendulous, there will be a considerable skin surplus that has to be reduced. The skin reduction may be planned as when doing a reduction mammoplasty with an inverted T-scar (Fig. 26.**5**). The areola-nipple complex has then to be transposed on a broad dermis-subcutaneous pedicle preferably based in

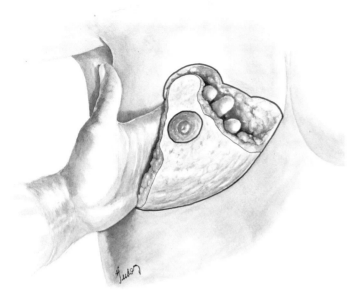

Fig. 26.**6**

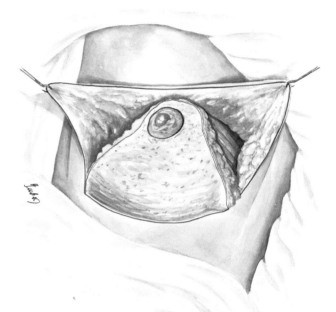

Fig. 26.**8**

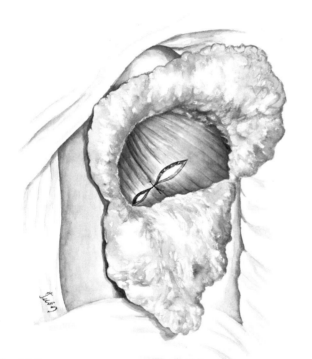

Fig. 26.**7**

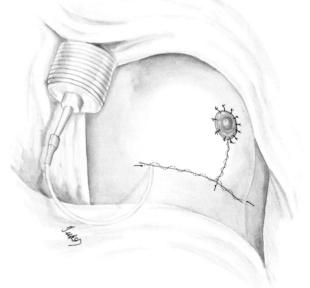

Fig. 26.**6**   The nipple-areolar region on a dermis-subcutaneous pedicle based inferiorly.

Fig. 26.**7**   Implant placed submuscularly.

Fig. 26.**8**   The pedicle is to be covered by the skin flaps.

Fig. 26.**9**   Closure completed.

Fig. 26.**9**

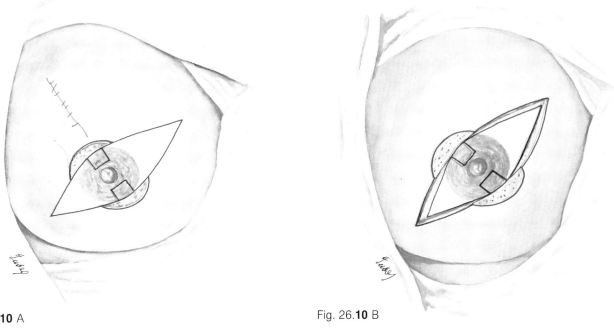

Fig. 26.**10** A

Fig. 26.**10** B

Fig. 26.**10** A, B Design of total mastectomy with immediate reconstruction utilizing part of the areolar skin for nipple reconstruction.

Fig. 26.**11** Skin is dissected off the gland.

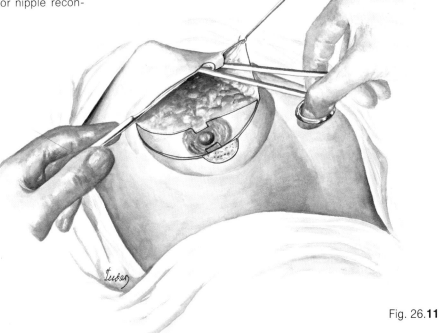

Fig. 26.**11**

the submammary fold (Fig. 26.**6**), an implant is introduced submuscularely (Fig. 26.**7**), and the skin flaps sutured on top of the pedicle (Figs. 26.**8**, 26.**9**). An alternative is to reduce the skin as a large horizontal ellipse leaving the areola based on a dermis-subcutaneous flap attached to the inferior skin border.

To avoid leaving any breast tissue underneath the areola complex, the nipple and subareolar region might be included in the specimen once the areolar skin has been dissected from the deep dermal layer (Figs. 26.**10**, 26.**11**). The excised areolar skin could then be used as a free graft in combination with small skin flaps to simulate a nipple (Figs. 26.**12**, 26.**13**). If the edges of the horizontal ellipse

is close to the original areola, these small flaps could in fact include areolar skin giving the fake nipple a normal color (Fig. 26.**14**).

The reconstruction with a prosthesis should be made in the same operation. To minimize the complication rate, the prosthesis should be placed in a separate submuscular pocket. The easiest way to prepare the pocket is from the upper lateral border of the major pectoral muscle, taking care that the pocket extends far enough in medial and caudal direction underneath the serratus and rectus sheath. The lateral entrance to the submuscular plane has to be carefully closed after a properly sized implant has been introduced. The submuscular pocket and the post-

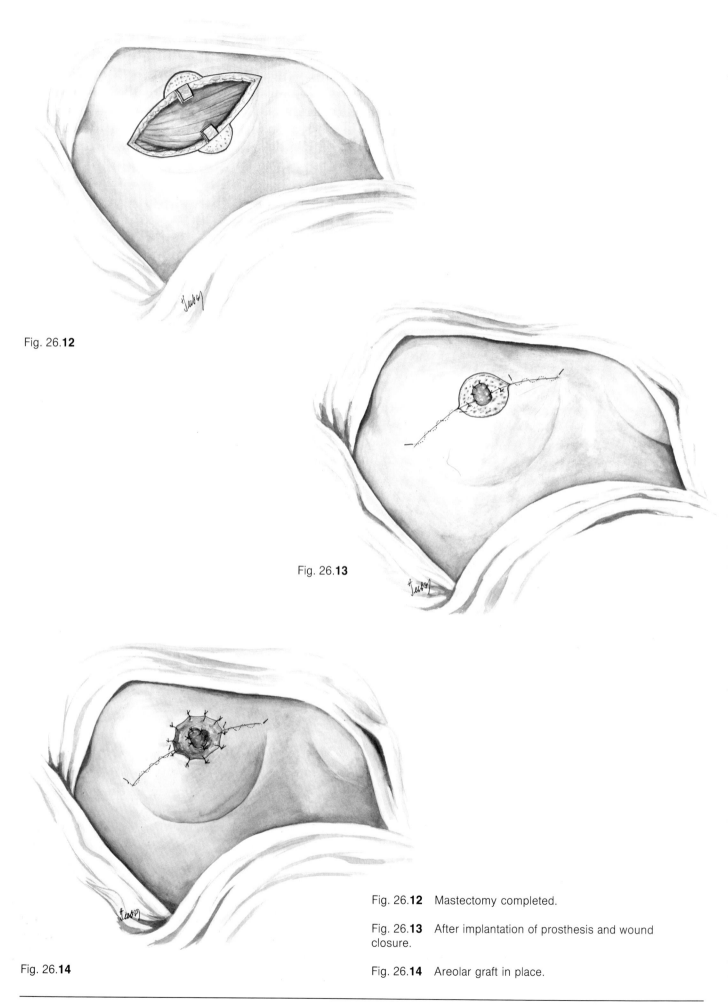

Fig. 26.**12**

Fig. 26.**13**

Fig. 26.**14**

Fig. 26.**12**   Mastectomy completed.

Fig. 26.**13**   After implantation of prosthesis and wound closure.

Fig. 26.**14**   Areolar graft in place.

mastectomy pocket are drained separately. By using the submuscular technique, cover of the prosthesis will be better and minor circulatory disturbances of the areola or skin will not lead to an extrusion of the prosthesis. The subcutaneous mastectomy is a difficult operation, which has to be performed most carefully and with a good atraumatic technique. But even so, complications may occur, such as circulatory disturbances with partial necrosis of areola or skin, especially if the mastectomy is combined with reduction of the skin envelope, asymmetry of the prosthesis, and capsular contracture. The preservation of the nipple areola complex, however, gives a better esthetic result than a faked one does (Figs. 26.**15**A, B; 26.**16**A, B). As mentioned above, the weak point of the subcutaneous mastectomy is the glandular rest beneath the areola. This could be avoided by excising the complete areola with the gland and reconstructing the areola-nipple complex in the same way as in reconstruction after mastectomy. This may give less satisfactory cosmetic results, but is in terms of mastectomy a safer procedure. This procedure we call total mastectomy with immediate reconstruction.

Total Mastectomy and Immediate Reconstruction

Over fifteen years ago, discouraged by the results of subcutaneous mastectomy, the authors attempted various techniques to change the operation. Because the nipple-areolar area was the most frequent area noted to have devascularization and because cancer of the breast frequently occurs in this site, we decided to incorporate an excision of this area in the removal of breast tissue.

The incision is planned to extend obliquely and slightly upward from just medial to each nipple, encompassing an ellipse of skin incorporating the nipple-areola complex and extending toward the axilla as far as necessary to allow direct visualization of the breast. This permits direct access to remove all breast tissue. It necessitates, however, leaving a direct scar over the nipple-areolar area. A pocket is made beneath the pectoral muscle and the serratus and rectus abdominis fascia to provide an adequate cover. A smooth-walled gel-filled prosthesis was difficult to secure in a fixed position. Because of this, a polyurethane foam-covered prosthesis was used. This prosthesis, although more difficult to insert, did not migrate and surpisingly did not cause excess breast capsule formation. It was found that the breast mound did not move, and therefore a proper nipple placement could be accomplished in the original operation with greater accuracy. Immediate nipple reconstruction, however, is not mandatory, and in certain cases we prefer to allow the breast reconstruction to heal and perform the nipple-areolar reconstruction at a second stage.

Patients who are not obese are the best candidates for total mastectomy (Fig. 26.**17**A, B, C). If a large layer of fat surrounds the depressed area where the breast has been removed, then the prosthesis must be extremely large in order to extend above the cavity in which it is placed. Ordinarily, obese patients have large breasts so that an extra large prosthesis is necessary to give breast symmetry to compare with the opposite large breast. In our experience extra large prosthesis do not do well. We recommend simple mastectomy for extremely obese women and later reconstruction if feasible, rather than immediate repair.

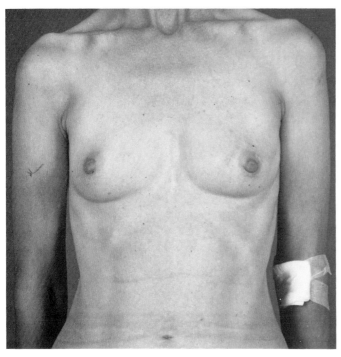

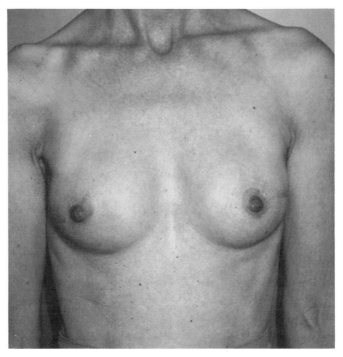

Fig. 26.**15**
A: 37-year-old patient with pronounced nodular mastopathy and atypia at biopsy.

B: One year after bilateral subcutaneous mastectomy from a curved incision along the cranial border of the areola and extended laterally.

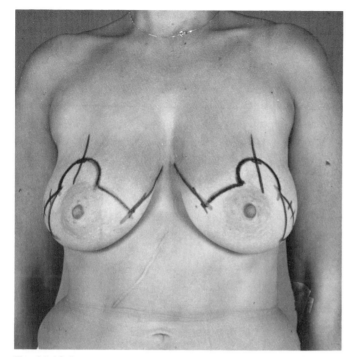

Fig. 26.**16** A

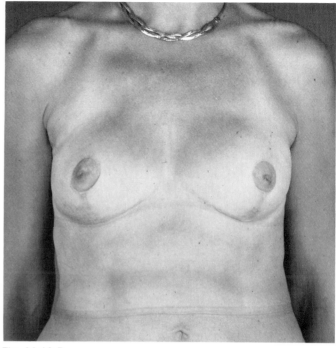

Fig. 26.**16** B

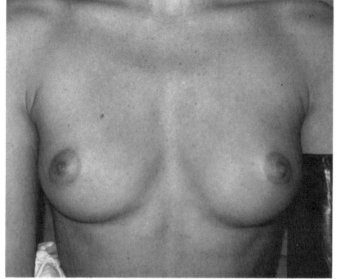

Fig. 26.**17** A

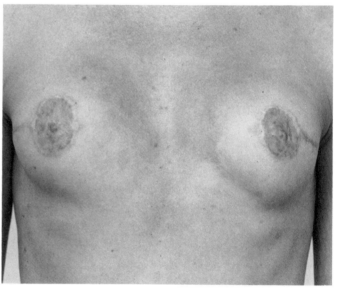

Fig. 26.**17** B

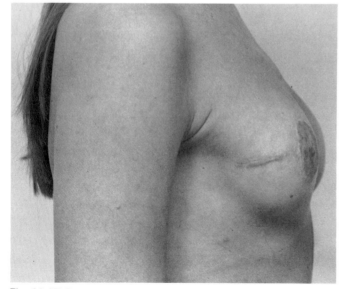

Fig. 26.**17** C

Fig. 26.**16**
A: 34-year-old patient with history of premenopausal breast cancer (mother). Nodular breasts. Atypia at biopsy.
B: Two years after subcutaneous mastectomy with simultaneous skin reduction. Nipple-areola based inferiorly.

Fig. 26.**17**
A: 23-year-old woman with family history of cancer of the breast. Mother, aunt, and sister died of breast cancer premenopausally. This patient did not want subcutaneous mastectomy because of her family history. She requested a total mastectomy.
B, C: After total mastectomy with reconstruction of the areola.

Correction of Subcutaneous Mastectomy Complication

The most common complications are experienced in patients having had their implant placed subcutaneously. If only a slight displacement of the prosthesis is at hand, an open localized capsulotomy might be sufficient. Mostly, however, there is a pronounced contracture. In these cases or if the prosthesis has eroded, it has to be removed and replaced in a new submuscular pocket. Depending on how meticulously the primary operation was performed, it might be necessary to raise the skin flaps to remove glandular remains left behind in continuity with the anterior part of the capsule. The posterior wall of the capsule lining the pectoralis could be left in place since no glandular rests are to be expected underneath. A new pocket for the implant is made retromuscularly.

The Norfolk group, when dealing with all types of complications after subcutaneous mastectomy, prefer to accomplish a total mastectomy using the same technique described above (Horton and Carraway 1976).

An incision is recommended beginning approximately 2 cm medial to the areola extending transversely across the breast, circumscribing the areola-nipple complex (if it is present), and extending laterally as far as necessary (usually to the anterior axillary line). If the prosthesis is present, it is removed. Generally there will be breast tissue around the capsule. In 18 consecutive biopsy cases of previous subcutaneous mastectomy having complications and later corrected with this technique, breast tissue was present in each specimen (Horton et al. 1978). The capsule should be excised with the specimen except over the pectoralis muscle, since no breast tissue exists beneath the capsule in this area. Occasionally, calcification has been noted within the capsule. In such cases we feel this should be excised. The nipple-areolar tissue if present is discarded, since a new nipple-areolar complex can be best reconstructed from the thigh.

Reconstruction is continued by opening the plane between the pectoralis major and the pectoralis minor muscle in the axilla. Dissection beneath the pectoralis major muscle will allow this muscle bulk to be used to cover the implant. An additional helpful technique has been to identify the medial edge of the pectoralis minor muscle and to undermine this muscle in a lateral direction. It can then be rotated laterally to produce secure coverage of the prosthesis at the top of the pocket. Careful but forceful dissection is essential to extend the submuscular pocket to at least 3 cm below the desired inframammary line. Lateral extension of the pocket by careful dissection beneath the serratus fascia is equally essential. If the dissection is difficult and the pectoralis muscle and serratus fascia thin, the latissimus muscle or rectus muscle may be used for additional coverage. We occasionally have used a superiorly based flap of rectus fascia which can be fashioned to cover the lower third of the prosthesis and will reinforce any pectoralis weakness in this area. A suction drain is inserted in the pocket prior to the implant placement. We ordinarily use a 250 to 350 cc polyethylene foam-covered gel prosthesis. The pocket is closed and the skin draped over the breast mound. All excess skin is trimmed. The new areola site ordinarily covers a portion of the incision line. At this point the material for the nipple reconstruction is accessed. Skin from the inner thigh is used to prepare full thickness areolar grafts (Broadbent et al. 1977). Local skin flaps or composite ear lobe grafts can be used to reconstruct the nipple. Occasionally, the tip of the normal discarded nipple might be used to provide a nipple graft.

The most difficult aspect of this operation is to properly position the nipple-areolar graft on the new breast mound. We recommend outlining the periphery of the new breast mound with marking solution and marking the area for the nipple-areolar complex on each apex. Measurements from the sternal notch and from the midline of the chest to each nipple are helpful. After selection of the appropriate areola recipient site, this area is denuded of epithelium and the nipple-areolar grafts applied. Bolster dressings are used and a light brassiere-type dressing is employed. Suction drains are removed in 24 to 48 hours.

In certain cases we have used rectus abdominis myocutaneous flaps to reconstruct subcutaneous mastectomy nipples. In most cases this flap can be constructed to carry enough skin and subcutaneous tissue to produce an adequate breast mound without the use of a prosthesis. In case skin is not needed in this repair, the epidermis can be excised, and the denuded flap placed beneath the breast area to reconstruct an adequately sized breast. Low rectus flaps produce a more desirable low abdominal scar, but occasionally will produce abdominal weakness unless the repair is reinforced with synthetic mesh. Upper rectus flaps produce more obvious scars, but better abdominal wall strength postoperatively.

Results

We have operated on many referred patients having severe complications after subcutaneous mastectomy. After total mastectomy and submuscular reconstruction, there has been no loss of implants or of the nipple-areola grafts. No migration of implants has been noted. The reconstructed breasts have remained soft and recurrent capsule contracture has been noted. No skin necrosis has been noted. Even in cases where the prosthesis is exposed and skin ulceration present, the skin excision can be extended to incorporate the area of ulceration. All of the patients have been more pleased with the total mastectomy than they were with the subcutaneous mastectomy result. Those patients who previously had capsular contracture with preoperative pain and discomfort have had soft nontender breasts (Horton et al. 1979). Our longest evaluation postoperatively is over 15 years. This technique allows excision of all excess skin and wrinkles and produces a tight skin envelope.

The cosmetic result of the "total prophylactic mastectomy" patient is not normal. Adequate nipple projection is not present, and a large central scar is present over the breast. The operation is not to be done inadvisably and patients must be carefully selected. It does, however, allow the conscientious surgeon to remove all breast tissue visible by direct inspection and does provide a padding of muscle that seems to prevent and/or disguise capsular contraction and later erosion of skin over the breast prosthesis.

Conclusions

1. An operation to remove premalignant breast tissue is needed to prevent breast cancer

2. The operation of meticulous subcutaneous mastectomy with submuscular implant is proposed as a technique to remove premalignant breast disease, the drawback being that it leaves some glandular tissue under the areola

3. The operation of total mastectomy with a free areolar nipple graft from the thigh and subpectoral implantation can be used to help patients with significant breast disease

References

Bandeian, J., F. E. Rosato, C. E. Horton: Evaluation of patients with augmented breasts. Surg. Gynecol. Obstet. 147: 596–598, 1978

Broadbent, T. R., R. M. Wolf, P. S. Metz: Restoring the mammary areola by a skin graft from the upper inner thigh. Br. J. Plast. Surg. 30: 220–222, 1977

Freeman, B. S.: Subcutaneous mastectomy for benign lesions with immediate or delayed prosthetic replacement. Plast. Reconstr. Surg. 30: 676–682, 1962

Goldman, L. D., R. M. Goldwyn: Some anatomic considerations of subcutaneous mastectomy. Plast. Reconstr. Surg. 51: 501–505, 1973

Horton, C. E., J. H. Carraway: Total mastectomy with immediate reconstruction for premalignant disease. In R. M. Goldburgh: Plastic and Reconstructive Surgery of the Breast. Little, Brown and Company, Boston 1976

Horton, C. E., F. E. Rosato, F. A. Schuler, J. B. McCraw: Postmastectomy reconstruction. Ann. Surg. 188: 773, 1978

Horton, C. E., F. E. Rosato, J. B. McCraw, R. V. Dowden: Immediate reconstruction following mastectomy for cancer. Clin. Plast. Surg. 6: 1979

Layton, J. J.: Pre-cancerous breast lesions. Proc. Natl. Cancer Cont. 5: 151, 1964

Lynch, J. B., J. J. Madden, J. D. Franklin: Breast reconstruction following mastectomy. Plast. Reconstr. Surg. 61: 371–376, 1978

Monson, Yen, Macmahon, Warren: Chronic mastitis and carcinoma of the breast. Lancet 224, 1976

Pennisi, V. R., A. Capozzi: Treatment of chronic cystic disease of the breast by subcutaneous mastectomy. Plast. Reconstr. Surg. 52: 520, 1973

Pennisi, V. R., A. Capozzi, F. M. Perez: The subcutaneous mastectomy date evaluation center. Breast 2: 1976

Potter, J. F., W. P. Slimbaugh, S. C. Woodward: Can breast cancer be anticipated? A follow-up of benign breast biopsies. Ann. Surg. 167: 829, 1968

Rice, C. O., J. H. Strickler: Adenomammectomy for benign lesions. Surg. Gynecol. Obstet. 93: 759, 1951

Rosato, F. E., C. E. Horton, G. P. Maxwell: Postmastectomy breast reconstruction. Curr. Probl. Surg. 17: 585–632, 1980

Schlenker, J. D., et al.: Loss of silicone implants after subcutaneous mastectomy and reconstruction. Plast. Reconstr. Surg. 62: 853–861, 1978

Strömbeck, J. O.: Subcutaneous mastectomy has to be a mastectomy. In H. Bohmert: Breast Cancer and Breast Reconstruction. G. Thieme Verlag, Stuttgart 1982

Wolfe, J. N.: Risk for breast cancer development determined by mammographic parenchymal pattern. Cancer 37: 2486–2492, 1976

Chapter 27

Reduction Mammaplasty

J. O. Strömbeck

Introduction

The size of the female breast is determined by the amount of glandular tissue and fat tissue. What is considered to be the normal size of the female breast varies from race to race. The variation in size depends to some degree on the amount of glandular tissue, but largely on the volume of fat tissue. As an average, 1 kg of weight gain gives an enlargement of each breast of about 20 g. This means that a weight gain of 7 to 8 kg gives a breast enlargement that about corresponds to an augmentation mammaplasty with implantation of a prosthesis of 150 cc (Strömbeck 1964).

Besides the increase in volume that occurs during pregnancy, the breast is subject to physiologic variations in size over a lifetime. For instance, an increase in volume is seen during the premenstrual period due to the accumulation of fluid in the breast. Changes of volume of about 20% during the menstrual cycle has been recorded by Döring (1953). During the climacteric period, a fatty transformation of the glandular components is seen that accounts for a certain reduction of the volume unless it is combined with a general increase in fat tissue. Thus, what could be regarded as a normal breast size is dependent on ethnic group, degree of adiposity, and on fashion trends as to what is considered to be beautiful. Similarly, as it is difficult to give the normal size of a breast, it is difficult to clearly define what is a pathologically enlarged breast. For this condition, the term *mammary hypertrophy* is often used. This term, however, implies hypertrophy in the glandular tissue, which is frequently not the case. It is, therefore, more logical to avoid this term and instead use the term *macromastia*, which is purely descriptive and means quite simply that the breasts are large and does not imply as to whether they consist of glandular tissue or fat. From a practical point of view, macromastia is a condition when the patient is so disturbed by the breast size or shape that there is a reason to perform a reduction mammaplasty. One could find all degrees from the almost normal-sized but ptotic breast to the extremely enlarged breasts that sometimes could perforate spontaneously and are called gigantomastia.

Etiology of Macromastia

It appears reasonable to believe that pronounced development of the breast is caused by an abnormal hormonal production. However, this does not seem to be the case. It is more probable that in these patients the mammary tissue has an increased sensitivity to hormonal stimulation.

Women with large breasts often have a hereditary disposition for this either on the fathers or mothers side. This is true for the type of breast enlargement that makes its debut during puberty and where the glandular component is especially prominent. The breast enlargement may also make its debut later in life, for instance, in connection with pregnancy. In these patients, there is only a slight reduction in the breast volume after delivery or nursing and the end result is a considerable enlargement in comparison with the condition before pregnancy. Adiposity is also a very common cause of macromastia. In these cases there is not an increase of the amount of glandular tissue, but only of fat tissue. Even if the deposition of fat tissue is different in different women, an average increase in weight of 1 kg gives an increase in breast weight of 20 g.

Symptoms

The major symptoms in macromastia are those directly connected with the size and weight of the breasts. The increased load on shoulder and cervical bones causes a sense of fatigue and pain in the cervical and upper thoracic spine. Just as common is shoulder grooving by brassiere. Apart from discomfort from local pressure and possibly ulceration, the shoulder straps may also cause pressure symptoms on the brachial plexus with neurologic symptoms from the arms.

Among other somatic symptoms are pains in the breasts. These pains may be independent of menstruation as especially seen in very large breasts or be premenstrual. The latter type is often associated with glandular fibroadenomatosis (fibrocystic disease). A further somatic symptom is intertriginous eczema around the inframammary fold. This symptom is most often seen in patients with general adiposity.

Another important part of the symptomatology is the psychosocial problem. Many women with large breasts consider their breasts as disgusting, always in the way, and a hindrance in their choice of clothes. They have difficulty in buying ready-made clothes, requiring one top-size and a different bottom-size. Macromastia is also a handicap in sport activities such as running, tennis, or golf. A further problem is that a large breast always becomes ptotic and if the ptoses becomes very pronounced, it could be experienced as esthetically less pleasing.

Indication for Operation

The indication for operation depends on the symptoms the patient experiences. Usually it is not difficult to decide on the appropriateness of a reduction mammaplasty. However, some advice as to the contraindications would not be out of place. A quite evident contraindication is poor anesthetic risk where the operation may endanger the life of the patient. Other contraindications that are much more difficult to evaluate are the psychological contraindications. It is quite evident that this type of operation should not be performed if the surgeon is not convinced that it will be of benefit to the patient.

There is a group of women, especially very young patients, who have a totally unrealistic expectations of a plastic surgeon being able to shape and reshape the breasts without leaving any scars. If the symptoms the patient specifies seem to be out of all proportion to the real deformity, one must be very cautious and even refuse to perform the operation. This might sometimes be difficult since this group of patients who are the least suited for the operation are those who are most eager to be operated on. To this group also the so-called dysmorphophobias belong. The patient channels all her problems to some minor deformity that would not even be noticeable to the uninitiated. Dysmorphophobics fixate on the breasts. Advoiding surgery on this type of patient could seem a simple task, but in practice I believe that all plastic surgeons have to learn the lesson by bitter experience.

Preoperative Information to the Patient

Having accepted a patient for reduction mammaplasty, some necessary information has to be given. Along with general information, such as the nature of the operation, anesthesia, the length of hospitalization, the convalescent period, it is especially important to carefully inform the patient of the scars that will result from surgery. It is necessary to point out that scar healing has a lengthy course. Sometimes there could initially be a period of hypertrophy with red, bulging scars that take a long time to pale and become atrophic. The risk for ugly scars is much higher in young patients than in older. Additional important preoperative information should concern the sensitivity of the nipple and areola as sensitivity might be impaired after the operation (see p. 307). Further information may involve the possibility of nursing after surgery. As an average, it could be said that about 50% of patients could nurse satisfactorily after a reduction mammaplasty (see p. 307).

Since macromastia could be caused by a general adiposity, it is most desirable that the patient should reduce her weight before the operation. This lessens the risk for complications and also makes it easier to decide on an adequate reduction. If the patient loses weight after the operation, there is risk that the breasts will become too small, and if she instead gains weight afterward, the breasts might be too big. It is wise to accept the patient for operation when she has the weight she will have in the future (satisfactory weight) and adapt the size of the reduction so that the breast will have a suitable size. Of course, the patient's own desire as to the future breast size has to be considered.

Very young patients should be considered with special caution since they have a tendency to get ugly scars at the same time as they have high demands on the esthetic result and the adequate postoperative size. A further difficulty is that one never knows how a future pregnancy will affect the breast and breast size. No fixed rules can be set and each case has to be judged individually, but generally speaking more reservations apply to the very young patient.

Preoperative Investigation

A careful history, physical examination, and laboratory tests have to be made before any major operation. In this context, the anesthesiologist often has special requirements. Preoperative mammography is to be recommended in patients over the age of 35. If any suspicious areas are found at palpation or mammography, an adequate biopsy has to be done (see p. 40).

Surgical Treatment

History and Principles

Since the 1920s, reduction and shaping of large breasts and ptoses has awakened a great interest and has become a more common operation. A great number of surgical techniques have been published and the literature is very extensive. A complete review is hardly possible or desirable in this chapter. A more extensive schematic review may be found in Lalardrie and Jouglard's book (1974).

Some comments on general principle, however, can be made. Reduction might be performed without taking any notice of the function of the breast and thus consist of a reduction and shaping in combination with a free nipple grafting (e. g., Thorek 1922). Operations preserving the function of the breast may be done by dissecting the skin from the gland, which is reduced followed by the tailoring of the skin to fit the size of the reduced gland (e. g., Passot 1925; Axhaussen 1926; Biesenberger 1931). The reduction may also be done by cutting skin and gland in one piece with transposition of the nipple area without any extensive undermining of the skin in the remaining part of the gland (e. g., Lexer 1931; Holländer 1924; Lessing 1953).

Depending on training and experience, the surgeon usually uses the technique that in his hands gives the best results. The techniques that are most commonly used are probably the following in order of publication date: horizontal glandular bipedical bridge or with only a medial pedicle, Strömbeck (1960); broad superior pedicle, Pitanguy (1961); oblique technique, Dufourmentel-Mouly (1961); vertical dermal flap, McKissock

(1972); B-plasty, Regnault (1974); inferior dermal pedicle, Robbins (1977); and modifications of those.

All of these techniques have in common that skin and gland could be shaped without any major undermining of the skin, that the areolar area remains connected with the remaining gland, and that the skin within the nipple-carrying glandular flap that is buried in the breast has the major part of the dermis left intact.

To facilitate the transposition of the nipple area complex, techniques have been described where the nipple-carrying flap has been dissected off from the gland and is thus being carried on a dermal subcutaneous pedicle (Skoog 1963; Weiner et al. 1973). Besides these techniques using transposition of the nipple complex, subtotal amputation with free grafting of the nipple area seems to be a fairly common procedure.

If the breast is regarded as a geometric figure that should be reduced with maintenance of the base of the breast and the geometric shape, this could be done in different ways.

Excision of a horizontal wedge from the inferior part of the breast is combined with a vertical wedge with the base facing the horizontal excision and the apex corresponding to the summit of the breast (Fig. 27.1A, B). This seems to be the natural way to do a resection since it is the prototype of the subtotal amputation with free nipple grafting where no concern has to be taken for the function of the breast. The scars left by this procedure form an inverted T. The planning starts with the point that should become the summit of the new breast and all reduction is made below this point.

In planning, one may start with the base of the breast. If the breast is considered as a rubber balloon filled with fluid, it would be possible to tie off the breast with a tourniquet somewhere in the middle so that a breast of suitable size and shape is created (Fig. 27.2A, B). What is outside the tourniquet corresponds to the volume of the breast that has to be resected and the position of the tourniquet on the surface of the breast corresponds to a circle, which in each point of its periphery corresponds to the distance of the areola to the base of the breast. The circumference of this circle, however, is considerably longer than what corresponds to the circumference of the areola (Fig. 27.3). If the skin had great elasticity, it would be possible to suture the circumference of the areola to the skin circle. That would give a perfect fitting of the skin capsule (Fig. 27.4A, B). Such a technique with gathering of the skin has been described by Padron (1972). It is possible to reduce this circumference of the skin in different ways:

1. By medially and laterally placed wedge excisions with the edge of the wedges in the medial respectively lateral corner of the mammary fold (Pers and Bretteville-Jensen 1972) (Fig. 27.5A, B).

2. By a rectangular excision above the submammary fold. This results in a T-shaped scar with a very short leg in the inframammary fold (Peixoto 1980) (Fig. 27.6A, B).

   In these techniques the shaping is performed starting from the midline of the breast.

3. The wedge excision could be done entirely on the lateral side (Dufourmentel-Mouly 1961) (Fig. 27.7A, B).

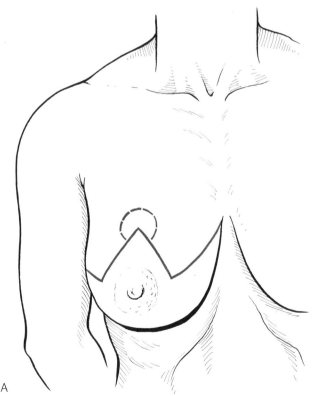

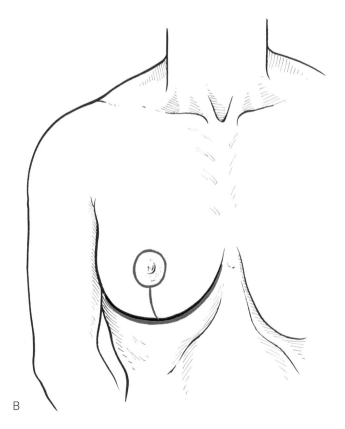

A

B

Fig. 27.1 A, B Pattern of excision of breast tissue from the inferior aspect of the breast using the upper part as the basis for reconstruction. This leaves an inverted T-shaped scar.

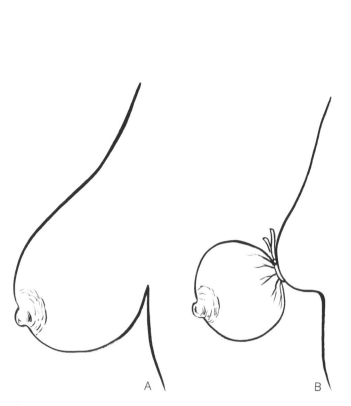

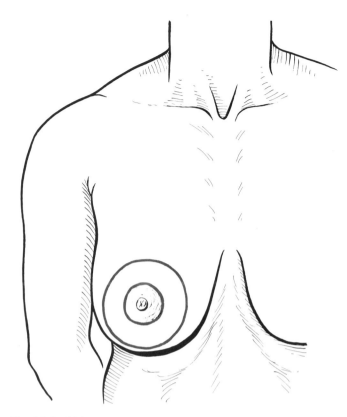

Fig. 27.**2** A, B   Reducing the breast by using the proximal portion of the breast as the basis for reconstruction.

Fig. 27.**3**   Using the base of the breast (fig. 27.2) results in a discrepancy between the areolar and skin circumferences.

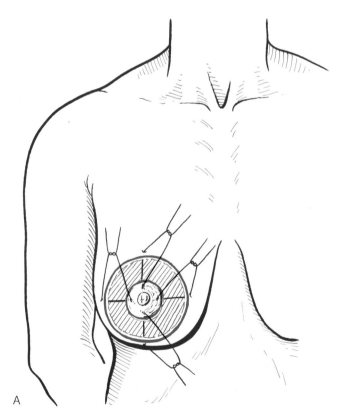

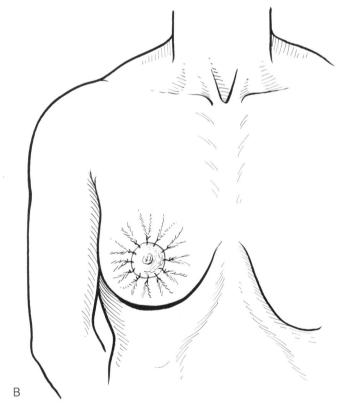

Fig. 27.**4** A, B   This discrepancy can be equalized by direct strategic placement of closing sutures utilizing the elastic properties of the skin. (Padron)

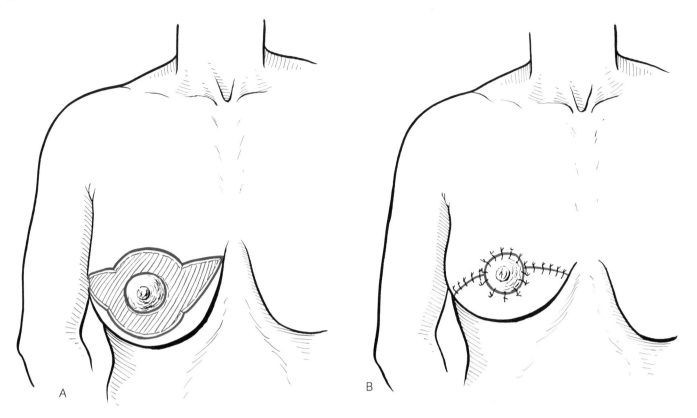

Fig. 27.5 A, B   Reduction of the outer circle by medial and lateral wedge excisions (Pers and Bretteville-Jensen).

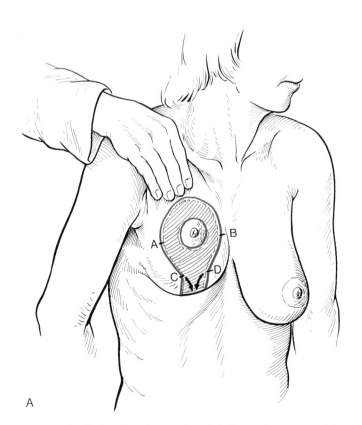

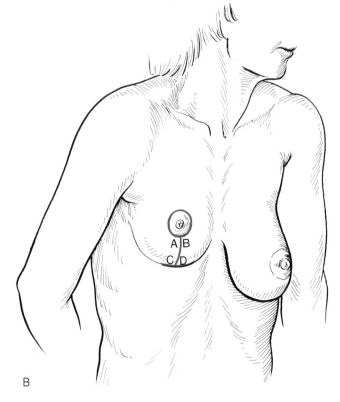

Fig. 27.6 A   Reduction of the outer circle by rectangular excision above the inframammary fold (Peixoto).

Fig. 27.6 B   Resulting scars are T-shaped with a very short horizontal component.

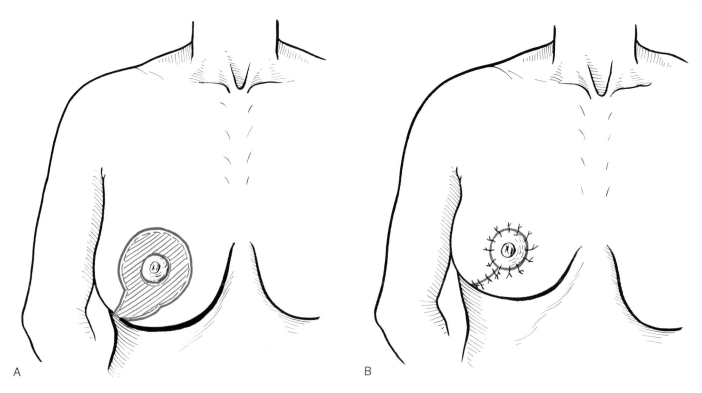

Fig. 27.**7** A, B Reduction of the outer circle by lateral wedge excision (Dufourmentel-Mouly). Resulting scars have no medial component.

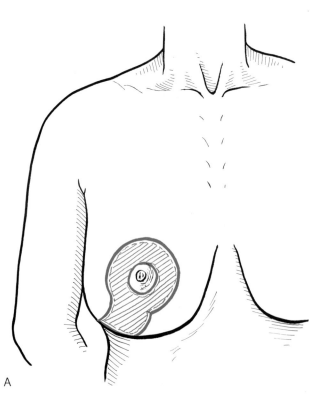
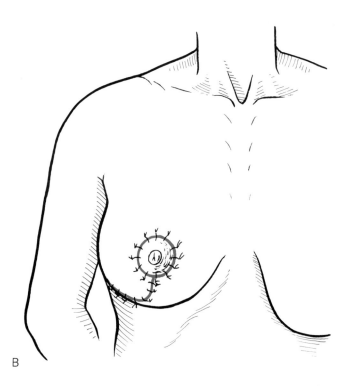

Fig. 27.**8** A, B Reduction of the outer circle by lateral-caudal excision (Regnault). Resulting scars are lateral and L-shaped.

4. Lateral and from the lower lateral quadrant so that the upper part of the breast is rotated laterally and downward. This results in an L-shaped scar (Regnault 1974) (Fig. 27.**8**A, B).

5. If the wedge excision is done in the midline with the edge pointing downward, the vertical line that is the distance from the areola to the inframammary fold will become too long and two wedges above the inframammary fold have to be added with the edges pointing medially and laterally (Schrudde 1972). This also results in an inverted T scar.

I am aware that the description given above is most schematic, but it has to be regarded as an attempt to illustrate what is done in the different techniques without taking any consideration of how the glandular pedicle is created or how the glandular resection is made. There are also interesting techniques that have not been mentioned which leave only a horizontal scar in the inframammary fold (Passot 1925; Ribeiro 1975). This is possible in patients with considerable ptoses where the upper horizontal incision line lies above the areola.

I will now describe in more detail some of the most common techniques. The selection is subjective and limited by the fact that I will deal only with techniques of which I have had personal experience.

Techniques Giving an Inverted T Scar

Preoperative Planning

The preoperative planning has to be performed carefully since the future symmetry of the breasts depends on the accuracy of the planning. The plan begins with an assessment of the patient sitting with her arms hanging down at her sides. An estimation is made of the amount of breast tissue to be removed. At this time, it is important to look for side differences in volume and to try to estimate the difference of volume in weight. With increased experience, the weight to be resected and side differences in grams can be fairly closely estimated by sight. There are instruments described and commercially available to more accurately measure the volume of the breast. The next step is that the midline of the breast is marked with a line dividing the breast in two equal parts that usually corresponds to the midclavicular line. The symmetrical position of the breast meridian could be checked with measuring tape from the midsternal line. The summit of the breast should be located on this breast meridian (Fig. 27.**9**), and different modalities have been used to decide the exact location, for example, in the level of the midpoint of the upper arm, sixth intercostal space, or a fixed distance from the upper sternal notch. The safest way of locating the nipple is to use the position of the inframammary fold since this is independent of the size of the patient and her configuration. The summit of the breast should be in a position corresponding to the projection of the submammary fold on the anterior surface of the breast (Fig. 27.**10**). An easy way to check this is to use a pair of calipers of the type used in obstetrics for measuring the pelvis. With such an instrument, it is easy to measure the distance from the point where the breast meridian meets the clavicle to the inframammary fold and project this distance on the anterior surface. Using this instrument, symmetry is easily achieved by determining the same distance on the other breast. With the apex in this point, a triangular resection of the central part of the breast should be calculated so that the remaining part of the breast medially and laterally could be joined without tension (Fig. 27.**11**). The angle in this triangle varies depending on the size of the breast. To decide the lower excision, one has to calculate from the summit of the breast along the legs of the triangle, a distance that should correspond to the length of the lower pole of the breast from nipple to inframammary fold (Fig. 27.**12**). If the distance between the areola and the submammary fold is approximately 6 cm and the diameter of the areola region some 4.5 cm, the distance from the summit along the legs of the triangle should be 8 to 9 cm. The horizontal excision is planned from the inframammary fold which represents the inferior border of the horizontal ellipse and from the respectively medial lateral corner of the submammary fold so that adaptation becomes possible and "dog ears" will be avoided (Fig. 27.**13**).

This planning should produce a conical breast with the summit in the right location. The skin in the top of the cone has to be removed to give room for the areola (Fig. 27.**14**). The skin excision can be planned either before the beginning of the operation or during the operation when the cone has been formed.

It is paramount for the result that a good symmetry is achieved. Personally I find it easier to get a good symmetry if I use a pattern with a fixed angle between the vertical lines and with a calculated placement of the areola (Fig. 27.**15**).

It should be pointed out that when using a pattern, the angle sometimes has to be changed. This is most easily done if the pattern is rotated so that a medial skin flap seems to be of sufficient length. The border of the pattern is marked on the skin and after that the accuracy of the markings is tested by first moving the breasts laterally so that the lower medial corner hits the inframammary fold and this point is marked (Fig. 27.**16**). The breast is then moved medially to see where the lateral corner hits the inframammary fold. If it does not easily reach the marking made in the inframammary fold, the length of the lateral skin flap has to be lengthened. This is easy to do freehand and in so doing the size of the key-hole in the upper circular part may be lengthend laterally (Fig. 27.**17**). Whatever technique is used, the end result is the same if the length of the skin flaps are checked so that they have sufficient length. Otherwise there will be too great tightness with risk for a wide scar.

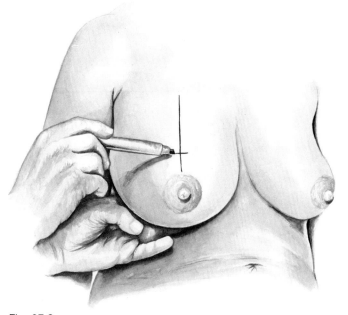

Fig. 27.**9**

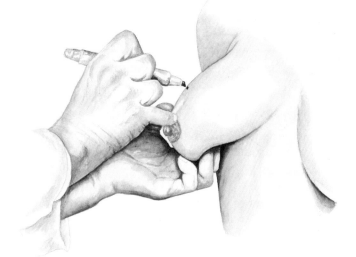

Fig. 27.**10**

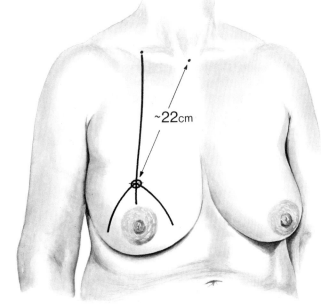

Fig. 27.**11**

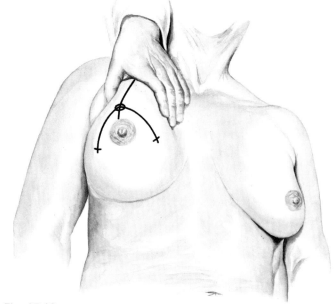

Fig. 27.**12**

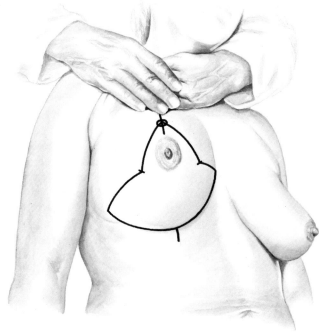

Fig. 27.**13**

Fig. 27.**9** Preoperative marking. Breast meridian and new location of the nipple on a level with the submammary fold.

Fig. 27.**10** The submammary fold ist the safest guide to avoid placing the nipple too high.

Fig. 27.**11** The distance from the supra sternal notch to the nipple is as an average 22 cm, but depends on the morphological type of the patient.

Fig. 27.**12** The legs of the triangular skin excision should be 8–9 cm. The angle is determined by manual trial.

Fig. 27.**13** Estimation of the horizontal excision.

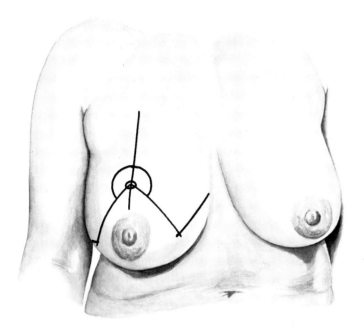

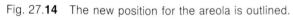

Fig. 27.**14** The new position for the areola is outlined.

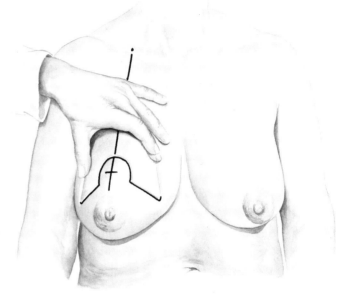

Fig. 27.**15** A pattern can be used to estimate the skin resection.

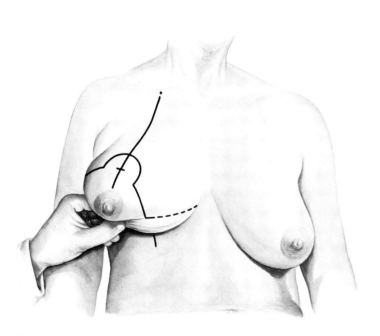

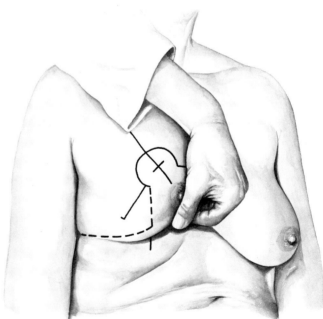

Fig. 27.**16** and 27.**17** The length of the marked skin flaps should be checked and if necessary corrected to avoid excessive stretching of the flaps.

Fig. 27.**17**

Operation According to Strömbeck

The preoperative planning of the skin incisions has to be made before scrubbing with, for example, a felt marking pen that is not easily scrubbed off. The operation is performed with the patient in horizontal position under general anesthesia. To lessen the blood loss, infiltration of local anesthesia with epinephrine is recommended. I use 0.25% lidocaine (Xylocaine) with epinephrine 1 : 400,000. The amount used varies from 40 to 100 ml/breast. The infiltration is done subcutaneously in areas to be incised and on the undersurface of the breast over the pectoral fascia, sometimes also in the parts of the breast tissue that should be incised. The operation starts by circular incision of the areola with a diameter of about 4 to 5 cm keeping the breast extended. The glandular flaps are designed basically as a horizontal bridge between the medial and lateral skin flaps (Fig. 27.**18**). The flaps could be made broader than the vertical part of the skin incisions. Depending on the shape of the breast, the flaps should be broadend either above or below the corners of the medial flap. The areola-carrying glandular flap is thus a horizontal bridge that has two bases to include the skin flap areas medially and laterally. The skin in these flaps between the skin flap and the circumcised areola is removed in superficial layer corresponding to the dermis (Fig. 27.**19**). Following this, resection of glandular tissue is made above the areola and horizontally below the skin flaps and the glandular bridge through skin and gland (Fig. 27.**20**). In smaller breasts it is not necessary to do an upper glandular resection. The resected tissue is weighed to check that it corresponds to the preoperative estimation and especially to determine that an adequate resection is done from the two breasts to provide good symmetry. When the vertical skin edges are sutured together and the borders of the horizontal incisions are adapted, the glandular bridge will fold automatically so that the nipple area will appear in the part of the key-hole

designed for it and the edges of the areola could be sutured to the skin (Fig. 27.**21**). This transposition of the nipple-carrying flap has to be made without any tension whatsoever. If the glandular flaps are short, this will be difficult. It is then most easily dealt with by cutting the lateral pedicle completely so that the nipple could rotate in place (Fig. 27.**22**). It is important to release all tension, and in patients with a short medial glandular bridge, it might be necessary to divide the dermis medially to such an extent that the areola becomes completely relaxed (Fig. 27.**23**). This could be done without any danger to the circulation since in these cases the medial pedicle is thick and fairly short. I leave a suction drain for 24 hours or longer if necessary (Fig. 27.**24**). Bleeding during operation varies considerably, and if the estimated blood loss exceeds 800 cc, it could be necessary to give a blood transfusion. Bleeding is usually reduced to a minimum by using infiltration with local anesthesia with epinephrine. In so doing, the total blood loss could be reduced to 100 to 200 cc.

For skin sutures I use some interrupted 3/0 sutures in the corners and subcuticulare and intracuticulare running 4/0 sutures with resorbable material (Dexon®) that does not have to be removed or monofilament nylon that is removed after 10 to 14 days.

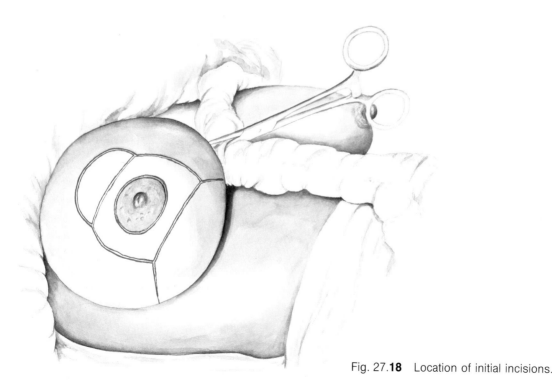

Fig. 27.**18**   Location of initial incisions.

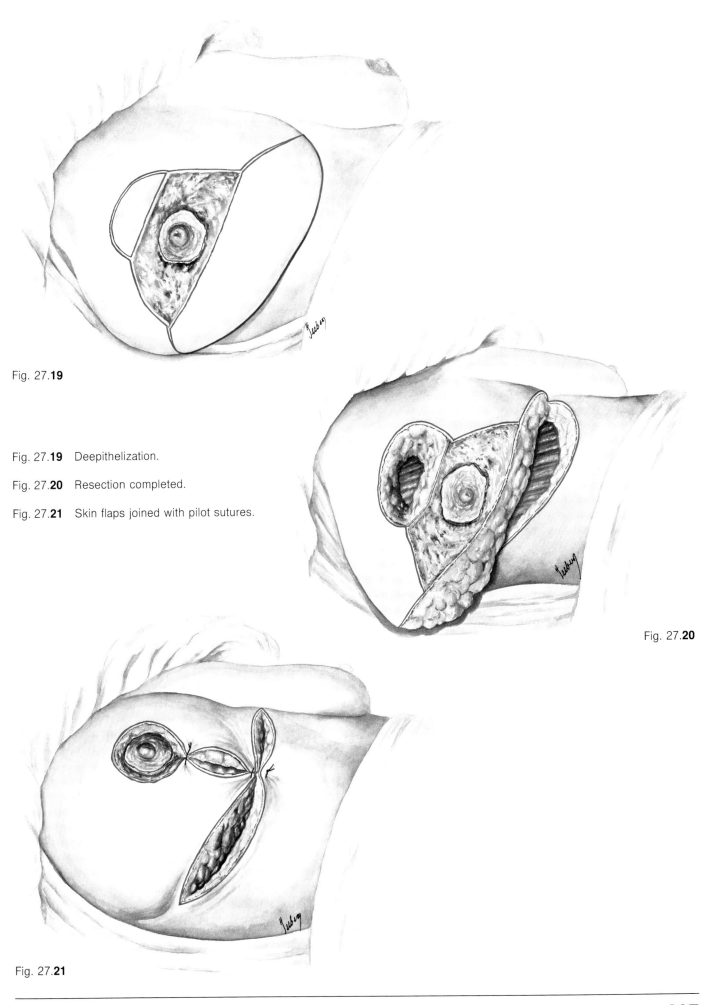

Fig. 27.**19**

Fig. 27.**19** Deepithelization.

Fig. 27.**20** Resection completed.

Fig. 27.**21** Skin flaps joined with pilot sutures.

Fig. 27.**20**

Fig. 27.**21**

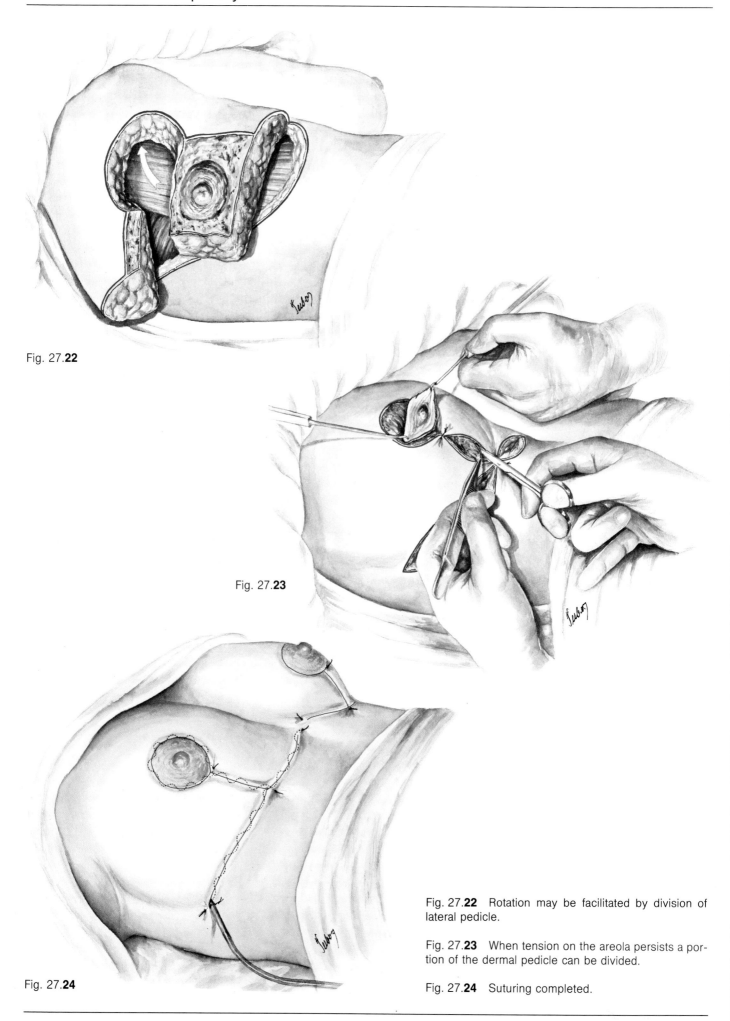

Fig. 27.**22**

Fig. 27.**23**

Fig. 27.**24**

Fig. 27.**22** Rotation may be facilitated by division of lateral pedicle.

Fig. 27.**23** When tension on the areola persists a portion of the dermal pedicle can be divided.

Fig. 27.**24** Suturing completed.

Operation According to Pitanguy

Dr. Pitanguy does the preoperative planning on the operating table with the patient in a supine position. The planning is otherwise identical with that described above with the exception that the opening for the areola is decided on after the shaping of the breasts. The areola is circumscribed with suitable diameter and the skin in the triangle around the areola is removed superficially in the dermal plane (Fig. 27.25). The glandular resection is made from the lower part of the breast and with excision of glandular tissue from the underside of the breast after the breast has been dissected off from the pectoral fascia (Fig. 27.26A, B). The glandular segments are approximated with catgut sutures in the midline so that a breast cone is created (Fig. 27.27). The skin is undermined slightly to the sides and the vertical skin edges opposed. Excess skin is excised above the inframammary fold so that a good adaptation is achieved. The shaping of the breast is now completed and the skin in the summit of the new breast is circularly excised to receive the areola that now is sutured in place (Fig. 27.28A, B).

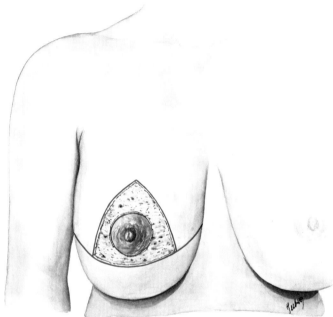

Fig. 27.**25**

Fig. 27.**25**   Pattern of deepithelization.

Fig. 27.**26** A, B   Resection completed.

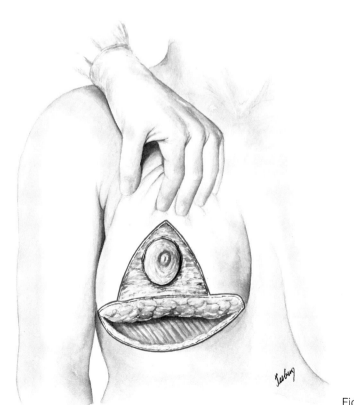

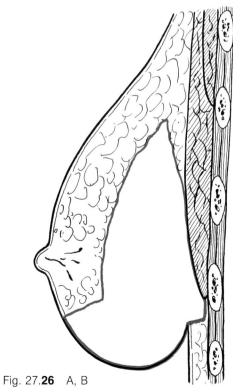

Fig. 27.**26**   A, B

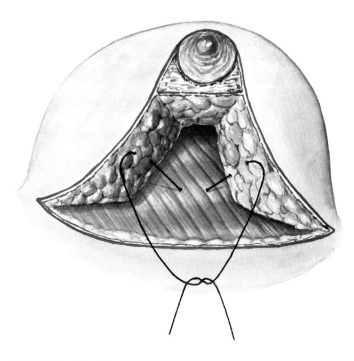

Fig. 27.**27**   Glandular suture.

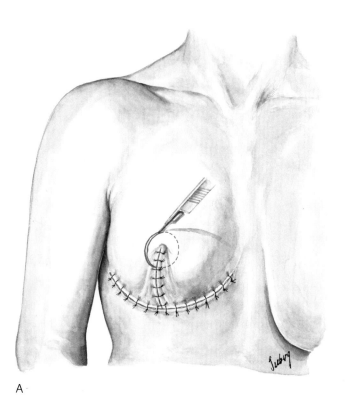

A

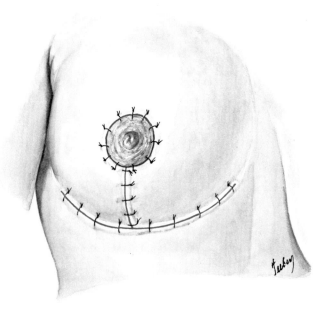

B

Fig. 27.**28** A, B   Circular excision of skin at the summit to permit delivery of the areola at the appropriate location.

Operation According to McKissock

The preoperative planning is basically identical with that described above using the key-hole technique. The nipple-carrying glandular flap is vertical extending from the upper parts of the key-hole down to the submammary fold (Fig. 27.**29**). This glandular flap is de-epithelized after the areola has been circumscribed to a suitable size. The borderlines of the flap are incised down to the pectoral muscle on both sides. The glandular resection is done medially and laterally between the skin flaps and the glandular bridge with some additional removal of tissue underneath the skin flaps (Fig. 27.**30**). If more tissue has to be removed, it can be taken underneath the vertical flap if only a 5-cm attachement to the chest wall is left above the inframammary fold area (Fig. 27.**31**). When the skin edges are sutured together the suturing starts with the horizontal incision from medial and lateral side towards the midline of the breast (Fig. 27.**32**A). It is now possible to see if the skin flaps are too long. Excessive skin can be removed before suturing the vertical line. The areolar segment can be sutured to achieve good projection (Fig. 27.**32**B, C).

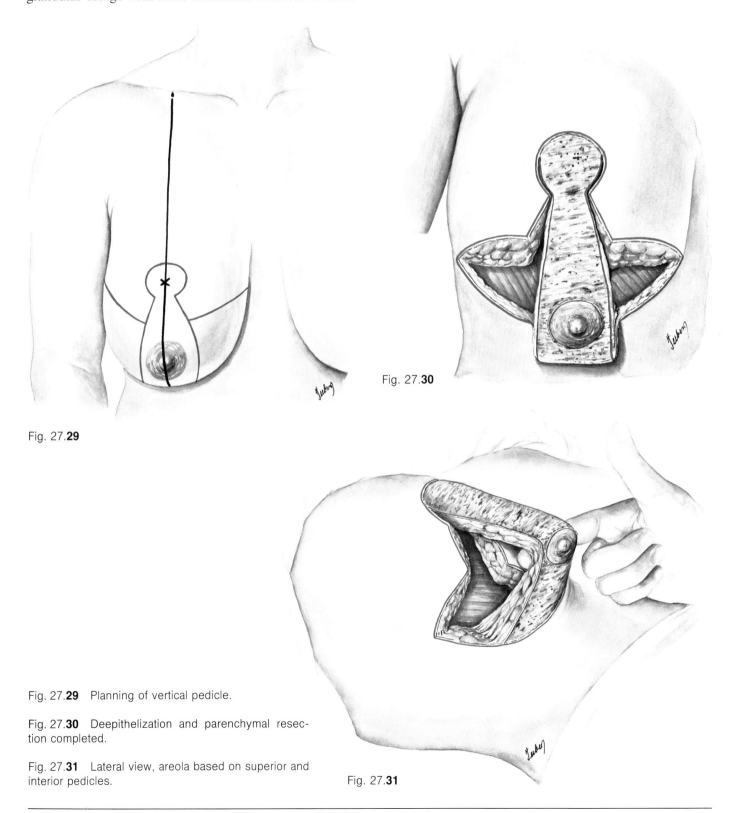

Fig. 27.**29**

Fig. 27.**30**

Fig. 27.**31**

Fig. 27.**29**   Planning of vertical pedicle.

Fig. 27.**30**   Deepithelization and parenchymal resection completed.

Fig. 27.**31**   Lateral view, areola based on superior and interior pedicles.

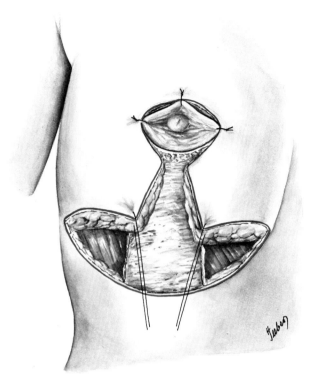

Fig. 27.**32** A

Fig. 27.**32** A–C Closure of medial and lateral flaps over the folded vertical pedicle.

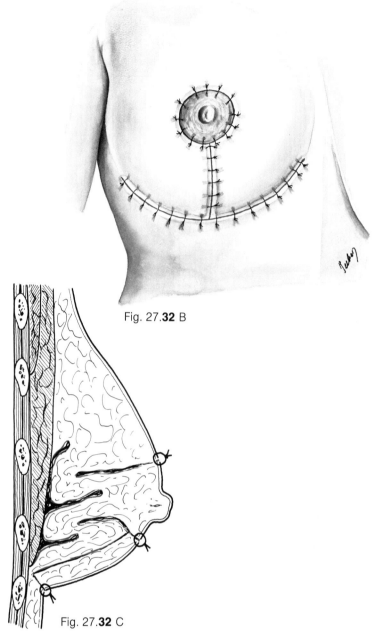

Fig. 27.**32** B

Fig. 27.**32** C

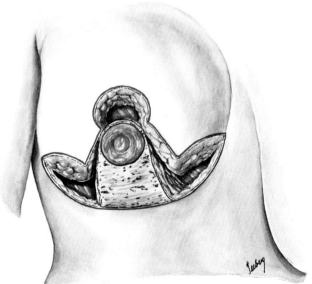

Fig. 27.**33** Inferior pedicle after resection.

Inferior Dermal Flap

This technique has been described by Robbins (1977) and by Courtiss and Goldwyn (1977). The preoperative planning is the same as described above (see p. 283). The areola-carrying glandular flap is based in the inframammary fold and somewhat broader than the vertical flap of McKissock. The resection is made outside the glandular flap above, medially and laterally extending underneath the skin flaps (Fig. 27.**33**). The incision lines are opposed and sutured (Figs. 27.**34**, 27.**35**). Even if it is easy to suture the areola in place, there may sometimes be a lack of projection of the areola region with a tendency for it to fall back. To prevent this, a dermal platform can be left in the circular part of the key-hole as advocated by Schultz and Marcus (1981).

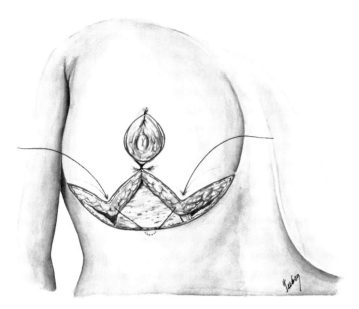

Fig. 27.**34**   The skin flaps sutured over the pedicle.

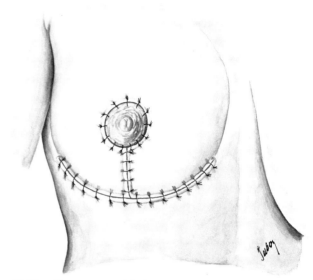

Fig. 27.**35**   Closure completed.

Subtotal Amputation with Free Nipple Grafting

Preoperative planning as described above (see p. 283). The areolar complex is excised as a free graft preserving a little parenchyma underneath the nipple. The skin in the circular part of the keyhole is de-epithelized (Fig. 27.**36**).

The breast is incised along the marked skin incision all the way through down to the chest wall leaving the necessary amount of breast tissue under the skin flaps to build up the contour (Fig. 27.**37**). When the resection has been completed, the skin edges are adapted (Fig. 27.**38**). The free nipple areolar graft is sutured in the denuded circle on the summit of the breast (Fig. 27.**39**).

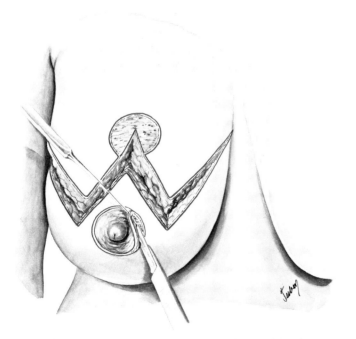

Fig. 27.**36**   Areola and nipple are removed as a full thickness composite graft.

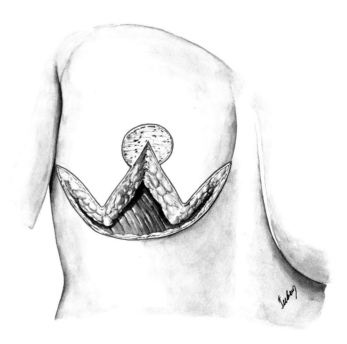

Fig. 27.**37**   Resection completed. Recipient area deepithelized.

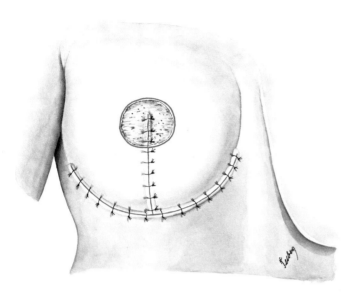

Fig. 27.**38**   Breast cone re-established.

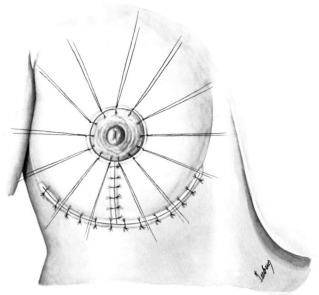

Fig. 27.**39**   Nipple areola graft sutured in place.

Techniques with Lateral Resection

Oblique Technique According to Dufourmentel and Mouly

For preoperative planning, the new position of the nipple is calculated starting from the periphery of the breast and three points are marked with the patient lying down:

1. 16 to 20 cm from the upper sternal notch on a line joining this point with the nipple
2. 8 to 9 cm from the midline of the sternum (lower sternal ridge) on a horizontal line through the nipple
3. 6 cm above the inframammary fold on a vertical line from the midpoint of the submammary fold to the nipple (Fig. 27.**40**).

These three points represent different points in the skin incision that should be sutured to the periphery of the areola. The size of the areola is calculated as a circle with a diameter of 4 to 5 cm. So that the skin incision that should border the areola should coordinate with the areola circumference, the length and position of the skin incision is established with help of a circular wire ring having the same diameter as the areola. The wire is applied on the breast and opened so that it hits all three of the above-mentioned points. The opening in the wire is localized so that it opens against the point where the inframammary fold meets the anterior axillary line, point 4 (Fig. 27.**41**). This point has to be marked with the patient sitting up before the other measurements are made. By joining the two endpoints of the open wire with the lateral corner of the inframammary fold (point 4), the lateral resection is designed (Fig. 27.**42**). These two lines should be of equal length and situated symmetrically in regards to the radius of the breast. In very large breasts the upper line becomes longer than the lower, and to compensate for that the incision in the inframammary fold has to be curved upward laterally so that a Burow's triangle could be removed (Fig. 27.**43**). This results in an L-shaped scar where one leg of the L will be situated lateral to the breasts.

The operation starts by circumscribing the areola and de-epithelizing the skin between areola and the skin incisions (Fig. 27.**44**). After that, the skin and gland are excised in one wedge-shaped piece between the lateral incision lines. Excessive tissue is then resected from the under surface of the breast underneath the glandular flap if needed. The areola-carrying flap has a broad pedicle medially and upward (Fig. 27.**45**A). The gland is adapted and the skin sutured. The areola is sutured in place (Fig. 27.**45**B).

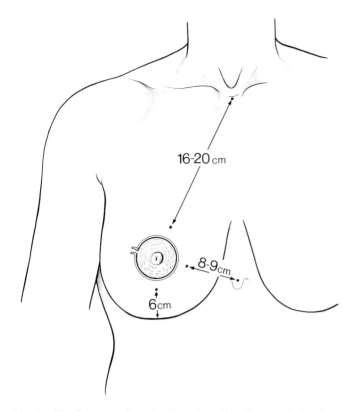

Fig. 27.**40** Preoperative planning. Locating the areola by three reference points and utilizing an open wire ring.

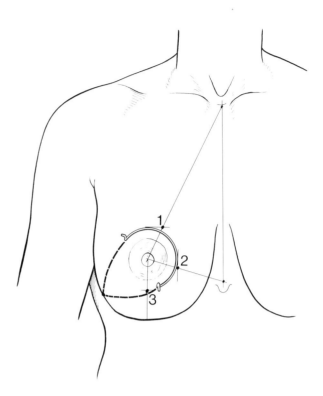

Fig. 27.**41** The wire ring is opened to meet the three reference points. The opening localized against the lateral end of the submammary fold.

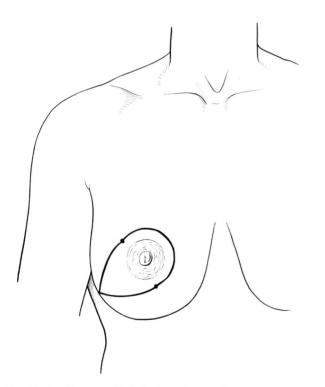

Fig. 27.**42** Pattern of inferio-lateral resection.

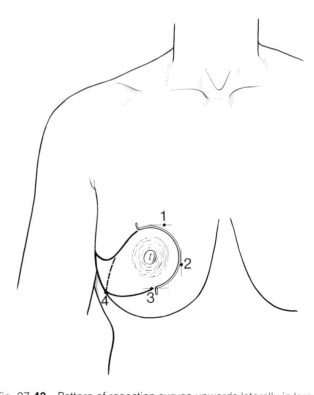

Fig. 27.**43** Pattern of resection curves upwards laterally in larger breasts.

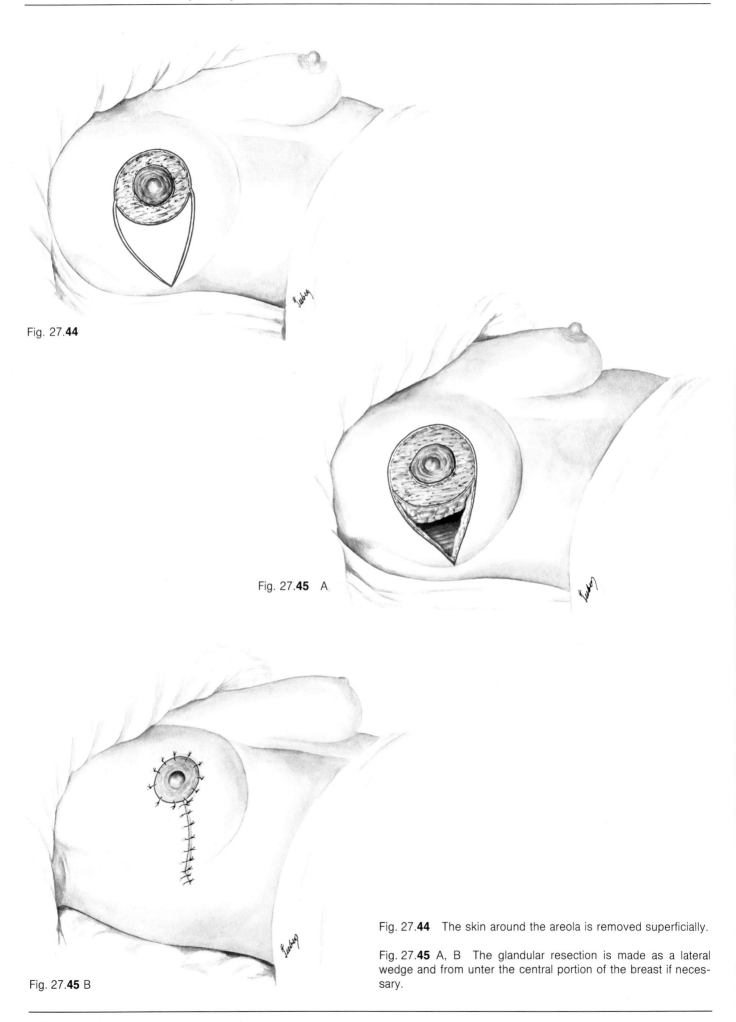

Fig. 27.**44**

Fig. 27.**45** A.

Fig. 27.**45** B

Fig. 27.**44**   The skin around the areola is removed superficially.

Fig. 27.**45** A, B   The glandular resection is made as a lateral wedge and from unter the central portion of the breast if necessary.

B-plasty According to Regnault

A variation of the lateral resection has been described by Paule Regnault (1974) where the resection lies more medially and results in a scar that will be L-shaped with one vertical leg from the areola to the inframammary fold and the other leg in the lateral part of the submammary fold. In this way, the long lateral scar that sometimes extends out below the new submammary fold will be avoided.

For preoperative planning, the points that have to be decided before the patient is placed on the operating table are the first two points as described in the oblique technique (Fig. 27.46A) (see p. 27.18). The lateral border of the circular incision around the areola is calculated freehand on the operating table so that good symmetry with the medial coordinates is achieved. After that, a line 1 to 2 cm above the inframammary fold in its lateral part is marked and from the midpoint of the inframammary fold the marking curves up in the direction of the areola. This vertical line extends about 4 cm above the horizontal line of the new submammary fold. This is point 3 which should be connected with point 2, forming the medial part of the circular line. The lateral incision line is then calculated as a slightly curved line against the lateral corner of the inframammary fold. The now-completed planning resembles the letter B (Fig. 27.46B).

The operation starts with a circumscription of the areola with a diameter of about 4 to 5 cm. The skin is then excised in the dermal level between the areola incision and the circular skin incision (Fig. 27.47). Skin and gland

in the inferior part of the marked area are excised and if necessary excessive tissue has to be removed so that the volume will be satisfactory (Fig. 27.48A). The skin edges are then adapted. When suturing the areola, the circumference of the circular skin incision is often longer than the areola incision. Because of this, a certain gathering of skin has to be made (Fig. 27.48B).

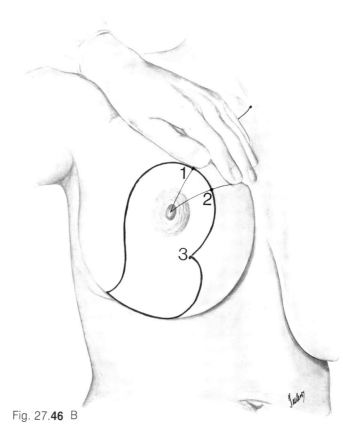

Fig. 27.**46** B

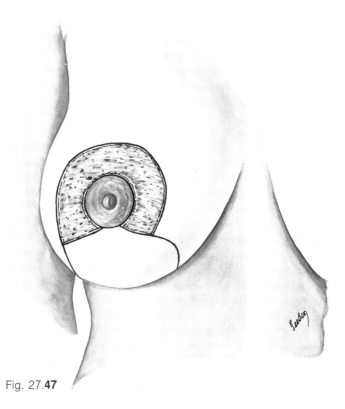

Fig. 27.**46** A

Fig. 27.**46** A, B   Location of incisional pattern by reference points (see text).

Fig. 27.**47**   Superficial skin excision.

Fig. 27.**47**

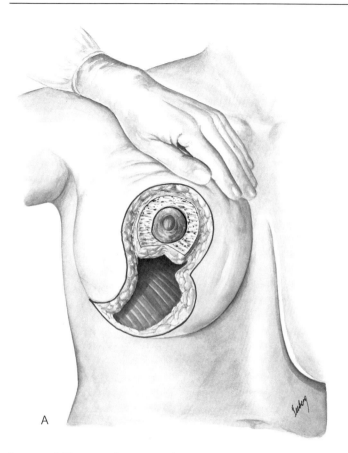

A

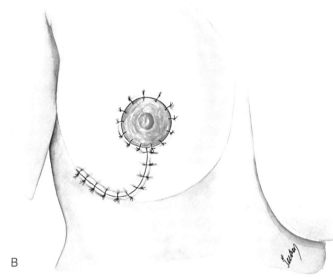

B

Fig. 27.**48** A, B   Glandular excision and suturing completed.

Lateral Resection and L-shaped Scar According to Strömbeck

It might seem unnecessarily confusing to describe one further variation of the lateral technique, but I think it would not be out of place to report how I apply the lateral technique (Fig. 27.**49**).

The preoperative planning that I described in 1976 and later in 1983 is done with the patient in the sitting position after identification of certain fixed points. The upper limit of the skin incision is localized at the projection of the submammary fold on the anterior surface of the skin, point A (Fig. 27.**50**A). Point B lies on a vertical line from the midpoint of the inframammary fold with the breast

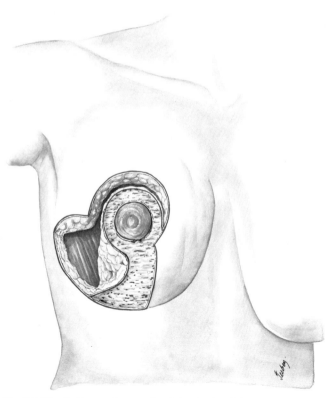

Fig. 27.**49**   Pattern of superior-lateral glandular resection and deepithelization of areolar pedicle.

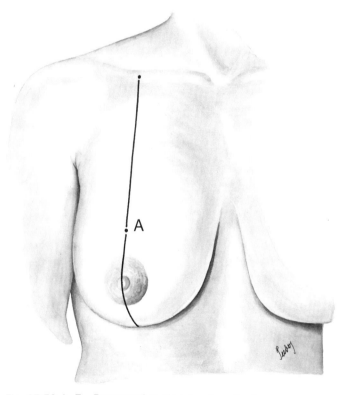

A

Fig. 27.**50** A–E   Preoperative planning (see text).

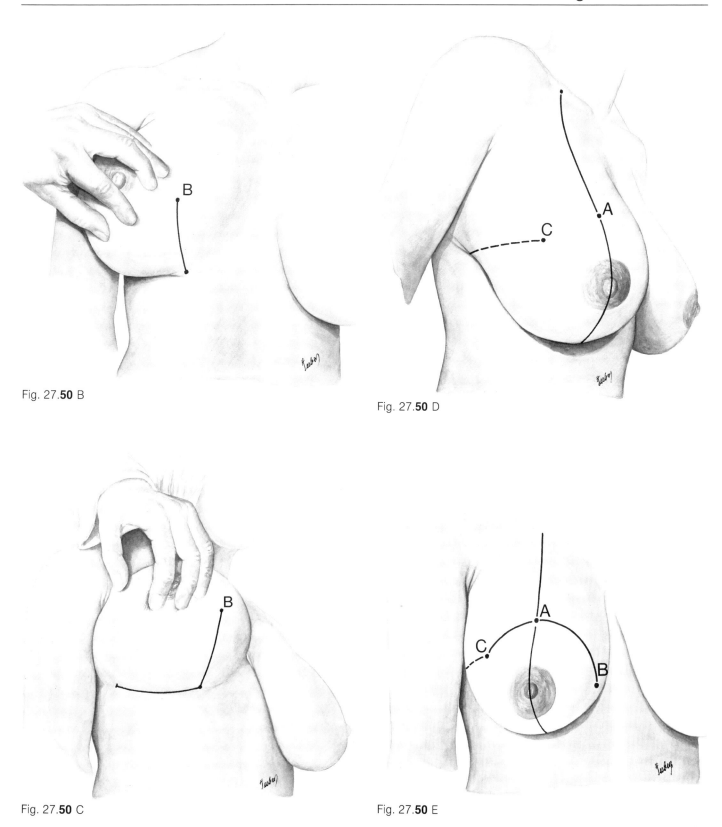

Fig. 27.**50** B

Fig. 27.**50** D

Fig. 27.**50** C

Fig. 27.**50** E

pressed laterally some 5 cm above the inframammary fold, which is marked in its lateral part (Fig. 27.**50**B, C). Point C is on a horizontal line from the lateral end of the inframammary fold the same distance from the lateral corner of the submammary fold as point B is from the medial (Fig. 27.**50**D).

These three points are joined with a curved line and represent the skin line around the areola (Fig. 27.**50**E). Even if the planning is made differently, the end result will be very similar to that described by Regnault. The difference lies more in the operative technique that gives a glandular pedicle based medially and downward and with a "double-breasted" suturing.

During the operation, the nipple-carrying glandular flap is outlined, having its base medially and downward, with its upper medial corner at the same level as the nipple and the lower lateral corner in the lateral end of the infra-mammary fold. After the areola has been circumscribed with a diameter of 5 cm the skin within the flap outside the medial skin incisions is de-epithelized (Fig. 27.**51**A). While pressing the breast caudally, the upper skin incision along the preoperative marking is made and brought through the gland down to the pectoral fascia (Fig. 27.**51**B). The glandular flap is incised around the borders straight down to the muscle (Fig. 27.**52**). Before the lateral resection is completed, the skin is dissected off the gland over the lateral part of the breast. The undermining has to be carried some centimeters above the level of point C (Fig. 27.**53**A). The lateral resection is now

completed in the area where the skin has been dissected off (Figs. 27.**53**B, 27.**54**). The shaping of the breasts starts with closing the skin circumference around the areola. That means that points B and C are joined with a suture. However, it is often possible to decrease the length of the skin line by suturing point B to a point some centimeters above point C. In spite of that, the skin circumference often becomes longer than what corresponds to the areola circumference. By pulling the undermined skin flap in a medial and downward direction an adaptation can be done after excision of the surplus skin (Fig. 27.**55**). Before closing the skin, the edges of the gland may be sutured together. I have found, however, that it es easier to get a good cosmetic result if no sutures are put in the gland (Fig. 27.**56**).

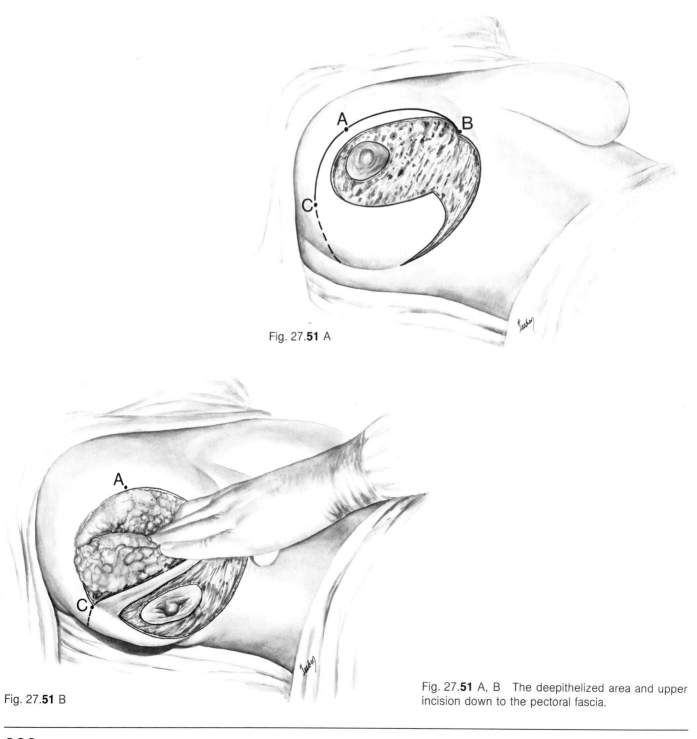

Fig. 27.**51** A

Fig. 27.**51** B

Fig. 27.**51** A, B   The deepithelized area and upper incision down to the pectoral fascia.

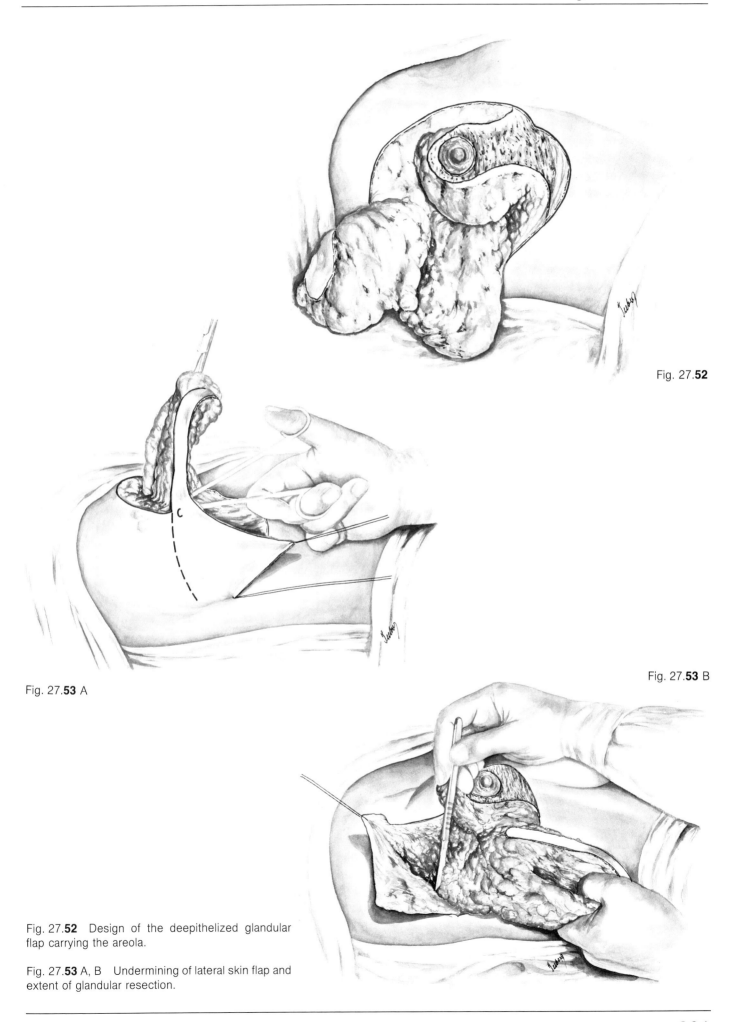

Fig. 27.**52**

Fig. 27.**53** B

Fig. 27.**53** A

Fig. 27.**52** Design of the deepithelized glandular flap carrying the areola.

Fig. 27.**53** A, B Undermining of lateral skin flap and extent of glandular resection.

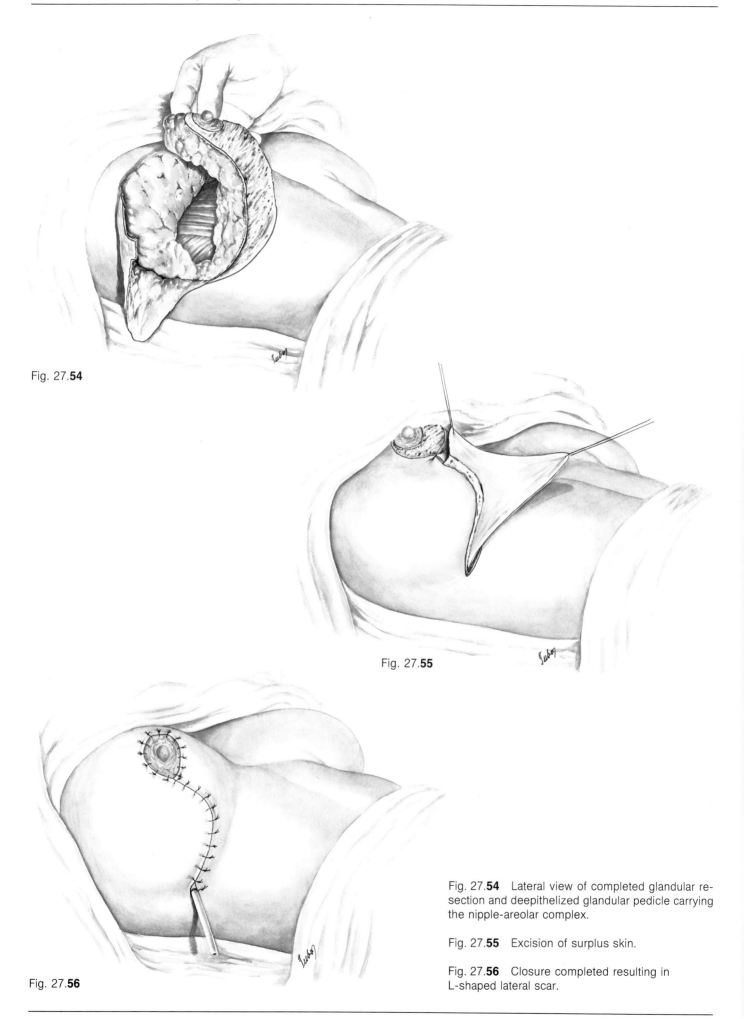

Fig. 27.**54**

Fig. 27.**55**

Fig. 27.**56**

Fig. 27.**54** Lateral view of completed glandular re-section and deepithelized glandular pedicle carrying the nipple-areolar complex.

Fig. 27.**55** Excision of surplus skin.

Fig. 27.**56** Closure completed resulting in L-shaped lateral scar.

Tennis-ball Technique According to Pers and Bretteville-Jensen

The prinicple is that the lower pole of the breast from the submammary fold as a triangle up to the lower edge of the new nipple site is kept intact, that the nipple-areola complex is transposed on a vertical dermal-glandular flap between the upper part of the lower triangular flap, and the upper border of the new areola incision and that resection is made as wedges medially and laterally and if necessary also underneath the nipple carrying glandular flap (Fig. 27.**57**). Preoperative planning can be made with a special pattern or freehand if the suitable distances are carefully calculated. The operation results in two long scars from the areola to the medial and lateral corners of the inframammary fold (Fig. 27.**58**).

Author's preferences

The abundance of different operative techniques could be confusing and raises the question whether one technique or the other is to be preferred in different types of macromastias. As a general principle, it could be said that all of the above techniques could be used with suitable modifications in all types of enlargements ranging from ptoses to very large breasts. Basically the skin incisions are the same, whereas the amount of resected tissue could vary from zero upward.

Personally I have some preferences. In moderate enlargements in combination with rather pronounced ptoses, I prefer to use a technique with a horizontal glandular bridge and often with only a medial pedicle (Fig. 27.**59**A–D). In smaller hypertrophies and especially in young patients, I prefer the lateral technique with L-shaped scar, whereas in very large and fat breasts, I prefer the inferiorly based dermal glandular flap (Fig. 27.**60**A–D).

Postoperative Complications

Hematoma

Postoperative hematoma is the most frequent complication. Small amounts of bleeding giving slight postoperative swelling and discoloration of the skin do not require any special treatment. Larger hematomas have to be evacuated and hemostasis obtained. The frequency of hematoma requiring evacuation was in a report of 670 patient 2.7% (Strömbeck 1976). Hematomas may prolong the convalescence time but does not affect the end result.

Glandular Complications

Complications caused by circulatory disturbances in the breast usually effect the fat tissue and are classified as fat necrosis even if part of the gland might be necrotic. This complication is correlated to the degree of obesity. An analysis of a group of 1,306 breasts gives the frequency of 1.4% in patient of normal weight, rising to 1.75% in moderately obese patient and to 8.9% in very obese patients (Strömbeck 1976). Major fat necrosis often produces a considerable temperature rise, up to 38 to 39°C during the first postoperative days, and a tense hard breast. If the breasts are not drained, there usually will be spontaneous perforation in the lower part of the operation field, which then drains until all necrotic tissue is gone. This could take months. It is therefore recommended that the wound be opened under general anesthesia and all nonviable tissue excised as soon as demarcation can be expected. This complication sometimes means a considerable lengthening of the postoperative period and in cases of major necroses may lead to an asymmetry since the affected side will be smaller than what was intended.

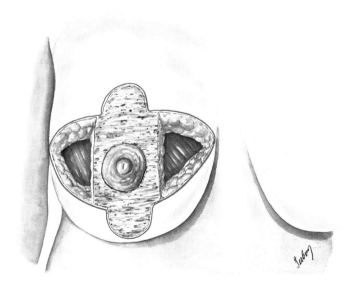

Fig. 27.**57** Medial and lateral glandular resection preserving the lower pole of the breast. Deepithelized vertical pedicle carries the areola.

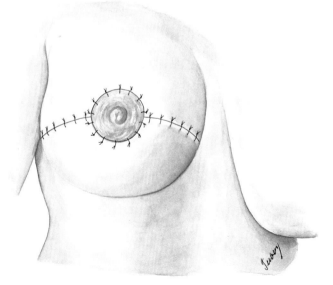

Fig. 27.**58** Closure completed, horizontal midglandular scar results.

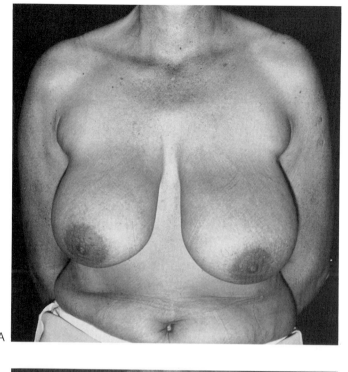

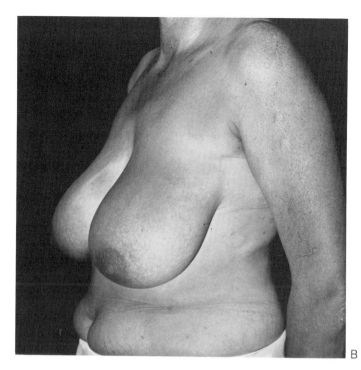

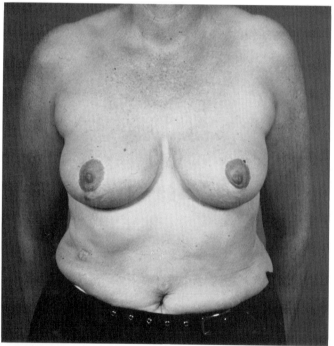

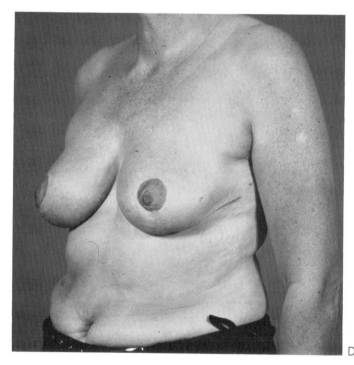

Fig. 27.**59** A, B: Preoperative photos of 37-year-old patient. C, D: Eight years after reduction mammaplasty with the Strömbeck bipedicle technique. 600 g removed from the right breast and 750 g from the left.

Minor fat necroses are noticed as local lumps that could remain for a long time. This might disturb both the patient and the doctor and malignancy should be excluded by needle aspiration biopsy. Sometimes it is better to remove the lump surgically. In the above-mentioned material, the total frequency of fat necrosis was 2.1%.

Nipple Complications

Circulatory disturbances leading to loss of the nipple-areola complex are extremly rare. They may be seen in very fat patients with excessive macromastia where the nipple-carrying glandular flap is unusually long and becomes strangulated. In the above-mentioned material,

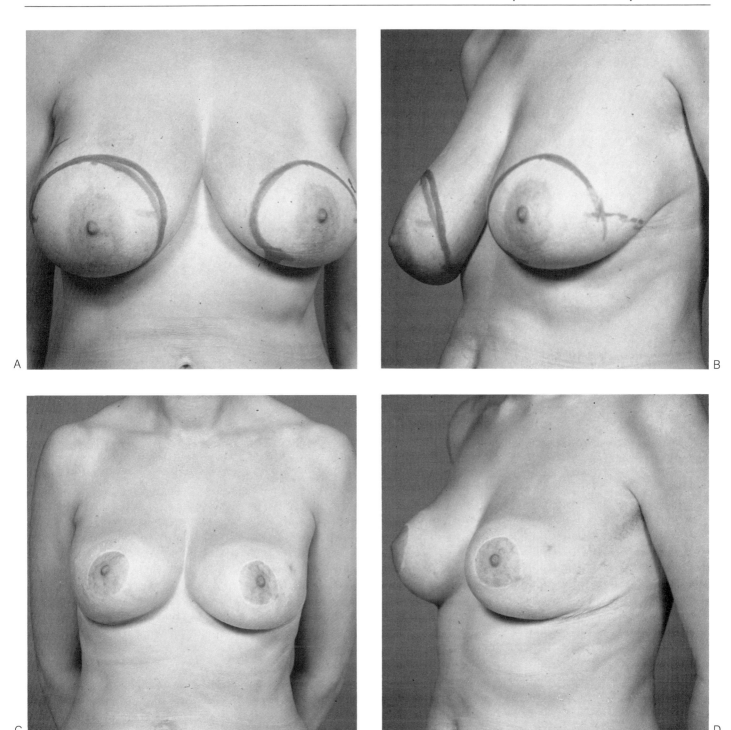

three complete nipple necroses were seen in 1,306 breasts. If impaired circulation in the areola is seen in the postoperative period, it is difficult to do anything about it. If, however, the circulation seems to be remarkably poor at the time of the operation, one could cut the areola free and use it as a free graft. The problem is then to have a good recipient area. As a safeguard, it might be an advantage to keep some of the deep dermis in the circular part of the key-hole to provide a suitable bed for a free graft if necessary.

Fig. 27.**60** A, B: 36-year-old patient preoperatively.
C, D: One year after lateral reduction with L-shaped scars. Resection weight right side, 500 g; left side, 350 g.

Skin Complications

Circulatory disturbances in the skin flaps are extremely rare and if smaller defects should appear, they heal by second intension. Separation in the scars might take place, especially if the suturing is done under tension. In the technique with an inverted T scar, it is usually the lower meeting point of the flaps where the separation might appear.

Results

Concerning results after reduction mammaplasty, it is primarily the opinion of the patient that is of major interest. The surgeon's judgment of the end result does not always correspond with the patient's.

Which factors affect the subjective result, that is, the patient's opinion of the operation? Whether the patient is satisfied or not depends on the expectations she had before the operation. Preoperative information is most important and should especially stress the disadvantages involved. Even adequate oral and written information does not always reach the patient. She has her own opinions and shuts off all information that does not fit into her own concepts. Besides her expectations are certain parameters of importance such as size, scars, sensitivity, cosmetic result, and function (e.g., nursing ability). But there is another factor of importance: The age of the patient at the time of operation. To gain an opinion on the patient's subjective views of the result, I have sent questionaires at three different times to patients I have operated on (Strömbeck 1964, 1976, 1983). This type of follow up is impaired by great weaknesses: Are the patients completely honest? Do they want to avoid displeasing the doctor? The drop-out rate is large (some 20%) and one does not know if it is the dissatisfied who don't want to answer or the satisfied. If the patients are asked to come for a personal follow up, the drop-out rate is even larger. Nonetheless, the infor-

mation gained might be of interest. If the three above-mentioned follow ups are combined, they show the following figures.

Degree of Satisfaction

The patients were asked about the degree of satisfaction by choosing one of four possibilities: extremely satisfied, satisfied, fairly satisfied, and dissatisfied. The answers given by 375 patients were: extremely satisfied 60%, satisfied 25%, fairly satisfied 14%, and dissatisfied 1%.

The question as to whether the patient regarded the scars as almost invisible, somewhat disturbing, or ugly was answered as follows: 56%, 33%, and 11%, respectively (Fig. 27.**61**). If they regarded the postoperative breast size as satisfactory 83%, too large 13% or too small 4% (Fig. 27.**62**). The patients were also asked their opinion on nipple sensitivity and 53% said that the sensitivity was just the same as before the operation, 31% that it was somewhat reduced in comparison with the preoperative condition, and 16% that it was poor (Fig. 27.**63**). Thus it seems that the size and the scars are of greater importance for the degree of satisfaction than the nipple sensitivity.

Nipple Sensitivity

In this context, erotic sensitivity is the most important. This is difficult to quantify and you have to ask the patient directly for her opinion. As could be seen from the above, disturbance in nipple sensitivity after the operation is very common. It is rare, however, that the patient complains about this. This is probably not because of shyness, but more from the fact that very large breasts often originally have poor nipple sensitivity. This has to be explained and discussed with the patient before the operation and if the nipple sensitivity is extremely important to the patient, it might be a partial contraindication for surgery, and if surgery is decided, it is better to choose a technique where the gland is not detached from the chest wall.

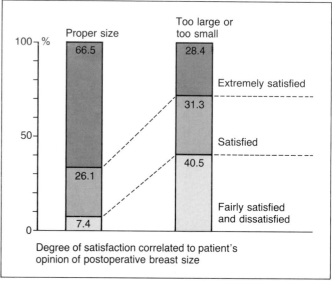

Fig. 27.**61**   Degree of satisfaction correlated to patient's subjective opinion of the scars. Questionnaires 377 patients.

Fig. 27.**62**   Degree of satisfaction correlated to patient's opinion of postoperative breast size. Questionnaires 377 patients.

Another interesting fact that could be gained from these follow ups is that patients younger than 25 years of age at the time of operation are the least satisfied with the result. This could also be seen from the answers to the question as to whether the result corresponded to their preoperative expectations and if they would choose to have the operation if they had a second choice. This showed once again that the indications for operating on very young patients should be very strict, (Fig. 27.**64**, Table 27.**1**).

Table 27.**1** Age at operation correlated to the answer "yes" to the questions "does the result correspond to your preoperative expectations?" and "if you had a second choice would you then like to have the operation?"

| | Age at operation (n = 377) | | |
	< 20	20–24	≧ 25 years
Result in compliance with patient's expectations	76.2%	81.2%	87.2%
If the patient had a second choice she would like to have the operation	76.2%	95.3%	94.9%

Postoperative Lactation

As in all the above techniques with the exception of the free-nipple grafting, the major part of the remaining gland remains connected with the areola. There is theoretically the capacity for lactation after the operation. The outcome, however, is not so favorable. I found that of my patients, roughly half of the women nurse with good capacity after reduction procedures. However, many of them never tried to nurse because they were afraid that it would impair the cosmetic result. Of the patients who had nursed both before and after surgery, I had eight patients of which two nursed better after the operation than before, two with less success than before the operation, and the remaining four just as good afterwards as before (Strömbeck 1983).

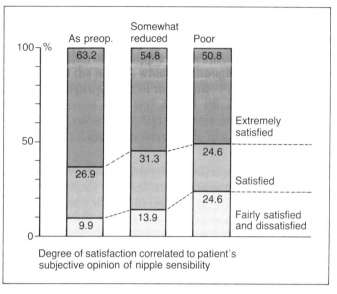

Fig. 27.**63** Degree of satisfaction correlated to patient's subjective opinion of nipple sensibility. Questionnaires 377 patients.

Special Types of Breast Deformities

Breast Asymmetries

Smaller asymmetries in basically normal-sized breasts rarely require any surgery. Sometimes the younger patients may be concerned about the difference since the nipples may lie at different heights. A very restrictive policy as to surgery is to be recommended. In more pronounced asymmetries, correction is indicated. If the smaller breast is about normal or of acceptable size to the patient, a reduction should be made of the larger breast. It is then important that the new nipple position becomes symmetrical with the normal side and that the reduction is adequate to give a size equal to the nonoperated side. Careful preoperative planning is paramount. Sometimes both breasts have to be reduced, for example, if the smaller breast is ptotic or too large to please the patient.

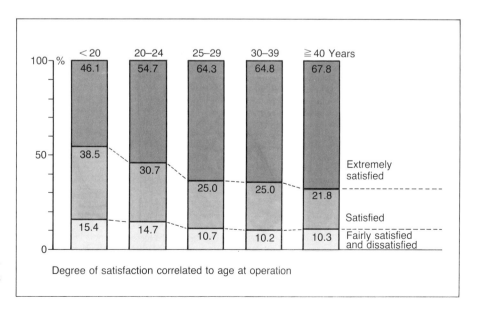

Fig. 27.**64** Degree of satisfaction correlated to age at operation. Questionnaires 377 patients.

If the larger breast is over-sized or ptotic and the smaller unacceptably small, both breasts have to be altered, one with reduction and the other with augmentation mammaplasty.

Poland's Syndrome

The patient with Poland's syndrome presents a special problem. This syndrome has the following characteristics: Amastia; deficient pectoralis major muscle; shorter upper limb; and hand anomalies including syndactyly. All defects are seen on the same side. Even if the hand and arm components of the syndrome are missing, the term Poland's syndrome is used.

The basic principle of treatment is augmentation of the amastic side with a breast prosthesis. The problem these patients offer is similar to that of a postmastectomy patient that should be reconstructed. The same considerations as to the use of a latissimus dorsi myocutaneous flap and mastopexy on the normal side have to be made (see p. 256). The nipple is of male type and sometimes after augmentation may become distended to match the normal side, but if the patient so wishes, an areolar reconstruction could be made (see p. 252).

Rare Deformities

A rare deformity that is seen mostly in rather small breasts are double-contoured breasts where the areola area protrudes like a bell (Fig. 27.**65**). Most of these patients are candidates for augmentation rather than reduction mammaplasty, but the bell deformity has to be dealt with separately. This is most easily done by a circular incision around the periphery of the natural areola and an inner incision concentric with the first and with a smaller diameter. In this way the size of the areola is reduced, and if necessary, part of the gland may be removed underneath the areola area to achieve flatness in this area.

This deformity could be even more pronounced with an extremely extended areola and a breast having the shape of a large pendulous sausage (Fig. 27.**66**). The principle of the operation for these patients is exactly the same, with a circular superficial excision of areola tissue and perhaps also skin around the reduced areola (Fig. 27.**67**) and undermining of the skin down to the breast periphery (Fig. 27.**68**) where the base of the protruding tissue is anchored (Fig. 27.**69**). Suturing of the two circles together, perhaps in combination with a little wedge-skin excison with the apex pointing to the inframammary fold, will give a pleasing result (Figs. 27.**65**B, 27.**70**B).

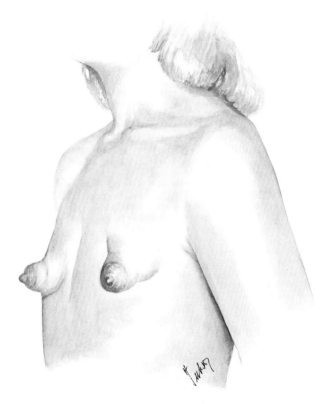

Fig. 27.**65** A   Bell-shaped breasts.

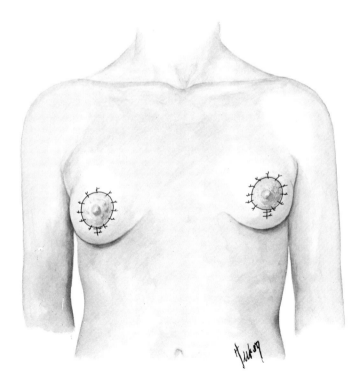

Fig. 27.**65** B   Appearance of breasts following completion of technique shown in figs. 27.66–70.

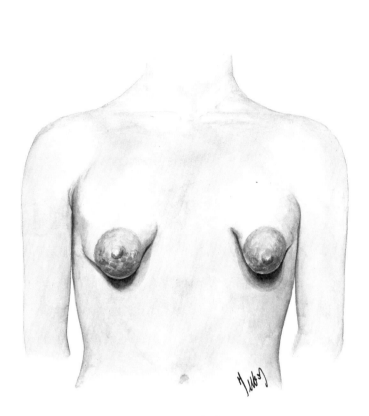
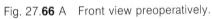

Fig. 27.**66** A   Front view preoperatively.

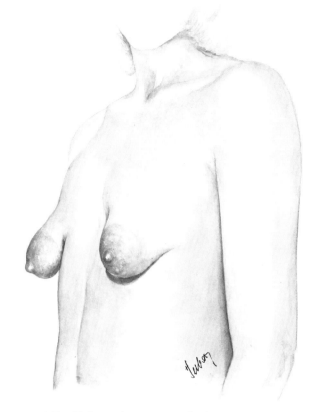

Fig. 27.**66** B   Oblique view preoperatively.

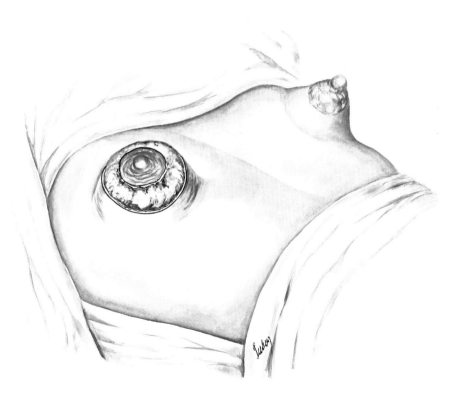

Fig. 27.**67**   The areola is reduced by peripheral circular excision in a superficial plane.

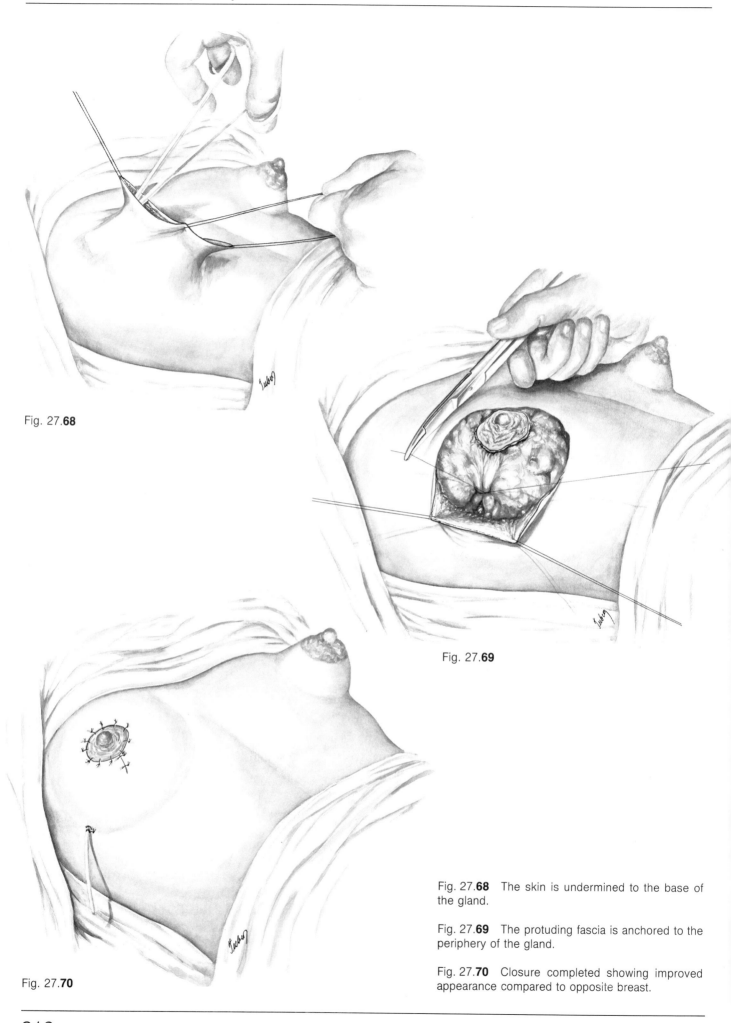

Fig. 27.**68**

Fig. 27.**69**

Fig. 27.**70**

Fig. 27.**68** The skin is undermined to the base of the gland.

Fig. 27.**69** The protuding fascia is anchored to the periphery of the gland.

Fig. 27.**70** Closure completed showing improved appearance compared to opposite breast.

References

Axhausen, G.: Über Mammaplastik. Med. Klin. 22: 1437–1449, 1926

Biesenberger, H.: Deformitäten und kosmetische Operationen der weiblichen Brust. W. Maudrich, Wien 1931

Courtiss, E. H., R. M. Goldwyn: Reduction mammaplasty by the inferior pedicle technique. Plast. Reconstr. Surg. 59: 500–507, 1977

Döring, G. K.: Über Veränderungen des Brustvolumens im Cyclus. Arch. Gynaek. 184: 51–58, 1953

Dufourmentel, C., R. Mouly: Plastie mammaire par la méthode oblique. Ann. Chir. Plast. 6: 45–58, 1961

Dufourmentel, C., R. Mouly: Reduction mammaplasty by the lateral Approach. In R. M. Goldwyn: Plastic and Reconstruction Surgery of the Breast. Little, Brown & Co., Boston 1976

Galtier, M.: Chirurgie Esthétique Mammaire. G. Doin & Cie, Paris 1955

Holländer, E.: Die Operation der Mammahypertrophie und der Hängebrust. Deutsch. Med. Wschr. 50: 1400–1402, 1924

Lalardrie, J. P. & Jonglard, J. P.: Chirurgie Plastique du Sein. Masson et Cie, Paris 1974

Lessing, M.: Eine neue Methode der Mammaplastik. Zbl. Gynaek. 75: 968–974, 1953

Lexer, E.: Die gesamte Wiederherstellungs-Chirurgie, Vol. 2. Johann Ambrosius Barth, Leipzig 1931

McKissock, P. K.: Reduction mammaplasty with a vertical dermal flap. Plast. Reconstr. Surg. 49: 245–252, 1972

Maliniac, J. W.: Breast Deformities and Their Repair. Grune & Stratton, New York 1950

Padron, J. G.: Mammareduktionsplastik. Transacta der III. Tagung der Vereinigung der Deutschen Plastischen Chirurgen, Köln 1972

Passot, R.: La correction esthétique du prolapsus mammaire par le procédé de la transposition du mamelon. Presse Méd. 33: 317–318, 1925

Peixoto, G.: Reduction mammaplasty: A personal technique. Plast. Reconstr. Surg. 65: 217–225, 1980

Pers, M., G. Bretteville-Jensen: Reduction mammaplasty based on a vertical vascular bipedicle and "tennis ball" assembly. Scand. J. Plast. Reconstr. Surg. 6: 61–68, 1972

Pitanguy, I.: Une nouvelle technique de plastie mammaire. Étude de 245 cas consécutifs et présentation d'une technique personelle. Ann. Chir. Plast. 7: 199–207, 1962

Ragnell, A.: Operative correction of hypertrophy and ptosis of the female breast. Acta Chir. Scand. Suppl. 113, 1946

Regnault, P.: Reduction mammaplasty by the B-technique. Plast. Reconstr. Surg. 53: 19–25, 1974

Ribeiro, L.: A new technique for reduction mammaplasty. Plast. Reconstr. Surg. 55: 330–334, 1975

Robbins, T. H.: A reduction mammaplasty with the areola nipple based on an inferior dermal pedicle. Plast. Reconstr. Surg. 59: 64–67, 1977

Schrudde, J.: Eine Methode der Mammaplastik. Transacta der III. Tagung der Vereinigung der Deutschen plastischen Chirurgen, Köln 1972

Schultz, R. C., N. J. Markus: Platform for nipple projection: Modification of the inferior pedicle technique for breast reduction. Plast. Reconstr. Surg. 68: 208–214, 1981

Schwarzmann, E.: Die Technik der Mammaplastik. Chirurg 2: 932–943, 1930

Skoog, T.: A technique of breast reduction. Acta Chir. Scand. 126: 453–465, 1963

Skoog, T.: Plastic Surgery. New Methods and Refinements. Almqvist & Wiksell International, Stockholm 1974

Strömbeck, J. O.: Mammaplasty: Report of a new technique based on the two-pedicle procedure. Br. J. Plast. Surg. 13: 79–90, 1960

Strömbeck, J. O.: Macromastia in women and its surgical treatment. Acta Chir. Scand. Suppl. 341, 1964

Strömbeck, J. O.: Reduction mammaplasty. Surg. Clin. North Am. 51: 453–469, 1971

Strömbeck, J. O.: Reduction mammaplasty by upper and lower glandular resections. In R. M. Goldwyn: Plastic and Reconstructive Surgery of the Breast. Little, Brown & Co., Boston 1976

Strömbeck, J. O.: Benign diseases of the female breast. Surgical treatment and cosmetic aspects. Excerpta Medica International Congress Series No 412. Proceedings of the VIII World Congress of Gynecology and Obstetrics, Mexico City, 17–22 October 1976. Excerpta Medica, Amsterdam 1977

Strömbeck, J. O.: Late results after reduction mammaplasty. In R. M. Goldwyn: Long-term Results in Plastic and Reconstructive Surgery. Little, Brown & Co., Boston 1980

Strömbeck, J. O.: Reduction mammaplasty. In N. G. Georgiade: Aesthetic Breast Surgery. Williams & Wilkins Co., Baltimore 1983

Thorek, M.: Plastic Surgery of the Breast and Abdominal Wall. C. C. Thomas, Springfield, Baltimore 1942

Weiner, D. L., A. E. Aiache, L. Silver, T. Tittiranonda: A single dermal pedicle for nipple transposition in subcutaneous mastectomy, reduction mammaplasty or mastopexy. Plast. Reconstr. Surg. 51: 115–120, 1973

Wise, R. J.: Breast reduction with nipple transposition. In R. M. Goldwyn: Plastic and Reconstructive Surgery of the Breast. Little, Brown & Co., Boston 1976

Chapter 28

Breast Augmentation

P. Regnault

The popularity of increasing the breast size by surgery, over the last few years, is due to the improvements in the surgical techniques as well as in the quality of the implants. It has become a relatively minor procedure that might even be performed without hospitalization and even under local anesthesia. The main complication, hardness due to fibrosis of the capsule, has been greatly reduced and its treatment improved.

History

Breast augmentation started around 1945 in the United States by a major procedure described by several authors that consisted in using a free dermafat graft from the buttocks (Bames 1953). The results were impaired by resorption and infection in such a large percentage that the operation was abandoned. In the late 1950s, the use of prosthetic material appeared: ivalon sponges and later etheron. The simplicity of inserting a foreign body, in comparison to grafting, and the good early results made the procedure quite popular, but the late results appeared very unsatisfactory in a large number of the cases. Since the 1960s, there appeared the silicone bags, filled with silicone gel introduced by Cronin (1964). With various useful modifications they remain the implants that we are using now: silicone bags either empty and filled with saline at time of surgery, or prefilled with silicone gel. The very late results are yet unknown, but the percentage of good results over a ten-year period is good enough to recommend the operation.

Indication

Augmentation is indicated whenever the breast size is not in an esthetic proportion with the body and the correction is desired by the woman. Most women who look for an increase in their breast volume simply want to be able to dress easily without adding padded brassieres. Some of them have been concerned for many years, before they come for consultation. The defect is obvious and they do not have any psychiatric disturbance.

There are few contraindications. Of course, as with any unnecessary procedure, it is contraindicated when it might be a threat to the patient's health. Anticoagulant therapy is obviously an important contraindication. Any undiagnosed lump should be treated first. Fibrocystic problems, if present, should also be evaluated. In patients with more severe ptosis of the breast, a simple breast augmentation does not give a satisfactory result, even though the patient would like to believe so. In these cases, a mastopexy has to be done either first or simultaneously, depending on the surgeon's judgement. Minor ptosis alone may be improved by augmentation. Occasionally, a young woman comes for breast augmentation with a beautiful breast in good proportion to her body, not knowing that she already has the best. She is most happy to be refused. The reasonable lower age limit is eighteen but there is no older limit, as long as the operation may bring happiness without harming (Regnault 1977).

Implants

The implants on the market today that are most widely used are the soft silicone gel bags of various shapes and sizes. Some surgeons recommend the nonprefilled or half filled ones. For the technique that I describe here, the most suitable implants have been the round prefilled ones with either a "regular profile" or "low profile," according to the patient's breast, thorax, and the projection desired (Fig. 28.**1**). Oval or elongated implants are used only in cases of some chest deformities or aplasia of the pectoralis muscles.

First Consultation

The first consultation and examination is extremely important for an appropriate decision and a happy result. The motivation for surgery should have been in the woman's mind for several years and her desire for a larger breast should come sincerely from herself alone, not being influenced by her family or friends.

The examination of the entire body is done for comparison of the various parts and an evaluation of the existing breast volume in relation to the hips, the shoulders and the waist line, as well as the woman's height and silhouette. The ideal "36–24–36" can rarely be predicted after surgery, since the great majority of women already have larger hips and waist. The brassiere cup size is what is easily understood and can be approximately predicted. The estimated increase in volume is a very important point to explain and discuss according to patient's desire and her physical condition. Measuring the thorax perimeter at the submammary fold and at the nipples automatically demonstrates the existing condition: for example, a person having 29 inches at the submammary fold and 35 at the nipples wears a 34A brassiere (see Table 28.**1, 2**). These measurements are used by most woman as a means to purchase appropriate sized brassieres.

The most esthetic cup size, and also the easiest for clothing is the B cup, whatever the thorax perimeter. It is obvious that to increase a cup size, the volume required is larger when the thorax perimeter is larger. By measuring patients before and after surgery, the results have shown that besides measurements, the tissue elasticity is also important to consider: softer and more elastic tissues seem to expand more than firm ones. Absence of the pectoralis muscle requires special custom made implants. The implants may be shown to the patient and inserted in her brassiere to explain the approximate change.

The breast itself is examined from the point of view of possible pathologic conditions. The position of the nipple location in relation to the submammary fold shows the degree of ptosis and is of the utmost importance, since the operative technique may be different. A minor ptosis (nipple at the fold level) may very well be corrected by a simple augmentation, whereas a moderate or major ptosis needs a mastopexy simultaneously or before the augmentation.

Asymmetry of volume is worth considering when the person is already aware of it. When it is hardly visible, a difference of 20 cc between the two implants is enough to correct this. When it is large enough to give clothing problems, it can be estimated by measuring the thoracic halfs separately at nipple level and comparing them. A 1 cm difference roughly corresponds to about 50 cc volume difference.

Abnormally protruding areolas may be noticed and it should be clear to the patient that a special correction is then necessary if desired since the augmentation will not improve this deformity.

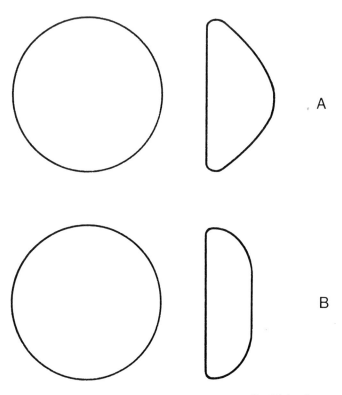

Fig. 28.**1** Comparison of regular (A) and low profile (B) implants to be used in relation to the physical conditions.

The quality of the skin and previous scars, if present, may be an indication about scarring problems. The presence or absence of subcutaneous fat may modify the result. Leanness is an absolute indication for the submuscular technique. Information about gynecologic or recent skin infection are important to obtain since such infections should be dealt with before surgery.

At the time of the first consultation, the choice of volume and shape of implants are marked on the patient's chart to be used at the time of surgery. However, it happens that at the last minute the patient may make some recommendations as to expected change ("please not too big" or "make sure it will be large enough to show") so that it is good policy to have various sizes available. It has always been rewarding to try to understand the patient's desire and remember that she will be the one who will have these implants for life. In esthetic surgery, patients should be pleased with the results (Brody 1981).

Table 28.**1** Table of average volume augmentation in the most common cases of small breast (with existing A cup brassiere)

		A	B	C	D	
32	before	140	180	220	(+ 40)
34	before	200	260	320	(+ 60)
36	before	260	340	420	(+ 80)
38	before	340	440	540	(+ 100)

Table 28.**2** Table of average volume augmentation in cases of complete aplasia (AA cup)

		AA	A	B	C	
32	before	120	180	240	(+ 60)
34	before	180	260	320	(+ 80)
36	before	260	360	460	(+ 100)
38	before	360	480	600	(+ 120)

Operative Planning

Prior to anesthesia it is important to examine the patient in the sitting position to remind one of the general contour of the breast in this position. Then the patient is placed in a supine position with elbows semiflexed, hands under her hips.

After scrubbing and draping, marking of the location of the submammary fold, the midline, and the area to be undermined is done. In cases of asymmetry, clear indication of the difference should be marked. It is very important to measure the distance of the submammary incision from the nipple center, for a symmetric location. The average distance is 6 cm and it may vary 1 cm more or less according to the thorax and augmentation required. The incision is marked under the vertical of the areola. The length varies from 3 to 6 cm according to the size of the implant (Fig. 28.**2**).

Anesthesia

No difference in results was found whether the patient was under complete general anesthesia or under sedation and local infiltration. So, when patients seem rather nervous, general anesthesia is better. Otherwise, preoperative sedation and intercostal block of the 3rd, 4th, and 5th nerves plus direct infiltration of the lower part of the operative field with 0.50% solution of xylocaine with epinephrine 1/200,000. The usual total amount of anesthetic solution is 100 cc for both sides. Even with general anesthesia, local infiltration may be used in the lower quadrants to help hemostasis, using the same solution.

Surgical Technique

I use a partially submuscular augmentation of the breast volume by inserting the implant behind the pectoralis major muscle, which covers the upper two thirds or three quarters of the implant only (Regnault 1977, 1978).

Anatomical reminder: The breast extends from the 2nd interspace to the 6th interspace, vertically and from the sternum to the anterior axillary line horizontally (Fig. 28.**3**). The deep surface of the gland lies on the pectoralis major almost entirely with its lateral portion on the serratus anterior. The pectoralis major is covered partially by the pectoralis fascia, which is thick at the insertions on the sternum, clavicle, and humerus; at the sternocostal and abdominal origins it blends with the rectus abdominis. The lateral edge of the pectoralis muscle lies on the serratus. The pectoralis major is a thick fanshaped muscle that may vary in its insertions on the ribs, as well as its thickness and tonicity.

The skin and fat are incised, following the planning. The muscle is identified. It is found at the upper medial region above the incision, sometimes quite higher than expected (Fig. 28.**4**). A few muscular fibers are clamped and severed and a finger is introduced under the muscle, in the cleavage plan, superficial to the rib cage and the pectoralis minor at the upper part. Once the blunt finger dissection of the upper portion is done, the lower attachments on the ribs and sternum are separated under direct vision by clamping and electrocoagulation. The muscular insertions are thus severed on the ribs and on the sternum as high as the third rib. Careful hemostasis is pursued until a dry field is obtained. The size of the pocket obtained should be larger than the implant.

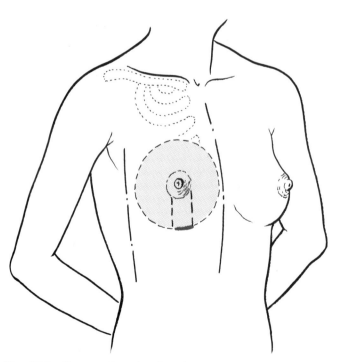

Fig. 28.**2** Preoperative planning drawn on the patient showing the submammary incision in the vertical of the areola and the undermining, which should be larger than the implant. Midsternal line and anterior axillary line are shown.

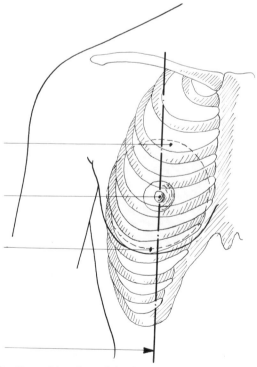

Fig. 28.**3** Normal location of the breast in relation to the thorax. The breast tissue lies between the sternum and anterior axillary line vertically and between the 2nd and 6th interspaces horizontally.

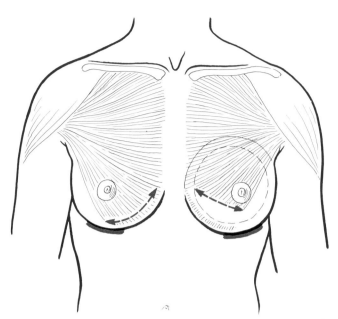

Fig. 28.**4** Location of the pectoralis major incision and dissection on the right side. Location of the implant, partially covered by the pectoralis muscle, on the left side. The implant circle is smaller than the undermining.

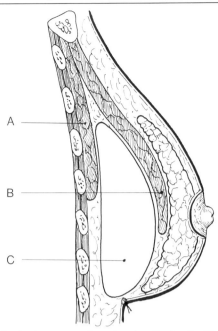

Fig. 28.**5** Sagittal cross section showing the implant between the muscles at the upper part. It lies between the pectoralis major and costal grill at the mid part and between the gland and costal grill at the lower part. A. Pectoralis minor B. Pectoralis major C. Implant

The implant is introduced by squeezing it into the pocket and it should then be hardly visible at the incision (Fig. 28.**5**). If it appears to bulge, the pocket should be enlarged by gentle blunt dissection of the periphery and by enlarging the anterior muscle opening. Additional hemostasis may be necessary.

Drainage is rarely used: only when some uncontrollable bleeding occurs. In these cases, a separate stab wound incision is made laterally and a Penroselike silicone drain is left for 48 hours.

Suturing is accomplished by layers: separate stitches on the fascia, not including the pectoralis, which is left free and does not cover the lower third or fourth of the implant. The skin is approximated by a subcuticular running suture. Paper adhesive strips cover the incision. No other dressing is applied unless a drain has been necessary.

Postoperative Instructions

It is recommended to restrict pectoralis major contractions for seven days, so that arm efforts are forbidden. Sport activities are not permitted for one month. Mild sedatives and analgesics are prescribed, although many patients do not need them. The patient is seen one week later. The breast is usually a little swollen, and the patient is told that it will be slightly smaller within a month or so. She is asked to start massaging her implant over the rib cage by moving it in all directions for a few minutes twice daily. The use of brassieres is forbidden for about three months to allow free movement of breasts and implants, which makes a constant massage and prevents the unnatural location of the implants which might occur if the straps were pulled too tight. Later, only the very soft type of brassiere is permitted, avoiding the underwire support.

Advantages and Disadvantages of the Partially Submuscular Technique with Submammary Approach

Advantages

The inframammary approach leaves a well-located scar in a natural fold, under the breast, in the vertical position where it is invisible and may be hidden by small brassieres. Some persons make hypertrophic scars, which need treatment and remain visible permanently.

This approach is the easiest being directly at the lower limit of the undermining. It allows a direct vision of the whole undermined area and easier hemostasis. In case of hematoma, reopening the wound is a simple way of complete evacuation. In case of fibrotic capsule, this location of the scar gives the best approach.

The partially subpectoral undermining allows an easily dissected pocket suitable for any size of implant. Hemostasis is easier than with the subglandular dissection, since it is an anatomical cleavage plan, and the upper part of the field is usually dry. Bleeding at the muscular insertions and split where the muscle is, is well visible and controllable. Postoperative pain is less evident with submuscular than with subglandular undermining.

In lean persons, the natural padding of the pectoralis major over the upper part of the implant is a great aesthetic advantage; it gives a much more natural appearance.

The percentage of fibrotic capsular formation is only about 15% as compared with the subglandular dissection. Where it is 60%, there might possibly be less foreign body reaction from the muscle than from the mammary gland and better-visualized pocket walls.

315

Disadvantages

An occasional adhesion of the pocket to the upper part of the muscle and lifting of the implant with contraction of the pectoralis will occur; this may be temporary for a few weeks after surgery, or permanent and may then be corrected by enlarging the upper half of the capsule.

Slipping of the implant below the submammary fold also happens occasionally on one side or both. It is easily corrected by resuturing the available tissue with stronger permanent sutures and supporting the breasts with a brassiere night and day for one month. These cases have a very thin and loose capsule as opposed to the fibrous ones.

Extrusion of the implant several years after surgery is rare, but may happen in cases of excessive prolonged efforts such as competitive sports with arm strain or ceiling painting. Normally, restriction of sports or arm exertions for one month are sufficient. Swimming and tennis are permitted after one month, at the same pace as before surgery.

Other Techniques

The technique just described is the one that the author uses in 99% of her cases, but it happens that some preferences or circumstances bring some change.

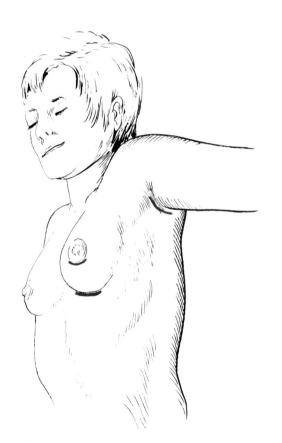

Fig. 28.**6** Possible skin incisions for periareolar, axillary, and submammary approaches.

Subglandular Undermining

Historically, this was the first approach for the placement of grafts or any kind of implant and it seems a very logical approach.

Once the cutaneous incision has been made, the undermining is done entirely above the pectoralis major and serratus, below the gland and fat tissue. Hemostasis may be much more tedious than with the submuscular dissection because of the many small vessels in this location. Sharp undermining is mostly necessary because blunt undermining tears and breaks muscular fibers. Drainage is often necessary. When a large implant is used, the pocket may have to be so wide that the gland vascularization is compromised.

In my opinion, the disadvantages are so numerous that the partially submuscular pocket is preferable in the great majority of the cases.

Other Approaches

Whatever the technique of undermining, incision, and the approach may vary according to the surgeon and the desire to please the patient (Fig. 28.**6**).

Periareolar

A semicircular incision is made at the inferior margin of the areola, about one third of its circumference. The fat and gland are then incised down to the pectoralis major. The undermining is then done, either subglandular or submuscular. Hemostasis may sometimes be a little difficult. A fiberoptic light is often used. Inserting a very large implant may be somewhat difficult. The scar may be excellent, almost invisible, but if it becomes hypertrophic, then it is much more visible than a submammary scar. Revision of these scars is very disappointing as they have a tendency to reform (Jones and Tauras 1973; Wilkinson 1978).

Abdominal Approach

When performing any esthetic procedure on the abdomen such as abdominoplasty or scar revision of the upper quadrants, it provides an opportunity to use the same incision to insert mammary implants. The undermining from the abdominal area to the breast area is done by blunt dissection. Once there, subpectoral undermining is the easiest way to create the pocket for the prosthesis. The undermining should, of course, be as wide as previously described. Separating the muscle from the ribs and sternum is done exclusively by tearing. Bleeding is rarely a problem. If necessary, a fiberoptic light is used with temporary packing and pressure. In case of doubt a small drain is left. When closing the pocket and suturing the fascia, one or two stitches are very important to prevent slipping of the implants, especially when they are small. These sutures should be symmetric and at the level of the submammary fold (Hinderer 1975).

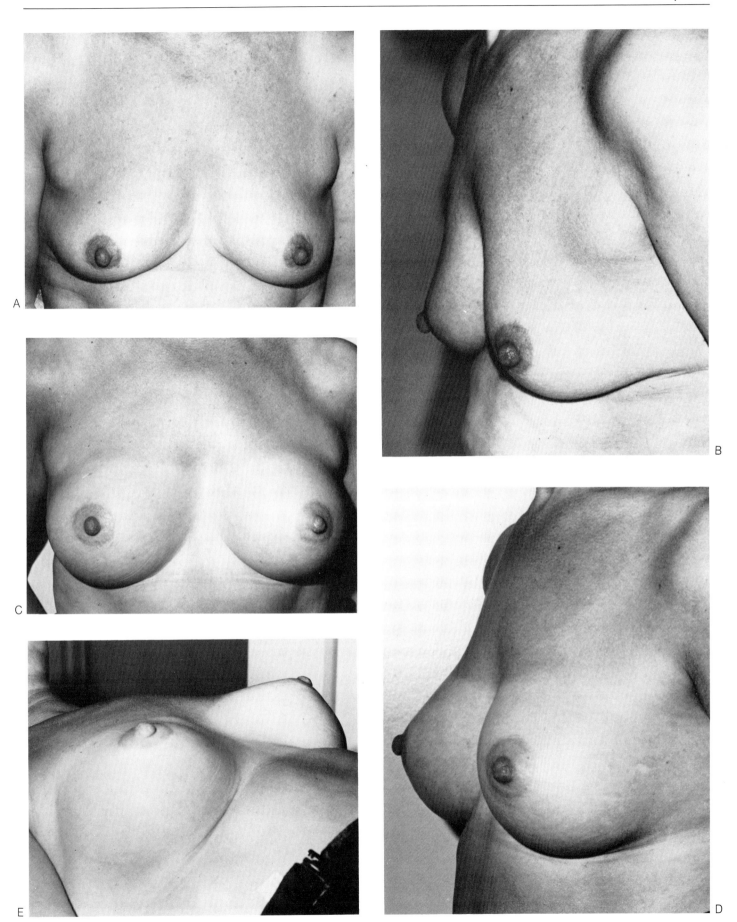

Fig. 28.**7** A, B: Preoperative appearance. C, D, E: Postoperative result after partial submuscular implantation.

Axillary approach

This is a good approach when dealing with highly placed breasts where only a small augmentation is required. Otherwise, the undermining down to the submammary fold may be difficult and would require the use of dissecting instruments. Bleeding is controllable by packing and pressure only. But when the local conditions are favorable, the result has the great advantage of leaving scars that are usually fine and easily concealed. The incision for such a procedure 4 to 6 cm long in the hair-bearing midaxillary area and should follow the direction of the normal crease lines. Sharp dissection of the subcutaneous tissue is done until the edge of the pectoralis major is identified and the dissection then continues either above or below the muscle. I personally prefer the submuscular undermining. The introduction of the implant might be more difficult and the postoperative dressing should provide some pressure on the upper part of the implant to prevent upward dislocation of the prosthesis (Virias 1966; Eiseman 1974; Agris et al. 1976).

Complications, Prevention, and Treatment

Operative Bleeding

Unnecessary bleeding may be prevented by careful attention to the patient's bleeding history and coagulation studies. Constant use of aspirin or even its moderate use within two weeks of surgery increase the risk of bleeding. Premenstrual operations are better to avoid.

The use of local infiltration anesthesia with epinephrine in the usual bleeding area, even when the patient is under general anesthesia, has become routine in my cases because it has proved to reduce bleeding and hematomas so effectively that they have practically disappeared.

When, in spite of previous precautions, more than usual bleeding occurs, then temporary packing and pressure are used. With a fiberoptic light some bleeding points may be seen in an unusual location, at the upper limit of the undermining or on the anterior wall. With diffuse difficult-to-control oozing, a stab wound incision is made at the lowest point to introduce a drain that is left for 24 to 72 hours. A pressure dressing is applied, the arms and shoulder immobilized, and vitamins K and C may be prescribed.

Hematoma

This is the most common complication that surgeons meet when doing breast augmentation. Its prevention is the same as for operative bleeding. Postoperative movements should be restricted and aspirin forbidden. It may happen that operative bleeding has been minimal and then one hour to ten days after surgery one or both breasts become extremely swollen and painful. Under these conditions, it is imperative to return the patient to the operating room within 24 hours, evacuate the hematoma, try to find the bleeding points, replace the implant, and leave a drain. This is usually done under local anesthesia. If bleeding seems too difficult to control, it may be wise to postpone the reinsertion of the implants for a few days, but certainly to reinsert them within the week. Otherwise fibrotic tissues will have already appeared.

Infection

Infection is extremely rare when surgery is done under the aseptic conditions of a modern operating room with sterilization equipment. Yet occasionally, within a month after surgery, pain and swelling with erythema of the lower part of the breast or the whole breast may appear. It usually is not bilateral, although this would not be impossible.

This may be prevented in a large percentage by investigating the patient's susceptibility to infection, particularly a history of recent gynecologic or skin infections.

The routine use of antibiotics is controversial, but if there is no known allergy, it has been the habit of a large number of surgeons to prescribe a broad-spectrum antibiotic. When infection is established on the skin, gynecologic area, or upper respiratory tract, it is safer to have it treated first and postpone the operation. When infections are recent, antibiotics should be started before surgery and continued for a minimum of ten days after the operation.

When preventive measures have not been taken or have been insufficient, treatment of the infected implants should be started immediately with energetic antibiotic therapy. Excision of the infected wound and reclosure may be tried, but is rarely successful. Most of the time the implant has to be removed and the wound left open. It may discharge for several weeks then close, leaving fibrotic tissue and retractions. It will be necessary to wait a minimum of three months before reinserting another implant. At that time all scar tissue should be well dissected and removed, to be able to obtain a good result symmetrical with the other breast.

Inflammatory reaction of the suture lines is a minor complication, but should not be neglected because it may cause bad scarring. When abnormal itchiness or pain appears early after surgery, the sutures should be removed immediately and replaced by a few sterile paper strips. This complication is somewhat prevented by the use of the most inert suture material possible and protecting the scar with a light permeable paper strip.

These local reactions should be treated immediately by cleaning with mild antiseptics and local application of antibiotics. It is better to avoid ointments which have a tendency to delay healing. Systemic antibiotic therapy should be continued until disappearance of the redness.

Mondor's disease occurs occasionally on one or both sides. The patient is aware of the painful red string that appears vertically under one or both breasts. Since this is a mild inflammation of the subcutaneous veins, local application of warm wet dressings and mild antibiotic therapy may be used and the patient should be assured that it will soon completely disappear (Fischl et al. 1975).

Fibrotic Capsular Formation

These remain the most frequent and most difficult complications encountered. It may be to a degree prevented by the strict observation of aseptic surgery, the submuscular technique, maintenance of a dry field, immediate postoperative immobility, early massaging of the implants over the thorax, avoidance of tight brassieres and clothes for a few months, and the avoidance of breast congestion by hormones. However, none of these precautions is mandatory and it is probably a foreign body reaction to the implant. That is the most important cause of the fibrotic reaction. Sponge material and fixating dacron nets are not used anymore, but reaction to the silicone of the implant's envelope and gel may continue, which transudes through the surface after a few months or years. The ideal implant has not yet been discovered, although new materials are under study.

In recent works trying to explain the pathogenesis of fibrotic capsular formation, the following factors have been discussed: foreign body reaction to the silicone bag, organized hematoma, "bleeding" of the silicone gel through the envelope, and low-grade infection (Wilflingseder et al. 1974; Williams et al. 1975; Jenny and Smahel 1980). Several authors have stated the presence of *Staphylococcus epidermidis* in the pocket surrounding the prosthesis. This bacteria could often be found in glandular ducts without having any clinical significance. If, however, the pocket around the prosthesis becomes contaminated with *Staphylococcus epidermidis*, a low-grade infection is caused, which after months or years could cause a fibrosis. This might explain why a contracture could be unilateral and why a contracture is less commonly seen with a submuscular pocket. The use of antibiotics started one day before surgery and continued for ten days may thus be a good preventive measure, although no proof has been confirmed. To add antibiotics (cephalothin) into the silicone envelope itself has been claimed to prevent capsular fibrosis. (Courtiss et al. 1979; Burkardt et al. 1981).

The prevention of capsule formation by the use of local steroids free in the pocket or in the inflatable implants is not recommended because of the risk of wound dehiscence or local atrophy of the tissues. I have, however, successfully used the preventive local infiltration of the upper pole and anterior muscular wall with 10% triamcilonone, taking care not to leave any free liquid in the cavity. Treatment of the fibrotic capsule varies when it is seen early and when it is relatively soft. In this case, treatment by external manual compression of the capsule may cause its rupture, and the whole area becomes suddenly as soft, as before. The patient should be advised to start massaging her implants several times daily. Very often the rupturing maneuver has to be repeated one or more times, which might be discouraging to the patient and the surgeon. Besides, this squeezing maneuver is painful and may provoke hematomas or rupture of the implant (Baker et al. 1976; Eisenberg and Bartels 1977).

When the capsule has become very hard, the only treatment is secondary surgery. The scar is incised and the capsule is opened with a cautery knife. The implant is removed and the capsule is incised peripherally; then it is enlarged by blunt finger dissection. The anterior wall may have to be incised in a few locations also. If the pectoralis seems to have reinserted or be insufficiently divided at its lower medial insertions, this should be corrected. The fibrotic tissue left is infiltrated with injections of triamcilonone, but none is left free in the cavity. The implant is carefully examined and only a perfect, recently inserted implant may be reutilized. A new one should always be available.

If calcifications are found in the capsule, it should be completely dissected and removed. This requires a larger incision, more hemostasis, and often drainage (Benjamin and Guy 1977).

When the implants have not been placed subpectorally at first, this should be done at this time by opening the submuscular space and forming a second pocket under the first. To make sure that the implant will remain in this subpectoral pocket, a few stitches are placed to close the previous one. Drainage is sometimes used. Recurrence of capsular fibrosis is rare after change of the pocket, or in those cases when it was already under the pectoralis. If recurrence does happen, one may try the same operation using smaller implants. Should this also prove unsuccessful, the only solution is removal of the implants, which is often requested by the patient because the breast is unesthetic, unpleasant to touch, and often painful.

Sensory changes

Sensory changes may occur in the nipple-areola complex and in the skin area laterally and above the suture line. Mostly these are a temporary anesthesia due to stretching of some sensory nerves, but sometimes they may be permanent when nerves have been cut. (Courtiss and Goldwyn 1976). The occurrence of this complication is much less with the subpectoral dissection than with the subglandular one.

Hypersensitivity of the nipple may occur, and although temporary, it is sometimes quite severe requiring nipple protection with lanolin cream, the use of a dressing, and loose clothing.

Scars

Scars are rarely hypertropic. Their formation might be reduced by the use of a careful running subcuticular suture and protection of the scar immediately after surgery and for several months with light paper strips that are changed only when nonadherent. Benzoin is recommended to secure the strips that protect the scar from local reaction. Irritation by brassieres is avoided. Nothing can prevent the formation of true cheloids.

Treatment of hypertropic scars may be carried out by local infiltration with steroids. This leaves a hypotrophic scar, which may be removed after a few months. Cheloids may be treated by repeated injections or steroids or by radiotherapy immediately after excision of the scars.

Unesthetic Result

This is avoided by careful preoperative planning and symmetrical dissection. It still happens that the breast becomes ptotic at a later time due to loss of weight, age, or pregancy and appears ptotic in front of the implant. Secondary mastopexy can then be done.

More frequently unesthetic results are due to fibrotic capsular formation and are treated accordingly.

Unhappy Patient

In spite of an excellent result, it may happen that a woman cannot get adapted to her new breasts. This usually happens when the patient has been motivated by a depressive state related to a completely different matter or when the operation has been sought under the influence of another. This can be avoided by questioning the patient's motivation for surgery and refusing those cases not sincerely motivated for a long time (Edgerton et al. 1961). When a patient says that she prefers her previous breast appearance, it is wise to try to postpone removal of the implants, hoping that her adaptation will come with time.

References

Agris, J., R. O. Dingman, R. J. Wilensky: A dissector for the transaxillary approach in augmentation mammaplasty. Plast. Reconstr. Surg. 57: 10, 1976

Baker, J. L. Jr., R. J. Bartels, W. M. Douglas: Closed compression technique for rupturing a contracted capsule around a breast implant. Plast. Reconstr. Surg. 58: 137, 1976

Bames, H. O.: Augmentation mammaplasty by lipo-transplant. Plast. Reconstr. Surg. 11: 404, 1953

Benjamin, J. L., C. Guy: Calcification of implant capsules following augmentation mammaplasty. Plast. Reconstr. Surg. 59: 432, 1977

Brody, G. S.: Breast implant, size selection and patient satisfaction. Plast. Reconstr. Surg. 68: 611, 1981

Burkhardt, B. R., M. Fried, P. L. Schnur, J. J. Tofield, et al.: Capsules, infection and intraluminal Antibiotics. Plast. Reconstr. Surg. 68: 43, 1981

Courtiss, E. H., R. M. Goldwyn: Breast sensation before and after plastic surgery. Plast. Reconstr. Surg. 58: 1, 1976

Courtiss, E. H., R. M. Goldwyn, G. W. Anastasi: The fate of breast implants with infections around them. Plast. Reconstr. Surg. 63: 812, 1979

Cronin, T. D., F. J. Gerow: Augmentation mammaplasty: A new "natural feel" prosthesis. Transactions of the Third International Congress of Plastic Surgery. Int. Congr. Series Nr. 66 Excerpta Medica Foundation, Amsterdam 1964

Edgerton, M. T., E. Meyer, W. E. Jacobson: Augmentation mammaplasty. II. Further surgical and psychiatric evaluation. Plast. Reconstr. Surg. 27: 279, 1961

Eiseman, G.: Augmentation mammaplasty by the transaxillary approach. Plast. Reconstr. Surg. 54: 229, 1974

Eisenberg, H. V., R. J. Bartels: Rupture of a silicone bag-gel breast implant by closed compression capsulotomy. Plast. Reconstr. Surg. 59: 849, 1977

Fischl, R. A., S. Kahn, B. E. Simon: Mondor's disease. An unusual complication of mammaplasty. Plast. Reconstr. Surg. 56: 319, 1975

Hinderer, U. T.: The dermolipectomy approach for augmentation mammaplasty. Clin. Plast. Surg. 2: 353, 1975

Jenny, H., J. Smahel: Clinico-pathological correlations in the pseudo-capsule formation after breast augmentation. Transactions of the Seventh International Congress of Plastic and Reconstructive Surgery. Sociedad Brasileira de Cirurgia Plastica Sao Paulo, p. 575 1980

Jones, F. R., A. P. Tauras: A periareolar incision for augmentation mammaplasty. Plast. Reconstr. Surg. 51: 641, 1973

Peterson, H. D., G. B. Burt: The role of steroids in prevention of circumferential capsular scaring in augmentation mammaplasty. Plast. Reconstr. Surg. 54: 28, 1974

Regnault, P.: The hypoplastic and ptotic breast: A combined operation with prosthetic augmentation. Plast. Reconstr. Surg. 37: 31, 1966

Regnault, P.: Breast Ptosis. Definition and treatment. Clin. Plast. Surg. 3: 193, 1975

Regnault, P.: Partially submuscular breast augmentation. Plast. Reconstr. Surg. 59: 72, 1977

Regnault, P.: Experience with augmentation mammaplasty. In: Symposium on Aesthetic Surgery of the breast. C. V. Mosby, New York 1978

Virias, J. C.: Protesis mamarias por via axilar. Rev. Actual. Med. 1: 1, 1966

Wilflingseder, P., A. Propst, G. Mikuz: Constrictive fibrosis following silicone implants in mammary augmentation. Chir. Plast. 2: 215, 1974

Wilkinson, T. S.: Gel mammary augmentation via minimal periareolar incisions. In: Symposium on Aesthetic Surgery of the Breast. C. V. Mosby, New York 1978

Williams, C., S. Aston, T. D. Rees: The effect of hematoma on the thickness of pseudosheaths around silicone implants. Plast. Reconstr. Surg. 56: 194, 1975

Chapter 29

The Inverted Nipple

J. O. Strömbeck and L. Wallenberg

Introduction

The inverted nipple is most often a congenital condition, but inversion may also be caused by cancer, operative procedures, trauma or postmastitic fibrosis. Inversion means that in place of the normal nipple, a hollow cavity of varying size is found surrounded by a more or less developed ring of contractile tissue to the border of the areola. The cylinder of musculofibrocollagenous elements forming the nipple is much thinner than normal and deeply attached to the glandular parenchyma by fibrous bands (Schwager et al. 1974) (Fig. 29.1). The glandular lactiferous ducts are short and underdeveloped (Broadbent and Woolf 1976).

The condition seems to have a hereditary background, can be seen unilaterally or bilaterally (Skoog 1952), and is said to be more common in women with large and pendulous breasts (Schwager et al. 1974). The incidence of inverted nipples in a consecutive series of 339 autopsy cases and mastectomy specimens for breast cancer, where the tumor was not localized in the vicinity of the nipple, was reported to be 1 in 57 (Schwager et al. 1974).

Embryology

During the fourth week in human embryos, two lines of thickened ectoderm, the mamillary ridges, are formed, extending from the axilla to the groin. They later disappear except for the spot of the future breast. During the sixth week, solid buds of epidermis grow down into the underlying mesenchyma. The solid gland buds are later branched into secondary buds, forming the lactiferous ducts. During the 8th and 9th months, the epidermal surface over the glandular buds will be depressed and a canalization of the buds completed. Later, the nipple is given its normal everted form by a proliferation of mesodermal tissue around the lactiferous ducts.

Symptoms

The inverted nipple produces three types of problems:

1. Feeding problems. The infant has no possibility to grasp the inverted nipple with his mouth. Occasionly the nipple may be pulled out with the fingers or by means of a pump. In the long run, however, the elastic resistance will make too great demands on the new-born infant.

2. Hygienic problems. The irregular crypts and the deeply positioned openings of the lactiferous ducts make it difficult to establish proper hygiene. Infections occur unless prevented by meticulous cleansing.

3. Cosmetic problems. For many women, the condition may be cosmetically disturbing and present a psychologic handicap.

These three problems, of course, may be assessed in different ways. Corrective surgical intervention, to re-establish as close as possible the normal anatomy, does not guarantee restoration of feeding capacity. Since the hygienic problem may be considered to be the least important, our conclusion is that the surgical treatment for inverted nipples should be regarded as a cosmetic procedure thereby placing special demands on the surgeon.

Survey of Operative Techniques

The techniques that are published for the surgical treatment of inverted nipples could roughly be divided into two groups. One group consists of mainly older techniques where the nipple is exposed by means of an adapta-

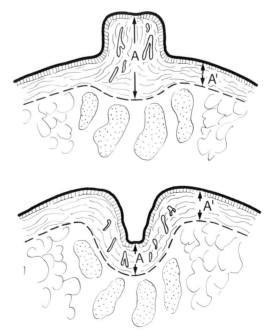

Fig. 29.1 Histology of normal and inverted nipple. (After Schwager et al.)

tion of skin to the base of the nipple sometimes by means of a resection of the total areolar area. In these techniques, the predominant aim is to establish feeding capacity. The nipple is left in a cavity at skin level, but it can be grasped by the infants mouth. No attempts are made to divide the fibrous bands that tie the nipple down and invert it.

The other group of more recent techniques takes a more cosmetic view on the problem. These methods are designed to create the lump of fibrocollagenous connective tissue that is situated under the nipple and is responsible for the normal projection of the nipple above skin level. The methods often include cutting the fibrous bands that tie the nipple down and also include a conscious dividing of lactiferous ducts.

Attempts have been made to surgically correct inverted nipples as early as 1873, when Kehrer described his mamilloplasty, which included a large horizontal oval excision of skin and fascia within the areola leaving the base of the nipple in the middle. After closure of the defect, the nipple was lying in a cavity, only reaching skin level.

In 1889, Axford tried to keep the nipple everted by putting a buried purse-string suture around the base of the nipple through three oval excisions of skin and fat, including the nipple and areolar skin. In this way, a folded fascial tissue support was established to the everted nipple.

Basch, in 1893, studied the circular areolomamillary muscular bundles surrounding the nipple. He thought that the constriction of these bundles made eversion of the nipple impossible and he cut them with a tenotome.

In 1917, Sellheim published a technique where the whole areolar skin was undermined up to the nipple. The nipple was everted by dividing the muscle fibers. The areolar skin, now hanging from the everted nipple like an umbrella, was draped around the nipple base and sutured there to prevent reinversion. The surrounding skin could be adapted directly to the nipple base by small triangular excisions. The areolar skin area itself was lost (Fig. 29.**2**).

Skoog (1952) varied the theme of Sellheim. He stressed the importance of a better adaptation of the skin edges to the mamilloplasty. His method included an undermining of areolar skin into the nipple base and a dissection of the fibrous bands inverting the nipple. Special care was taken not to jeopardize the lactiferous ducts. With the areolar skin hanging like an umbrella from the everted nipple, four large and four small triangular excisions were made matching each other geometrically (Fig. 29.**3**).

In his monograph, Galtier (1955) reported a method focusing on the necessity of filling out the dead space that is created by everting the nipple. Via a small curved incision in the areolar skin about 1 cm from the nipple base, he divided all tight bands attached to the nipple skin including the lactiferous ducts. Then a small glandular flap was designed and brought into the dead space under the everted nipple and the defects were closed. This method reconstituted the missing bulk of tissue under the nipple after it was everted (Fig. 29.**4**).

The technique of Spina (1957) was another variation of Sellheim's method. To begin with, the method of Spina was identical with that of Sellheim consisting of an undermining of the areolar skin and redraping it around the mamillary base. But Spina then substituted the lost

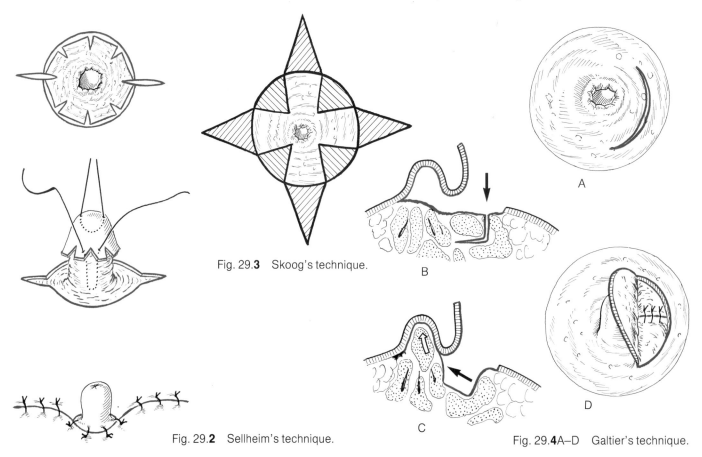

Fig. 29.**3**   Skoog's technique.

Fig. 29.**2**   Sellheim's technique.

Fig. 29.**4**A–D   Galtier's technique.

areolar skin with a labial skin graft. A small marginal peripheral zone of normal areolar skin was saved in place in order to get a natural transition from the graft to normal skin.

Lamont (1973) returned to Axford's principle of a purse-string suture around the nipple base to prevent reinversion of the nipple. He exposed the nipple base via a semicircular periareolar incision and all fibrous bands inverting the nipple were cut.

Schwager et al. (1974) published a paper on the treatment of 13 cases of inverted nipples. The technique was a combination of those of Axford and Lamont. Via a periareolar incision, the nipple base was explored and all fibrous bands inverting the nipple were cut. Efforts were made not to impair the lactiferous ducts. A deep purse-string suture was placed at the nipple-areolar border in order to condense the subcutaneous tissue supporting the nipple. The paper also included a substantial histologic examination of the submamillary tissue. The study concluded that the cone of tissue consisting of dense fibrocollagenous connective tissue under the nipple plays a major role in the achievement of the normal projection of the nipple. In cases with inverted nipples, the thickness of this cone of tissue did not exceed that of normal areolar skin.

Pitanguy (1974) was the first to make an approach to the inverted nipple via a transmamillary incision. This allowed a more direct visualization of the tight fibrous bands that inserted deep in the dermis of the nipple and caused inversion of the nipple. The fibrous bands were shown to run parallel to the lactiferous ducts. When the two halves of the nipple were split, the fibrous bands could be cut under direct visualization. The wound was closed in multiple layers. Broadbent (1976), in his method, adopted the transmamillary incision to explore the inverted nipple. However, he deepened the incision considerably

down into the glandular tissue. All lactiferous ducts and fibrous bands were consciously divided at right angles to the incision and the nipple was everted. He tried to stop any reinversion of the nipple by reconstituting the cone of tissue under the nipple, which he thought to be important for a normal projection of the nipple. For that purpose, a glandular tissue flap was raised on each side of the incision and turned 180 degrees to fill out the dead space. Suturing of all incisions were made from in and out (Fig. 29.**5**).

Finally, the method of Morris (1980) represents a mixture of the methods of Axford, Schwager, and Lamont. Through a stab wound in the areolar skin on each side of the nipple while pulling the nipple out, all fibrous bands were cut and the nipple could be everted. To stop reinversion, the dead space under the nipple was obliterated by means of one or two buried absorbable sutures.

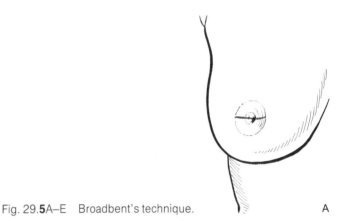

Fig. 29.**5**A–E Broadbent's technique.

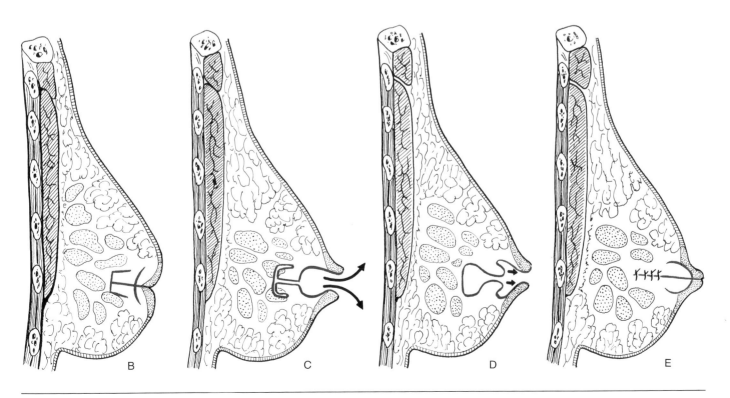

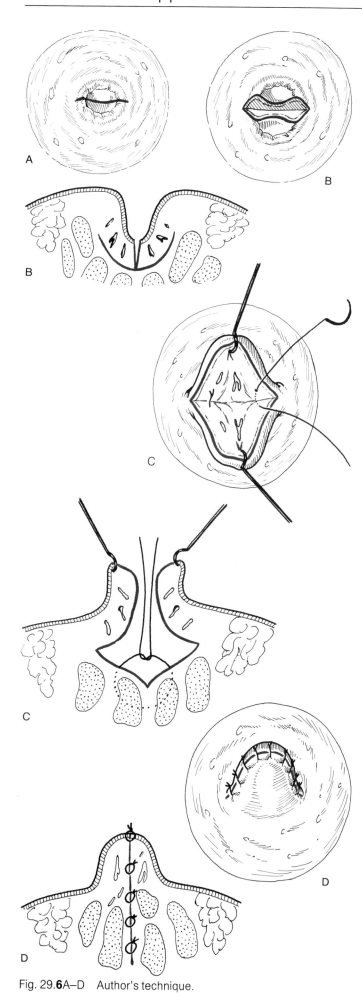

Fig. 29.**6**A–D   Author's technique.

Author's Material

During the past four years, 28 patients with 47 inverted nipples have been referred to the Plastic Surgery Unit at Sabbatsberg Hospital in Stockholm, Sweden. The majority of the patients were in the range of 26 to 35 years of age, with two cases under 20 years and six cases over 40.

Since inversion of the nipple might be a symptom of carcinoma of the breast, so a careful history must be taken to exclude this as a cause of the inversions.

Since it is assumed that there is a correlation between inverted nipples and macromastia it was interesting to note that seven patients earlier had a reduction mammoplasty.

Five of the cases became pregnant after surgery for inverted nipples, but none were able to breast feed their infants.

We have been using a method comparable to the method of Pitanguy including a deep splitting of the nipple via a transmamillary incision. All lactiferous ducts and obvious fibrous bands that tie the nipple down are cut under direct vision. The dead space is obliterated by suturing all incisions in layers (Fig. 29.**6**). In one case with a strong, intraoperative tendency to reinversion, the glandular flaps according to Broadbent were used.

The overall recurrence rate among the seven surgeons involved was 11 nipples (23%). Since the overall recurrence rate in our material seems to be high, we want to stress some points that we regard to be of importance. All inward traction of the nipple has to be completely released. The eversion of the nipple creates an empty space underneath, which has to be eliminated, either by careful adaptation of the walls or by filling it with a glandular flap. Without a good support of sutures or flap, the tissue will fall back in its earlier position resulting in a recurrence.

References

Axford, W. L.: Mamillaplasty. Ann. Surg. 9: 277–279, 1889

Basch, K.: Beiträge zur Kenntnis des menschlichen Milchapparats. Arch. Gynaekol. 44: 36, 1893

Broadbent, T. R., R. M. Woolf: Benign inverted nipple: Trans-nipple-areolar correction. J. Plast. Reconstr. Surg. 58: 673–677, 1976

Galtier, M.: Chirurgie esthétique mammaire. G. Doin et Cie, Paris p. 192–195. 1955

Kehrer, F. A.: Zur plastischen Chirurgie der Hohlwarzen. Zentralbl. Med. Wiss. 17: 259–261, 1873

Lamont, E.: Congenital inversion of the nipple in identical twins. Br. J. Plast. Surg. 26: 178, 1973

Morris, A. M., Y. S. Rai, P. M. Lamont: A method for correcting the inverted nipple. Br. J. Plast. Surg. 33: 41–42, 1980

Pitanguy, I., S. R. Matta, A. F. Filho: Inverted nipple. Rev. Bras. Cir. 64: 199–207, 1974

Schwager, R. G., J. W. Smith, G. F. Gray, D. Jr. Goulian: Inversion of the human female nipple, with a simple method of treatment. Plast. Reconstr. Surg. 54: 564–569, 1974

Sellheim, H.: Brustwarzenplastik bei Hohlwarzen. Zentralbl. Gynäkol. 41: 305–311, 1917

Skoog, T.: An operation for inverted nipple. Br. J. Plast. Surg. 5: 65–69, 1952

Spina, V.: Inverted nipple – Contribution to the surgical treatment. Plast. Reconstr. Surg. 19: 63–66, 1957

Chapter 30

Male Breast Carcinoma

W. H. Messerschmidt and F. E. Rosato

Introduction

The incidence of carcinoma of the male breast is low; consequently most published series are small, making retrospective studies difficult at best. Prospective randomized investigations are virtually impossible. In addition, because of its rarity, recognition and treatment of the disease are often delayed.

Male breast cancer was first reported by the English physician John of Arderne in the early 14th century. A priest is described who had a slow-growing lesion on his right nipple. A barber had promised him cure; however, the priest sought another opinion from John of Arderne. John, with popular disrespect for barber-surgeons, cautioned that the barber's treatment "would bring him to the death without recovery" (Scheike 1975). This might be the first recorded instance of a formally sought "second opinon."

The actual recognition that cancer occurs in the male breast, however, was not until Franciscus Arcaneus (1493–1573) and Ambroise Pare (1510–1590) described the disease separately but at nearly the same time (Scheike 1975). Fabricus Hildanus (1537–1619) is credited with the first documented case report (Meyskens 1976). Early in the 18th century, carcinoma of the male breast was the topic of Lorenz Heister's (1683–1758) inaugural address to the German Surgical Society. In 1883, Velpeau reported 14 cases and Paul Poirier wrote a thorough study of the disease (Holleb 1968 Part I).

Clinical features of the disease and details and results of surgical treatment were described by Wainwright in 1927 and other investigators in the 1930s and 1940s. More recently, larger series have been reported and the benefits of endocrine ablative therapy have been well documented (Meyskens 1976).

Epidemiology

Breast cancer occurs infrequently in the male. Most series report that carcinoma of the breast appears in about one male for every 100 females. Data from the 3rd National Cancer Survey show that 194 cases were diagnosed between 1969 and 1971 in the United States. These cases accounted for only 0.2% of malignant diseases in males and the female to male ratio was 136 to 1. The incidence was similar for black and white males (Cutler and Young 1975). The age distribution is depicted in Fig. 30.1. Although the disease is very rare before the age of 30, it has been reported in males as young as five years of age and as old as 93 years (Crichlow 1972). A five- to ten-year difference in the average age at diagnosis between male and females with breast cancer, males being older at diagnosis has been well documented (Table 30.1).

The annual incidence of male breast cancer varies geographically. Highest incidences are reported in West Germany and Connecticut with one case per 100,000 males and lowest are in Yugoslavia, Uganda, and Singapore with only 0.1 case per 100,000 males. The overall inci-

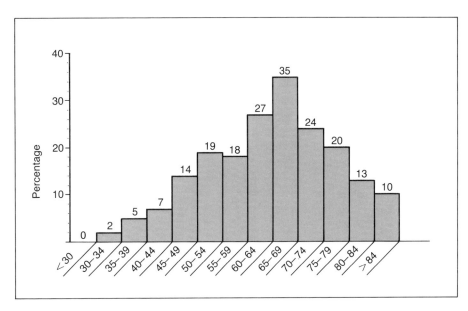

Fig. 30.1 Age distribution of carcinoma of the male breast in the United States (Cutler 1975)

Table 30.1 Average age at diagnosis for males and females with breast cancer

Author	Male (yr.)	Female (yr.)
Holleb (1968, Part I)	64	58
Chrichlow (1972)	59.6	
McGuire (1979)	64.6	59.8
Scheike (1975)	65.2	
Donegan (1979)	71.2	60.6
Haagensen (1971)	60	50
Norris (1969)	59	
Mausner (1969)	64	56.1
Cortese (1971)	59.1	

dence in the United States is 0.7/100,000. Countries with low rates for female breast carcinoma, such as Japan and Finland, are also seen to have low breast cancer rates for males (McGuire 1979).

Data from several studies have suggested that mortality rates are higher for nonwhite males and that widowed and divorced males have higher mortality rates than single or married men. These results, however, are refuted by others. Other investigators report an apparently high incidence and mortality of male breast carcinoma in Jewish males as compared with Catholics or Protestants. Review of these studies, however, suggest that these differences are due to the population examined and may be deceptive (Crichlow 1972).

Etiologic Considerations

Although the cause of breast cancer in males, as in females, is unknown, several factors have been implicated in its pathogenesis. Among these are hormonal influences, heredity, gynecomastia, Klinefelter's syndrome, radiation, trauma, and bilharziasis.

Male breast cancer offers a unique opportunity to study differences in hormonal effects in males and females. Many studies have reported data suggesting an alteration of estrogen metabolism in males with breast cancer. Urinary excretion and plasma levels of estrone, estradiol, and estriol have been shown to be higher in these patients than in controls. However, the fact that some breast tumors can synthesize estrogens from androgens has to be considered in interpreting these results (McGuire 1979).

Development of breast carcinoma after exogenous estrogen administration or endocrine ablative procedures in the treatment of advanced prostatic carinoma is described in several case reports. However, a survey of urologists identified only two cases of breast cancer in over 17,000 patients receiving estrogen therapy (Holleb 1968 Part I). Another series of 3,000 such patients found only one case of breast carcinoma (McGuire 1979). In a review of 457 cases of male breast cancer, only two patients had received estrogens. It has also been suggested that cases of breast cancer in males being treated for advanced prostatic carcinoma may actually represent metastases,

since up to 5% of males with prostate cancer have metastases to the breast at autopsy (Crichlow 1972).

The effect of estrogens on the male breast, however, cannot be ignored. The breasts of males given estrogens have clearly been shown to develop lobules and acini indistinguishable from those in female breasts (Crichlow 1972). Also of significant interest is a case report of the development of breast cancer in two British males who had transsexual procedures with castration and administration of large doses of estrogens (McGuire 1979).

A group of patients of particular interest in the study of male breast cancer are those with Klinefelter's syndrome or seminiferous tubule dysgenesis. This disorder is characterized by hypogonadism, aspermia, increased gonadotrophic hormones, positive sex chromatin, and male phenotype. Changes in the breast tissue include gynecomastia and the formation of true lobules (Sandison 1961). The incidence of breast carcinoma is definitely increased in Klinefelters patients. In a series of 242 males with breast cancer, nine were found to have positive sex chromatin. This is significant since the expected occurrence was only 0.5 given a 2 per 1,000 incidence of sex chromatin positivity in normal males. It appears that the incidence of breast cancer with Klinefelter's disease is at least 20 times the incidence in normal males (Scheike 1975).

Gynecomastia has been proposed as an etiologic factor and even a premalignant condition in male breast cancer. Gynecomastia is described as an enlargement of the breast that is characterized by proliferation of ductal elements and connective tissue, without the development of acini accompanied by some degree of inflammatory cell infiltration (Sandison 1961). The finding of severe cellular atypia of the ductal epithelium in breast with both gynecomastia and carcinoma supports the theory of premalignancy. Some investigators have even reported a histologic transformation from gynecomastia to cancer. An earlier age of onset of breast cancer associated with gynecomastia (55 vs 65 years in one series) has also been found (Scheike 1975). In a collected review, however, only ten of 585 patients with breast cancer also had gynecomastia if one series with an incidence of seven out of 40 is excluded (Crichlow 1972). Thus, although patients with gynecomastia probably have an increased incidence of breast cancer, the establishment of gynecomastia as a premalignant condition is not well documented.

The influence of heredity, which is unquestionable in female breast cancer, appears to be present in male breast cancer as well. There are a number of reported occurrences of breast cancer in two or three males, as well as in males and females in the same family. Examination of prophylactic mastectomy specimens from the sons of one of these patients suggested mild dysplasia. Elevation of urinary estrogens has been reported in apparently healthy relatives as well (McGuire 1979).

Older literature mentioned trauma as a possible cause of carcinoma in the male breast. Only 30 reports of antecedent trauma, however, were noted in 532 patients in a more recent review (Crichlow 1972). Trauma is not currently thought to have any causal relationship to breast cancer, but may bring attention to an existing malignant lesion.

The evidence for the involvement of radiation injury in the development of male breast cancer is more convincing. Increased incidences of breast cancer in females have been reported in patients treated for pulmonary tuberculosis who were exposed to significant radiation via multiple fluoroscopies. Breast cancer also occurred more frequently in female survivors of the atomic explosions at Hiroshima and Nagasaki. Several case reports have documented the development of breast cancer in males 20 to 35 years after chest wall irradiation for mediastinal lymphoma and several benign conditions (Crichlow 1972). Males who have had such radiation treatment should be followed for the development of breast cancer.

An interesting possible association between bilharziasis and male breast cancer has been noted in Egypt where up to 6% of breast cancer occurs in males. This relationship is probably due to liver damage with resultant increases in estrogen production caused by this parasitic infection, which is very prevalent in Egypt. A similar mechanism is proposed in the reported increased incidences of gynecomastia and breast malignancy in association with starvation (Haagensen 1979). It is evident that hormonal influences have an integral role in the etiology of breast cancer.

Clinical Findings

Symptoms

The first symptom in the vast majority of male breast cancer patients is a painless mass. The mass is nearly always discovered by the patient himself in part due to the infrequent examination of the male breast during a routine physical examination. Pain or tenderness is uncommon.

Nipple discharge is an early symptom in up to 15% of patients. Bloody nipple discharge indicates malignancy in about 75% of males (Crichlow 1972). Serous discharge is generally associated with benign disease but occasionally does occur with cancer. Other presenting complaints include nipple or skin ulceration, nipple retraction, and occasionally an axillary mass (Table 30.2).

Table 30.2 Initial symptom of males with breast carcinoma (Scheike 1975)

Symptom	Percent of patients
Mass	71
Ulceration	7
Pain	7
Nipple discharge	4
Nipple retraction	4
Mass in axilla	1.5
Other	5.5

The duration of symptoms tends to be longer in males than in females, although the delay seems to be decreasing in recent years. Average durations as short as three months (Panettiere 1974) and as long as 2.4 years in an early series (Haagensen 1971) have been reported, but generally are between six and 21 months (Crichlow 1972; Scheike 1975; and Holleb 1978 Part I). Patients with bloody nipple discharge tend to present earlier than those with only a mass (Holleb 1968 Part I).

Physical Findings

At the time of presentation, a subareolar mass is nearly always palpable. The tumor is generally hard, poorly defined, and nontender. It is unusual, however, for a mass to be the only finding (Table 30.3). Nipple retraction, nipple or skin ulceration, and skin fixation are each found in about one third of patients (Scheike 1975; Holleb 1968 Part I). The frequency of these findings is probably related to the smaller mass of the normal male breast as well as the longer delay in seeking treatment as compared with females. Fixation of the tumor to the fascia, muscle, or chest wall, which was present in 22% of patients in a Danish series (Scheike 1975), probably has a similar explanation. Nipple discharge is a less common but important finding and is bloody in about 80% of cases associated with malignancy (Holleb 1968 Part I).

Ipsilateral axillary lymph nodes are clinically positive in about 50% of males with breast cancer, although their clinical presence or absence does not correlate well with the pathologic findings in many cases (Crichlow 1972; Holleb 1968 Part I). Higher percentages of axillary node involvement in males than in females reported in earlier literature probably reflected longer delays in treatment and more recent studies show little or no such difference (Crichlow 1972).

In a large series, about 85% of tumors were less than 5 cm in diameter in at presentation and there was good correlation between tumor size and frequency of ulceration. A significant relationship also existed between size and duration of symptoms (Scheike 1975).

Table 30.3 Physical findings with male breast cancer at the time of presentation (Scheike 1975; Holleb 1968, Part I)

Physical finding	Frequency (%)
Breast mass	96
(breast mass only)	(15)
Axillary nodes clinically positive	39
Ulceration or encrustation	37
(ulceration only)	(2)
Skin fixation	37
Nipple retraction	33
Muscle or chest wall fixation	22
Tenderness	13
Nipple discharge	6
(nipple discharge only)	(1)

There appears to be a slightly greater tendency for carcinoma to develop in the left breast than the right breast in males as in females. In a collected series of 1,142 patients, 51.7% of cancers were left sided (Crichlow 1972). This tendency remains without logical explanation.

Paget's carcinoma has been reported occasionally in males. This disease appears to be clinically and pathologically identical to the disease in females. The prognosis, however, appears to be quite poor (Haagensen 1971). Inflammatory carcinoma of the male breast has also been reported and also mimics the variant in females (Crichlow 1972).

Differential Diagnosis

In evaluating a mass in the male breast, the physician must differentiate between carcinoma of the breast and other conditions that have similar characteristics. These include gynecomastia, other benign lesions, and other malignancies that may present in the area of the breast such as sarcomas and metastatic tumors.

The most frequent and important of these lesions is gynecomastia. Gynecomastia occurs much more frequently than male breast cancer (McGuire 1979) and is usually distinguishable by its epidemiologic and physical characteristics (Table 30.4). Gynecomastia is more likely to be tender, tends to occur at a younger age, is more often bilateral, and sometimes accompanies estrogen administration or liver disease (Crichlow 1972). Patients with heart disease, especially those taking digitalis, may develop gynecomastia (McGuire 1979), but these older patients must also be considered candidates for carci-

noma. Carcinoma is unilateral, painless, and rare before the age of 30.

Gynecomastia may present in one of two ways. It may appear as a diffuse hypertrophy that is soft and on examination is very similar to the female breast. More often there is a tender, movable, discoid tumor that is centrally located. This type occurs at puberty, with liver disease, or as senile benign hypertrophy, which tends to be very tender and disappears in three to six months (Haagensen 1971). Although either carcinoma or gynecomastia may adhere to the areola, only carcinoma will show ulceration or fixation to the muscle or chest wall. Nipple discharge, especially sanguinous, is more likely to indicate the presence of carcinoma (Crichlow 1972). Mammography occasionally may give additional information (McGuire 1979).

Staging

The staging of carcinoma of the breast in males is the same as in females and should be completed prior to the initiation of definitive treatment. A complete history and physical examination are the most useful diagnostic maneuvers. A chest radiograph should be performed to rule out pulmonary metastases and a blood count and chemistry profile should be obtained. Bone and liver scans are rarely useful in the absence of bone pain or liver enzyme elevations respectively.

In the large Danish series, 35% of the patients were stage I when they presented, 11% were stage II, 42% were stage III, and 12% were stage IV using the TNM classication (Scheike 1975). The high percentage of stage III patients as compared with females is explained by the increased frequency of fixation and ulceration. A similar distribution was noted in other series. In the United States, the percentage of patients with carcinoma limited to breast and axilla at presentation increased from 38% in 1950 to 1954 to 58% in 1970 to 1973 (McGuire 1979).

Second Cancers

Considering the advanced age of the patients with male breast cancer, it is not surprising that a significant number of these patients develop a nonmammary carcinoma at some time before, after, or during the time when they have breast cancer. An incidence of second primary cancers of up to 13% has been reported (Donegan 1979). The distribution of these malignancies appears to be no different than in the general population.

Pathology

The male breast is essentially identical to the female breast at birth and through childhood. At puberty the female breast begins to develop rapidly, whereas the male breast may enlarge slightly and then regress somewhat. After puberty, the normal male breast consists of dense stroma with sparse simple ducts and no periductal fibrillary stroma. Lobules normally do not form (Sandison 1961).

Table 30.4 Characteristics of male breast cancer and gynecomastia helpful in differential diagnosis (Chrichlow 1972; Haagensen 1971; McGuire 1979)

Carcinoma	Gynecomastia
Incidence increasis with age	Occurs at any age, higher incidences in adolescents and elderly males
Nontender	Tender
Unilateral	Significant percentage bilateral
Hard	Firm to soft
Irregular mass	Well-defined, discoid mass
Muscle and chest wall fixation	May adhere to areola
May be associated with: nipple discharge (especially bloody) axillary lympadenopathy ulceration	May be associated with: other medical conditions – especially chronic liver disease, heart disease, and endocrine disorders drugs – especially estrogens, corticosteroids, cimetydine, digitalis, thiazides, reserpine, phenothiazines, and marijuana

Virtually all histologic types of breast cancers known to occur in females have been reported in males (Table 30.**5**). As in the female, carcinomas arising from the ductal elements are the most common type and account for over three quarters of all male breast cancers. Other histologic types including papillary, medullary, and mucinous carcinomas are uncommon. Lobular carcinomas, which are reported in about 9% of female cases, have been only rarely reported in males (Crichlow 1972). This is felt to be due to the fact that the normal male breast does not contain lobules. Grossly, male breast cancers mimic those in females, being grayish white with yellow streaks and occasional hemorrhage and having a firm granular consistency (Norris 1969).

Histologic grading is based on a point system assigned to three criteria tubule formation, number of mitoses and hyperchromatism, and nuclear irregularities. In the Danish series, 150 tumors were graded using this system and 54% were grade II. Grades I and III accounted for 29% and 17%, respectively. Prognosis is correlated with the histologic grade (Scheike 1975).

Estrogen and progesterone receptor activities have been measured in male breast cancer as in females. Positive estrogen receptors have been reported in 84% of tumors and positive progesterone receptors in 73% (McGuire 1979). It has not been possible to predict response to hormonal therapy on the basis of these assays.

Treatment

Males with breast cancer in whom evaluation and staging have found the disease to be localized (i. e., limited to the breast and axilla) are candidates for curative surgery. In large series, approximately 75% to 80% of male breast cancer patients are deemed resectable (Crichlow 1972). These patients are usually treated by radical mastectomy. The technique of this procedure in males is identical to that in females. It is generally thought that skin grafting in males undergoing radical mastectomy allows the surgeon to perform a wider resection for a better cancer operation and probably should be used routinely. It is also observed that with grafting, wound complications due to tension, such as skin flap necrosis, are lessened (Holleb 1968 Part II).

Table 30.**5** Frequency of histological types of male vs female breast cancer (McGuire 1979)

Histologic type	Male (%)	Female (%)
infiltrating ductal, intraductal	78	78.1
Papillary	5	1.2
Medullary	4	4.3
Mucinos	2	2.6
Lobular	< 1	8.7
Adenocarcinoma, type not specified	7	–
Other	4	4.6

More recently, some surgeons feel that modified radical or simple mastectomy is adequate treatment in most cases of male breast cancer, especially in older patients (Scheike 1975). Because of the lack of randomized studies, it is difficult to evaluate the results of these procedures as patients undergoing simple mastectomy often have particularly favorable or unfavorable prognoses and may have received adjuvant treatment (Crichlow 1972). Simple mastectomy at this point cannot be considered the procedure of choice, but clearly has its place in treating patients with advanced disease and possibly elderly patients or those with very favorable pathology.

Adjuvant Therapy

Radiation therapy has been used as an adjuvant to the surgical treatment of male breast carcinoma to a limited extent. It has been given preoperatively or postoperatively and some surgeons have used radiotherapy whenever axillary metastases were present (Crichlow 1972). At this time, the numbers of patients are too small to adequately evaluate this modality as adjuvant treatment. Chemotherapy and hormonal manipulation have also been used as adjuvant therapy, but their use has been based on experience in treating female patients and data concerning males are insufficient to recommend or discourage their use (McGuire 1979).

Treatment of Advanced Disease

Breast cancer in males tends to metastasize to the same sites as in females. In order of decreasing frequency, the most common sites are bone, lung, pleura, liver, and brain (Scheike 1974). Bone metastases are nearly always osteolytic. A localized metastasis, especially one which is symptomatic, may occasionally be treated by radiation or even surgical excision (Crichlow 1972). More often, however, the disease is more widely disseminated and systemic treatment is needed.

Endocrine Ablation

Endocrine ablative procedures have become the most important modalities in the treatment of metastatic breast carcinoma in males. Orchiectomy is the first line of treatment. Complete responses, usually defined as the disappearance of all lesions for at least three to six months, have been reported in 43% (Kraybill 1971) to 67% (McGuire 1979) of patients. In those patients who respond, the median duration of the response was 22 months and median survival of 56 months in a large series (Meyskens 1976). These figures are significantly higher than those for female breast cancer patients undergoing oophorectomy.

Adrenalectomy is the second most commonly used endocrine ablation and usually follows orchiectomy. Good response rates and durations are reported even after orchiectomy failure (Table 30.**6**). Hypophysectomy has been performed less frequently but also has a significant response rate (Meyskens 1976). Current data do not

Procedure	Responses (%)	Median duration of response (mo)	Median survival (mo)
Orchiectomy	67	22	56 (nonresponders: 38)
Adrenalectomy (total) after orchiectomy	76	–	–
response after orchiectomy	91	32	74
nonresponse	50	16	–
Hypophysectomy	59	20	90

Table 30.**6** Response of advanced male breast cancer to endocrine ablative procedurs (Meyskens 1976)

support the ability of hormone receptor assays to predict responses to endocrine ablation and these procedures should not be withheld on the basis of such study (Kraybill 1981)

Additive Hormonal Therapy

The response of metastatic breast cancer to additive hormonal treatment is significantly poorer in males than in females. Although response rates of up to 38% have been reported with the use of diethylstilbestrol (DES), other reports are much less encouraging and the results in treating bony metastases with DES are dismal (McGuire 1979). Responses to progestational hormone administration have been reported (Kraybill 1981). Corticosteroids have occasionally been given, but although they may improve the patient's sense of well-being, they have no effect on tumor growth (Crichlow 1972).

Chemotherapy

Treatment with cytotoxic agents has been used with little success. Combination chemotherapy with cytoxan and prednisone, or adriamycin, cytoxan, 5-fluorouracil, methotrexate, and thiotepa seems to be the most useful treatment (Kraybill 1981). Chemotherapy should be reserved for patients who have failed after endocrine ablation.

Prognosis

Male breast cancer has long been considered to have a much worse prognosis than female breast cancer. More recent data with shorter delays in treatment and adjusting for age, however, suggest that this may not be true (Scheike 1974). Prognosis is affected by many factors including histologic type, histologic grade, and clinical staging (Table 30.**7**).

Overall five-year survival rates of about 35% are reported (Crichlow 1972). Certain histologic types of tumors have better prognoses than others. Papillary carcinoma, for example, is associated with five-year survivals approaching 100%, whereas Paget's disease of the breast, which has a favorable prognosis in females, has a poor prognosis in males (Meyskens 1976).

The presence or absence of axillary node involvement and distant metastases are very significant factors in determining prognosis. Five-year survival rates with or without positive nodes are 28% and 80%, respectively and ten-year rates are 4% and 62%, respectively (Meyskens 1976). Patients with distant metastases at the time of diagnosis (clinical stage IV) have five- and ten-year survivals of only 4% and 0% compared with those in patients without distant metastases of 41% and 20% (Scheike 1974).

Histologic grade also has a definite effect on survival with ten-year rates of 39%, 9%, and 0% for grades I, II, and III, respectively (Meyskens 1976). Ulceration and fixation have also been shown to decrease survival (Scheike 1974).

The prognosis is slightly poorer for males than females, but not nearly as significantly as originally thought. Although the survival of males with positive nodes seems to be slightly less than for similar females, the overall survival is nearly equal if adjusted for age (Crichlow 1972).

Table 30.**7** Relationship of survival to clinical and pathologix features in male breast cancer (Meyskens 1976; Scheike 1974)

Feature	5-year survival (%)	10-year survival (%)
Axillary node status		
positive	28	4
negative	80	62
Distant metastases (at time of diagnosis)		
present	4	0
absent	41	20
Histologic grade		
I	55	39
II	54	9
III	5	0
Tumor size (cm)		
< 2	55	n/a
2–3	39	n/a
3–4	36	n/a
> 4	16	n/a

n/a = not available

Summary

Carcinoma of the breast in the male is a relatively rare disease representing only 0.2% of malignant diseases in males and less than 1% of all breast cancer. A number of etiologic factors have been proposed including heredity, gynecomastia, Klinefelter's syndrome, radiation, and liver disease. Although the exact role these other conditions play in the development of male breast cancer is uncertain, it appears evident that some alteration in estrogen metabolism is involved in many cases.

Male breast cancer most often appears as a painless mass in the breast that is usually discovered by the patient. Nipple discharge is occasionally present and bloody nipple discharge in a male generally indicates malignancy. The duration of symptoms in males is generally longer than in females, which may lead to a worse prognosis. Clinically a subareolar mass is nearly always present and is often associated with ulceration or fixation to the skin or fascia. At the time of presentation, axillary node metastases are present in about 50% of patients and metastatic disease in about 10% to 20%. The vast majority of cancers of the breast in males are ductal carcinomas; however, nearly all histologic types of tumors known to occur in females have been reported in males.

The treatment of choice for the majority of male breast cancers is radical mastectomy. Skin grafting is nearly always considered necessary. Adjuvant therapy is not currently in routine use. The most effective treatment for advanced breast cancer in the male is endocrine ablation. Orchiectomy is the initial treatment for metastatic disease and adrenalectomy or hypophysectomy should be considered in those patients who either fail or relapse after orchiectomy. In general, the prognosis is poor with five-year survival rates of 35% and lower ten-year survival rates. In matched populations, the prognosis is probably only very slightly poorer in males than in females. Earlier diagnosis and improved treatment modalities hopefully will improve this prognosis.

References

Cortese, A. F., G. N. Cornell: Carcinoma of the male breast. Ann. Surg. 173: 275–80, 1971

Crichlow, R. W.: Carcinoma of the male breast. Surg. Gynecol. Obstet. 134: 1011–19, 1972

Cutler, S. J., J. L. Young (eds.): Third National Cancer Survey Incidence Data. DHEW Publication No. (NIH) 75–787. U.S. Dept. of Health, Education, and Welfare, (Tables 5, 7, 19) 1975

Donegan, W. L.: Cancer of the Breast. 2nd ed. WB Saunders Co., Philadelphia: 1979

Haagensen, C. D.: Disease of the Breast. 2nd ed. WB Saunders Co., Philadelphia: 1971

Holleb, A. L., H. P. Freeman, J. H. Farrow: Cancer of the male breast, Part I. N. Y. State J. Med. 68: 544–53, 1968

Holleb, A. L., H. P. Freeman, J. H. Farrow: Cancer of the male breast, Part II. N. Y. State J. Med. 68: 656–63, 1968

Kraybill, W. G., R. Kaufman, D. Kinne: Treatment of advanced male breast cancer. Cancer 47: 2185–89, 1981

Mauser, J. S., M. B. Shimkin, N. H. Moss, G. P. Rosemond: Cancer of the breast in Philadelphia hospitals 1951–1964. Cancer 23: 260–74, 1969

McGuire, W. L. (ed.): Breast Cancer 3: Advances in Research and Treatment: Current Topics. Plenum Medical Book Co., New York 1979

Meyskens, F. L., D. C. Tormey, J. P. Neifield: Male breast cancer: A review. Cancer Treat. Rev. 3: 83–93, 1976

Norris, H. J., H. B. Taylor: Carcinoma of the male breast. Cancer 23: 1428–35, 1969

Panettiere, F. J.: Cancer in the male breast. Cancer 34: 1324–27, 1974

Sandison, A. T.: An Autopsy Study of the Adult Human Breast. NCI Monograph No. 8 U. S. Government Printing Office, 1961

Scheike, O.: Male breast cancer 6: Factors influencing prognosis. Br. J. Cancer 30: 261–70, 1974

Scheike, O.: Male breast cancer. Acta Pathol. Microbiol. Scand. 251 (suppl.): 13–35, 1975

Subject Index

Abbreviations

AASH	Adrenal Androgen Stimulating Hormone
ABC	Aspiration Biopsy Cytology
ACS	American Cancer Society
AG	Aminoglutethemide
AID	Automatic Interaction Detection
BCDDP	Breast Cancer Detection Demonstration Project
BSE	Breast Self Examination
CAF	Cytoxan Adriamycin Fluorouracil
CAT	Computerized Axial Tomography
CBC	Complete Blood Count
CBCG	Cooperative Breast Cancer Group
CBG	Corticosteroid Binding Globulin
CDP	Cystic Disease Protein
CDSP	Collaborative Drug Surveillance Program
CEA	Carcinoembryonic Antigen
CMF	Cyclophosphamide Methotrexate Fluoracil
CMFVP	Cyclophosphamide Methotrexate Fluoracil Vincristine Prednisone
CRT	Cathode-Ray Tube
DCIS	Ductal Carcinoma In Situ
DES	Diethylstilbestrol
DMBA	Dimethylbenzantrazene
DY	Dense Parenchymal Pattern
EDTA	Ethylene Diamine Tetra Acetic Acid
ER	Estrogen receptor
FAC	Fluoracil Adrenamycin Cyclophosphamide
FSH	Follicle Stimulating Hormone
GCDFP	Gross Cystic Disease Fluid Pattern
HC	Hydrocortisone
HCG	Human Chorionic Gonadotropin
HIP	Health Insurance Plan of Greater New York
ICSH	Interstitial Cellstimulating Hormone
LCIS	Lobular Carcinoma In Situ
LDH	Lactic Dehydrogenase
LH	Luteinizing Hormone
L-PAM	L+Phenylalanine Mustard
MGG	May-Grünwald-Giemsa
MOPP	Mustardgen-Oncovin Procarbazine Prednisone
MTV	Mouse Tumor Virus
NCI	National Cancer Institute
NG	Nuclear grade
NIH	National Institute of Health
NOS	Not Otherwise Specified
NSABP	National Surgical Adjuvant Breast Project
P_2	Prominent Duct Pattern
PAP	Perioxidase Antiperioxidase
PAS	Periodic Acid Schiff
PEV	Peritumor Edema Evolving Cancer
PR	Progesterone Receptor
RT	Radio Therapy
SHBG	Sex Hormone Bindung Globulin
SMA-18	Sequential Multiple Analyses
SONAR	Sound Navigation Ranging
TNM	Tumor Nodes Metastases
pTNM	Postoperative TNM Classification
TRAM	Transverse Rectus Abdominis Musculocutaneous Flap
UICC	Union International Contre le Cancer